BLANCHARD & LOEB PUBLISHERS
Nurse's Choice for Better Care™

Nurse's Handbook of I.V. Drugs

Second Edition

Blanchard & Loeb
PUBLISHERS, LLC
Nurse's Choice for Better Care™

Blanchard & Loeb
PUBLISHERS, LLC
Nurse's Choice for Better Care™

Publishers: Ross Blanchard, Stanley E. Loeb
Clinical Director: Marlene Ciranowicz-Steenburg, RN, MSN, CDE
Book Editor: Catherine E. Harold
Copy Editor: Jenifer F. Walker
Interior Illustrations: Rolin Graphics, Inc.

The information and recommendations in this book must be considered in light of each patient's clinical condition and of details provided by the drug manufacturer in the latest package insert. The publisher disclaims responsibility for the reader's misuse or misunderstanding of information published in this book, as well as for undetected errors in the information.

Printed in the United States of America

Blanchard & Loeb Publishers, LLC
454 Railroad Avenue
Shiremanstown, PA 17011

Contents

Reviewers and Clinical Consultants

Karen T. Bruchak, RN, MSN, MBA
Director, Medical-Surgical Nursing
The Chester County Hospital
Chester, PA

Terri Corbo, PharmD, BCPS
Clinical Specialist, Cardiology
Christiana Care Health System
Newark, DE

Kimberly Anne Boykin Couch, PharmD
Clinical Specialist
Christiana Care Health System
Adjunct Faculty
University of Delaware School of Nursing
Newark, DE

How to Use This Book

Blanchard & Loeb Publishers Nurse's Handbook of I.V. Drugs, second edition, gives you what today's nurses and nursing students need: accurate, concise, and reliable facts about I.V. drug administration. This book emphasizes the vital information you need to know before, during, and after drug administration. And the information is presented in easy-to-understand language and organized alphabetically, so you can find what you need quickly.

What's Special

In addition to the drug information you expect to find in each entry (see "Drug Entries" below for details), *Nurse's Handbook of I.V. Drugs,* second editon, boasts these special features:

- **Practical trim size and good-size type** give you a book that's easy to carry, easy to read, and easy to handle. You can hold the book in one hand, see complete pages at a glance, and use your other hand to document or perform other activities.
- **Introductory material** reviews essential general information you need to know to administer I.V. drugs safely and effectively, including an overview of pharmacology and the principles of I.V. drug administration. In addition, the five steps of the nursing process are reviewed and related specifically to drug therapy.
- **Useful illustrations** throughout the text help you visualize selected mechanisms of action by showing how drugs work at the cellular, tissue, and organ levels. In addition, the inside front cover features a chart listing all the drugs whose mechanisms of action are illustrated—along with other drugs that have similar mechanisms of action.
- **No-nonsense writing style** that uses the terms and abbreviations you typically encounter in your practice and your studies (although a few abbreviations may not be used in certain facilities). (See *Abbreviations,* pages 778 to 780.) And to avoid sexist language, we alternate male and female pronouns as we move from letter to letter throughout the book.
- **Up-to-date drug information,** including the latest FDA-approved drugs, new and changed indications, new warnings, and newly reported adverse reactions.
- **Dosage adjustment,** highlighted in color, alerts you to expected dosage changes for patients with a specific condition or disorder, such as advanced age or renal impairment.

- **Warning,** highlighted in color, calls attention to important facts that you need to know before, during, and after drug administration. For example, in the alatrofloxacin entry, the Warning reports that the drug usually is reserved for hospitalized patients and is given for no longer than 2 weeks because of the high risk of severe liver damage.
- **Easy-to-use tables** for route, onset, peak, and duration provide a timesaving way to track and check this important data. (See pages viii to ix for details on route, onset, peak, and duration charts.)
- **Useful appendices** provide you with even more handy information you can use every day in your practice and studies, such as the *I.V. Antineoplastic Drugs* appendix, where you can review generic and trade antineoplastic drug names and their indications, and dosages. You'll also find help with calculating solution strengths, parenteral dosages, and flow rates. Plus, on the inside back cover, you'll find a handy table that shows which drugs are compatible in a syringe.

Drug Entries

Nurse's Handbook of I.V. Drugs, second editon, clearly and concisely presents all the vital facts on the drugs that you'll typically administer. To help you find the information you need quickly, drug entries are organized alphabetically by generic drug name—from abatacept to zoledronic acid. For ease of use, every drug entry follows a consistent format. However, if specific details are unknown or don't apply, that heading isn't included so you can go right to the next section. (Exceptions are the headings "Adverse Reactions" and "Interactions," where "None with the usual dosages" and "None known" may be used.)

Generic and Trade Names

First, each entry identifies the drug's main generic name as well as alternate generic names. (For drugs prescribed by trade name, you can quickly check the comprehensive index, which refers you to the appropriate generic name and page.) Next, the entry lists the most common U.S. trade names for each drug. It also includes common trade names available only in Canada, marked (CAN).

Class, Category, and Schedule

Each entry lists the drug's chemical and therapeutic classes. With this information, you can compare drugs in the same chemical class but in different therapeutic classes and vice versa.

FDA PREGNANCY RISK CATEGORIES

Each drug may be placed in a pregnancy risk category based on the FDA's estimate of risk to the fetus. If the FDA hasn't provided a category, the *Nurse's Handbook of I.V. Drugs* notes that the drug is "Not rated." The categories range from A to X, signifying least to greatest fetal risk.

A Controlled studies show no risk

Adequate, well-controlled studies with pregnant women have failed to demonstrate a risk to the fetus in any trimester of pregnancy.

B No evidence of risk in humans

Adequate, well-controlled studies with pregnant women haven't shown increased risk of fetal abnormalities despite adverse findings in animals, or—in the absence of adequate human studies—animal studies show no fetal risk. The chance of fetal harm exists but is remote.

C Risk can't be ruled out

Adequate, well-controlled human studies are lacking, and animal studies are lacking as well or have demonstrated a risk to the fetus. A chance of fetal harm exists if the drug is administered during pregnancy, but the potential benefits may outweigh the potential risk.

D Positive evidence of risk

Studies in humans, or investigational or post-marketing data, have demonstrated fetal risk. Nevertheless, potential benefits from the drug's use may outweigh potential risks. For example, the drug may be acceptable if needed in a life-threatening situation or serious disease for which safer drugs can't be used or are ineffective.

X Contraindicated in pregnancy

Studies in animals or humans, or investigational or post-marketing reports, have demonstrated positive evidence of fetal abnormalities or risks; these risks clearly outweigh any possible benefit to the patient.

The entry also lists the FDA's pregnancy risk category, which categorizes drugs based on their potential to cause birth defects. (For details, see *FDA pregnancy risk categories.*) Where appropriate, the entry also includes the drug's controlled substance schedule. (For details, see *Controlled substance schedules,* page viii.)

CONTROLLED SUBSTANCE SCHEDULES

The Controlled Substances Act of 1970 mandated that certain prescription drugs be categorized in schedules based on their potential for abuse. The greater their abuse potential, the greater the restrictions on their prescription. The controlled substance schedules range from I to V, signifying highest to lowest abuse potential.

I High potential for abuse

No accepted medical use exists for Schedule I drugs, which include heroin and lysergic acid diethylamide (LSD).

II High potential for abuse

Use may lead to severe physical or psychological dependence. Prescriptions must be written in ink or typewritten and must be signed by the prescriber. Oral prescriptions must be confirmed in writing within 72 hours and may be given only in a genuine emergency. No renewals are permitted.

III Some potential for abuse

Use may lead to low-to-moderate physical dependence or high psychological dependence. Prescriptions may be oral or written. Up to five renewals are permitted within 6 months.

IV Low potential for abuse

Use may lead to limited physical or psychological dependence. Prescriptions may be oral or written. Up to five renewals are permitted within 6 months.

V Subject to state and local regulation

Abuse potential is low; a prescription may not be required.

Indications and Dosages

This section lists FDA-approved therapeutic indications. For each indication, you'll find the applicable drug form or route, age-group (adults, adolescents, or children), and dosage (which includes amount per dose, timing, and duration).

Route, Onset, Peak, and Duration

Quick-reference charts show the drug's onset, peak, and duration (when known) for the appropriate administration route. The *onset of action* is the time a drug takes to be absorbed, reach a therapeutic blood level, and elicit an initial therapeutic response. The *peak therapeutic effect* occurs when a drug reaches its highest blood concentration and the greatest amount of drug reaches the site of action to produce the maximum therapeutic response. The *duration of action* is the amount of time that a drug remains at a blood concentration that produces a therapeutic response.

Mechanism of Action

Set off by a box, this section concisely describes how a drug achieves its therapeutic effects at the cellular, tissue, or organ level, as appropriate. Illustrations of selected mechanisms of action lend exceptional detail and clarity to sometimes complex processes.

Incompatibilities

This section alerts you to drugs or solutions that are incompatible with the topic drug when mixed in a syringe or solution or infused through the same I.V. line.

Contraindications

An alphabetical list details the conditions and disorders that preclude administration of the topic drug.

Interactions

This section presents the drugs, foods, and activities (such as alcohol use and smoking) that can cause important, problematic, or life-threatening interactions with the topic drug. For each interacting drug, food, or activity, you'll learn the effects of the interaction.

Adverse Reactions

Organized by body system, this section highlights common, serious, and life-threatening adverse reactions in alphabetical order.

Nursing Considerations

Warnings, general precautions, and key information that you must know before, during, and after drug administration are detailed in this section. Examples include whether or not you need to take special precautions when preparing a drug for administration and how to properly reconstitute, dilute, store, handle, or dispose of a drug.

Patient teaching information is also included here. You'll find important guidelines for patients, such as how to spot and manage adverse reactions, when to report them, which cautions to observe, and more. To save you time, however, this section doesn't repeat basic patient-teaching points. (For a summary of those, see *Teaching your patient about I.V. drug therapy,* pages x and xi.)

TEACHING YOUR PATIENT ABOUT I.V. DRUG THERAPY

Your teaching about I.V. drug therapy will vary with your patient's needs and your practice setting. To help guide your teaching, each drug entry provides key information that you must teach your patient about that drug. For all patients, however, you should also:

- Teach the generic and trade names for each prescribed drug that he'll take after discharge—even if he took the drug before admission.
- Clearly explain why each drug was prescribed, how it works, and what it's supposed to do. To help your patient understand the drug's therapeutic effects, relate its action to her disorder or condition.
- Review the I.V. administration process, and inform the patient how often the drug will be administered. If the patient will be switched from an I.V. drug to another drug form (for example, from I.V. methyldopate hydrochloride to oral methyldopa for continuing treatment of hypertension), teach him how to administer the new form correctly. Also instruct him how often to take the drug and for what length of time. Emphasize that he should take the drug exactly as prescribed.
- If the patient is being switched to an oral drug, describe the drug's appearance. Explain that she may break scored tablets in half for safe, accurate dosing but *should not* break unscored tablets because doing so may alter the drug dosage. If the patient has difficulty swallowing capsules, explain that she can open ones that contain sprinkles and take them with food or a drink but that she shouldn't do this with capsules that contain powder. Also, warn her not to crush or chew enteric-coated, extended-release, sustained-release, or similar drug forms.
- Teach the patient common adverse reactions associated with his drug therapy, and advise him to immediately report any dangerous ones, such as syncope. Also instruct the patient to report changes at the I.V. site, such as pain, redness, or leaking fluid.
- If the patient experiences unpleasant adverse reactions, such as a rash or mild itching, inform her that her prescriber may adjust the dosage or substitute a drug that causes fewer adverse reactions. Tell her which adverse reactions resolve with time.
- Caution the patient that some adverse reactions, such as dizziness and drowsiness, can impair his ability to perform activities requiring alertness, such as driving a car or operating machinery. If the drug is known to have CNS effects, advise the pa-

tient to avoid such activities until the drug's full CNS effects are known or as directed by the prescriber.

- ☑ If your patient will be self-administering a drug, teach her how to store the drug properly. Let her know if the drug is sensitive to light or temperature and how to protect it from these elements. Instruct the patient to store the drug in its original container, if possible, with the drug's name and dosage clearly printed on the label.
- ☑ Inform the patient which devices are available for drug administration and which ones to avoid. For example, advise him to ask the prescriber about using an infusion control device for administering I.V. morphine sulfate infusions.
- ☑ Teach your patient who will be self-administering a drug what to do if she misses a dose. Generally, she should administer a once-daily drug as soon as she remembers—provided that she remembers within the first 24 hours. If 24 hours has elapsed, she should administer the next scheduled dose, but not double the dose. If she has questions or concerns about missed doses, advise her to contact the prescriber.
- ☑ Provide information that is specific to the prescribed drug. For example, if your patient takes a diuretic to manage heart failure, instruct him to weigh himself daily at the same time of day, using the same scale and wearing the same amount of clothing; or if the patient takes digoxin or an antihypertensive, teach him how to measure his pulse and blood pressure and how to record the measurements. Then instruct him to bring the diary to his regular appointments so that the prescriber can monitor his response to the drug.
- ☑ Advise the patient to refill prescriptions promptly, unless she no longer needs the drug. Also instruct her to discard expired drugs because they may become ineffective or even dangerous over time.
- ☑ Warn the patient to keep all drugs out of the reach of children at all times.

In short, *Nurse's Handbook of I.V. Drugs,* second edition, is designed expressly to give you more of what you need in a versatile and highly useful format. It puts vital drug information at your fingertips and helps you remain ALWAYS CURRENT in this critical part of your practice or studies.

Foreword

As you know, administering I.V. drug therapy safely and effectively is a top priority for nurses in today's health care environment. In the past, I.V. drug therapy was administered primarily in acute care settings. However, as health care has expanded to include multiple specialties, the practice settings for I.V. drug therapy have also broadened. Today, nurses care for a diverse population of patients in hospitals, outpatient clinics, extended care facilities, surgical centers, and the patient's own home.

The types of drugs that can be administered by I.V. injection or infusion are wide ranging and include antibiotics, antivirals, antineoplastics, and narcotics. New drugs are continually becoming available to manage various health problems, such as HIV infection and cancer, and to manage or prevent drug-induced complications. In addition, many patients have more than one health problem and are taking multiple medications.

Your Responsibilities in I.V. Drug Therapy

Your basic responsibilities in drug therapy—whether enteral or parenteral—include:

- administering the right drug in the right dose by the right route at the right time to the right patient
- knowing the therapeutic use, dosage, interactions, adverse effects, and warnings of each administered drug
- being aware of newly approved drugs that may be prescribed
- knowing about changes to existing drugs, such as new indications and dosages and recently reported adverse reactions and interactions
- concentrating fully when preparing and administering drugs
- responding promptly and appropriately to serious or life-threatening adverse reactions, interactions, and other complications.

Beyond these basic responsibilities, however, you also need additional nursing knowledge and skills to meet the demands of today's I.V. drug therapy—for example, knowing when and how to observe the I.V. insertion site and surrounding area for signs and symptoms of complications. *Blanchard & Loeb Publishers Nurse's Handbook of I.V. Drugs,* second edition, provides all this information in an accurate and easy-to-use reference that has been developed specifically for you.

Meeting Your Needs

This book offers a wealth of reliable and easy-to-understand information on virtually all of the I.V. drugs you're likely to administer. For example, you'll find:

- instructions on how to prepare a drug dose, including directions for reconstitution and further dilution when appropriate
- appropriate storage information, including specific temperatures required for storing drugs before preparation and, if indicated, after reconstitution and dilution, as well as recommended lighting conditions, if applicable
- important facts on drug stability, such as how long the drug remains stable after reconstitution and dilution, and drug compatibility
- instructions on which drugs require special equipment, such as specific filters or a diluent supplied directly by the manufacturer
- recommended administration rate, when applicable, and whether the drug is administered as a continuous infusion, an intermittent infusion, or an injection.
- appropriate guidelines for patient monitoring after drug administration—for example, for adverse reactions, such as tissue sloughing and necrosis.

You can depend on the accuracy and reliability of the information contained in *Nurse's Handbook of I.V. Drugs,* second edition, because each entry has been reviewed by experts in nursing and pharmacology. What's more, every drug fact has been checked against the most respected drug references today, including the *American Hospital Formulary Service Drug Information, Drug Facts and Comparisons, The Physician's Desk Reference,* and the USP DI's *Drug Information for the Health Care Professional.*

Nurse's Handbook of I.V. Drugs, second edition, is also more practical and convenient than many other drug references on the market. For example, it's organized alphabetically by generic drug name, each entry follows a consistent format, and the writing throughout is concise and clear. And its Nursing Considerations are rich in advice and guidance specific to your responsibilities.

Whether you work in a hospital, a clinic, or another setting, you face greater challenges than ever before: more patients who are acutely ill, tighter budgets and staffing, and more complex drug therapy. But your ultimate goal must remain to provide your patients with the best and safest care possible. That's why we highly recommend the new second edition of *Blanchard & Loeb Publishers*

Nurse's Handbook of I.V. Drugs to help you provide that optimal care. We have found the information in this book so valuable and practical that we use it every day—in our practice and in the classroom. Just slip it in your pocket and take it with you. We're confident that you'll refer to this book again and again and that it will become one of your most essential tools.

Joseph P. Zbilut, RN,C, DNSc, PhD, ANP
Professor, Adult Health Nursing
Rush University College of Nursing
Professor, Molecular Biophysics and Physiology
Rush Medical College
Chicago, IL

Kimberly Anne Boykin Couch, PharmD
Clinical Specialist
Christiana Care Health System
Adjunct Faculty
University of Delaware School of Nursing
Newark, DE

Overview of Pharmacology

Understanding the basics of pharmacology is an essential nursing responsibility. Pharmacology is the science that deals with the physical and chemical properties, and the biochemical and physiologic effects, of drugs. It includes the areas of pharmacokinetics, pharmacodynamics, pharmacotherapeutics, pharmacognosy, and toxicodynamics.

Blanchard & Loeb Publishers Nurse's Handbook of I.V. Drugs, second edition, deals primarily with pharmacokinetics, pharmacodynamics, and pharmacotherapeutics—the information you need to administer drug therapy safely and effectively (discussed below). *Pharmacognosy* is the branch of pharmacology that deals with the biological, biochemical, and economic features of naturally occurring drugs. *Toxicodynamics* is the study of the harmful effects that excessive amounts of a drug produce in the body; in a drug overdose or drug poisoning, large drug doses may saturate or overwhelm normal mechanisms that control absorption, distribution, metabolism, and excretion.

Drug Nomenclature

Most drugs are known by several names—chemical, generic, trade, and official—each of which serves a specific function. (See *How drugs are named,* page xvi.) However, multiple drug names can also contribute to medication errors. You may find a familiar drug packaged with an unfamiliar name if your institution changes suppliers or if a familiar drug is newly approved in a different dose or for a new indication.

Drug Classification

Drugs can be classified in various ways. Most pharmacology textbooks group drugs by their functional classification, such as psychotherapeutics, which is based on common characteristics. Drugs can also be classified according to their therapeutic use, such as antibiotics and sedative-hypnotics. Drugs within a certain therapeutic class may be further divided into subgroups based on their mechanisms of action. For example, the therapeutic class antineoplastics can be further classified as alkylating agents, antibiotic antineoplastics, antimetabolites, antimitotics, biological response modifiers, and hormonal antineoplastics.

HOW DRUGS ARE NAMED

A drug's chemical, generic, trade, and official names are developed at different phases of the drug development process and serve different functions. For example, the various names of the commonly prescribed diuretic chlorothiazide sodium are:

- Chemical name: 6-chloro-*2H*–1,2,4-benzothiadiazine-7-sulfonamide 1,1-dioxide monosodium salt, or $C_7H_5ClN_3NaO_4S_2$
- Generic name: chlorothiazide sodium
- Trade name: Diuril
- Official name: Chlorothiazide Sodium for Injection, USP

A drug's *chemical name* describes its atomic and molecular structures. The chemical name of chlorothiazide sodium indicates that the drug is a substituted ring structure with a sulfonamide group as well as a sodium salt.

Once a drug successfully completes several clinical trials, it receives a *generic name,* also known as the nonproprietary name. The generic name is usually derived from, but shorter than, the chemical name. The United States Adopted Names Council is responsible for selecting generic names, which are intended for unrestricted public use.

Before submitting the drug for FDA approval, the manufacturer creates and registers a *trade name* (or brand name) when the drug appears ready to be marketed. Trade names are copyrighted and followed by the symbol ® to indicate that they're registered and that their use is restricted to the drug manufacturer. Once the original patent on a drug has expired, any manufacturer may produce the drug and market it with its own trade name.

A drug's *official name* is the name under which it's listed in the United States Pharmacopoeia (USP) and the National Formulary (NF).

Pharmacokinetics

Pharmacokinetics is the study of a drug's actions—or fate—as it passes through the body during absorption, distribution, metabolism, and excretion.

Absorption

Before a drug can begin working, it must be transformed from its pharmaceutical dosage form to a biologically available (bioavailable) substance that can pass through various biological cell membranes to reach its site of action. This process is known as absorption. A drug's absorption rate depends on its route of administration, its circulation through the tissue into which it's administered, and its solubility—that is, whether it's more water-soluble (hydrophilic) or fat-soluble (lipophilic).

Although drugs may penetrate cellular membranes either actively or passively, most drugs do so by *passive diffusion,* moving inertly from an area of higher concentration to an area of lower concentration. Passive diffusion may occur through water or fat. Passive diffusion through water—*aqueous diffusion*—occurs within large water-filled compartments, such as interstitial spaces, and across epithelial membrane tight junctions and pores in the epithelial lining of blood vessels. Aqueous diffusion is driven by concentration gradients. Drug molecules that are bound to large plasma proteins, such as albumin, are too large to pass through aqueous pores in this way. Passive diffusion through fat—*lipid diffusion*—plays an important role in drug metabolism because of the large number of lipid barriers that separate the aqueous compartments of the body. The ability of a drug to move through lipid layers between aqueous compartments often depends on the pH of the medium—that is, the ability of the water-soluble or fat-soluble drug to form weak acid or weak base.

Drugs whose molecules are too large to readily diffuse may rely on *active diffusion,* in which special carriers on molecules, including peptides, amino acids, and glucose, transport the drug through the membranes. However, some molecules with selective membrane carriers can expel foreign drug molecules; this is why many drugs can't cross the blood-brain barrier.

Drug absorption begins at the administration route. The three main administration route categories are parenteral (consisting of I.M., I.V., S.C., and intradermal routes), enteral (consisting of oral, nasogastric, and rectal routes), and transcutaneous. Depending on its nature or chemical makeup, a drug may be better absorbed from one site than from another.

I.V. drug administration allows for rapid distribution throughout the body because a drug is injected or infused directly into the blood circulation. This route usually provides the greatest bioavailability and may be used whenever other routes are contraindicated or inadequate. Drug absorption is much faster and more predictable after parenteral administration than after enteral administration.

Distribution

Distribution is the process by which a drug is transported by the circulating fluids to various sites, including its sites of action. To ensure maximum therapeutic effectiveness, the drug must permeate all membranes that separate it from its intended site of action. Drug distribution is influenced by blood flow, tissue availability, and protein binding.

Metabolism

Drug metabolism is the enzymatic conversion of a drug's structure into substrate molecules or polar compounds that are either less active or inactive and are readily excreted. Drugs can also be synthesized to larger molecules. Metabolism may also convert a drug to a more toxic compound. Because the primary site of drug metabolism is the liver, children, the elderly, and patients with impaired hepatic function are at risk for altered therapeutic effects.

Biotransformation is the process by which a drug changes into its active metabolite. Compounds that require metabolic biotransformation for activation are known as *prodrugs*. During phase I of biotransformation, the parent drug is converted into an inactive or partially active metabolite. Much of the original drug may be eliminated during this phase. During phase II, the inactive or partially active metabolite binds with available substrates, such as acetic acid, glucuronic acid, sulfuric acid, or water, to form its active metabolite. When biotransformation leads to synthesis, larger molecules are produced to create a pharmacologic effect.

Excretion

The body eliminates drugs by both metabolism and excretion. Drug metabolites—and, in some cases, the active drug itself—are eventually excreted from the body, usually through bile, feces, and urine. The primary organ for drug elimination is the kidney. Impaired renal function may cause excessive drug accumulation in the body, thus increasing the patient's risk of adverse drug reactions and toxicity. Other excretion routes include evaporation through the skin, exhalation from the lungs, and secretion into saliva and breast milk.

A drug's elimination *half-life* is the amount of time required for half of the drug to be eliminated from the body. The half-life roughly correlates with the drug's duration of action and is based on normal renal and hepatic function. Typically, the longer the half-life, the less often the drug has to be given and the longer it remains in the body after it's discontinued.

Pharmacodynamics

Pharmacodynamics is the study of the biochemical and physiologic effects of drugs and their mechanisms of action. A drug's actions may be structurally specific or nonspecific. Structurally specific drugs combine with cell receptors, such as proteins or glycoproteins, to enhance or inhibit cellular enzyme actions. Drug receptors are the cellular components affected at the site of action. Many drugs form chemical bonds with drug receptors, but a drug can bond with a receptor only if it has a similar shape—much the same way that a key fits into a lock. When a drug combines with a receptor, channels are either opened or closed and cellular biochemical messengers, such as cyclic adenosine monophosphate or calcium ions, are activated. Once activated, cellular functions can be turned either on or off by these messengers. Structurally nonspecific drugs, such as biological response modifiers, don't combine with cell receptors; rather, they produce changes within the cell membrane or interior.

The mechanisms by which drugs interact with the body are not always known. Drugs may work by physical action (such as the protective effects of a topical ointment) or chemical reaction (such as an antacid's effect on the gastric mucosa), or by modifying the metabolic activity of invading pathogens (such as an antibiotic) or replacing a missing biochemical substance (such as insulin).

Agonists

Agonists are drugs that interact with a receptor to stimulate a response. They alter cell physiology by binding to plasma membranes or intracellular structures. *Partial agonists* can't achieve maximal effects even though they may occupy all available receptor sites on a cell. *Strong agonists* can cause maximal effects while occupying only a small number of receptor sites on a cell. *Weak agonists* must occupy many more receptor sites than strong agonists to produce the same effect.

Antagonists

Antagonists are drugs that attach to a receptor but don't stimulate a response; instead, they inhibit or block responses that would normally be caused by agonists. *Competitive antagonists* bind to receptor sites that are also compatible with an agonist, thus preventing the agonist from binding to the site. *Noncompetitive antagonists* bind to receptor sites that aren't occupied by an agonist; this changes the receptor site so that it's no longer recognized by the agonist. *Irreversible antagonists* work in much the same way that noncompetitive ones do, except that they permanently bind with the receptor.

Antagonism plays an important role in drug interactions. When two agonists that cause opposite therapeutic effects, such as a vasodilator and a vasoconstrictor, are combined, the effects cancel each other out. When two antagonists, such as morphine and naloxone, are combined, both drugs may become inactive.

Pharmacotherapeutics

Pharmacotherapeutics is the study of how drugs are used to prevent or treat disease. Understanding why a drug is prescribed for a certain disease can assist you in prioritizing drug administration with other patient care activities. Knowing a drug's desired and unwanted effects may help you uncover problems not readily apparent from the admitting diagnosis. This information may also help you prevent such problems as adverse reactions and drug interactions.

A drug's *desired effect* is the intended or expected clinical response to the drug. This is the response you start to evaluate as soon as a drug is given. Dosage adjustments and the continuation of therapy often depend on your accurate evaluation and documentation of the patient's response.

An *adverse reaction* is any noxious and unintended response to a drug that occurs at therapeutic doses used for prophylaxis, diagnosis, or therapy. Adverse reactions associated with excessive amounts of a drug are considered drug overdoses. Be prepared to follow your institution's policy for reporting adverse drug reactions.

An *idiosyncratic response* is a genetically determined abnormal or excessive response to a drug that occurs in a particular patient. The unusual response may indicate that the drug has saturated or overwhelmed mechanisms that normally control absorption, distribution, metabolism, or excretion, thus altering the expected response. You may be unsure whether a reaction is adverse or idiosyncratic. Once you report the reaction, the pharmacist usually determines the appropriate course of action.

An *allergic reaction* is an adverse response that results from previous exposure to the same drug or to one that is chemically similar to it. The patient's immune system reacts to the drug as if it were a foreign invader and may produce a mild hypersensitivity reaction, characterized by localized dermatitis, urticaria, angioedema, or photosensitivity. Allergic reactions should be reported to the prescriber immediately and the drug should be discontinued. Follow-up care may include giving drugs, including antihistamines and corticosteroids, to counteract the allergic response.

An *anaphylactic reaction* is an immediate hypersensitivity response characterized by urticaria, pruritus, and angioedema. Left untreated, an anaphylactic reaction can lead to systemic involvement, resulting in shock. It's often associated with life-threatening hypotension and respiratory distress. Be prepared to assist with emergency life support measures, especially if the reaction occurs in response to I.V. drugs, which have the fastest rate of absorption.

A *drug interaction* occurs when one drug alters the pharmacokinetics of another drug—for example, when two or more drugs are given concurrently. Such concurrent administration can increase or decrease the therapeutic or adverse effects of either drug. Some drug interactions are beneficial. For example, when taken with penicillin G, probenecid decreases the excretion rate of penicillin G, resulting in higher blood levels of penicillin G. Drug interactions may also occur when a drug's metabolism is altered, often owing to the induction of or competition for metabolizing enzymes. For example, H_2-receptor agonists, which reduce secretion of the enzyme gastrin, may alter the breakdown of enteric coatings on other drugs. Drug interactions due to carrier protein competition typically occur when a drug inhibits the kidneys' ability to reduce excretion of other drugs. For example, probenecid is completely reabsorbed by the renal tubules and is metabolized very slowly. It competes with the same carrier protein as sulfonamides for active tubular secretion and so decreases the renal excretion of sulfonamides. This particular competition can lead to an increased risk of sulfonamide toxicity.

Special Considerations

Although every drug has a usual dosage range, certain factors—such as a patient's age, weight, culture and ethnicity, gender, pregnancy status, and renal and hepatic function—may contribute to the need for dosage adjustments. When you encounter special considerations such as these, be prepared to reassess the prescribed dosage to make sure that it's safe and effective for your patient.

Culture and Ethnicity

Certain drugs are more effective or more likely to produce adverse effects in particular ethnic groups or races. For example, blacks with hypertension respond better to thiazide diuretics than do patients of other races; on the other hand, blacks also have an increased risk of developing angioedema associated with angiotensin-converting enzyme (ACE) inhibitors. A patient's religious or cultural background may also call for special consideration. For example, a drug made from porcine products may be unacceptable to a Jewish or Muslim patient.

Elderly Patients

Because aging produces certain changes in body composition and organ function, elderly patients present unique therapeutic and dosing problems that require special attention. For example, the weight of the liver, the number of functioning hepatic cells, and hepatic blood flow all decrease as a person ages, resulting in slower drug metabolism. Renal function may also decrease with aging. These processes can lead to the accumulation of active drugs and metabolites as well as increased sensitivity to the effects of some drugs in elderly patients. Because they're also more likely to have multiple chronic illnesses, many elderly patients take multiple prescription drugs each day, thus increasing the risk of drug interactions.

Children

Because their bodily functions are not fully developed, children—particularly those under age 12—may metabolize drugs differently than adults. In infants, immature renal and hepatic function delay metabolism and excretion of drugs. As a result, pediatric drug dosages are very different from adult dosages.

The FDA has provided drug manufacturers with guidelines that define pediatric age categories. Use these categories as a guide when administering drugs, unless the manufacturer provides a specific age range:

- neonates—birth up to age 1 month
- infants—ages 1 month to 2 years
- children—ages 2 to 12
- adolescents—ages 12 to 16.

Pregnancy

The many physiologic changes that take place in the body during pregnancy may affect a drug's pharmacokinetics and alter its effectiveness. Additionally, exposure to drugs may pose risks for the developing fetus. Before administering a drug to a pregnant patient, be sure to check its assigned FDA pregnancy risk category and intervene appropriately.

PRINCIPLES OF I.V. DRUG ADMINISTRATION

Because there are thousands of drugs and hundreds of facts about each one, taking responsibility for drug administration can seem overwhelming. Administering I.V. drugs requires a combination of skills—not only knowing how to administer drugs safely but also knowledge of anatomy (such as the location of veins in the body) and of assessment (for example, when and how to observe the insertion site, surrounding area, and the patient for complications).

In I.V. drug administration, a drug enters the circulatory system through a single, small-volume injection or a slow, large-volume infusion rather than through GI absorption. Because drugs injected I.V. don't encounter absorption barriers, this route produces the most rapid drug action, making it vital in emergency situations. The I.V. route is also used when the patient is uncooperative, unconscious, or unable to accept medication by the oral or I.M. route or when a drug is ineffective by other routes. Although it's the preferred route for certain situations, I.V. administration has several disadvantages: I.V. drugs are generally more expensive to administer than other dosage forms because they require strict sterility, and once the drug has been injected, it can't be removed and the dosage can't be reduced.

One way that you can enhance your understanding of the principles of I.V. drug administration is to *associate, ask,* and *predict* during the critical thinking process. For example, *associate* each drug with general information you may already know about the drug or drug class. *Ask* yourself why a drug may be given by the I.V. route or why it's given multiple times throughout the day rather than only once. Learn to *predict* a drug's actions, uses, adverse effects, and possible drug interactions based on your knowledge of the drug's mechanism of action. As you apply these principles to I.V. drug administration, you'll begin to intuitively know which facts you need to make rational clinical decisions.

Each facility or agency has its own protocols for I.V. drug administration, including care of the I.V. site. Many of them use the Intravenous Nurses Society's Standards of Practice to formulate their policies. Individual state nursing practice guidelines are another component that may be used to develop I.V. administration protocols.

"Rights" of Drug Administration

Always keep in mind the following "rights" of drug administration, which apply to all forms of drug administration, including I.V.: the right drug, right time, right dose, right patient, right route, and right preparation and administration.

Right Drug

Many drugs have similar spellings, a variety of concentrations, and several generic forms. Before administering any drug, compare the exact spelling and concentration of the prescribed drug that appears on the label with the information contained in the medication administration record or drug profile. Regardless of which drug distribution system your facility uses, you should read the drug label and compare it to the medication administration record at least three times:

- before removing the drug from the dispensing unit or unit-dose cart
- before reconstituting, diluting, or measuring the prescribed dose
- before opening a unit-dose package (just prior to administering the drug to the patient).

Right Time

Various factors can affect the time a drug is given, such as the timing of meals, other drugs, or scheduled diagnostic tests; standardized times used by the institution; and factors that may alter the consistency of blood levels and drug absorption. Before giving any p.r.n. drug, check the patient's chart to ensure that no one else has already administered it and that the specified time interval has passed. Also, document administration of a p.r.n. drug immediately.

Right Dose

Whenever you're dispensing an unfamiliar drug or in doubt about a dosage, check the prescribed dose against the range specified in a reliable reference. In addition, because many I.V. drugs come in different concentrations—such as urokinase, which is available in concentrations ranging from 5,000 to 250,000 international units—you must examine the label closely to ensure that you're administering the proper strength. Also make sure that you're using the appropriate concentration for the method of administration. For example, the 5,000– and 9,000–international unit concentrations of urokinase are used *only* for clearing I.V. catheter occlusions, *not* for I.V. or intracoronary drug administration. Conversely, the 250,000–international unit concentration is used *only* for I.V. and intracoronary drug administration.

Be sure to consider any reasons for which your patient might need a dosage adjustment, such as age, preexisting medical conditions, or response to the drug. Also, be familiar with the standard abbreviations your institution uses for writing prescriptions.

Right Patient

Always compare the name of the patient on the medication record with the name on the patient's identification bracelet. When using a unit-dose system, compare the name on the drug profile with that on the identification bracelet.

Right Route

Each prescribed drug should specify the administration route. If the administration route is missing, consult the prescribing physician. Never substitute one route for another unless you obtain a prescription for the change. Severe adverse reactions can result from administering a parenteral drug by the wrong route. For example, the antineoplastic drug vinblastine can cause potentially fatal paralysis when administered intrathecally and requires special labeling when it's being prepared.

Right Preparation and Administration

Be sure to maintain aseptic technique when handling drugs that need to be reconstituted, diluted, and measured. Follow any specific directions included in the manufacturer's insert regarding diluent type and amount and the use of filters, if needed. Clearly label any drug that you've reconstituted with the patient's name, the strength or dose, the date and time that you prepared the drug, the amount and type of diluent that you used, the expiration date, and your initials. Be aware that certain drugs and diluents contain additives that have been known to cause adverse reactions. One example is benzyl alcohol, a preservative found in some drugs and diluents, which may cause a fatal toxic syndrome in neonates and premature infants, characterized by CNS, respiratory, circulatory, and renal impairment and metabolic acidosis. Also, determine whether your patient has an allergy to a prescribed drug or its components, to similar drugs, or to a recommended diluent; if so, report it to the prescriber. If the patient is allergic to a diluent, discuss possible alternative diluents with the pharmacist.

Become familiar with the I.V. administration method being used. For example, if you're using an I.V. administration set, find out the accurate flow rate—usually between 10 and 60 drops/ml. If you're using an infusion device, know how to use it correctly. Also, check the infusion rate periodically to ensure that the appropriate amount of drug is being administered.

Types of Venous Access

I.V. drugs can be administered through a peripheral or central venous access. The type of access depends on such factors as the patient's overall medical condition, the type of drug to be administered, and the amount of time the patient requires I.V. drug therapy.

Once I.V. access has been established, it is used for either continuous or intermittent injection or infusion. Intermittent infusion typically involves the use of a saline, or heparin, lock. This device is advantageous because it allows for immediate venous access and doesn't require continuous administration of fluids to maintain its patency.

Peripheral I.V. Drug Administration

In peripheral I.V. administration, a drug is injected or infused through a peripheral vein, usually one in the forearm. Peripheral access is used to administer various fluids and solutions, including antibiotics, chemotherapeutic drugs, blood products, and hydrating fluids. It is typically used for short-term drug administration in the hospital and in outpatient settings. For longer periods of drug administration, a midline catheter may be used. This is a longer catheter that remains in the peripheral venous system, typically in the larger veins of the arm below the axilla. A peripheral insertion site may also be used for a peripherally inserted central catheter (PICC), which delivers drugs directly into the central venous system.

Veins in the distal part of the upper extremity are typically selected first, but the choice of vein depends on the type of drug being administered, possible adverse effects, the patient's age and medical condition, which hand is dominant, and the length of time the I.V. line will be in place. These factors also influence the choice of a venipuncture device, which may range from a winged infusion set to an over-the-needle catheter made of polyethylene, silicone, or other materials. Use the shortest needle and the smallest gauge that meet the needs of the drug or solution to be infused.

Central Venous Administration

Central venous therapy is commonly used to administer long-term drug therapy to patients whose condition contraindicates the placement of a peripheral I.V. line. Central venous access may be achieved by the placement of centrally or peripherally inserted catheters or implantable ports.

If venous access is placed in the upper part of the body, the central venous catheter tip lies in the superior vena cava; if femoral venous access is used, the catheter tip lies in the inferior superior vena cava. Common sites for centrally inserted catheters are the subclavian vein and the internal or external jugular veins. Common sites for PICCs are the basilic, cephalic, and median cubital veins in the upper extremity. Surgically implanted central venous ports have a self-sealing septum with a catheter attached that leads to the superior vena cava. Ports may be accessed using noncoring needles from above or at the side of the port, depending on the type used.

The type of central catheter used varies, depending on such factors as the type and number of drugs to be administered and the amount of time the central access will be in place. Single-lumen or multi-lumen catheters may be used, depending on the patient's needs. Tunneled catheters, such as the Hickman catheter, are used when long-term use is anticipated. These catheters are radiopaque and have a cuff at the end, near the body entrance site. Part of the tunneled catheter lies within subcutaneous tissue, which over time turns into a collagenous matrix that gradually adheres to the cuff, thus helping to secure the catheter and protect against infection.

Alternative Infusion Methods

Although the focus of this book is I.V. drug therapy, you should be aware of other methods used to infuse drugs, such as subcutaneous (S.C.) and intraosseous infusion. One of the most common uses of the S.C. route is insulin administration. A programmed insulin pump administers small amounts of regular insulin throughout the day through a needle or catheter inserted into the patient's abdomen. Intraosseous infusions are administered by a needle inserted into the bone marrow. They are used in such conditions as shock, anaphylaxis, or trauma when venous access is not available.

Infusion Devices

I.V. drug therapy commonly requires the use of an infusion device to ensure that the appropriate dose is being administered—for example, when administering I.V. antiarrhythmics (such as lidocaine hydrochloride or procainamide hydrochloride) or when administering drugs to children. The type of infusion device can vary, depending on the drug used, the amount of fluid to be given, and the setting at which the drug is being administered.

Electronic infusion devices (also known as electronic infusion pumps and controllers) are powered by electricity or battery packs. These devices come in various sizes, from compact ambulatory versions designed for portable use to multidrug infusion pumps commonly used in acute care settings. Controller devices don't assist in drug delivery; rather they monitor the drop flow based on a programmed rate. Electronic infusion pumps provide a positive pressure flow to assist with drug delivery.

Electronic infusion devices may be equipped with alarms to signal increased pressure or air in the I.V. line or the completion of an infusion. Some devices prevent free flow of the solution if the I.V. line becomes disconnected from the device, which can prevent serious complications. Others contain a free-flow alarm, which can signal an uncontrolled rate of fluid administration stemming from accidental disconnection.

Patient-Controlled Analgesia

Patient-controlled analgesia (PCA) allows the patient to be actively involved in his own drug delivery. First, you administer the loading dose and program the pump to deliver additional bolus doses of the drug within predetermined limits for amount and frequency. The patient then presses a button when he wants to activate a bolus dose. You must clearly explain the drug delivery system to the patient, making sure he understands that there is a "lock-out" period during which he won't be able to administer additional doses.

Complications of I.V. Therapy

Because I.V. drug administration requires a break in the skin, it poses an increased risk of infection, ranging from local infection of surrounding tissues to sepsis. To prevent infection or detect it early, monitor the I.V. site, change dressings and tubing, and rotate the I.V. site in accordance with your facility's policy. Administration sets are typically changed every 24 to 48 hours (every 24 hours for intermittent infusion), and I.V. sites are rotated every 48 to 72 hours.

Two other potential complications of I.V. therapy are infiltration—the leakage of nonvesicant solution into surrounding tissues—and extravasation—the leakage of a vesicant solution, such as certain chemotherapeutic drugs, into surrounding tissues. To detect these complications, frequently assess the I.V. site and surrounding area. If you observe either of these conditions, restart the I.V. line at another site. Extravasation can cause tissue necrosis, gangrene, and other reactions around the injection site. If extravasation occurs, expect to use a drug such as phentolamine to antagonize vasoconstriction and minimize sloughing and tissue necrosis.

Other risks associated with I.V. drug therapy include catheter occlusion, circulatory overload, phlebitis, thrombosis, hematoma, pulmonary or air embolism, and venous spasm. Some potential complications are specific to the I.V. access route. For example, central venous catheters increase the risk of arterial puncture, pneumothorax, and hemothorax during catheter placement.

The rapid drug distribution and greater bioavailability associated with I.V. therapy mean that you must be vigilant in monitoring for adverse drug reactions. Too-rapid administration of a drug can result in a type of reaction known as speed shock. Anaphylactic reactions can occur within a few minutes of drug administration or several days afterward. Become familiar with the potential adverse effects of each drug you administer.

Safe Handling of Toxic Agents

I.V. drug administration may expose you to toxic agents, such as many antineoplastic drugs. To protect yourself from potential carcinogenic, mutagenic, and teratogenic effects of these drugs, learn how to handle them safely. Because no standard procedure exists, follow your facility's protocols for preparation and handling of antineoplastic drugs and for appropriate disposal of used equipment. In addition, before you prepare a toxic drug, consult the manufacturer's package insert for specific recommendations, such as the use of a biological containment cabinet, gloves, and gown.

Preventing Needlestick Injuries

Take steps to avoid needlestick injuries when you administer I.V. drugs and when you handle certain preparations, such as immune globulin intravenous, which is made from human plasma and therefore may contain infectious agents such as viruses. Needleless administration systems have been developed to decrease the risk of needlestick injuries and exposure to such viruses as HIV.

Other Uses for I.V. Access

In addition to drug administration, I.V. access is also used for infusions of hydrating fluids, blood and blood products, and total parenteral nutrition (TPN).

Parenteral Fluids

Parenteral fluids may be infused at a slow rate to maintain an I.V. access, to treat certain medical conditions (such as the administration of normal saline to treat hyperparathyroidism), or to restore fluid volume in patients with hypovolemic shock or burns. (See *Selected water and electrolyte solutions,* page xxx.)

SELECTED WATER AND ELECTROLYTE SOLUTIONS

The chart below provides electrolyte contents for some common solutions you may administer in your clinical practice.

I.V. Solution	Electrolyte Contents
0.5% dextrose in water	No electrolytes
Dextrose 2.5% with ½ strength lactated Ringer's injection	1.4 mEq/L of calcium 54 to 55 mEq/L of chloride 14 mEq/L of lactate 2 mEq/L of potassium 65 mEq/L of sodium
Dextrose 5% with lactated Ringer's injection	2.7 to 3 mEq/L of calcium 109 to 112 mEq/L of chloride 28 mEq/L of lactate 4 mEq/L of potassium 130 mEq/L of sodium
Lactated Ringer's injection	2.7 to 3 mEq/L of calcium 109 to 110 mEq/L of chloride 28 mEq/L of lactate 4 mEq/L of potassium 130 mEq/L of sodium
⅙ M Sodium lactate	167 mEq/L of lactate 167 mEq/L of sodium
0.45% Sodium chloride	77 mEq/L of chloride 77 mEq/L of sodium
0.9% Sodium chloride	154 mEq/L of chloride 154 mEq/L of sodium
3% Sodium chloride	513 mEq/L of chloride 513 mEq/L of sodium
5% Sodium chloride	855 mEq/L of chloride 855 mEq/L of sodium

Blood Products

I.V. access is used for transfusion of blood and blood products, including whole blood, packed red blood cells, platelets, and plasma. Learn your facility's protocols and the techniques required for administering blood products. Before you administer blood, verify the prescriber's order and that the patient has an appropriate I.V. access, typically an 18G or 20G catheter (smaller for children). Ensure that no solution other than normal saline is infusing in the I.V. line to be used. Two other critical steps are verifying the patient's ABO blood and Rh types and verifying his identity to ensure that the right product is given to the right patient. (See *Understanding blood types and Rh factor,* page xxxii.) Observe the patient continuously during the first 10 to 15 minutes because the majority of anaphylactic and ABO incompatibility reactions occur during that time. Blood infusions are generally not administered for longer than 4 hours because of the risk of septicemia.

Total Parenteral Nutrition

Also referred to as I.V. hyperalimentation, total parenteral nutrition (TPN) provides nutrition for patients who are unable to eat, digest, or absorb a sufficient amount of nutrients. TPN is typically administered by a central venous catheter, usually a subclavian catheter; however, PICC lines or tunneled catheters may also be used. Administer TPN as a continuous infusion, using an infusion pump. Monitor the patient for adverse reactions, including infection, sepsis, and venous thrombosis from the I.V. access; hyperglycemia if the patient can't metabolize the glucose in the TPN fast enough; or hypoglycemia if the infusion is stopped abruptly.

UNDERSTANDING BLOOD TYPES AND Rh FACTOR

Verification of ABO blood and Rh types is vital if you'll be administering blood products. Administering the wrong blood type or Rh factor to a patient could set off an immune response that results in the destruction of red blood cells (RBCs). Understanding the role that antigens and antibodies play in blood typing will help you understand the importance of transfusing the correct blood product.

Antigens are glycoproteins or glycolipids found on the membrane surface of RBCs. Specific antigens on the RBC designate an individual's ABO blood type. The four major blood types are A, B, AB, and O. Individuals inherit antigens and blood types from their parents. Within a few months of birth, a child develops antibodies against the antigens he doesn't have. The antigens and antibodies for the specific blood types are as follows:

Type	Antigen	Antibody
A	A	Anti-B
B	B	Anti-A
AB	A and B	None
O	None	Anti-A and Anti-B

Each patient should ideally receive his own specific blood type. However, in an emergency, type O blood can be administered to anyone because it contains no A or B antigens. For this reason, people with type O blood are called *universal donors.* Conversely, persons with type AB blood, which has both antigens, can receive any blood type and are called *universal recipients.*

Antigens are also a component of the Rh factor; one of them—the D antigen—is of particular significance. Patients who have the D antigen are considered Rh-positive, whereas patients who lack the D antigen are Rh-negative. Antibodies to the D antigen don't develop automatically; they can form if a person has received a previous transfusion or delivered a child who has the antigen. If a person with antibodies to the D antigen receives a transfusion of Rh-positive blood, he can develop a transfusion reaction that results in RBC destruction.

I.V. Drug Therapy and the Nursing Process

A systematic approach to nursing care, the nursing process helps guide you as you develop, implement, and evaluate your care and ensures that you'll deliver safe, consistent, and effective I.V. drug therapy to your patients. The nursing process consists of five steps: assessment, nursing diagnosis, planning, implementation, and evaluation. Even though documentation is not a step in the nursing process, you're legally and professionally responsible for documenting all aspects of your care before, during, and after drug administration.

Assessment

The first step in the nursing process, assessment involves gathering information that is essential to guide your patient's drug therapy. This information includes the patient's drug history, present drug use, allergies, medical history, and physical examination findings. Assessment is an ongoing process that serves as a baseline against which to compare any changes in your patient's condition; it's also the basis for developing and individualizing the patient's plan of care.

Drug History

The patient's drug history is critical in your planning of drug-related care. Ask about his previous use of OTC and prescription drugs as well as herbal remedies. For each drug, determine:

- the reason the patient took it
- the prescribed dosage
- the administration route
- the frequency of administration
- the duration of the drug therapy
- any adverse reactions the patient may have experienced and how he handled them.

If the patient received previous I.V. therapy, ask him the type of vascular access that was used and how he tolerated the therapy.

Also, determine if the patient has a history of drug abuse or addiction; if he has, find out the administration route he used. Depending on his physical and emotional state, you may need to obtain the drug history from other sources, such as family members, friends, or other caregivers, and from the medical record.

Present Drug Use

Ask about the patient's current use of OTC and prescription drugs as well as herbal remedies. As you did in the drug history, find out the specific details for each drug (dosage, route, frequency, and reason for taking). Also ask the patient if he thinks the drug has been effective and when he took the last dose.

If the patient uses herbal remedies, similarly explore the use of these products because herbs may interact with certain drugs. Also ask about the patient's use of recreational drugs, such as alcohol and tobacco, as well as illegal drugs, such as marijuana and heroin. Again, be sure to ascertain the administration route he used. If the patient acknowledges use of these drugs, be alert for possible drug interactions. This information may also provide you with insight about the patient's response—or lack of response—to his current drug treatment plan.

Try to find out if the patient has any other problems that might affect his compliance with the drug treatment plan, and intervene appropriately. For instance, a patient who is unemployed and has no health insurance may fail to fill a needed prescription. In such a case, contact an appropriate individual in your facility who may be able to help the patient obtain financial assistance.

Be sure to ask the patient if his drug treatment plan requires special monitoring or follow-up laboratory tests. For example, patients who take antihypertensives need to have their blood pressure checked routinely, and those who take warfarin must have their prothrombin time tested regularly. Other patients must undergo periodic blood tests to assess their hepatic and renal function. Determine whether the patient has complied with this part of his treatment plan, and ask him if he knows the results of the latest monitoring or laboratory tests.

Allergies

Find out if the patient is allergic to any drugs or foods. If he has an allergy, explore it further by determining the type of drug or food that triggers a reaction, the first time he experienced a reaction, the characteristics of the reaction, and other related information. Keep in mind that some patients consider annoying symptoms, such as indigestion, an allergic reaction. However, be sure to document a true allergy according to your facility's policy to ensure that the patient doesn't receive that drug or any related drug that may cause a similar reaction. Also, document allergies to foods because they may lead to drug interactions or adverse drug reactions. For example, sulfite is a food additive as well as a drug additive, so a patient with a known allergy to sulfite-containing foods is likely to react to sulfite-containing drugs.

Medical History

While reviewing your patient's medical history, determine if he has any acute or chronic conditions that may interfere with his drug therapy. Certain disorders involving major body systems, such as the cardiovascular, GI, hepatic, and renal systems, may affect a drug's absorption, transport, metabolism, or excretion and interfere with its action; they may also increase the incidence of adverse reactions and lead to toxicity. For each disorder identified, try to determine when the condition was diagnosed, what drugs were prescribed, and who prescribed them. This information can help you determine whether the patient is receiving incompatible drugs and whether more than one prescriber is managing his drug therapy.

Ask a female patient if she is or may be pregnant or if she's breast-feeding. Many drugs are safe to use during pregnancy, but others may harm the fetus. Also, some drugs are distributed into breast milk. If your patient is or might be pregnant, check the FDA's pregnancy risk category for the prescribed drug and notify the prescriber if the drug may pose a risk to the fetus. If the patient is breast-feeding, find out if the drug is distributed in breast milk and intervene appropriately.

In addition, ask the patient about any preexisting conditions or procedures that may have implications for the I.V. site selection, such as a history of lymphatic or superior vena caval obstruction, lymph node dissection, mastectomy, or radiation therapy to the upper torso, or the presence of an internal arteriovenous fistula for hemodialysis.

Physical Examination Findings

As part of the physical examination, note the patient's age and weight. Be aware that age determines the dosage of certain drugs, such as sedatives and hypnotics, whereas weight determines the dosage of others, including some I.V. antibiotics and anticoagulants. As you perform the physical examination, note any abnormal findings that may point to body organ or system dysfunction. For example, if you detect liver enlargement and ascites, the patient may have impaired hepatic function, which can affect the metabolism of a drug he's taking and lead to harmful adverse or toxic effects. Also note whether a body organ or system appears to be responding to drug treatment. For example, if a patient has been taking an antibiotic to treat chronic bronchitis, thoroughly evaluate his respiratory status to measure his progress. And be sure to assess the patient for possible adverse reactions to the drugs he's taking.

Also assess the condition of potential vascular access sites, and evaluate their suitability for I.V. drug administration.

Assess the patient's neurologic function to ensure that he can understand his drug regimen and carry out required tasks, such as performing a finger stick to obtain blood for glucose measurement. If a patient can't understand essential drug information, you'll need to identify a family member or another person who is willing to become involved in the teaching process.

Nursing Diagnosis

Based on information derived from the assessment and physical examination findings, the nursing diagnoses are statements of actual or potential problems that a nurse is licensed to treat or manage alone or in collaboration with other members of the health care team. They're worded according to guidelines established by the North American Nursing Diagnosis Association.

One of the most common nursing diagnoses related to drug therapy is *knowledge deficit,* which indicates that the patient doesn't have sufficient understanding of his drug regimen. However, adverse reactions are the basis for most nursing diagnoses related to drug administration. For example, a patient receiving an opioid analgesic might have a nursing diagnosis of *constipation* related to decreased intestinal motility or *ineffective breathing pattern* related to respiratory depression. Many antiarrhythmics cause orthostatic hypotension and thus may place an elderly patient at *high risk for injury* related to possible syncope. Broad-spectrum antibiotics, such as penicillin G, may lead to the overgrowth of *Clostridium difficile,* a bacterium that is normally present in the intestines. This overgrowth, in turn, may lead to pseudomembranous enterocolitis, characterized by abdominal pain and severe diarrhea. The nursing diagnoses in such a case might include *risk for infection* related to bacterial overgrowth, *alteration in comfort* related to abdominal pain, and *fluid balance deficit* related to diarrhea.

Planning

During the planning phase, you'll establish expected outcomes—or goals—for the patient and then develop specific nursing interventions to achieve them. Expected outcomes are observable or measurable goals that should occur as a result of nursing interventions and sometimes in conjunction with medical interventions. Developed in collaboration with the patient, the outcomes should be realistic and objective and should clearly communicate to other nurses the direction of the plan of care. They should be written as behaviors or responses for the patient, not the nurse, to achieve and should include a time frame for measuring the patient's progress. An example of a typical expected outcome is: "The patient will accurately demonstrate self-administration of insulin before discharge." Based on each outcome statement that you establish, you'll then develop appropriate nursing interventions, which may include drug administration techniques, patient teaching, monitoring of vital signs, calculation of drug dosages based on weight, and recording of intake and output.

Implementation

As you implement the nursing interventions, be sure to stringently follow the classic rule of drug administration: administer the right dose of the right drug by the right route to the right patient at the right time. Also, keep in mind that you have a legal and professional responsibility to follow institutional policy regarding standing orders, prescription renewal, and the use of nursing judgment. During the implementation phase, you'll also begin to evaluate the patient's expected outcomes and nursing interventions and make necessary changes to the plan of care.

Evaluation

Evaluation is an ongoing process rather than a single step in the nursing process. During this phase, you evaluate each expected outcome to determine whether or not it has been achieved and whether the original plan of care is working or needs to be modified. In evaluating a patient's drug treatment plan, you should determine whether or not the drug is controlling the signs and symptoms for which it was prescribed. You should also evaluate the patient for psychological or physiologic responses to the drug, especially adverse reactions. This constant monitoring allows you to make appropriate and timely suggestions for changes to the plan of care, such as dosage adjustments or changes in delivery routes, until each expected outcome has been achieved.

Documentation

You're responsible for documenting all your actions related to the patient's drug therapy, from the assessment phase to evaluation. Each time you administer a drug, document the drug name, dose, time given, and your evaluation of its effect. Also document the condition of the I.V. insertion site, including the presence (be specific) or absence of any I.V.-related complications, specific interventions that were required, and the patient's response. When you administer drugs that require additional nursing judgment, such as those prescribed on an as-needed basis, document the rationale for administering the drug and follow-up assessment or interventions for each dose administered.

If you decide to withhold a prescribed drug based on your nursing judgment, document your action and the rationale for it, and notify the prescriber of your action in a timely manner. Whenever you notify a prescriber about a significant finding related to drug therapy, such as an adverse reaction, document the date and time, the person you contacted, what you discussed, and how you intervened.

A

abatacept

Orencia

Class and Category

Chemical: Human cytotoxic T-lymphocyte–associated antigen 4
Therapeutic: T-cell activation blocker
Pregnancy category: C

Indications and Dosages

▶ *To reduce signs and symptoms, slow the progression of structural damage, and improve physical function in patients with moderate to severe active rheumatoid arthritis and an inadequate response to one or more disease-modifying anti-rheumatic drugs (DMARDs)*

I.V. INFUSION

Adults. 30-minute infusion of 500 mg for patients weighing less than 60 kg; 750 mg for patients weighing 60 to 100 kg; and 1,000 mg for patients weighing more than 100 kg. Repeat in 2 and 4 wk and then q 4 wk thereafter.

Route	Onset	Peak	Duration
I.V.	Unknown	60 days	Unknown

Mechanism of Action

Inhibits T-cell activation by binding to CD80 and CD86, blocking their interaction with CD28. Interaction with CD28 normally provides a co-stimulatory signal needed for T-cell activation. Without this signal, T cells aren't activated, which slows the structural damage in rheumatoid arthritis and improves physical function.

Contraindications

Hypersensitivity to abatacept and its components

Interactions

DRUGS

live vaccines: Effects of vaccine may be blunted

tumor necrosis factor (TNF) antagonists: Increased risk of serious infections

Adverse Reactions

CNS: Dizziness, headache
CV: Hypertension, hypotension
EENT: Nasopharyngitis, rhinitis, sinusitis
GI: Diverticulitis, nausea
GU: Acute pyelonephritis, UTI
MS: Back or limb pain
RESP: Bronchitis, cough, dyspnea, upper respiratory tract infection, pneumonia, wheezing
SKIN: Cellulites, flushing, pruritus, rash, urticaria
Other: Anaphylaxis, abatacept antibody formation, herpes simplex or localized infection, influenza, malignancies

Nursing Considerations

- Before starting abatacept, screen patient for latent tuberculosis, as ordered. If tuberculosis is detected, expect to delay abatacept therapy until after effective tuberculosis treatment has been given.
- Use cautiously in patients with a history of recurrent infections or underlying medical conditions that increase the risk of infection.
- Be aware that drug may be given with other DMARDs. Expect to avoid giving abatacept with TNF antagonists because of an increased risk of infection or with anakinra because combined effects are unknown.
- Reconstitute each abatacept vial with 10 ml of sterile water for injection using only the silicone-free disposable syringe provided and an 18G to 21G needle. If drug is accidentally reconstituted with siliconized syringe, discard the solution. To minimize foaming during reconstitution, rotate the vial by swirling it gently until contents are dissolved. Don't shake the vial. Once the powder is dissolved completely, vent the vial with a needle to dissipate any foam before withdrawal.
- Further dilute to 100 ml by withdrawing a volume equal to the volume of reconstituted drug from a 100-ml infusion bag or bottle of 0.9% sodium chloride solution. For example, for two vials, remove 20 ml; for three vials, remove 30 ml, and for four vials, remove 40 ml. Slowly add the reconstituted solution from each vial prepared using the same silicone-free disposable syringe provided with each vial. Gently mix.

- Administer each abatacept dose over 30 minutes using an infusion set and a sterile, non-pyrogenic, low-protein–binding filter. Discard any unused solution after 24 hours. Don't infuse abatacept concurrently in the same intravenous line with other drugs.
- Monitor patient closely for infusion-related reactions, such as dizziness, headache, and hypertension, especially during the first hour of the infusion. Notify prescriber if they occur.
- **WARNING** Monitor patient closely for hypersensitivity reactions, changes in blood pressure, dyspnea, nausea, flushing, urticaria, cough, pruritus, rash, and wheezing. While most reactions are not life-threatening, notify prescriber and prepare to discontinue infusion and provide supportive care if reaction is severe.
- If patient has COPD, assess him often for respiratory dusfunction during abatacept therapy because adverse respiratory reactions are more likely in patients with COPD.
- Notify prescriber and expect to stop drug if patient develops a serious infection during abatacept therapy.
- Avoid giving live vaccines during and within 3 months after abatacept therapy because abatacept may decrease the vaccine's effectiveness.

PATIENT TEACHING

- Review signs and symptoms of a possible allergic reaction, including rash and dyspnea. Urge patient to report any such symptoms immediately.
- Urge patient to immediately report signs of infection, such as cough, fever, chills, dyspnea, or headache.
- Explain that patient should receive no live vaccines during and for 3 months after abatacept therapy.
- If patient has COPD, caution about the increased risk of adverse respiratory effects. Tell him to notify prescriber immediately if they occur.

abciximab

ReoPro

Class and Category

Chemical: Fab fragment of chimeric 7E3 antibody
Therapeutic: Platelet aggregation inhibitor
Pregnancy category: C

Indications and Dosages

▶ *To prevent acute myocardial ischemic complications after percutaneous transluminal coronary angioplasty (PTCA) in patients at high risk for abrupt closure of treated coronary artery*

I.V. INFUSION OR INJECTION

Adults. 250 mcg/kg bolus 10 to 60 min before PTCA. *Maintenance:* 0.125 mcg/kg/min by continuous infusion for 12 hr. *Maximum:* 10 mcg/min.

▶ *To treat unstable angina in patients who haven't responded to conventional therapy and are scheduled for PTCA within 24 hr*

I.V. INFUSION OR INJECTION

Adults. 250 mcg/kg bolus, then 10 mcg/min continuous infusion over 18 to 24 hr, concluding 1 hr after PTCA.

Route	Onset	Peak	Duration
I.V.	Unknown	Unknown	48 hr

Mechanism of Action

Binds to glycoprotein IIb/IIIa receptor sites on surface of activated platelets. Circulating fibrinogen can bind to these receptor sites and link platelets together, forming a clot that eventually blocks a coronary artery. By binding to receptor sites, abciximab prevents normal binding of fibrinogen and other factors and inhibits platelet aggregation.

Incompatibilities

Don't mix abciximab with other drugs. Administer it through a separate I.V. line, whenever possible.

Contraindications

Active internal bleeding, arteriovenous malformation or aneurysm, bleeding disorders, CVA in past 2 years or that caused significant neurologic deficit at any time, GI or GU bleeding in past 6 weeks, hypersensitivity to abciximab, intracranial neoplasm, I.V. dextran therapy before or during PTCA, oral anticoagulant therapy in past 7 days unless PT is less than 1.2 times the control, severe uncontrolled hypertension, surgery in past 6 weeks, thrombocytopenia, vasculitis

Interactions

DRUGS

cefamandole, cefoperazone, cefotetan, dipyridamole, heparin, NSAIDs, oral anticoagulants, thrombolytic drugs, ticlopidine: Increased risk of bleeding

Adverse Reactions

CNS: Confusion, dizziness, hyperesthesia
CV: Atrial fibrillation or flutter, bradycardia, embolism, hypotension, peripheral edema, pseudoaneurysm, supraventricular tachycardia, third-degree AV block, thrombophlebitis, weak pulse
GI: Dysphagia, hematemesis, nausea, vomiting
GU: Dysuria, hematuria, renal dysfunction, urinary frequency, urinary incontinence, urine retention
HEME: Anemia, bleeding, leukocytosis, thrombocytopenia
RESP: Bronchitis, bronchospasm, crackles, dyspnea, pleural effusion, pneumonia, pulmonary edema, pulmonary embolism, wheezing
SKIN: Pruritus, rash, urticaria
Other: Development of human antichimeric antibodies

Nursing Considerations

- Be aware that abciximab may be used with heparin and aspirin therapy.
- Obtain PT, APTT, and platelet count before initiating therapy.
- Inspect abciximab for particles; don't use if opaque particles are present. Don't shake container.
- Administer I.V. bolus over at least 1 minute, using a sterile, nonpyrogenic, low protein-binding 0.2- to 0.22-micron filter.
- For continuous I.V. infusion, withdraw 4.5 ml from 2-mg/ml solution and inject prescribed amount into 250-ml bag of normal saline solution or D_5W, using an in-line sterile, nonpyrogenic, low protein-binding 0.2- to 0.22-micron filter. Discard unused portion.
- Infuse prescribed amount, using a continuous infusion pump.
- Avoid I.M. injections, venipunctures, and use of indwelling urinary catheters, NG tubes, and automatic blood pressure cuffs during abciximab therapy to prevent bleeding. If appropriate, insert an intermittent I.V. access device to obtain blood samples.
- Monitor for GI, GU, and retroperitoneal bleeding and for bleeding at all puncture sites.
- **WARNING** If hemorrhage occurs, prepare to discontinue infusion immediately. Expect to treat severe thrombocytopenia with platelet transfusions if needed.
- Monitor for hypersensitivity reactions, such as rash, pruritus, wheezing, and dysphagia from laryngeal edema. If such reactions occur, discontinue infusion and notify prescriber immedi-

ately. If anaphylaxis occurs, administer epinephrine, antihistamines, and corticosteroids, as prescribed.
- Monitor PT, APTT, and activated clotting time during and after therapy.
- Obtain platelet count 2 to 4 hours after initial bolus and every 24 hours thereafter during abciximab therapy as ordered. Expect platelet function to return to normal within 48 hours of conclusion of therapy.
- Monitor vital signs and continuous ECG tracings during treatment.
- Store drug at 2° to 8° C (36° to 46° F). Protect from freezing.

PATIENT TEACHING
- Teach patient about possible adverse reactions associated with abciximab, including bleeding and hypersensitivity reactions, such as rash, urticaria, and dyspnea.
- Tell patient to prevent injury from falls by maintaining bed rest and from bleeding by keeping limb immobile while catheter sheath is in place.

acetazolamide sodium
acetazolamide

Acetazolam (CAN), Ak-Zol, Apo-Acetazolamide (CAN), Dazamide, Diamox, Diamox Sequels, Storzolamide

Class and Category

Chemical: Sulfonamide derivative
Therapeutic: Anticonvulsant, antiglaucoma agent, diuretic
Pregnancy category: C

Indications and Dosages

▶ *As short-term therapy to treat secondary glaucoma and preoperatively to treat acute congestive (angle-closure) glaucoma*

I.V. INJECTION, TABLETS

Adults. 250 mg I.V. or P.O. b.i.d. or q 4 hr; or 500 mg I.V. or P.O. initially, followed by 125 to 250 mg q 4 hr for severe acute glaucoma. To initially lower intraocular pressure rapidly, 500 mg I.V.; may repeat in 2 to 4 hours in acute cases, depending on patient response. Oral therapy usually initiated after initial I.V. dose.

S.R. CAPSULES

Adults. 1 S.R. capsule (500 mg) b.i.d.

I.V. INJECTION

Children. 5 to 10 mg/kg/dose q 6 hr.

S.R. CAPSULES, TABLETS
Children. 10 to 15 mg/kg daily in divided doses q 6 to 8 hr.

▶ *To treat chronic simple (open-angle) glaucoma*

I.V. INJECTION, E.R. CAPSULES, TABLETS
Adults. 250 to 1,000 mg daily (in divided doses for dosages above 250 mg).

▶ *To induce diuresis in heart failure*

I.V. INJECTION, TABLETS
Adults. *Initial:* 250 to 375 mg or 5 mg/kg daily in morning. *Maintenance:* 250 to 375 mg or 5 mg/kg on alternate days or for 2 days, followed by a drug-free day.

▶ *To treat drug-induced edema*

I.V. INJECTION, TABLETS
Adults. 250 to 375 mg daily for 1 to 2 days.
I.V. INJECTION, TABLETS
Children. 5 mg/kg/dose daily in morning.

▶ *To treat seizures, including generalized tonic-clonic, absence, and mixed seizures, and myoclonic jerk patterns*

I.V. INJECTION, TABLETS
Adults and children. 8 to 30 mg/kg daily in divided doses. *Optimal:* 375 to 1,000 mg daily; when used with other anticonvulsants, 250 mg daily.

Route	Onset	Peak	Duration
I.V.*	2 min	15 min	4 to 5 hr

Mechanism of Action

Inhibits the enyzme carbonic anhydrase, which normally appears in the eyes' ciliary processes, brain's choroid plexes, and kidneys' proximal tubule cells. In the eyes, enzyme inhibition decreases aqueous humor secretion, which lowers intraocular pressure. In the brain, inhibition may delay abnormal, intermittent, and excessive discharge from neurons that cause seizures. In the kidneys, it increases bicarbonate excretion, which carries out water, potassium, and sodium, thus inducing diuresis and metabolic acidosis. This acidosis counteracts respiratory alkalosis.

Contraindications

Chronic noncongestive angle-closure glaucoma; cirrhosis; hyperchloremic acidosis; hypersensitivity to acetazolamide; hypokale-

* Effects on intraocular pressure.

mia; hyponatremia; severe pulmonary obstruction; severe renal, hepatic, or adrenocortical impairment

Interactions

DRUGS

amphetamines, methenamine, phenobarbital, procainamide, quinidine: Decreased excretion and possibly toxicity of these drugs
corticosteroids: Increased risk of hypokalemia
cyclosporine: Increased blood cyclosporine level, possibly nephrotoxicity or neurotoxicity
diflunisal: Possibly significantly decreased intraocular pressure
lithium: Increased excretion and decreased effectiveness of lithium
primidone: Decreased blood and urine primidone levels
salicylates: Increased risk of salicylate toxicity

Adverse Reactions

CNS: Ataxia, confusion, depression, disorientation, dizziness, drowsiness, fatigue, fever, flaccid paralysis, headache, lassitude, malaise, nervousness, paresthesia, seizures, tremor, weakness
EENT: Altered taste, tinnitus, transient myopia
GI: Anorexia, constipation, diarrhea, hepatic dysfunction, melena, nausea, vomiting
GU: Crystalluria, decreased libido, glycosuria, hematuria, impotence, nephrotoxicity, phosphaturia, polyuria, renal calculi, renal colic, urinary frequency
HEME: Agranulocytosis, hemolytic anemia, leukopenia, pancytopenia, thrombocytopenia, thrombocytopenic purpura
SKIN: Photosensitivity, pruritus, rash, Stevens-Johnson syndrome, urticaria
Other: Acidosis, hyperuricemia, hypokalemia, weight loss

Nursing Considerations

- Be aware that I.V. acetazolamide may be used if patient cannot take oral drugs. I.M. injection is painful.
- Be aware that acetazolamide may increase the risk of hepatic encephalopathy in patients with hepatic cirrhosis.
- Reconstitute each 500-mg vial with at least 5 ml sterile water for injection. Use within 24 hours; drug has no preservative.
- Monitor blood test results during acetazolamide therapy to detect electrolyte imbalances.
- Monitor blood and urine glucose levels in patients with diabetes mellitus because acetazolamide may lead to elevated levels.
- Monitor patients with a history of calcium-containing calculi for drug-induced calculi.

- Monitor patients with gout or respiratory impairment for exacerbation of these conditions.
- Monitor fluid intake and output every 8 hours and body weight daily to detect excessive fluid and weight loss.

PATIENT TEACHING

- Instruct patient to take acetazolamide exactly as prescribed. Tell him to take a missed dose as soon as he remembers but not to take a double dose.
- Inform patient that tablets may be crushed and suspended in chocolate or other sweet syrup. Or, one tablet may be dissolved in 10 ml of hot water and added to 10 ml of honey or syrup.
- Advise patient to avoid potentially hazardous activities if dizziness or drowsiness occurs.
- Urge patient who takes high doses of salicylates to notify prescriber immediately if signs of salicylate toxicity, such as anorexia, tachypnea, and lethargy, occur.

acetylcysteine

Mucomyst, Mucosil

Class and Category

Chemical: N-acetyl derivative of cysteine
Therapeutic: Antidote (for acetaminophen overdose), mucolytic
Pregnancy category: B

Indications and Dosages

▶ *To treat acetaminophen overdose*

I.V. INFUSION

Adults and children. 300 mg/kg over 21 hours as follows: 150 mg/kg in 200 ml 5% dextrose over 60 min; followed by 50 mg/kg in 500 ml 5% dextrose over 4 hours; followed by 100 mg/kg in 1,000 ml 5% dextrose over 16 hours.

DOSAGE ADJUSTMENT Total volume adjusted individually for patients weighing less than 40 kg (88 lb) and for those who need fluid restriction.

Incompatibilities

Don't give acetylcysteine with nebulization equipment if drug may contact iron, copper, or rubber. Don't give drug with amphotericin B, ampicillin sodium, chlortetracycline, chymotrypsin, erythromycin, hydrogen peroxide, iodized oil, oxytetracycline, tetracycline, or trypsin.

Mechanism of Action

Decreases viscosity of pulmonary secretions by breaking disulfide links that bind glycoproteins in mucus. Reduces liver damage from acetaminophen overdose. Usually, acetaminophen's toxic metabolites bind with glutathione in the liver, which detoxifies them. When acetaminophen overdose depletes glutathione stores, toxic metabolites bind with protein in liver cells, killing them. Acetylcysteine maintains or restores levels of glutathione or acts as its substitute, which reduces liver damage from acetaminophen overdose.

Contraindications

Hypersensitivity to acetylcysteine; no contraindications when used as antidote

Interactions

DRUGS

activated charcoal: Possibly adsorption and decreased effectiveness of acetylcysteine

nitroglycerin: Increased effects of nitroglycerin and possibly significant hypotension and headache

Adverse Reactions

CNS: Chills, dizziness, drowsiness, fever, headache
CV: Hypertension, hypotension, tachycardia
EENT: Rhinorrhea, stomatitis, tooth damage
GI: Anorexia, constipation, hepatotoxicity, nausea, vomiting
RESP: Bronchospasm, chest tightness, hemoptysis
SKIN: Clammy skin, pruritus, rash, urticaria
Other: Angioedema

Nursing Considerations

- Be aware that acetylcysteine should be used cautiously in patients with asthma or a history of bronchospasm because drug may adversely affect respiratory function.
- To avoid fluid overload and possibly fatal hyponatremia or seizures, adjust total volume, as ordered, for patients who weigh less than 40 kg and for those who need fluid restriction.
- If needed, dilute 20% instillation or inhalation solution with normal saline solution or sterile water. The 10% solution may be used undiluted.
- To treat acetaminophen overdose, dilute 20% oral solution with cola or other soft drink to a concentration of 5%, and use within 1 hour. Acetylcysteine is most effective if given within

24 hours of acetaminophen ingestion.
- If patient vomits loading dose or any maintenance dose within 1 hour of administration, repeat dose as prescribed.
- Keep in mind that a suicidal patient may not provide reliable information about vomiting. Watch such a patient to ensure that he receives all of prescribed dose.
- During treatment for acetaminophen overdose, monitor patient for signs of hepatotoxicity, such as prolonged bleeding time, altered coagulation, and easy bruising.
- Be aware that acetylcysteine may have a disagreeable odor, which disappears as treatment progresses.
- Because nebulization causes sticky residue on face and in mouth, have patient wash his face and rinse his mouth at the end of each treatment.
- Be aware that an open vial of solution may turn light purple; this change doesn't alter effectiveness.
- Refrigerate opened vials, and discard them after 96 hours.
- Assess type, frequency, and characteristics of patient's cough. Particularly note sputum. If cough doesn't clear secretions, prepare to perform mechanical suctioning.
- Monitor patient for tachycardia.

PATIENT TEACHING
- Instruct patient to notify prescriber immediately about nausea, rash, or vomiting.
- Warn patient about acetylcysteine's unpleasant smell; reassure him that it subsides as treatment progresses.
- To decrease mucus viscosity, encourage patient to consume 2 to 3 L of fluid daily unless contraindicated by another condition.

acyclovir sodium

Zovirax

Class and Category

Chemical: Synthetic purine nucleoside analogue
Therapeutic: Antiviral
Pregnancy category: B

Indications and Dosages

▶ *To treat an initial episode of severe genital herpes infection*

I.V. INFUSION

Adults and children age 12 and over. 5 mg/kg q 8 hr for 5 days. *Maximum:* 20 mg/kg q 8 hr.

Infants and children up to age 12. 250 mg/m² q 8 hr for 5 days. *Maximum:* 20 mg/kg q 8 hr.

▶ *To treat mucocutaneous herpes simplex (HSV-1 and HSV-2) infections in immunocompromised patients*

I.V. INFUSION

Adults and children age 12 and over. 5 mg/kg q 8 hr for 7 days. *Maximum:* 20 mg/kg q 8 hr.

Infants and children up to age 12. 10 mg/kg q 8 hr for 7 days. *Maximum:* 20 mg/kg q 8 hr.

▶ *To treat herpes simplex encephalitis*

I.V. INFUSION

Adults and children age 12 and over. 10 mg/kg q 8 hr for 10 days. *Maximum:* 20 mg/kg q 8 hr.

Children ages 3 months to 12 years. 20 mg/kg q 8 hr for 10 days. *Maximum:* 20 mg/kg q 8 hr.

▶ *To treat herpes zoster caused by varicella zoster virus in immunocompromised patients*

I.V. INFUSION

Adults and children age 12 and over. 10 mg/kg q 8 hr for 7 days. *Maximum:* 20 mg/kg q 8 hr.

Children up to age 12. 20 mg/kg q 8 hr for 7 days. *Maximum:* 20 mg/kg q 8 hr.

▶ *To treat neonatal herpes simplex infections*

I.V. INFUSION

Infants up to age 3 months. 10 mg/kg q 8 hr for 10 days. *Maximum:* 20 mg/kg q 8 hr.

DOSAGE ADJUSTMENT Dosing interval increased to q 12 hr if patient's creatinine clearance is 25 to 50 ml/min/1.73 m² or to q 24 hr if creatinine clearance is 10 to 25 ml/min/1.73 m²; dosage reduced by 50% and dosing interval increased to q 24 hr if creatinine clearance is 10 ml/min/1.73 m² or less. Hemodialysis patients require an extra dose after each hemodialysis session. Dosage for obese patients should be based on ideal body weight.

Incompatibilities

Don't mix acyclovir sodium with biological or colloidal solutions, such as blood products or protein-containing solutions. Don't mix with parabens because a precipitate may form.

Contraindications

Hypersensitivity to acyclovir or valacyclovir

Mechanism of Action

Prevents viral DNA replication of herpes simplex types 1 and 2 and varicella zoster virus. Infected cells selectively take up acyclovir, which is ultimately converted by virus-induced enzyme thymidine kinase to acyclovir triphosphate. Acyclovir triphosphate stops replication of viral DNA by incorporation into and termination of the growing DNA chain, and by inhibition and inactivation of the viral DNA polymerase, an enzyme used in the viral DNA replication process.

Interactions

DRUGS

nephrotoxic drugs (such as aminoglycosides, penicillin, tacrolimus): Increased risk of nephrotoxicity
probenecid: Increased and prolonged blood acyclovir level
zidovudine: Increased lethargy and fatigue

Adverse Reactions

CNS: Agitation, coma, confusion, delirium, dizziness, fever, hallucinations, light-headedness, obtundation, psychosis, seizures, somnolence, tiredness, tremor, weakness
GI: Anorexia, diarrhea, elevated liver function test results, nausea, thirst, vomiting
GU: Elevated BUN and serum creatinine levels, hematuria, renal failure
HEME: Anemia, leukocytosis, leukopenia, neutropenia, neutrophilia, thrombotic thrombocytic purpura or hemolytic-uremic syndrome, thrombocytopenia, thrombocytosis
SKIN: Pruritus, rash, urticaria
Other: Injection site edema, pain, or redness

Nursing Considerations

- For initial drug reconstitution, add 10 or 20 ml of sterile water for injection to each 500-mg or 1-g vial of acyclovir, respectively, to yield a concentration of 50 mg/ml. Shake well. Don't mix with bacteriostatic water for injection containing parabens to avoid precipitation.
- **WARNING** Don't mix acyclovir with bacteriostatic water for injection containing benzyl alcohol because neonates and immature infants may develop a fatal toxic syndrome characterized by CNS, respiratory, circulatory, and renal impairment and metabolic acidosis.

- Use reconstituted acyclovir within 12 hours when stored at room temperature of 15° to 25° C (59° to 77° F). If a precipitate forms during refrigeration, allow reconstituted acyclovir to warm to room temperature to dissolve the precipitate.
- Further dilute reconstituted acyclovir with 60 to 150 ml of standard electrolyte or dextrose solution to a concentration of 7 mg/ml or less. Concentrations greater than 10 mg/ml may produce phlebitis or inflammation at injection site if extravasation occurs.
- Use final solution within 24 hours when stored at 15° to 25° C.
- Obtain baseline BUN and serum creatinine levels before and during therapy, as ordered.
- **WARNING** Administer acyclovir at a constant rate over at least 1 hour. Be aware that rapid administration may cause renal tubular damage and result in acute renal failure.
- Expect to hydrate patient during acyclovir administration to avoid precipitation of drug in renal tubules; maximum urinary concentrations are reached within 2 hours.
- Monitor BUN and serum creatinine levels and assess input and output of patients who are dehydrated, are using other nephrotoxic drugs, or have preexisting impaired renal function because acyclovir increases the risk of nephrotoxicity. Be aware that drug may precipitate in renal tubules if maximum solubility of free acyclovir (2.5 mg/ml at 37° C in water) is exceeded.
- Evaluate for altered LOC, confusion, and psychosis in patients with neurologic abnormalities or a prior neurologic reaction to cytotoxic drugs and in immunocompromised and elderly patients because of potential for neuropsychiatric toxicity.
- Be aware that immunocompromised patients receiving acyclovir may be at risk for thrombotic thrombocytopenic purpura/hemolytic-uremic syndrome. Monitor such patients for signs and symptoms, including petechiae, fever, confusion, hematuria, and acute renal failure.
- Be aware that acyclovir therapy may need to be prolonged in an immunocompromised patient because lesions take longer to heal.
- Notify prescriber if patient doesn't improve within a few days of beginning acyclovir therapy.
- Before reconstituting drug, store it at 15° to 25° C (59° to 77° F).

PATIENT TEACHING

- Inform patient that acyclovir won't prevent transmission of herpes simplex virus to sexual partners or cure the condition but

that condom use may help prevent transmission. Instruct patient to avoid sexual activity if he or his partner exhibits signs or symptoms of genital herpes. However, explain that he may be contagious even before the first sign of a herpetic lesion.
- To decrease irritation to genital area, encourage patient to wear loose-fitting clothes during acyclovir therapy and to keep this area clean and dry.

adenosine

Adenocard, Adenoscan

Class and Category

Chemical: Monophosphorylated adenine riboside
Therapeutic: Antiarrhythmic
Pregnancy category: C

Indications and Dosages

▶ *To convert paroxysmal supraventricular tachycardia (PSVT) to normal sinus rhythm*

I.V. INJECTION

Adults and children weighing 50 kg (110 lb) or more. *Initial:* 6 mg by rapid peripheral I.V. bolus over 1 to 2 sec. If PSVT continues after 1 to 2 min, 12 mg given as rapid bolus and repeated in 1 to 2 min if needed.

WARNING Don't give single doses of more than 12 mg.

Children weighing less than 50 kg. *Initial:* 0.05 to 0.1 mg/kg as rapid central or peripheral I.V. bolus followed by saline flush. If PSVT continues after 1 to 2 min, additional bolus injections are given, incrementally increasing dose by 0.05 to 0.1 mg/kg. Follow each bolus with saline flush. Injections continue until PSVT converts to normal sinus rhythm or until patient reaches maximum single dose of 0.3 mg/kg.

Route	Onset	Peak	Duration
I.V.	Immediate	Immediate	Unknown

Mechanism of Action

Slows conduction time through the AV node and can interrupt reentry pathways through the AV node to restore normal sinus rhythm.

Incompatibilities

Don't mix adenosine with other drugs.

Contraindications

Atrial fibrillation or flutter; hypersensitivity to adenosine; second- or third-degree heart block or sick sinus syndrome, except in patients with a functioning artificial pacemaker; ventricular tachycardia

Interactions

DRUGS

carbamazepine: Increased heart block
digoxin, verapamil: Possibly increased depressant effect on SA or AV node
dipyridamole: Increased effects of adenosine
methylxanthines, such as theophylline: Antagonized effects of adenosine

FOODS

caffeine: Antagonized effects of adenosine

Adverse Reactions

CNS: Apprehension, dizziness, headache, heaviness in arms, light-headedness, nervousness, paresthesia, seizures
CV: Atrial fibrillation, bradycardia, chest pain or pressure, heart block, hypertension, hypotension, MI, palpitations, prolonged asystole, sinus exit block or pause, torsades de pointes, transient hypertension, ventricular fibrillation, ventricular tachycardia
EENT: Blurred vision, metallic taste, throat tightness
GI: Nausea, vomiting
MS: Jaw, neck, and back pain
RESP: Bronchoconstriction, bronchospasm, dyspnea, hyperventilation, respiratory arrest
SKIN: Diaphoresis, facial flushing
Other: Injection site reaction

Nursing Considerations

- Before use, inspect adenosine for crystals. If solution isn't clear, don't give it.
- Give adenosine by rapid I.V. bolus over 1 to 2 seconds. Slower administration can cause systemic vasodilation and reflex tachycardia.
- Expect prescriber to inject adenosine directly into a vein, if appropriate, to ensure that it reaches systemic circulation. If administered into an I.V. line, give as close to insertion site as possible and follow with rapid saline flush.

- Monitor heart rate and rhythm, blood pressure, and respiratory status frequently during adenosine therapy.
- Be aware that at the time of conversion to normal sinus rhythm, arrhythmias (such as PVCs, premature atrial contractions, sinus bradycardia, sinus tachycardia, and AV block) may occur for a few seconds but don't require intervention.
- WARNING Discontinue use and notify prescriber immediately if severe respiratory difficulties develop.
- Store adenosine at room temperature. Discard unused portion.

PATIENT TEACHING

- Instruct patient to report chest pain, palpitations, difficulty breathing, or severe headache during adenosine therapy.
- Warn patient that he may temporarily experience mild reactions, such as flushing, nausea, and dizziness.

alatrofloxacin mesylate

Trovan I.V.

trovafloxacin mesylate

Trovan

Class and Category

Chemical: Fluoroquinolone
Therapeutic: Antibacterial
Pregnancy category: C

Indications and Dosages

▶ *To treat life-threatening nosocomial pneumonia*

I.V. INFUSION, TABLETS

Adults. 300 mg I.V. q 24 hr, followed by 200 mg P.O. q 24 hr when patient is stabilized, for 10 to 14 days.

▶ *To treat life-threatening community-acquired pneumonia*

I.V. INFUSION, TABLETS

Adults. 200 mg I.V. q 24 hr, followed by 200 mg P.O. q 24 hr when patient is stabilized, for 7 to 14 days; or 200 mg P.O. q 24 hr for 7 to 14 days.

▶ *To treat complicated, life-threatening intra-abdominal infections, including postsurgical, gynecologic, and pelvic infections*

I.V. INFUSION, TABLETS

Adults. 300 mg I.V. q 24 hr, followed by 200 mg P.O. q 24 hr when patient is stabilized, for 7 to 14 days.

▶ *To treat complicated, life- or limb-threatening skin and soft-tissue infections, including diabetic foot infections*

I.V. INFUSION, TABLETS

Adults. 200 mg I.V. q 24 hr, followed by 200 mg P.O. q 24 hr when patient is stabilized, for 10 to 14 days; or 200 mg P.O. q 24 hr for 10 to 14 days.

DOSAGE ADJUSTMENT For patients with mild to moderate cirrhosis, 300-mg dosage reduced to 200 mg and 200-mg dosage reduced to 100 mg.

Mechanism of Action

Interferes with DNA gyrase, the enzyme necessary for DNA replication in aerobic and anaerobic bacteria. May be active against pathogens that are resistant to such antibiotics as penicillins, cephalosporins, aminoglycosides, macrolides, and tetracyclines.

Incompatibilities

Don't mix alatrofloxacin with or infuse it simultaneously through the same I.V. line as other drugs or any solutions containing multivalent cations, such as magnesium. Don't dilute alatrofloxacin with normal saline solution or lactated Ringer's solution.

Contraindications

Hypersensitivity to alatrofloxacin, quinolone antibiotics, trovafloxacin, or their components

Interactions

DRUGS

aluminum-, citric acid–, magnesium-, or sodium citrate–containing antacids; iron; morphine sulfate; sucralfate: Decreased absorption of oral trovafloxacin

Adverse Reactions

CNS: Dizziness, headache, light-headedness, seizures
CV: Hypotension
EENT: Hoarseness, throat tightness
GI: Abdominal pain, acute hepatic failure (evidenced by anorexia, dark urine, dysphagia, fatigue, jaundice, pale stools, and vomiting)
GU: Vaginitis
RESP: Dyspnea
SKIN: Erythema, photosensitivity, pruritus, rash, urticaria
Other: Angioedema, infusion site pain

Nursing Considerations

- Using aseptic technique, withdraw appropriate amount of alatrofloxacin concentrate from vial and dilute further with appropriate I.V. solution to a final concentration of 1 to 2 mg/ml. Compatible I.V. solutions are D_5W, 0.45 normal saline, D_5/0.45 normal saline, D_5/0.2 normal saline, and D_5/lactated Ringer's solutions.
- If you're using the same I.V. line to give other drugs sequentially, flush line with a compatible solution before and after administering alatrofloxacin. Though it can't be used to dilute alatrofloxacin, normal saline solution can be used to flush I.V. line.
- Refrigerate diluted solution for up to 7 days or store at room temperature for 3 days in glass bottles or polyvinyl chloride I.V. containers.
- **WARNING** Infuse alatrofloxacin over 60 minutes; rapid or bolus I.V. injection may cause hypotension.
- Periodically assess liver function test results. Results may be elevated for up to 21 days after alatrofloxacin administration.
- **WARNING** Be aware that alatrofloxacin may cause severe liver damage, which may lead to death or need for liver transplantation. Expect therapy to last no longer than 2 weeks because more prolonged therapy increases the risk of liver damage. Alatrofloxacin is reserved for hospitalized patients with life- or limb-threatening infections.
- Protect vial from light before use. Store at room temperature; don't freeze.

PATIENT TEACHING

- Instruct patient to report rash; urticaria; trouble swallowing; swelling of lips, face, or tongue; hoarseness; throat tightness; abdominal pain; or nausea and vomiting.
- Advise patient to avoid potentially hazardous activities if he experiences dizziness or lightheadedness.
- Instruct patient to avoid exposure to direct sunlight and ultraviolet light (such as tanning beds).

alefacept

Amevive

Class and Category

Chemical: Recombinant leukocyte function–related antigen-3 immunoglobulin GI fusion protein

Therapeutic: Immunosuppresant
Pregnancy category: B

Indications and Dosages

▶ *To treat moderate to severe chronic plaque psoriasis in patients who are candidates for systemic therapy or phototherapy*

I.V. INJECTION

Adults. *Initial:* 7.5 mg q wk for 12 wk. After at least 12 wk in which drug isn't given, a second 12-wk course may be given, if needed and if patient's CD4 and T-lymphocyte counts are within normal ranges.

Mechanism of Action

Binds to the lymphocyte antigen and CD2 and inhibits LFA-3/CD2 interaction to interfere with T-lymphocyte activation. Alefacept also reduces the subsets of CD2+ T lymphocytes. Because activation of T lymphocytes plays a role in the pathophysiology of chronic plaque psoriasis, interference with lymphocytic activity helps to prevent plaque formation.

Incompatibilities

Don't add other drugs to solutions containing alefacept.

Contraindications

Breast-feeding, hypersensitivity to alefacept or its components

Interactions

DRUGS

None reported

Adverse Reactions

CNS: Chills, dizziness, headache
CV: Coronary artery disease, MI
EENT: Pharyngitis
GI: Nausea
HEME: Lymphopenia
MS: Myalgia
RESP: Increased cough
SKIN: Pruritus, urticaria
Other: Angioedema, injection site pain or inflammation, infection, malignancies

Nursing Considerations

• Use alefacept cautiously in patients at high risk for cancer because this drug increases the risk. Know that alefacept isn't recommended for use in patients with a history of a systemic malignancy.

- Also use cautiously in patients with chronic infection or a history of recurrent infections. Drug may increase risk of infection because of its immunosuppressive action.
- Obtain a CD4+ and T-cell count before starting drug therapy, as ordered. If counts are below normal, expect to delay therapy. After therapy starts, monitor patient's CD4+ and T-cell counts weekly throughout therapy. If levels drop below 250 cells/mm^3, notify prescriber because drug will need to be withheld. If counts remain below 250 cells/mm^3 for 1 month, therapy should be stopped.
- Reconstitute drug with 0.6 ml of the supplied diluent (sterile water for injection) before administration. With the needle pointed at the side wall of the vial, slowly inject the diluent into the alefacept vial. Expect some foaming. To prevent excessive foaming, don't shake or vigorously agitate vial. Instead, swirl vial gently during dissolution, which usually takes less than 2 minutes.
- Give drug as soon as possible after reconstitution. Discard solution if not used within 4 hours.
- Don't filter reconstituted solution during preparation or administration.
- For I.V. use, prepare two syringes containing 3 ml normal saline solution to be used for flushing before and after giving drug. Then prime the winged infusion set with 3 ml normal saline solution and insert into the vein. Attach the filled syringe to the infusion set and administer the solution over no more than 5 seconds. Finish by flushing the set with 3 ml normal saline solution.
- Be aware that alefacept shouldn't be started in a patient with a serious infection. Monitor patient closely during and after therapy for signs and symptoms of infection. If these occur, report them to the prescriber immediately and start treatment, as prescribed, to reduce the risk of serious infection. If infection becomes serious, expect drug to be discontinued.
- Monitor patient for allergic reactions. If these occur, stop drug and notify prescriber immediately.

PATIENT TEACHING

- Advise patient that weekly blood tests will be needed to monitor his WBC during alefacept therapy.

- Teach patient the signs and symptoms of infection and common warning signs of malignancy. Emphasize the importance of complying with follow-up visits and promptly reporting to prescriber any unusual or sudden evidence of malignancy or infection.
- Inform female patient to notify prescriber if she becomes pregnant during alefacept therapy or 8 weeks afterward.

alglucerase

Ceredase

Class and Category

Chemical: Glucocerebrosidase beta-glucosidase
Therapeutic: Enzyme replacement
Pregnancy category: C

Indications and Dosages

▶ *To treat chronic nonneuropathic Gaucher's disease in patients with moderate to severe anemia, thrombocytopenia with bleeding tendencies, bone disease, or significant hepatomegaly or splenomegaly*

I.V. INFUSION

Adults and children age 2 and over. Highly individualized. 2.5 units/kg up to 60 units/kg infused over 1 to 2 hr, usually q 2 wk.

DOSAGE ADJUSTMENT Highly individualized dosage based on body size and disease severity. Some patients may need infusion once every other day; others may need it once q 4 wk. Maintenance dosage progressively reduced every 3 to 6 mo to as low as 1 units/kg.

Route	Onset	Peak	Duration
I.V.	Up to 60 min	Unknown	Variable

Mechanism of Action

Catalyzes hydrolysis of glucocerebroside to glucose and ceramide in membrane lipids. Gaucher's disease results from deficiency of the enzyme beta-glucocerebrosidase and causes the lipid glucocerebroside to accumulate in tissue macrophages.

Contraindications

Hypersensitivity to alglucerase

Adverse Reactions
CNS: Chills, dizziness, fatigue, fever, headache
CV: Transient peripheral edema, vasomotor irritability
EENT: Oral ulcerations
GI: Abdominal discomfort, diarrhea, nausea, vomiting
MS: Backache
Other: I.V. site burning, itching, or swelling

Nursing Considerations
- If patient is hypersensitive to alglucerase, expect to give antihistamines before starting alglucerase therapy.
- On day of dose, use aseptic technique to dilute alglucerase with normal saline solution to final volume of no more than 200 ml.
- Don't shake drug; doing so could inactivate it.
- Don't use alglucerase if it's discolored or contains precipitate.
- Be aware that drug doesn't contain preservatives. Discard unused portion.
- Infuse alglucerase with in-line I.V. particle filter.

PATIENT TEACHING
- Tell patient that he may experience flulike symptoms with each dose of alglucerase.
- Instruct patient to report headache, hot flashes, nausea, and other adverse reactions.
- Inform patient that alglucerase is derived from pooled human placental tissue and poses a slight risk of viral contamination.
- Advise patient to keep appointments for scheduled doses of alglucerase.

allopurinol sodium
Aloprim

Class and Category
Chemical: Hypoxanthine derivative, xanthine oxidase inhibitor
Therapeutic: Antihyperuricemic
Pregnancy category: C

Indications and Dosages
▶ *To treat increased serum and urine uric acid levels in patients with leukemia, lymphoma, and solid tumors when chemotherapy has increased those levels and patient can't tolerate oral therapy*

I.V. INFUSION

Adults. 200 to 400 mg/m^2 q day as a single infusion or in equal divided infusions q 6, 8, or 12 hr. *Maximum:* 600 mg q day.

Children. 200 mg/m^2 q day as a single infusion or in equally divided infusions q 6, 8, or 12 hr.

DOSAGE ADJUSTMENT Dosage adjusted to 200 mg daily if creatinine clearance is 10 to 20 ml/min/1.73 m^2, to 100 mg daily if creatinine clearance is 3 to 10 ml/min/1.73 m^2, or to 100 mg q other day if creatinine clearance falls below 3 ml/min/1.73 m^2.

Mechanism of Action

Inhibits uric acid production by inhibiting xanthine oxidase, the enzyme responsible for converting hypoxanthine and xanthine to uric acid. Allopurinol is metabolized to oxipurinol, which also inhibits xanthine oxidase.

Incompatibilities

Don't combine allopurinol in solution with amikacin, amphotericin B, carmustine, cefotaxime sodium, chlorpromazine hydrochloride, cimetidine hydrochloride, clindamycin phosphate, cytarabine, dacarbazine, daunorubicin hydrochloride, diphenhydramine hydrochloride, doxorubicin hydrochloride, doxycycline hyclate, droperidol, floxuridine, gentamicin sulfate, haloperidol lactate, hydroxyzine hydrochloride, idarubicin hydrochloride, imipenem and cilastatin sodium, mechlorethamine hydrochloride, meperidine hydrochloride, methylprednisolone sodium succinate, metoclopramide hydrochloride, minocycline hydrochloride, nalbuphine hydrochloride, netilmicin sulfate, ondansetron hydrochloride, prochlorperazine edisylate, promethazine hydrochloride, sodium bicarbonate, streptozocin, tobramycin sulfate, vinorelbine tartrate.

Contraindications

Hypersensitivity to allopurinol

Interactions

DRUGS

ACE inhibitors: Increased risk of hypersensitivity reactions
amoxicillin, ampicillin: Increased risk of rash
azathioprine, mercaptopurine: Inactivation of these drugs
chlorpropamide: Increased risk of hypoglycemia in patients with renal insufficiency
cyclophosphamide, other cytotoxic drugs: Enhanced bone marrow suppression

dicumarol: Increased half-life and anticoagulant action of dicumarol
thiazide diuretics: Possibly increased risk of allopurinol toxicity
uricosuric drugs: Increased urinary excretion of uric acid
vitamin C (large doses): Possibly urine acidification and increased risk of renal calculus formation

Adverse Reactions

CNS: Chills, coma, drowsiness, fever, headache, mental status changes, neuritis, paresthesia, peripheral neuropathy, seizures, somnolence
CV: Arrhythmias, cardiopulmonary arrest, hypertension, hypotension, vasculitis
EENT: Epistaxis, loss of taste
GI: Abdominal pain, diarrhea, elevated liver function test results, GI bleeding, granulomatous hepatitis, hepatic necrosis, hepatomegaly, intestinal obstruction, nausea, vomiting
GU: Exacerbation of renal calculi, hematuria, renal failure, UTI
HEME: Anemia, bone marrow depression, eosinophilia, leukocytosis, leukopenia, neutropenia, thrombocytopenia
MS: Arthralgia, exacerbation of gout, myopathy
SKIN: Alopecia; ecchymosis; jaundice; maculopapular, scaly, or exfoliative rash (sometimes fatal); pruritus; urticaria
Other: Septic shock

Nursing Considerations

- As ordered, obtain and review results of baseline CBC, uric acid levels, and renal and hepatic function studies before starting allopurinol therapy. Continue to monitor test results during therapy.
- Reconstitute and dilute to 6 mg/ml or less. To reconstitute, add 25 ml sterile water for injection to 30-ml vial of allopurinol powder. Dilute to desired concentration with normal saline solution or D_5W.
- Don't use if solution is discolored or contains particles.
- Store prepared solution at 20° to 25° C (68° to 77° F); don't refrigerate. Administer within 10 hours of reconstitution.
- Expect allopurinol therapy to begin 24 to 48 hours before start of chemotherapy.
- **WARNING** Discontinue allopurinol and notify prescriber immediately at first sign of a hypersensitivity reaction, such as a rash, which may precede more severe reactions.

- To decrease the risk of calculus formation, maintain fluid intake of up to 3 L daily and monitor patient for output of 2 L daily. Also, don't give patient vitamin C.

PATIENT TEACHING

- Instruct patient receiving allopurinol to drink at least 10 large glasses of water daily.
- Advise patient to report unusual bleeding or bruising, fever, chills, gout attack, numbness, and tingling.
- Inform patient that acute gout attacks may occur more frequently early in allopurinol treatment and that results may not be noticeable for 2 weeks or longer.
- Instruct patient not to drive or perform potentially hazardous tasks if allopurinol causes drowsiness.

alpha$_1$-proteinase inhibitor (human)

Prolastin, Zemaira

Class and Category

Chemical: Plasma protein
Therapeutic: Enzyme replacement
Pregnancy category: C

Indications and Dosages

▶ *To treat congenital alpha$_1$-antitrypsin deficiency in patients with signs of panacinar emphysema (Prolastin); to augment and maintain patients with emphysema who are deficient in alpha$_1$-proteinase inhibitor*

I.V. INFUSION

Adults. 60 mg/kg infused over 30 min for Prolastin and 15 min for Zemaira at a rate of at least 0.08 ml/kg/min once weekly.

Mechanism of Action

Replaces the enzyme alpha$_1$-antitrypsin, which normally inhibits the proteolytic enzyme elastase in patients with alpha$_1$-antitrypsin deficiency. Without alpha$_1$-proteinase inhibitor, elastase attacks and destroys alveolar membranes and causes emphysema.

Contraindications

Hypersensitivity to alpha$_1$-proteinase inhibitor, its components, or other alpha$_1$-proteinase products; selective immunoglobulin A (IgA) deficiency in patients with anti-IgA antibodies

Interactions

ACTIVITIES

smoking: Inactivation of alpha$_1$-proteinase inhibitor

Adverse Reactions

CNS: Asthenia, dizziness, fever, headache, paresthesia

EENT: Sinusitis

HEME: Mild, transient leukocytosis

RESP: Exacerbation of existing COPD, upper respiratory tract infection

SKIN: Pruritus

Other: Flulike symptoms, infusion site pain

Nursing Considerations

- Use alpha$_1$-proteinase inhibitor cautiously in patients at risk for circulatory overload because drug is a colloid solution that increases plasma volume.
- Before reconstituting alpha$_1$-proteinase inhibitor, remove drug and diluent from refrigerator and let it warm to room temperature.
- To reconstitute, remove caps from vials and cleanse rubber stoppers with antiseptic solution. After stoppers are dry, remove protective cover from diluent end of transfer device and insert into center of upright diluent vial. Then remove protective cover from drug end of transfer device, invert the diluent vial with attached transfer device, and, using minimal force, insert drug end of transfer device into center of rubber stopper of upright drug vial. Make sure flange of transfer device rests on stopper surface so that diluent flows into drug vial.
- During diluent transfer, wet lyophilized cake completely by gently tilting the drug vial. Don't allow air inlet filter to face downward. (Take care not to lose the vacuum because this will prolong reconstitution.) Once diluent transfer is complete, pull transfer device along with attached diluent vial out of drug vial and discard. Gently swirl drug vial until powder is completely dissolved. Avoid shaking because doing so may cause drug to foam and degrade.
- If you need more than one vial of alpha$_1$-proteinase inhibitor, use aseptic technique to transfer reconstituted solution from each vial into a sterile I.V. administration container.
- Within 3 hours of reconstitution, administer at room temperature as an I.V. infusion using the large-volume 5-micron conical filter provided. Place filter between distal end of I.V. administra-

tion set and infusion set, and infuse at 0.08 ml/kg/min or as determined by patient response and comfort. Expect the infusion to take about 15 minutes per vial.

- **WARNING** Alpha$_1$-proteinase inhibitor is made from human plasma and may contain infectious agents, such as viruses. Ensure that patient is immunized against hepatitis B before giving drug. If time doesn't allow for antibody formation, give a single dose of hepatitis B immune globulin with hepatitis B vaccine, as prescribed.
- Monitor patient for delayed fever, which may occur up to 12 hours after therapy. Fever usually resolves within 24 hours.

PATIENT TEACHING

- Tell patient to immediately report early evidence of an allergic reaction, such as chest tightness, difficult breathing, faintness, hives, wheezing, and any other unusual symptoms.
- Advise patient to notify prescriber if signs or symptoms of viral infection (chills, drowsiness, fever, and runny nose, followed 2 weeks later by joint pain and a rash) occur after receiving drug.
- Stress the importance of receiving weekly doses to maintain an adequate antielastase barrier in the lungs. Explain that treatment must continue for life.
- Warn patient not to smoke.

alteplase, recombinant

(tissue plasminogen activator, recombinant)

Activase, Activase rt-PA (CAN)

Class and Category

Chemical: Purified glycoprotein
Therapeutic: Thrombolytic
Pregnancy category: C

Indications and Dosages

▶ *To treat acute MI*

ACCELERATED I.V. INFUSION

Adults weighing more than 67 kg (148 lb). 15-mg bolus, followed by 50 mg infused over next 30 min and then by 35 mg infused over next 60 min.

Adults weighing 67 kg or less. 15-mg bolus, followed by 0.75 mg/kg (up to 50 mg) infused over next 30 min and then 0.5 mg/kg (up to 35 mg) infused over next 60 min.

I.V. INFUSION

Adults weighing more than 65 kg (143 lb). 100 mg infused over 3 hr as follows: 6 to 10 mg by bolus over first 1 to 2 min, 50 to 54 mg over remainder of first hr, 20 mg over second hr, and 20 mg over third hr.

Adults weighing 65 kg or less. 1.25 mg/kg infused over 3 hr on similar administration schedule for those weighing more than 65 kg.

▶ *To treat acute ischemic CVA*

I.V. INFUSION

Adults. 0.9 mg/kg infused over 60 min, with 10% of total dose given as bolus over first min. *Maximum:* 90 mg.

WARNING To avoid acute bleeding complications, expect to treat patient for acute ischemic CVA within 3 hr after onset of CVA symptoms and only after computed tomography or other diagnostic imaging method rules out intracranial hemorrhage.

▶ *To treat pulmonary embolism*

I.V. INFUSION

Adults. 100 mg infused over 2 hr.

Route	Onset	Peak	Duration
I.V.	Immediate	20 to 120 min	4 hr

Mechanism of Action

Binds to fibrin in a thrombus and converts trapped plasminogen to plasmin. Plasmin breaks down fibrin, fibrinogen, and other clotting factors, which dissolves the thrombus.

Incompatibilities

Don't add other drugs to solution that contains alteplase or infuse other drugs through same I.V. line.

Contraindications

For all indications: Active internal bleeding, arteriovenous malformation or aneurysm, bleeding diathesis, intracranial neoplasm, severe uncontrolled hypertension

For acute MI and pulmonary embolism only: History of CVA, intracranial or intraspinal surgery or trauma in past 2 months

For acute ischemic CVA only: Recent head trauma, recent intracranial surgery, recent previous CVA, seizure activity at onset of

CVA, subarachnoid hemorrhage, suspicion or history of intracranial hemorrhage

Interactions

DRUGS

drugs that alter platelet function (such as abciximab, acetylsalicylic acid, and dipyridamole), heparin, vitamin K antagonists: Increased risk of bleeding

Adverse Reactions

CNS: Cerebral edema, cerebral herniation, CVA, fever, seizures
CV: Arrhythmias (including bradycardia and electromechanical dissociation), cardiac arrest, cardiac tamponade, cardiogenic shock, cholesterol embolism, coronary thrombolysis, heart failure, hypotension, mitral insufficiency, myocardial reinfarction or rupture, pericardial effusion, pericarditis, venous thrombosis and embolism
EENT: Epistaxis, gingival bleeding, laryngeal edema
GI: GI bleeding, nausea, retroperitoneal bleeding, vomiting
GU: GU bleeding
RESP: Pleural effusion, pulmonary edema, pulmonary reembolization
SKIN: Bleeding at puncture sites, ecchymosis, rash, urticaria
Other: Anaphylaxis

Nursing Considerations

- If possible, obtain appropriate coagulation tests, such as PT, APTT, platelet count, and fibrin-fibrinogen degradation product titer, as ordered, before initiating alteplase therapy. Monitor coagulation test results during and after therapy.
- Immediately before using alteplase, reconstitute it only with sterile water for injection provided by manufacturer. Swirl gently to dissolve powder; don't shake.
- Be aware that 50-mg vials have a vacuum and should not be used if vacuum isn't present.
- Use a large-bore (18G) needle when reconstituting 50-mg vial and the transfer device provided when reconstituting 100-mg vial to direct the flow of sterile water for injection.
- When using transfer device, hold vial of alteplase upside down while pushing down onto transfer device connected to sterile water for injection. Then invert the vials to allow the sterile water for injection to flow into the alteplase.
- Store reconstituted solution at 2° to 30° C (36° to 86° F). Use reconstituted solution within 8 hours or discard.

- Use normal saline solution or D_5W immediately before drug administration if further dilution to a concentration of 0.5 mg/ml is desired. Mix by gently swirling or slowly inverting polyvinyl chloride bag or glass vial.
- Monitor for bleeding, especially at arterial puncture sites.
- Monitor blood pressure and heart rate and rhythm frequently during and after alteplase therapy.
- **WARNING** Alteplase therapy may cause arrhythmias from sudden reperfusion of the myocardium. Monitor continuous ECG for arrhythmias during drug therapy.
- Minimize bleeding from noncompressible sites by avoiding internal jugular and subclavian venous puncture sites. Avoid I.M. injection.
- Use a small-gauge (23G or smaller) needle for venipunctures. Use a distal arm vessel for venipunctures and for arterial punctures if needed. Apply pressure for 30 minutes after an arterial puncture, then apply a pressure dressing. Evaluate site frequently for signs of bleeding.
- Discontinue alteplase infusion immediately if serious bleeding occurs.
- After administering alteplase, apply pressure for at least 30 minutes and then apply a pressure dressing.
- Protect alteplase from excessive exposure to light.

PATIENT TEACHING

- Instruct patient beginning alteplase therapy to immediately report bleeding, including bleeding from the nose or gums.
- Advise patient to limit physical activity during alteplase administration to reduce the risk of injury and bleeding.

amikacin sulfate

Amikin

Class and Category

Chemical: Aminoglycoside
Therapeutic: Antibiotic
Pregnancy category: D

Indications and Dosages

▶ *To treat serious gram-negative bacterial infections (including septicemia; neonatal sepsis; respiratory tract, bone, joint, CNS, skin, soft-tissue, intra-abdominal, burn, and postoperative infections; and serious, complicated, and recurrent UTI) caused by* Acinetobacter, Enterobacter, Escherichia coli, Klebsiella, Proteus, Providencia, Pseudomonas, *and* Serratia; *and staphylococcal infections when penicillin is contraindicated*

I.V. INFUSION

Adults and children. 15 mg/kg daily in equal doses at equally spaced intervals (7.5 mg/kg q 12 hr or 5 mg/kg q 8 hr) for 7 to 10 days. *Maximum:* 1,500 mg daily.

Neonates. *Loading dose:* 10 mg/kg. *Maintenance:* 7.5 mg/kg q 12 hr for 7 to 10 days.

DOSAGE ADJUSTMENT For patients with impaired renal function, loading dose of 7.5 mg/kg daily, followed by maintenance dosage based on creatinine clearance and serum creatinine level and given q 12 hr. For morbidly obese patients, dosage not to exceed 1.5 g daily.

▶ *To treat uncomplicated UTI*

I.V. INFUSION

Adults. 250 mg b.i.d. for 7 to 10 days.

Route	Onset	Peak	Duration
I.V.	Immediate	Unknown	Unknown

Mechanism of Action

Binds to negatively charged sites on bacteria's outer cell membrane, disrupting cell integrity. Amikacin also binds to bacterial ribosomal subunits and inhibits protein synthesis. Both actions lead to cell death.

Incompatibilities

Don't mix or infuse amikacin with other drugs.

Contraindications

Hypersensitivity to amikacin or other aminoglycosides

Interactions

DRUGS

cephalosporins, enflurane, methoxyflurane, vancomycin: Increased nephrotoxic effects

general anesthetics: Increased risk of neuromuscular blockade

loop diuretics: Increased risk of *ototoxicity*

neuromuscular blockers: Possibly increased neuromuscular blockade and prolonged respiratory depression

penicillins: Possibly inactivation of or synergistic effects with amikacin

Adverse Reactions

CNS: Drowsiness, headache, loss of balance, neuromuscular blockade, tremor, vertigo
EENT: Hearing loss, ototoxicity, tinnitus
GI: Nausea, vomiting
GU: Azotemia, dysuria, nephrotoxicity, oliguria or polyuria, proteinuria
MS: Acute muscle paralysis; arthralgia; muscle fatigue, spasms, and weakness
RESP: Apnea
Other: Hyperkalemia

Nursing Considerations

- Expect to obtain results of culture and sensitivity tests before amikacin therapy begins.
- Prepare amikacin by adding contents of 500-mg vial to 100 to 200 ml of sterile diluent, such as normal saline solution or D_5W. Adjust amount of diluent proportionately for pediatric patients. Then infuse drug over 30 to 60 minutes.
- Don't use dark-colored solution. Solution color should range from colorless to light straw or pale yellow.
- Use 0.25- and 5-mg/ml I.V. solutions within 24 hours when stored at room temperature if they've been mixed with D_5W, D_5/normal saline, normal saline, lactated Ringer's, or other solutions noted in manufacturer's insert. These solutions remain potent for 60 days if stored at 4° C (39° F) and for 30 days if frozen at −15° C (5° F).
- Monitor patient for evidence of ototoxicity, such as tinnitus and vertigo, especially during high-dosage or prolonged amikacin therapy.
- **WARNING** Because amikacin may produce nephrotoxic effects, assess renal function before and daily during therapy, as ordered. To minimize renal tubule irritation, maintain patient hydration during therapy.
- Be aware that amikacin may exacerbate muscle weakness in such conditions as myasthenia gravis and Parkinson's disease.
- Measure serum amikacin concentrations as ordered, usually 30 to 90 minutes after injection (for peak concentration) and just before administering next dose (for trough concentration).
- Be aware that amikacin may be administered by I.M. injection into a large muscle mass at same dosages used for I.V. administration.

PATIENT TEACHING
- Inform patient that daily laboratory tests are necessary during amikacin treatment.
- Instruct patient to report ringing in ears, hearing changes, headache, nausea, vomiting, and changes in urination.

aminocaproic acid

Amicar

Class and Category

Chemical: Aminohexanoic acid
Therapeutic: Antifibrinolytic, antihemorrhagic
Pregnancy category: C

Indications and Dosages

▶ *To treat excessive bleeding caused by fibrinolysis*

I.V. INJECTION

Adults. 4 to 5 g in 250 ml of diluent over 1 hr, followed by continuous infusion of 1 g/hr in 50 ml of diluent. Continue for 8 hr or until bleeding stops.

Route	Onset	Peak	Duration
I.V.	Immediate	Unknown	Under 3 hr

Mechanism of Action

Inhibits the breakdown of blood clots by interfering with plasminogen activator substances and producing antiplasmin activity.

Contraindications

Hypersensitivity to aminocaproic acid; signs of active intravascular clotting, as in disseminated intravascular coagulation; upper urinary tract bleeding

Interactions

DRUGS

activated prothrombin, prothrombin complex concentrates: Increased risk of thrombosis
estrogens, oral contraceptives: Increased risk of hypercoagulation

Adverse Reactions

CNS: CVA, delirium, dizziness, hallucinations, headache, malaise, weakness

CV: Bradycardia, cardiomyopathy, edema, elevated serum CK level, hypotension, ischemia, thrombophlebitis
EENT: Nasal congestion, tinnitus
GI: Abdominal cramps and pain, diarrhea, elevated AST level, nausea, vomiting
GU: Elevated BUN level, intrarenal obstruction, renal failure
HEME: Agranulocytosis, leukopenia, thrombocytopenia
MS: Myopathy, rhabdomyolysis
RESP: Dyspnea, pulmonary embolism
SKIN: Pruritus, rash
Other: Anaphylaxis, elevated serum aldolase level

Nursing Considerations

- Mix aminocaproic acid solution with sterile water for injection, normal saline solution, D_5W, or Ringer's solution.
- **WARNING** Avoid rapid administration because of increased risks of hypotension and bradycardia.
- Monitor neurologic status for drug-induced changes. Note that increased clotting may lead to CVA.
- Be aware that dosage adjustment may be needed for patient with impaired renal function.
- Store between 15° and 30° C (59° and 86° F).

PATIENT TEACHING

- Inform patient that he will be closely monitored during aminocaproic acid therapy and will have blood drawn for laboratory tests before, during, and after treatment.

aminophylline
(theophylline ethylenediamine)

Class and Category

Chemical: Xanthine
Therapeutic: Bronchodilator
Pregnancy category: C

Indications and Dosages

▶ *To relieve acute bronchospasm*

I.V. INFUSION

Adults (nonsmokers) not taking theophylline products. *Initial:* 6 mg/kg (equal to 4.7 mg/kg anhydrous theophylline), not to exceed 25 mg/min. *Maintenance:* 0.7 mg/kg/hr for first 12 hr; then 0.5 mg/kg/hr.

Children ages 9 to 16 not taking theophylline products. *Ini-*

tial: 6 mg/kg (equal to 4.7 mg/kg anhydrous theophylline), not to exceed 25 mg/min. *Maintenance:* 1 mg/kg/hr for first 12 hr; then 0.8 mg/kg/hr.

Children ages 6 months to 9 years and young adult smokers not taking theophylline products. *Initial:* 6 mg/kg (equal to 4.7 mg/kg anhydrous theophylline), not to exceed 25 mg/min. *Maintenance:* 1.2 mg/kg/hr for first 12 hr; then 1 mg/kg/hr.

Adults and children taking theophylline products. *Initial:* If possible, determine the time, amount, administration route, and form of last dose. Loading dose is based on principle that each 0.63 mg/kg (0.5 mg/kg anhydrous theophylline) administered as a loading dose raises serum theophylline level by 1 mcg/ml. Defer loading dose if serum theophylline level can be readily obtained. If this isn't possible and patient has no obvious signs of theophylline toxicity, prescriber may order 3.1 mg/kg (2.5 mg/kg anhydrous theophylline), which may increase serum theophylline level by about 5 mcg/ml. *Maintenance:* For adults (nonsmokers), 0.7 mg/kg/hr for first 12 hr, and then 0.5 mg/kg/hr. For children ages 9 to 16, 1 mg/kg/hr for first 12 hr, and then 0.8 mg/kg/hr. For children ages 6 months to 9 years and young adult smokers, 1.2 mg/kg/hr for first 12 hr, and then 1 mg/kg/hr.

DOSAGE ADJUSTMENT For elderly patients and those with cor pulmonale, dosage reduced to 0.6 mg/kg for 12 hr, then to 0.3 mg/kg. For patients with heart failure and hepatic disease, dosage reduced to 0.5 mg/kg for 12 hr, then to 0.1 to 0.2 mg/kg.

Route	Onset	Peak	Duration
I.V.	Immediate	Unknown	4 to 8 hr

Mechanism of Action

Inhibits phosphodiesterase enzymes, causing bronchodilation. Normally, these enzymes inactivate cAMP and cGMP, which are responsible for bronchial smooth-muscle relaxation. Other mechanisms of action may include translocation of calcium, prostaglandin antagonism, stimulation of catecholamines, inhibition of cGMP metabolism, and adenosine receptor antagonism.

Incompatibilities

Don't add other drugs to prepared bag or bottle of aminophylline. Don't mix aminophylline in same syringe as doxapram. Avoid administering amiodarone, ciprofloxacin, diltiazem, dobutamine, hydralazine, or ondansetron into the Y port of a continuous infusion of aminophylline.

Contraindications

Active peptic ulcer disease, hypersensitivity to aminophylline, underlying seizure disorder

Interactions

DRUGS

activated charcoal, aminoglutethimide, barbiturates, ketoconazole, rifampin, sulfinpyrazone, sympathomimetics: Decreased blood theophylline level

allopurinol, calcium channel blockers, cimetidine, corticosteroids, disulfiram, ephedrine, influenza virus vaccine, interferon, macrolides, mexiletine, nonselective beta blockers, oral contraceptives, quinolones, thiabendazole: Increased blood theophylline level

benzodiazepines: Antagonized sedative effects of benzodiazepines

beta agonists: Increased effects of aminophylline and beta agonist

carbamazepine, isoniazid, loop diuretics: Increased or decreased blood theophylline level

halothane: Increased risk of cardiotoxicity

hydantoins: Decreased blood hydantoin level

ketamine: Increased risk of seizures

lithium: Decreased blood lithium level

neuromuscular blockers: Reversed neuromuscular blockade

propofol: Antagonized sedative effects of propofol

tetracyclines: Enhanced adverse effects of theophylline

FOODS

high-carbohydrate, low-protein diet: Decreased theophylline elimination and prolonged aminophylline half-life

low-carbohydrate, high-protein diet; charcoal-broiled beef: Increased theophylline elimination and shortened aminophylline half-life

ACTIVITIES

alcohol abuse: Increased effects of aminophylline

smoking (at least 1 pack daily): Decreased effects of aminophylline

Adverse Reactions

CNS: Dizziness, fever, headache, insomnia, irritability, restlessness, seizures

CV: Arrhythmias (including sinus tachycardia and life-threatening ventricular arrhythmias), hypotension, palpitations

ENDO: Hyperglycemia, syndrome of inappropriate ADH secretion

GI: Anorexia, diarrhea, epigastric pain, heavy feeling in stomach, hematemesis, indigestion, nausea, vomiting

GU: Diuresis, proteinuria, urine retention in men with prostate enlargement
MS: Muscle twitching
RESP: Respiratory arrest, tachypnea
SKIN: Alopecia, exfoliative dermatitis, flushing, rash, urticaria

Nursing Considerations

- Dilute aminophylline with D_5W, normal saline solution, or a dextrose and sodium chloride combination.
- **WARNING** Because aminophylline has a narrow therapeutic window (10 to 20 mcg/ml), closely monitor serum theophylline level and observe for signs of toxicity, such as tachycardia, tachypnea, nausea, vomiting, restlessness, and seizures. Keep in mind that acetaminophen, furosemide, phenylbutazone, probenecid, theobromine, coffee, tea, soft drinks, and chocolate can produce an inaccurate serum theophylline level.
- To determine peak serum theophylline level, draw blood sample 15 to 30 minutes after administering I.V. loading dose.
- Store between 15° and 30° C (59° and 86° F). Don't freeze; protect from light.

PATIENT TEACHING

- Advise patient to avoid excessive intake of caffeine (in coffee, tea, soft drinks, and chocolate), which can falsely elevate theophylline level.
- Inform patient that blood tests may be needed to monitor the effects of aminophylline.

amiodarone hydrochloride

Cordarone, Pacerone

Class and Category

Chemical: Iodinated benzofuran derivative
Therapeutic: Class III antiarrhythmic
Pregnancy category: D

Indications and Dosages

▶ *To treat life-threatening, recurrent ventricular fibrillation and hemodynamically unstable ventricular tachycardia when these arrhythmias don't respond to other drugs or when patient can't tolerate other drugs*

I.V. INFUSION

Adults. *Loading:* 150 mg over 10 min (15 mg/min) followed by 360 mg infused over 6 hr (1 mg/min). *Maintenance:* 540 mg infused over 18 hr (0.5 mg/min); then after the first 24 hr, 720 mg infused over 24 hr (0.5 mg/min), continued up to 96 hr or until rhythm is stable. Change to oral form as soon as possible.

Route	Onset	Peak	Duration
I.V.	Hours to 3 days	1 to 3 wk	Weeks to months

Mechanism of Action

Acts on cardiac cell membranes, prolonging repolarization and the refractory period and raising ventricular fibrillation threshold. Drug relaxes vascular smooth muscles, mainly in coronary circulation, and improves myocardial blood flow. It relaxes peripheral vascular smooth muscles, decreasing peripheral vascular resistance and myocardial oxygen consumption.

Incompatibilities

Amiodarone is incompatible with heparin. To prevent precipitation, don't add amiodarone admixed with D_5W to aminophylline 4 mg/ml, cefamandole nafate, cefazolin sodium, or mezlocillin sodium, and don't mix amiodarone 3 mg/ml with sodium bicarbonate.

Contraindications

Bradycardia that causes syncope (unless pacemaker is present), cardiogenic shock, hypersensitivity to amiodarone or its components, hypokalemia, hypomagnesemia, SA node dysfunction, second- and third-degree AV block (unless pacemaker is present)

Interactions

DRUGS

anticoagulants: Increased anticoagulant response, which can result in serious bleeding

azole antifungals, fluoroquinolones, macrolide antibiotics: Increased risk of prolonged QT interval and life-threatening arrhythmias

beta blockers: Increased serum levels of beta blockers with increased risk of AV block, hypotension, and bradycardia

calcium channel blockers: Increased serum levels of these drugs and increased risk of AV block, bradycardia, and hypotension

cholestyramine, phenytoin, rifampin, St. John's wort: Decreased serum amiodarone level

cimetidine: Increased serum amiodarone level

cyclosporine: Increased serum cyclosporine level

dextromethorphan, methotrexate, phenytoin: Increased serum levels of these drugs and increased risk of toxicity if amiodarone is taken orally for more than 2 weeks
digoxin: Increased serum digoxin level and risk of digitalis toxicity
diltiazem, propranolol, verapamil: Increased risk of hemodynamic and electrophysiologic abnormalities
disopyramide: Increased serum disopyramide level with QT prolongation and increased risk of arrhythmias
fentanyl: Increased serum fentanyl level with increased risk of bradycardia, decreased cardiac output, and hypotension
flecainide: Increased serum flecainide level
hydantoins: Increased serum hydantoin level with long-term use and reduced serum amiodarone level
lidocaine: Increased serum lidocaine level and increased risk of seizures and bradycardia
potassium- and magnesium-depleting drugs: Increased risk of hypokalemia and hypomagnesemia
procainamide: Increased serum procainamide or N-acetylprocainamide level
quinidine: Increased serum quinidine level with risk of life-threatening arrhythmias
ritonavir: Increased serum amiodarone level with increased risk of cardiotoxicity
simvastatin: Possibly increased risk of myopathy and rhabdomyolysis
theophylline: Increased serum theophylline level; increased risk of theophylline toxicity
warfarin: Increased PT and risk of bleeding
FOODS
grapefruit juice: Increased serum amiodarone level

Adverse Reactions

CNS: Abnormal gait, ataxia, confusion, delirium, disorientation, dizziness, fatigue, hallucinations, headache, insomnia, involuntary motor activity, lack of coordination, malaise, paresthesia, peripheral neuropathy, sleep disturbances, tremor
CV: Arrhythmias (including bradycardia, electromechanical dissociation, torsades de pointes, and ventricular tachycardia or fibrillation), cardiac arrest, cardiogenic shock, edema, heart failure, hypotension, vasculitis
EENT: Abnormal salivation, abnormal taste and smell, blurred vision, corneal microdeposits, dry eyes, halo vision, lens opacities,

macular degeneration, optic neuritis, optic neuropathy, papilledema, permanent blindness, photophobia, scotoma
ENDO: Hyperthyroidism, hypothyroidism, syndrome of inappropriate antidiuretic hormone secretion, thyrotoxicosis
GI: Abdominal pain, anorexia, cirrhosis, constipation, diarrhea, elevated liver function test results, hepatitis, nausea, pancreatitis, vomiting
GU: Acute renal failure, decreased libido, epididymitis, impotence, renal impairment or insufficiency
HEME: Agranulocytosis, aplastic or hemolytic anemia, coagulation abnormalities, neutropenia, pancytopenia, spontaneous bruising, thrombocytopenia
MS: Muscle weakness, myopathy, rhabdomyolysis
RESP: Acute respiratory distress syndrome; bronchospasm; infiltrates that lead to dyspnea, cough, pulmonary fibrosis, pulmonary interstitial pneumonitis, crackles, and wheezing; pleuritis; pneumonia
SKIN: Alopecia, bluish gray pigmentation, erythema multiforme, exfoliative dermatitis, flushing, photosensitivity, pruritus, rash, Stevens-Johnson syndrome, toxic epidermal necrolysis
Other: Anaphylactic shock, angioedema

Nursing Considerations

- WARNING Be aware that I.V. amiodarone may cause or worsen pulmonary disorders that may develop days to weeks after therapy and progress to respiratory failure or even death.
- Monitor vital signs and oxygen levels often during and after giving amiodarone. Keep emergency equipment and drugs nearby.
- WARNING Monitor continuous ECG; check for increased PR and QRS intervals, arrhythmias, and heart rate below 60 beats/min because amiodarone toxicity may cause or worsen arrhythmias.
- Monitor serum amiodarone level, which normally ranges from 1.0 to 2.5 mcg/ml.
- Assess liver enzyme and thyroid hormone levels; drug inhibits conversion of T_4 to T_3 and may cause drug-induced hyperthyroidism that may in turn lead to thyrotoxicosis and arrhythmia breakthrough or increased severity of arrhythmia.

PATIENT TEACHING

- Explain that frequent monitoring and laboratory tests will be needed during treatment.

- Advise patient to report swollen hands and feet, wheezing, dyspnea, cough, nausea, vomiting, dark urine, fatigue, yellow skin or sclerae, stomach pain, light-headedness, fainting, or a rapid, slow, pounding, or irregular heartbeat.
- Instruct patient to report abnormal bleeding or bruising.

ammonium chloride

Class and Category

Chemical: Ammonium ion
Therapeutic: Acidifier
Pregnancy category: C

Indications and Dosages

▶ *To treat hypochloremia and metabolic alkalosis*

I.V. INFUSION

Adults. Individualized, based on serum bicarbonate level. *Usual:* 100 to 200 mEq added to 500 or 1,000 ml of normal saline solution, infused at 5 ml/min or less (about 3 hr for an infusion of 1,000 ml).

Route	Onset	Peak	Duration
I.V.	1 to 3 min	3 to 6 hr	Unknown

Mechanism of Action

Is converted to urea and hydrochloric acid in the liver. During the conversion, the drug is dissociated into ammonium and chloride ions, and hydrogen ions are released. These ions enter into the blood and extracellular fluid, where hydrogen reacts with bicarbonate ions to form water and carbon dioxide. This process decreases bicarbonate ions and increases chloride ions in the blood and extracellular fluid, which decreases blood and urine pH and corrects alkalosis.

Incompatibilities

Don't mix ammonium chloride with alkalies and their carbonates, codeine, lead or silver salts, levorphanol, methadone, or strong oxidizing agents such as potassium chlorate.

Contraindications

Hypersensitivity to ammonium chloride or its components, markedly impaired renal or hepatic function, metabolic alkalosis caused by vomiting of hydrochloric acid and accompanied by sodium loss caused by sodium bicarbonate excretion in urine

Interactions

DRUGS

amphetamines, salicylates, sulfonylureas, tricyclic antidepressants: Decreased therapeutic blood ammonium level
chlorpropamide: Increased effects of ammonium

Adverse Reactions

CNS: Fever, headache
CV: Phlebitis or thrombosis extending from injection site
GI: Indigestion, nausea, severe hepatic dysfunction, vomiting
RESP: Hyperventilation
SKIN: Extravasation
Other: Injection site infection, irritation, or pain; hypovolemia; severe metabolic acidosis (with large doses)

Nursing Considerations

- Before using ammonium chloride solution, warm it to room temperature by placing infusion in warm water to dissolve crystals.
- During I.V. administration, keep sodium bicarbonate or sodium lactate nearby to treat overdose.
- Infuse ammonium chloride slowly to avoid I.V. site pain and irritation.
- **WARNING** Monitor for signs and symptoms of ammonia toxicity, including arrhythmias, such as bradycardia; coma; irregular breathing; pallor; retching; seizures; diaphoresis; and twitching.
- Monitor for signs of metabolic acidosis, such as increased respirations, increased serum pH, restlessness, and diaphoresis.
- Monitor serum bicarbonate level and results of urinalysis and renal and liver function tests as appropriate.
- Store drug below 40° C (104° F). Don't freeze.

PATIENT TEACHING

- Tell patient who's taking ammonium chloride to consume more potassium-rich foods, such as bananas, oranges, cantaloupe, spinach, dried fruit, and potatoes.

amobarbital sodium

Amytal

Class, Category, and Schedule

Chemical: Barbiturate

Therapeutic: Anticonvulsant, sedative-hypnotic
Pregnancy category: D
Controlled substance: Schedule II

Indications and Dosages

▶ *To produce sedation*

I.V. INJECTION

Adults. 30 to 50 mg b.i.d. or t.i.d. and may range from 15 to 120 mg b.i.d or t.i.d. *Maximum:* 1,000 mg/dose.

Children over age 6. 65 to 500 mg/dose for preoperative sedation.

▶ *To induce a hypnotic state*

I.V. INJECTION

Adults. 65 to 200 mg/dose. *Maximum:* 1,000 mg/dose.

Children age 6 and older. 65 to 500 mg/dose.

▶ *To manage seizures*

I.V. INJECTION

Adults. *Usual:* 65 to 500 mg up to a maximum of 1,000 mg. Dosage for acute seizures determined by response. Doses of 200 to 500 mg are typically required to control seizures.

Children age 6 and older. 65 to 500 mg.

Children up to age 6. 3 to 5 mg/kg/dose.

WARNING Use I.V. route only when other routes aren't appropriate. Inject slowly—at a rate of 50 mg/min or less—to prevent sudden respiratory depression, apnea, laryngospasm, or hypotension.

Route	Onset	Peak	Duration
I.V.	Unknown	Unknown	10 to 12 hr

Mechanism of Action

Nonselectively acts on the CNS to depress the sensory cortex, decrease motor activity, alter cerebellar function, and produce drowsiness, sedation, and hypnosis. Appears to reduce wakefulness and alertness by acting in the thalamus, where it depresses the reticular activating system and interferes with impulse transmission from the periphery to the cortex. Produces CNS depressant effects ranging from mild sedation and anxiety reduction to anesthesia and coma.

Incompatibilities

Don't mix amobarbital in solution with other drugs.

Contraindications
Alcoholism, history of porphyria, history of sedative or barbiturate addiction, hypersensitivity to barbiturates, renal or hepatic disease, severe respiratory disease, sleep apnea, suicidal tendency, uncontrolled pain

Interactions
DRUGS

acetaminophen: Increased blood acetaminophen level and risk of hepatotoxicity

antihistamines, CNS depressants, phenothiazines, tranquilizers: Increased CNS depression

beta blockers, carbamazepine, clonazepam, corticosteroids, digitoxin, doxycycline, estrogens, griseofulvin, metronidazole, oral anticoagulants, oral contraceptives, phenylbutazones, quinidine, theophyllines, tricyclic antidepressants: Decreased blood levels and effects of these drugs

chloramphenicol: Inhibited amobarbital metabolism; enhanced chloramphenicol metabolism

MAO inhibitors: Increased blood level and sedative effects of amobarbital

methoxyflurane: Increased nephrotoxicity

phenytoin: Altered effects of phenytoin

rifampin: Decreased blood level and effects of amobarbital

valproic acid: Increased amobarbital effects

ACTIVITIES

alcohol use: Increased blood level of amobarbital and additive CNS depressant effects

Adverse Reactions
CNS: Agitation, anxiety, ataxia, CNS depression, confusion, dizziness, hallucinations, hangover, headache, hyperkinesia, insomnia, nightmares, nervousness, paradoxical stimulation, psychiatric disturbance, somnolence, syncope, vertigo

CV: Bradycardia, hypotension, shock

EENT: Laryngospasm

GI: Constipation, diarrhea, epigastric pain, nausea, vomiting

RESP: Apnea, bronchospasm, hypoventilation, respiratory depression

SKIN: Exfoliative dermatitis, rash, Stevens-Johnson syndrome, urticaria

Other: Angioedema, gangrene of arm or leg from accidental injection into artery, injection site tissue damage and necrosis, physical and psychological dependence, potentially fatal withdrawal syndrome, tolerance

Nursing Considerations

- Be aware that amobarbital shouldn't be given during third trimester of pregnancy because repeated use can cause dependence in neonate. It also shouldn't be given to breast-feeding women because it may cause CNS depression in infants.
- Prepare amobarbital using sterile water for injection.
- Closely monitor blood pressure, pulse, and respirations during administration. Keep emergency equipment and drugs nearby in case respiratory depression or adverse hemodynamic effects occur. Be aware that patients with cardiovascular disease are at increased risk for adverse circulatory reactions, particularly when drug is administered too fast, and that those with pulmonary diseases associated with obstruction or dyspnea are at increased risk for ventilatory depression. Anticipate the risk of hypotension, even when giving drug at recommended rate.
- Monitor for hypersensitivity reactions, such as bronchospasm, difficulty breathing, facial edema, and urticaria, especially in patients with a history of asthma, angioedema, or urticaria.
- **WARNING** Don't administer solution after 30 minutes of exposure to air. Solution quickly becomes unstable because amobarbital sodium hydrolyzes in solution.
- **WARNING** To prevent tissue damage and necrosis at peripheral insertion sites, monitor closely for signs of extravasation. Be aware that accidental arterial injection may cause gangrene of arm or leg.
- Anticipate that amobarbital's CNS effects may exacerbate major depression, suicidal tendencies, or other mental disorders.
- Closely monitor debilitated or elderly patients, as appropriate, because they're more likely to experience such adverse CNS reactions as confusion, depression, and excitement. Take safety precautions.
- Be aware that amobarbital may cause paradoxical stimulation (excitement, euphoria, restlessness) in patients with acute pain and in children.
- Evaluate for signs of intensified or prolonged hypnotic effect in patients with shock or uremia.
- Assess hyperthyroid patients for exacerbated symptoms, such as increased nervousness and palpitations, due to amobarbital use.
- Be aware that barbituate-induced respiratory depression may cause complications in patients with severe anemia.

- Be aware that drug may trigger signs and symptoms in patients with acute intermittent porphyria.
- To prevent withdrawal symptoms, such as diaphoresis, insomnia, irritability, nightmares, and tremors, expect to taper amobarbital dosage gradually after long-term use, especially for epileptic patients.

PATIENT TEACHING

- Instruct patient to report severe dizziness, persistent drowsiness, rash, or skin lesions during amobarbital therapy.

amphotericin B

Amphocin, Fungizone Intravenous

amphotericin B cholesteryl sulfate complex

Amphotec

amphotericin B lipid complex

Abelcet

amphotericin B liposomal complex

AmBisome

Class and Category

Chemical: Amphoteric polyene macrolide
Therapeutic: Antifungal
Pregnancy category: B

Indications and Dosages

▶ *To treat severe fungal infections, using amphotericin B*

I.V. INFUSION

Adults and adolescents. *Initial:* 1-mg test dose in 20 ml of D_5W infused over 20 to 30 min; if test dose is tolerated, administer 0.25 to 0.3 mg/kg daily prepared as a 0.1-mg/ml infusion and given over 2 to 6 hr. Increased in 5- to 10-mg increments up to 50 mg daily, based on patient tolerance and infection severity, not to exceed a total daily dose of 1.5 mg/kg. *Maximum:* 50 mg daily infused over 2 to 6 hr.

Children. *Initial:* 0.25 mg/kg daily in D_5W infused over 6 hr; then increased in 0.125- to 0.25-mg/kg increments daily or every other day as tolerated. *Maximum:* 1 mg/kg or 30 mg/m^2 of body surface daily.

▶ *To treat aspergillosis, using amphotericin B cholesteryl sulfate complex*

I.V. INFUSION

Adults and children. Test dose of 1.6 to 8.3 mg in 10 ml of

D_5W infused over 15 to 30 min; if test dose is tolerated, then 3 to 4 mg/kg once daily infused at 1 mg/kg/hr.

▶ *To treat invasive amphotericin B–resistant fungal infections, using amphotericin B lipid complex*

I.V. INFUSION

Adults and children. 5 mg/kg daily infused at 2.5 mg/kg/hr.

▶ *To treat severe aspergillosis, candidiasis, or cryptococcosis, using amphotericin B liposomal complex*

I.V. INFUSION

Adults and children. 3 to 5 mg/kg daily infused over 2 hr. Infusion time may be decreased to 1 hr if tolerated, or increased if patient experiences discomfort.

▶ *To treat leishmaniasis, using amphotericin B liposomal complex*

I.V. INFUSION

Immunocompetent adults and children. 3 mg/kg daily infused over 2 hr on days 1 through 5 and on days 14 and 21. Infusion time may be decreased to 1 hr if tolerated, or increased if patient experiences discomfort.

Immunocompromised adults and children. 4 mg/kg daily infused over 2 hr on days 1 through 5 and on days 10, 17, 24, 31, and 38. Infusion time may be decreased to 1 hr if tolerated, or increased if patient experiences discomfort.

▶ *To treat presumed fungal infections in patients with febrile neutropenia, using amphotericin B lipid complex*

I.V. INFUSION

Adults and children. 3 mg/kg daily infused over 2 hr. Infusion time may be decreased to 1 hr if tolerated, or increased if patient experiences discomfort.

Route	Onset	Peak	Duration
I.V.	Immediate	Unknown	Unknown

Mechanism of Action

Binds to sterols in fungal cell plasma membranes, which changes membrane permeability and allows loss of potassium and small molecules from cells. This action results in cell impairment or death.

Incompatibilities

Don't reconstitute amphotericin B with diluents other than those recommended because solutions containing sodium chloride or bacteriostatic agents (such as benzyl alcohol) may cause drug precipitation.

Contraindications

Hypersensitivity to amphotericin B or its components

Interactions

DRUGS

antineoplastics: Increased risk of bronchospasm, hypotension, and nephrotoxicity
corticosteroids, corticotropin: Increased risk of hypokalemia and subsequent cardiac dysfunction
cyclosporine, nephrotoxic drugs: Increased risk of nephrotoxicity
digitalis glycosides: Possibly hypokalemia and more severe digitalis toxicity
flucytosine: Possibly increased flucytosine toxicity
leukocyte transfusion: Possibly dyspnea, hypoxemia, and pulmonary infiltrates
skeletal muscle relaxants: Possibly hypokalemia and subsequent increased muscle relaxation
zidovudine: Possibly myelotoxicity and nephrotoxicity

Adverse Reactions

CNS: Chills, fever, headache, tiredness, weakness
CV: Chest pain, hypotension, irregular heartbeat
EENT: Pharyngitis
GI: Abdominal pain, anorexia, diarrhea, dysphagia, hepatic failure, indigestion, nausea, vomiting
GU: Decreased or increased urine output, impaired renal function
HEME: Anemia, leukopenia, thrombocytopenia, unusual bleeding or bruising
MS: Arthralgia, muscle spasms, myalgia
RESP: Apnea, dyspnea, hypoxia, pulmonary edema, tachypnea
SKIN: Flushing, jaundice, maculopapular rash, pruritus and redness especially around ears, urticaria
Other: Anaphylaxis, hypocalcemia, hypokalemia, hypomagnesemia, infusion site pain and thrombophlebitis

Nursing Considerations

- To prepare amphotericin B, add 10 ml of sterile water for injection (without a bacteriostatic agent) to vial containing 50 mg of amphotericin B. For I.V. infusion, dilute the solution containing 5 mg/ml to 0.1 mg/ml by adding 1 ml (5 mg) of solution to 49 ml of D_5W with a pH above 4.2.

- Before using D_5W to dilute amphotericin B solution, aseptically determine injection's pH. If pH is below 4.2, follow manufacturer's instructions for buffering it.
- Because reconstituted amphotericin B is a colloidal suspension, avoid using an in-line membrane filter or use one with a mean pore diameter of more than 1 micron to prevent significant drug removal.
- To prepare amphotericin B cholesteryl sulfate complex, reconstitute it with sterile water for injection. Using a sterile syringe and a 20G needle, rapidly add 10 or 20 ml of sterile water for injection to a 50- or 100-mg vial, respectively, to obtain a solution containing 5 mg of amphotericin B per milliliter. Then shake gently by hand, rotating vial until all solids are dissolved. The fluid may be clear or opalescent. For infusion, further dilute reconstituted solution to about 0.6 mg/ml. Don't filter the solution. Flush existing line with D_5W or use a separate line. Don't use an in-line filter.
- To prepare amphotericin B lipid complex, shake vial gently until you see no yellow sediment. Using an 18G needle, withdraw prescribed dose from required number of vials into one or more 20-ml syringes. Replace needle with 5-micron filter needle that's supplied with each vial. Empty syringe contents into bag of D_5W so that final concentration is 1 mg/ml. Expect to use a concentration of 2 mg/ml for pediatric patients and patients with cardiovascular disease. Before infusion, shake bag until contents are mixed thoroughly. Flush existing line with D_5W or use a separate line. Don't use an in-line filter. If infusion exceeds 2 hours, shake infusion bag every 2 hours.
- To prepare amphotericin B liposomal complex, add 12 ml of sterile water for injection (without a bacteriostatic agent) to each 50-mg vial to achieve a concentration of 4 mg amphotericin B per milliliter. Immediately shake vial vigorously for at least 30 seconds until all particles completely disperse. Withdraw prescribed dose of amphotericin B liposomal complex suspension. Then use a 5-micron filter to inject it into D_5W to provide a final concentration of 1 to 2 mg/ml. Expect to use a lower concentration (0.2 to 0.5 mg/ml) for infants and young children. Flush existing line with D_5W or use a separate line. You may use an in-line filter with a mean pore diameter of at least 1 micron.

- To help minimize fever and shaking chills, expect to administer an antipyretic, an antihistamine, meperidine, or a corticosteroid just before infusing amphotericin B.
- Assess I.V. insertion site regularly to detect extravasation of amphotericin B, which may cause severe local irritation. To minimize local thrombophlebitis, plan to add heparin to infusion or to administer amphotericin on alternate days, which also may help prevent anorexia. Alternate-day dose shouldn't exceed 1.5 mg/kg.
- Monitor renal function closely because of risk of renal impairment. Plan to assess serum creatinine level every other day while amphotericin B dosage is increasing and then at least twice weekly during continued therapy. If serum creatinine or BUN level increases significantly, expect to discontinue amphotericin B until renal function improves. Be aware that a cumulative dose of more than 4 g may cause irreversible renal dysfunction.
- Expect to monitor CBC and platelet count weekly throughout therapy to detect adverse hematologic effects. Also monitor serum calcium, magnesium, and potassium levels twice weekly throughout therapy to detect abnormalities.
- Before drug reconstitution, store amphotericin B at 2° to 8° C (36° to 46° F), and protect from light. Use reconstituted amphotericin B within 24 hours if stored at room temperature or within 1 week if refrigerated. Use immediately if solution was reconstituted and diluted in D_5W.
- Before drug reconstitution, store amphotericin B cholesteryl sulfate complex at 15° to 30° C (59° to 86° F) unless otherwise specified. After reconstitution, store at 2° to 8° C (36° to 46° F). Use reconstituted amphotericin B cholesteryl sulfate complex within 24 hours.
- Before drug dilution, store amphotericin B lipid complex at 2° to 8° C, and protect from light. Use amphotericin B lipid complex within 6 hours if stored at room temperature or within 48 hours if stored at 2° to 8° C. Don't freeze.
- Before drug reconstitution, store amphotericin B liposomal complex at 2° to 8° C. Use reconstituted amphotericin B liposomal complex within 24 hours if stored at 2° to 8° C. Begin infusion of diluted drug within 6 hours. Don't freeze.

PATIENT TEACHING

- Instruct patient to report pain or discomfort at I.V. insertion site of amphotericin.

- Advise patient to report adverse reactions immediately, especially shortness of breath, chest pain, or wheezing.

ampicillin sodium

Ampicin (CAN), Omnipen-N, Polycillin-N, Totacillin-N

Class and Category

Chemical: Semisynthetic aminopenicillin
Therapeutic: Antibiotic
Pregnancy category: B

Indications and Dosages

▶ *To treat GI and GU infections (other than gonorrhea) caused by susceptible strains of* Shigella, Salmonella typhi *and other species,* Escherichia coli, Proteus mirabilis, *and enterococci*

I.V. INFUSION

Adults and children weighing 20 kg (44 lb) or more. 500 mg P.O. q 6 hr or 250 to 500 mg I.V. q 6 hr.

Children weighing less than 20 kg. 50 to 100 mg/kg daily in divided doses P.O. q 6 hr or 12.5 mg/kg I.V. q 6 hr.

▶ *To treat gonorrhea caused by susceptible strains of non–penicillinase-producing* Neisseria gonorrhoeaea

I.V. INFUSION

Adults and children weighing 45 kg (99 lb) or more. 500 mg q 6 hr.

Children weighing less than 40 kg (88 lb). 50 mg/kg daily in divided doses q 6 to 8 hr.

▶ *To treat respiratory tract infections caused by susceptible strains of non–penicillinase-producing* Haemophilus influenzae, *staphylococci, and streptococci, including* Streptococcus pneumoniae

I.V. INFUSION

Adults and children weighing 40 kg or more. 250 to 500 mg I.V. q 6 to 8 hr.

Children weighing less than 40 kg. 25 to 50 mg/kg daily I.V. in divided doses q 6 to 8 hr.

Children weighing less than 20 kg. 12.5 mg/kg I.V. q 6 hr.

▶ *To treat septicemia*

I.V. INFUSION

Adults. 8 to 14 g I.V. daily in divided doses q 3 to 4 hr for at least 3 days; then I.M.

Children. 150 to 200 mg/kg daily I.V. in divided doses q 3 to 4 hr for at least 3 days; then I.M.

▶ *To prevent bacterial endocarditis from dental, oral, or upper respiratory tract procedures*
I.V. INFUSION
Adults. 2 g within 30 min of procedure
Children. 50 mg/kg within 30 min of procedure
▶ *To treat bacterial meningitis caused by susceptible strains of* Neisseria meningitidis
I.V. INFUSION
Adults. 8 to 14 g daily or 150 to 200 mg/kg daily I.V. in equally divided doses q 3 to 4 hr for at least 3 days; then I.M. at same dosage and schedule.
Children. 100 to 200 mg/kg daily I.V. in equally divided doses q 3 to 4 hr for at least 3 days; then I.M. at same dosage and schedule.
▶ *To treat listeriosis*
I.V. INFUSION
Adults and children weighing 20 kg or more. 50 mg/kg q 6 hr.
Children weighing less than 20 kg. 12.5 mg/kg q 6 hr.

Route	Onset	Peak	Duration
I.V.	Immediate	Unknown	Unknown

Mechanism of Action
Inhibits bacterial cell wall synthesis. The rigid, cross-linked cell wall is assembled in several steps. Ampicillin exerts its effects on susceptible bacteria in the final stage of the cross-linking process by binding with and inactivating penicillin-binding proteins (enzymes responsible for linking the cell wall strands). This action causes bacterial cell lysis and death.

Incompatibilities
Don't mix ampicillin and any aminoglycoside in the same I.V. bag, bottle, or tubing; otherwise, both drugs will be inactivated. If patient must receive both drugs, administer them in separate sites at least 1 hour apart.

Contraindications
Hypersensitivity to any penicillin, infection caused by penicillinase-producing organism

Interactions
DRUGS
allopurinol: Increased risk of rash, particularly with hyperuricemia

aminoglycosides: Possibly inactivated action of aminoglycoside and ampicillin when given together
heparin, oral anticoagulants: Increased risk of bleeding
oral contraceptives: Possibly reduced contraceptive effectiveness and breakthrough bleeding
probenecid: Possibly increased serum ampicillin level and ampicillin toxicity
tetracyclines: Possibly impaired action of ampicillin

Adverse Reactions

CNS: Chills, fatigue, fever, headache, malaise
CV: Chest pain, edema, thrombophlebitis
EENT: Epistaxis, glossitis, laryngeal stridor, mucocutaneous candidiasis, stomatitis, throat tightness
GI: Abdominal distention, diarrhea, enterocolitis, flatulence, gastritis, nausea, pseudomembranous colitis, vomiting
GU: Dysuria, urine retention, vaginal candidiasis
HEME: Agranulocytosis, anemia, eosinophilia, leukopenia, thrombocytopenia, thrombocytopenic purpura
SKIN: Erythema multiforme; erythematous, mildly pruritic maculopapular rash or other types of rash; exfoliative dermatitis; pruritus; urticaria
Other: Anaphylaxis, facial edema, injection site pain

Nursing Considerations

- Avoid giving ampicillin to patients with mononucleosis because of increased risk of rash.
- Expect to give ampicillin for 48 to 72 hours after patient becomes asymptomatic. For streptococcal infection, expect to give ampicillin for at least 10 days after cultures show streptococcal eradication to reduce risk of rheumatic fever or glomerulonephritis.
- To dilute ampicillin for intermittent infusion, add 5 ml of sterile water or bacteriostatic water for injection to each 125-, 250-, or 500-mg vial or 7.4 to 10 ml of diluent to each 1- or 2-g vial. Infuse in suitable diluent at less than 30 mg/ml.
- WARNING Infuse I.V. solution for 3 to 5 minutes for each 125 or 500 mg or 10 to 15 minutes for each 1 or 2 g. More rapid infusion may cause seizures.
- Monitor patient closely for anaphylaxis, which may be life-threatening. Patients at greatest risk are those with a history of multiple allergies, hypersensitivity to cephalosporins, or a history of asthma, hay fever, or urticaria.

- Notify prescriber if patient has evidence of superinfection; expect to stop drug and provide appropriate treatment.
- WARNING In an anaphylactic reaction, stop drug, notify prescriber immediately, and provide immediate treatment with epinephrine, airway management, oxygen, and I.V. corticosteroids, as needed.
- If long-term or high-dose ampicillin therapy is required, closely monitor results of renal and liver function tests and CBCs.

PATIENT TEACHING

- Review signs of allergic reaction; if they occur, tell patient to contact prescriber immediately.

ampicillin sodium and sulbactam sodium

Unasyn

Class and Category

Chemical: Aminopenicillin, beta-lactamase inhibitor
Therapeutic: Broad-spectrum antibiotic
Pregnancy category: B

Indications and Dosages

▶ *To treat skin and soft-tissue infections caused by beta-lactamase–producing strains of* Staphylococcus aureus, Escherichia coli, Klebsiella *sp. (including* K. pneumoniae*),* Proteus mirabilis, Bacteroides fragilis, Enterobacter *sp., and* Acinetobacter calcoaceticus; *intra-abdominal infections caused by beta-lactamase–producing strains of* E. coli, Klebsiella *sp. (including* K. pneumoniae*),* Bacteroides *sp. (including* B. fragilis*), and* Enterobacter *sp.; gynecologic infections caused by beta-lactamase–producing strains of* E. coli *and* Bacteroides *sp. (including* B. fragilis*)*

I.V. INFUSION

Adults and children age 12 and over weighing 40 kg (88 lb) or more. 1.5 (1 g of ampicillin and 0.5 g of sulbactam) to 3 g (2 g of ampicillin and 1 g of sulbactam) q 6 hr, up to a maximum of 8 g of ampicillin and 4 g of sulbactam daily.

Children age 1 and over weighing less than 40 kg. 300 mg/kg (200 mg of ampicillin and 100 mg of sulbactam) daily in divided doses q 6 hr.

DOSAGE ADJUSTMENT Dosing frequency reduced to q 6 to

8 hr for patients with creatinine clearance of 30 ml/min/1.73 m^2 or more, to q 12 hr for patients with creatinine clearance of 15 to 29 ml/min/1.73 m^2, and to q 24 hr for patients with creatinine clearance of 5 to 14 ml/min/1.73 m^2.

Route	Onset	Peak	Duration
I.V.	Immediate	Unknown	Unknown

Mechanism of Action

Inhibits bacterial cell wall synthesis. The rigid, cross-linked cell wall is assembled in several steps. The drug exerts its effects on susceptible bacteria in the final stage of the cross-linking process by binding with and inactivating penicillin-binding proteins (enzymes responsible for linking the cell wall strands). This action causes bacterial cell lysis and death. When ampicillin is administered alone, beta-lactamases may degrade it, making it ineffective. When combined with sulbactam, degradation can't occur. So sulbactam extends ampicillin's bactericidal effects to beta-lactamase–producing bacteria.

Incompatibilities

To prevent mutual inactivation, don't mix ampicillin sodium and sulbactam sodium in the same I.V. bag, bottle, or tubing with an aminoglycoside. If patient must receive both drugs, administer them in separate sites at least 1 hour apart.

Contraindications

Hypersensitivity to ampicillin sodium and sulbactam sodium, its components, or any penicillin

Interactions

DRUGS

allopurinol: Increased risk of rash, particularly in hyperuricemic patient

aminoglycosides: Possibly inactivation of both drugs when given together

heparin, oral anticoagulants: Increased risk of bleeding

oral contraceptives: Possibly reduced contraceptive effectiveness and breakthrough bleeding

probenecid: Possibly increased blood ampicillin level and risk of ampicillin toxicity

tetracyclines: Possibly impaired action of ampicillin sodium and sulbactam sodium

Adverse Reactions

CNS: Chills, fatigue, fever, headache, malaise
CV: Chest pain, edema, thrombophlebitis
EENT: Black "hairy" tongue, epistaxis, glossitis, laryngeal stridor, mucocutaneous candidiasis, stomatitis, throat tightness
GI: Abdominal distention, diarrhea, enterocolitis, flatulence, gastritis, nausea, pseudomembranous colitis, vomiting
GU: Dysuria, urine retention, vaginal candidiasis
HEME: Agranulocytosis, anemia, eosinophilia, leukopenia, thrombocytopenia, thrombocytopenic purpura
SKIN: Erythema multiforme; erythematous, mildly pruritic maculopapular rash or other rash; exfoliative dermatitis; mucosal bleeding; pruritus; urticaria
Other: Anaphylaxis, facial edema

Nursing Considerations

- Avoid administering ampicillin sodium and sulbactam sodium to patients with mononucleosis because of increased risk of a rash.
- Add 3.2 ml of sterile water for injection to each 1.5-g vial or 6.4 ml to each 3-g vial. This provides a total concentration of 375 mg/ml (250 mg/ml of ampicillin and 125 mg/ml of sulbactam). Using a suitable diluent and the concentrations recommended in manufacturer's insert (including sterile water for injection, lactated Ringer's, or D_5/0.45 normal saline solution), further dilute to a final concentration of 3 to 45 mg/ml (2 to 30 mg/ml of ampicillin and 1 to 15 mg/ml of sulbactam).
- Let solution stand to allow foaming to dissipate; inspect for complete solubility before administering.
- Administer I.V. dose by slow injection over 10 to 15 minutes or by infusion over 15 to 30 minutes when diluted further.
- Monitor patient closely for anaphylaxis, which may be life-threatening. Patients at greatest risk are those with a history of hypersensitivity to penicillin, multiple allergies, hypersensitivity to cephalosporins, or a history of asthma, hay fever, or urticaria.
- **WARNING** If drug triggers an anaphylactic reaction, discontinue drug, notify prescriber immediately, and provide appropriate therapy. Anaphylaxis requires immediate treatment with epinephrine as well as airway management and administration of oxygen and I.V. corticosteroids, as needed.
- Monitor patient closely for diarrhea, which may signal pseudomembranous colitis. If diarrhea occurs, notify prescriber. If pseudomembranous colitis is diagnosed, expect to discontinue

drug and, possibly, administer fluids, electrolytes, protein, and antibiotic effective against *Clostridium difficile.*

- Keep in mind that each 1.5-g dose of ampicillin and sulbactam contains 5 mEq of sodium; take this into account when calculating patient's daily sodium intake.
- Be aware that drug's potency varies, depending on amount and type of diluent used and how solution is stored. For example, dilution with normnal saline solution for a final concentration of 45 mg/ml (30/15 mg/ml) retains potency for 8 hours when stored at 25° C (77° F) and for 48 hours when stored at 4° C (39° F). A dilution with normal saline solution for a final concentration of 30 mg/ml (20/10 mg/ml) retains potency for 72 hours when stored at 4° C. See manufacturer's insert for further details.

PATIENT TEACHING

- Instruct patient receiving ampicillin sodium and sulbactam sodium to immediately report sudden or unusual symptoms, such as shortness of breath, wheezing, rash, chest pain, or facial swelling. Tell him to notify prescriber immediately if diarrhea occurs.

anidulafungin

Eraxis

Class and Category

Chemical: Semi-synthetic echinocandin
Therapeutic: Antifungal
Pregnancy category: C

Indications and Dosages

▶ *To treat candidemia and other forms of* Candida *infection, such as intra-abdominal abscess and peritonitis*

I.V. INFUSION

Adults. 200 mg on day 1, followed by 100 mg daily, continued for at least 14 days after the last positive culture.

▶ *To treat esophageal candidiasis*

I.V. INFUSION

Adults. 100 mg on day 1, followed by 50 mg daily for at least 14 days and for at least 7 days following resolution of symptoms.

Contraindications

Hypersensitivity to anidulafungin, its components, or other echinocandins

Mechanism of Action

Inhibits glucan synthase, an enzyme needed for formation of 1,3-beta-D glucan, a substance essential for construction of the fungal cell wall. Because the fungus cannot exist without a cell wall, the infection resolves.

Interactions

DRUGS

None reported.

Adverse Reactions

CNS: Headache, dizziness, seizures
CV: Artial fibrillation, deep vein thrombosis, hypertension, hypotension, right bundle branch block, sinus arrhythmia, ventricular extrasystoles
ENDO: Hyperglycemia
GI: Diarrhea, elevated liver enzymes, dyspepsia, heptic necrosis, nausea
HEME: Leukopenia, neutropenia, thrombocytopenia
RESP: Dyspnea
SKIN: Flushing, pruritus, rash, urticaria
Other: Angioneurotic edema, hypercalcemia, hypokalemia, hyperkalemia, hypernatremia, hypomagnesemia

Nursing Considerations

- Reconstitute each 50-mg vial with 15 ml of the supplied diluent (20% dehydrated alcohol in water for injection) to provide a concentration of 3.33 mg/ml. Use within 24 hours after reconstitution.
- Further dilute the reconstituted solution with either 5% dextrose or normal saline solution. For a 50-mg dose, dilute with 100 ml; for a 100-mg dose, dilute with 250 ml; and for a 200-mg dose, dilute with 500 ml.
- Administer as an intravenous infusion at no more than 1.1 mg/minute.
- Monitor patient's liver function, as ordered. If abnormalities occur or hepatic funciton worsens, notify prescriber and expect to discontinue anidulafungin.

PATIENT TEACHING

- Inform patient that anidulafungin therapy will last 2 or more weeks. If the patient has esophageal candidiasis, explain that therapy will last at least 1 week after symptoms resolve. If the

patient has an abdominal abscess or peritonitis, explain that therapy will last 2 weeks after culture is negative.
- Tell patient to promptly report any histamine-related symptoms, such as rash, pruritus, or urticaria.

anistreplase
(anisoylated plasminogen-streptokinase activator complex)
Eminase

Class and Category
Chemical: p-Anisoylated derivative of the Lys-plasminogen-streptokinase activator complex
Therapeutic: Thrombolytic enzyme
Pregnancy category: C

Indications and Dosages
▶ *To treat acute MI (to lyse thrombi obstructing coronary arteries, reduce infarct size, improve ventricular function, and reduce mortality)*
I.V. INFUSION
Adults. 30 units injected over 2 to 5 min.

Route	Onset	Peak	Duration
I.V.	Immediate	20 min to 2 hr	4 to 6 hr

Mechanism of Action
Indirectly promotes the conversion of plasminogen to plasmin, an enzyme that breaks down fibrin clots, fibrinogen, and other plasma proteins, including procoagulant factors V and VIII.

Incompatibilities
Don't add other drugs to anistreplase solution or infuse other drugs through same I.V. line.

Contraindications
Active internal bleeding, arteriovenous malformation or aneurysm, bleeding diathesis, history of CVA, hypersensitivity to anistreplase or streptokinase, intracranial neoplasm, intracranial or intraspinal surgery or trauma within past 2 months, severe uncontrolled hypertension

Interactions

DRUGS

aspirin, dipyridamole, and other drugs that alter platelet function; heparin; vitamin K antagonists: Possibly increased risk of bleeding if administered before anistreplase

Adverse Reactions

CNS: Dizziness, fever, headache, intracranial hemorrhage
CV: Ankle edema, arrhythmias (especially accelerated idioventricular rhythm, conduction disorders, premature ventricular beats, sinus bradycardia, ventricular fibrillation, ventricular tachycardia), hypotension, vasculitis
EENT: Epistaxis
GI: Abdominal pain or swelling, constipation, GI bleeding, nausea, vomiting
GU: Hematuria, proteinuria, vaginal bleeding
HEME: Bleeding tendency, eosinophilia, mild to severe hemorrhage
MS: Arthralgia, back pain, joint stiffness, myalgia
RESP: Bronchospasm, dyspnea, hemoptysis
SKIN: Flushing, pruritus, rash, urticaria
Other: Anaphylaxis, angioedema

Nursing Considerations

- Obtain appropriate coagulation studies (such as PT, APTT, platelet count, and fibrin-fibrinogen degradation product titer) before initiating anistreplase treatment, if possible.
- To reconstitute anistreplase, slowly direct 5 ml of sterile water for injection or sodium chloride for injection against side of vial. Then gently roll vial to mix dry powder and fluid and minimize foaming. Don't shake vial. The resulting solution should be colorless to pale yellow and transparent.
- Before administering solution, inspect it for particles and discoloration. If present, discard and reconstitute drug from a new vial. Then withdraw entire contents of vial. Don't dilute reconstituted solution further before administration; don't add it to I.V. fluid. Don't add other drugs to vial or syringe that contains anistreplase. Discard drug if it isn't administered within 30 minutes of reconstitution.
- For maximum effectiveness, expect to administer anistreplase as soon as possible after onset of MI symptoms.
- Closely monitor all puncture sites, such as catheter insertion and needle puncture sites, for bleeding.

- Monitor the following patients for evidence of bleeding or hemorrhage because they're at increased risk during anistreplase therapy: those with acute pericarditis (risk of hemopericardium, possibly leading to cardiac tamponade); cerebrovascular disease; hemorrhagic ophthalmic conditions; history of major surgery, GI or GU bleeding, or trauma within past 10 days; hypertension; mitral stenosis with atrial fibrillation (risk of embolism); pregnancy; septic thrombophlebitis; severe hepatic or renal disease; or subacute bacterial endocarditis.
- Avoid giving I.M. injections and handling patient unnecessarily during anistreplase therapy. Perform venipuncture only when necessary, using a 23G or smaller needle.
- If the patient needs an arterial puncture after anistreplase administration, use an arm vessel that allows easy manual compression. Apply pressure for 30 minutes. Then apply a pressure dressing and check puncture site frequently for bleeding.
- Use continuous cardiac monitoring because arrhythmias may occur during reperfusion. Keep antiarrhythmics on hand during anistreplase therapy, and manage arrhythmias according to facility policy.
- Keep epinephrine, glucocorticoids, and antihistamines nearby to treat anaphylaxis.
- Know that anistreplase may be less effective if given more than 5 days after previous anistreplase or streptokinase administration. This occurs because patient may have developed antistreptokinase antibodies, which make him more resistant to the drug and make drug therapy less effective. Elevated serum antistreptokinase antibody levels and reduced drug effectiveness can persist for 5 days to 12 months.
- Store drug between 2° and 8° C (36° and 46° F).

PATIENT TEACHING

- Instruct patient receiving anistreplase to report adverse reactions immediately, especially bleeding, dizziness, and chest pain.

antihemophilic factor (recombinant), plasma/albumin-free method (rAHF-PFM)

Advate

Class and Category

Chemical: Recombinant protein
Therapeutic: Antihemophilic factor

Pregnancy category: C

Indications and Dosages

▶ *To prevent and control bleeding episodes in patients with hemophilia A and patients with Factor VIII inhibitors not exceeding 10 Bethesda Units/ml*

I.V. INJECTION

Adults and children. Highly individualized. *For early hemarthrosis, muscle bleeding episode, or mild oral bleeding episode:* Dose administered to achieve peak post-infusion Factor VIII activity in blood (determined by multiplying dose administered/kg body weight by 2) between 20% and 40% of normal with infusions q 12 to 24 hr for 1 to 3 days until bleeding episode resolved. *For more extensive hemarthrosis, muscle bleeding episode, or hematoma:* Dose administered to achieve peak post-infusion Factor VIII activity in blood between 30% and 60% of normal with infusions q 12 to 24 hr for 3 or more days until pain and disability are resolved. *For life-threatening bleeding episodes:* Dose administered to achieve peak post-infusion Factor VIII activity in blood between 60% and 100% with infusions q 8 to 24 hr until bleeding episode stops.

▶ *To prevent and control perioperative bleeding in patients with hemophilia A*

I.V. INJECTION

Adults and children. Highly individualized. *For minor surgery, including tooth extraction:* Dose administered to achieve peak post-infusion Factor VIII activity in blood (determined by multiplying dose administered/kg body weight by 2) between 60% and 100% of normal, given as a single bolus infusion within 1 hr of operation, with optional additional dose q 12 to 24 hr, as needed. *For major surgery:* Dose administered to achieve peak post-infusion Factor VIII activity in blood between 80% and 100% preoperatively and postoperatively with infusions q 8 to 24 hr.

Route	Onset	Peak	Duration
I.V.	Immediate	5 min	Unknown

Mechanism of Action

Provides supplemental Factor VIII, the coagulation factor needed for blood to clot that is missing in patients with hemophilia A and diminished in patients with Factor VIII inhibitors. After blood clots, bleeding stops.

Contraindications

Life-threatening, immediate hypersensitivity reactions, including anaphylaxis, with previous use of drug or exposure to mouse or hamster proteins

Interactions

DRUGS

None reported.

Adverse Reactions

CNS: Dizziness, fever, headache, rigidity
CV: Chest pain
EENT: Taste perversion
GI: Abdominal pain, diarrhea, nausea
HEME: Bleeding tendency, decreased coagulation Factor VIII, decreased hematocrit, hematoma, hemolytic anemia
MS: Joint swelling, lower limb edema
RESP: Dyspnea
SKIN: Diaphoresis, pruritus
Other: Anaphylaxis, catheter-related infection, hot flashes

Nursing Considerations

- Check to confirm that clotting defect is Factor VIII deficiency before administering antihemophilic factor (recombinant) because drug isn't effective in treating other coagulation factor deficiencies.
- Reconstitute drug using sterile water for injection. Bring both drug and diluent to room temperature; then clean stoppers with antiseptic solution and allow to dry. Remove protective covering from one end of double-ended needle and insert through center of diluent stopper. Remove protective covering from other end of double-ended needle. Invert diluent bottle over upright drug bottle; then rapidly insert free end of needle through drug stopper at center. The vacuum in bottle will draw in the diluent. Then disconnect the two bottles by removing needle from diluent bottle stopper, and remove the needle from drug bottle. Swirl gently until all drug is dissolved. Avoid shaking to prevent foaming and degradation of drug. Administer in a separate line within 3 hours of reconstitution.
- Take patient's pulse before and periodically during drug administration. If rate increases significantly, reduce administration rate or temporarily halt the injection to allow pulse rate to return to basline before resuming administration.

- To administer, use only plastic material because protein in drug will adhere to glass. Attach filter needle to syringe and draw back plunger to draw air into syringe. Insert needle into reconstituted drug vial. Inject air into bottle and then withdraw drug from vial. Remove and discard filter needle from syringe, attach a suitable needle, and inject I.V. bolus at no greater than 10 ml/min over no more than 5 min.
- Monitor patient's plasma Factor VIII level during and after treatment to ensure an adequate level has been reached and is being maintained, as ordered.
- Monitor patient for anaphylaxis, and have emergency equipment nearby.
- After giving drug, monitor patient for formation of neutralizing antibodies to Factor VIII, a known complication in the treatment of hemophilia A that may be evidenced by continued bleeding. Obtain laboratory analysis to detect the neutralizing antibodies, as ordered.
- Monitor patients with blood types A, B, and AB for hemolysis when giving large doses.

PATIENT TEACHING

- Teach patient and caregivers how to administer drug at home in an emergency situation.
- Instruct patient to discontinue drug and seek emergency help immediately if he has an acute allergic reaction, such as hives, chest tightness, wheezing, low blood pressure, or fainting during or after drug administration.

antithrombin III, human
(AT-III, heparin co-factor I)

ATnativ, Thrombate III

Class and Category

Chemical: Alpha$_2$-globulin
Therapeutic: Anticoagulant, antithrombotic
Pregnancy category: C

Indications and Dosages

▶ *To treat patients with hereditary antithrombin III (AT-III) deficiency who are undergoing surgery or obstetric procedures or who have thromboembolism*

I.V. INJECTION

Adults and children. *Initial:* Individualized dosage (based on weight, degree of AT-III deficiency, and desired level of AT-III to be achieved) sufficient to increase AT-III activity to 120% of normal, administered at 50 to 100 international units/min. *Maintenance:* Individualized dosage sufficient to keep AT-III activity at 80% or more of normal, administered q 24 hr for 2 to 8 days, depending on patient's condition and history and prescriber's judgment. A pregnant, immobilized, or postsurgical patient may need more prolonged therapy.

Route	Onset	Peak	Duration
I.V.	Immediate	Unknown	4 days

Mechanism of Action

Inhibits blood coagulation by inactivating thrombin; activated forms of factors IX, X, XI, and XII; and plasmin.

Incompatibilities

Don't mix AT-III with other drugs or solutions.

Interactions

DRUGS

heparin: Enhanced anticoagulant effect

Adverse Reactions

CNS: Chills, dizziness, fever, light-headedness
CV: Chest pain or tightness, hypotension, vasodilation
EENT: Unpleasant taste
GI: Abdominal cramps, bowel fullness, nausea
GU: Diuresis
HEME: Hematoma
RESP: Dyspnea
SKIN: Oozing lesions, urticaria

Nursing Considerations

- Reconstitute AT-III with 10 ml of sterile water for injection (provided by manufacturer) or alternate solution, such as normal saline solution or D_5W injection. Don't shake vial during reconstitution. Let solution come to room temperature before administration. If desired, dilute reconstituted solution further, using same diluent.
- **WARNING** Don't use diluent that contains benzyl alcohol to reconstitute AT-III for a neonate. This can cause a fatal toxic

syndrome characterized by metabolic acidosis, CNS depression, respiratory problems, renal failure, hypotension, seizures, and intracranial hemorrhage.
- Don't refrigerate reconstituted solution. Use it within 3 hours and discard unused solution.
- If after 30 minutes the initial dose doesn't increase AT-III activity to 120% of normal, expect prescriber to increase dosage.
- If patient requires a dosage increase, monitor AT-III activity more frequently and expect to adjust dosage accordingly.
- Expect to reduce heparin dosage to prevent bleeding during AT-III therapy.
- If mild adverse reactions occur, decrease infusion rate, as prescribed. If severe reactions occur, discontinue infusion, as prescribed, until they subside.
- Evaluate serum AT-III level twice a day until dosage is stabilized. After that, evaluate level once daily, immediately before administering a dose.
- Store drug between 2° and 8° C (36° and 46° F).

PATIENT TEACHING
- Inform patient that blood will be drawn periodically during AT-III therapy to guide dosage adjustments.

aprotinin

Trasylol

Class and Category

Chemical: Protease inhibitor
Therapeutic: Antifibrinolytic
Pregnancy category: B

Indications and Dosages

▶ *To reduce blood loss and the need for blood transfusion in patients undergoing repeat coronary artery bypass graft surgery and for those undergoing first-time surgery who are at high risk for bleeding or when blood transfusion is unavailable or unacceptable*

I.V. INFUSION

Adults. *High-dose regimen:* Test dose of 10,000 KIU (kallikrein inactivator units, 1 ml) 10 min before initial dose. If test dose is tolerated, give 2,000,000 KIU (200 ml) over 20 to 30 min with patient in a supine position, followed by maintenance dosage of 500,000 KIU/hr (50 ml/hr). To the priming fluid of the cardiopulmonary bypass circuit (pump prime dose), add 2,000,000 KIU

(200 ml). *Low-dose regimen:* Test dose of 10,000 KIU (1 ml) given 10 min before initial dose. If test dose is tolerated, give 1,000,000 KIU (100 ml) over 20 to 30 min followed by maintenance dosage of 250,000 KIU/hr (25 ml/hr). Add pump prime dose of 1,000,000 KIU (100 ml) to priming fluid.

Incompatibilities

Don't administer aprotinin with corticosteroids, heparin, tetracyclines, or nutrient solutions that contain amino acids or fat emulsions. Don't administer I.V. aprotinin through same I.V. line as any other drug; use a different I.V. line or catheter.

Mechanism of Action

Reduces bleeding, possibly by affecting plasmin and kallikrein, which prevents fibrinolysis and may inhibit the early phase of the intrinsic clotting cascade. Aprotinin also increases the resistance of platelets to damage from elevated plasmin levels and mechanical injury during cardiopulmonary bypass surgery.

Contraindications

Hypersensitivity to aprotinin or other aprotinin-containing product within previous 12 months

Interactions

DRUGS

captopril: Reduced antihypertensive effect
fibrinolytics, such as anistreplase and streptokinase: Inhibited fibrinolysis
heparin: Prolonged activated clotting time

Adverse Reactions

CNS: Confusion, CVA, fever
CV: Arrhythmias, cardiac arrest, heart failure, hypertension, hypotension, increased CK level, MI, pericarditis, peripheral edema
ENDO: Hyperglycemia
GI: Diarrhea, elevated liver function test results, nausea, vomiting
GU: Renal failure, UTI
HEME: Leukocytosis, thrombocytopenia
RESP: Apnea, asthma, dyspnea, pleural effusion, pneumonia, pneumothorax
Other: Anaphylaxis, infection, sepsis, shock

Nursing Considerations

- Administer aprotinin cautiously to patient with multiple allergies or history of previous aprotinin treatments. Also use drug cautiously in patient undergoing deep hypothermic circulatory arrest, especially one over age 65.
- If aprotinin is cloudy or contains precipitate or particles, discard it and obtain a new vial.
- Use aprotinin immediately after opening vial. Discard unused portion.
- To reduce risk of anaphylaxis, expect to administer a H_1-receptor antagonist, such as diphenhydramine, shortly before giving a loading dose of aprotinin to patient who has received aprotinin previously.
- Give aprotinin through a central line and only in an operative setting.
- After anesthesia induction and before sternotomy, expect the initial aprotinin dose to be given with patient supine. Maintenance dosage is given by constant infusion until patient leaves operating room. Before cardiopulmonary bypass begins, the pump prime dose is added to priming fluid of cardiopulmonary bypass circuit by replacing an aliquot of priming fluid with aprotinin.
- If anaphylaxis occurs, discontinue aprotinin immediately and notify prescriber. Then administer oxygen and I.V. epinephrine, antihistamines, and corticosteroids, as prescribed, and maintain a patent airway.

PATIENT TEACHING

- Inform patient that he'll receive aprotinin during surgery and explain its purpose.

argatroban

Acova

Class and Category

Chemical: N2-substituted derivative of arginine
Therapeutic: Anticoagulant
Pregnancy category: B

Indications and Dosages

▶ *To prevent or treat thrombosis in patients with heparin-induced thrombocytopenia*

I.V. INFUSION

Adults. 2 mcg/kg/min as a continuous infusion. *Maximum:* 10 mcg/kg/min.

DOSAGE ADJUSTMENT Dosage adjusted as prescribed to maintain a therapeutic APTT of 1.5 to 3 times the initial baseline value, not to exceed 100 sec. Initial dosage reduced to 0.5 mcg/kg/min for patients with moderate hepatic impairment.

Route	Onset	Peak	Duration
I.V.	Immediate	3 to 4 hr	Unknown

Mechanism of Action

Forms a tight bond with thrombin, neutralizing this enzyme's actions, even when the enzyme is trapped within clots. Thrombin causes fibrinogen to convert to fibrin, which is essential for clot formation.

Incompatibilities

Don't mix argatroban with other drugs.

Contraindications

Active major bleeding, hypersensitivity to argatroban or its components

Interactions

DRUGS

alteplase, antineoplastic drugs, antiplatelets, antithymocyte globulin, heparin, NSAIDs, reteplase, salicylates, streptokinase, strontium chloride Sr 89, warfarin: Increased risk of bleeding

porfimer: Possibly decreased efficacy of porfimer photodynamic therapy

Adverse Reactions

CNS: Cerebrovascular bleeding, fever, headache

CV: Atrial fibrillation, cardiac arrest, hypotension, unstable angina, ventricular tachycardia

GI: Abdominal pain, anorexia, diarrhea, elevated liver function test results, GI bleeding, nausea, vomiting

GU: Elevated BUN and serum creatinine levels, hematuria (microscopic), UTI

HEME: Hypoprothrombinemia

RESP: Cough, dyspnea, hemoptysis, pneumonia

SKIN: Bleeding at puncture site, rash

Other: Sepsis

Nursing Considerations

- Using normal saline solution, D_5W, or lactated Ringer's solution, dilute argatroban to 1 mg/ml before administration.
- Use diluted solution within 24 hours if it has been stored at 15° to 30° C (59° to 86° F), protected from direct sunlight, and kept in ambient indoor light. Use solution within 48 hours if it has been stored between 2° and 8° C (36° and 46° F) and kept in the dark.
- **WARNING** Monitor patients with thrombocytopenia or those receiving daily doses of salicylates greater than 6 g for signs and symptoms of bleeding because they're at increased risk of bleeding from hypoprothrombinemia.
- **WARNING** Expect to perform blood coagulation tests before and 2 hours after start of therapy because of the major risk of bleeding associated with argatroban. Be aware that coagulopathy must be ruled out before therapy starts.
- Monitor the following patients for evidence of bleeding because they're at increased risk during argatroban therapy: actively menstruating females; patients with known vascular or organ abnormalities, such as severe uncontrolled hypertension, advanced renal disease, infective endocarditis, dissecting aortic aneurysm, diverticulitis, hemophilia, hepatic disease (especially if associated with a deficiency of vitamin K–dependent clotting factors), inflammatory bowel disease, or peptic ulcer disease; and those who have recently had a CVA, major surgery (including eye, brain, or spinal cord surgery), large vessel puncture or organ biopsy, lumbar puncture, spinal anesthesia, or major bleeding (including intracranial, GI, intraocular, retroperitoneal, or pulmonary bleeding).
- Whenever possible, avoid I.M. injections in patients receiving argatroban to decrease the risk of bleeding.
- Be aware that thrombin times may not be helpful for monitoring argatroban activity because all thrombin-dependent coagulation tests are affected by the drug.
- Monitor APTT periodically, as ordered, during treatment to verify therapeutic drug levels.
- Expect drug dosage to be tapered before discontinuation to prevent the risk of rebound hypercoagulopathy; drug's effects last for only a short time once drug is discontinued.
- Store unopened vials between 15° and 30° C (59° and 86° F); protect from freezing and light.

PATIENT TEACHING
- Explain to patient receiving argatroban that heparin-induced thrombocytopenia is an antigen-antibody immunologic response that isn't related to dosage of heparin he may have received.
- Inform patient that argatroban is a blood thinner that is administered in the hospital by infusion into a vein. Explain that he'll be switched to another drug before discharge if he requires long-term anticoagulation.
- Advise patient to immediately report unusual or unexplained bleeding, such as blood in urine, easy bruising, nosebleeds, tarry stools, and vaginal bleeding.
- Instruct patient to be careful to avoid injury while receiving argatroban. For example, suggest that he brush his teeth gently, using a soft-bristled toothbrush, and take special care when flossing.
- Inform patient that the risk of bleeding associated with argatroban lasts for only a short time once drug is discontinued.

atenolol

Apo-Atenol (CAN), Novo-Atenol (CAN), Tenormin

Class and Category

Chemical: Beta-adrenergic blocker ($beta_1$ and at high doses $beta_2$)
Therapeutic: Antianginal, antihypertensive
Pregnancy category: D

Indications and Dosages

▶ *To treat acute MI*

I.V. INFUSION, TABLETS

Adults. *Initial:* 5 mg I.V. slowly over 5 min, followed by another 5 mg I.V. 10 min later. After an additional 10 min (if tolerated), 50 mg P.O., followed by another 50 mg P.O. 12 hr later. *Maintenance:* 50 mg P.O. b.i.d. or 100 mg P.O. daily for 6 to 9 days or until discharge from hospital.

DOSAGE ADJUSTMENT Dosage reduced to 50 mg daily P.O. for patients with creatinine clearance of of 15 to 35 ml/min/1.73 m^2 and to 25 mg daily for patients with creatinine clearance of less than 15 ml/min/1.73 m^2.

Route	Onset	Peak	Duration
I.V.	Immediate	5 min	12 hr
P.O.	1 hr	2 to 4 hr	24 hr

Mechanism of Action

Inhibits stimulation of $beta_1$-receptor sites, located primarily in the heart, causing a decrease in cardiac excitability, cardiac output, and myocardial oxygen demand. At high doses, atenolol inhibits stimulation of $beta_2$ receptors in the lungs, which may cause bronchoconstriction.

Contraindications

Cardiogenic shock, heart block greater than first degree, hypersensitivity to beta blockers, overt heart failure, sinus bradycardia

Interactions

DRUGS

calcium channel blockers (such as verapamil and diltiazem): Possibly symptomatic bradycardia and conduction abnormalities
catecholamine-depleting drugs (such as reserpine): Additive antihypertensive effect
clonidine: Rebound hypertension

Adverse Reactions

CNS: Depression, disorientation, dizziness, drowsiness, emotional lability, fatigue, fever, lethargy, light-headedness, short-term memory loss, vertigo
CV: Arrhythmias, including bradycardia and heart block; cardiogenic shock; cold arms and legs; heart failure; mesenteric artery thrombosis; mitral insufficiency; myocardial reinfarction; orthostatic hypotension; Raynaud's phenomenon
EENT: Dry eyes, laryngospasm, pharyngitis
GI: Diarrhea, ischemic colitis, nausea
GU: Renal failure
HEME: Agranulocytosis
MS: Leg pain
RESP: Bronchospasm, dyspnea, pulmonary emboli, respiratory distress, wheezing
SKIN: Erythematous rash
Other: Allergic reaction

Nursing Considerations

- Be aware that although its exact mechanism of action is unknown, atenolol improves survival rate in patients with a known or suspected acute MI.
- Dilute atenolol with dextrose, sodium chloride, or dextrose and sodium chloride solution.

- Inspect solution for particles or discoloration before administration.
- During I.V. atenolol therapy, monitor vital signs and cardiac rhythm closely.
- Expect to administer digoxin, a diuretic, or both at first sign of heart failure, and monitor patient closely. If heart failure continues, expect to discontinue atenolol.
- Closely monitor patient with hyperthyroidism because atenolol may mask some signs of thyrotoxicosis. Avoid abrupt withdrawal of atenolol, which may precipitate thyrotoxicosis.
- Assess diabetic patients for signs of hypoglycemia other than tachycardia (such as dizziness and sweating) because atenolol may mask tachycardia caused by hypoglycemia. Unlike other beta-adrenergic blockers, atenolol doesn't mask other signs of hypoglycemia, cause hypoglycemia, or delay the return of blood glucose to a normal level.
- Monitor patients with heart failure controlled by digitalis glycosides or diuretics for exacerbation of heart failure.
- Monitor for adverse effects, such as symptomatic bradycardia or hypotension, in patients with conduction abnormalities or left ventricular dysfunction who are receiving verapamil or diltiazem.
- Monitor for signs of reduced peripheral circulation, such as cold hands and feet, in patients with Raynaud's syndrome or other peripheral vascular disease.
- Because atenolol is excreted by the kidneys, monitor patients with impaired renal function for increased atenolol effects.
- Discard atenolol solution if it isn't used within 48 hours.
- Stop atenolol therapy and notify prescriber if patient develops bradycardia, hypotension, or another serious adverse reaction.
- If patient also receives clonidine, expect to discontinue atenolol several days before gradually withdrawing clonidine. Then expect to restart atenolol therapy several days after clonidine has been discontinued.
- Store drug between 20° and 25° C (68° and 77° F); protect from freezing and light.

PATIENT TEACHING

- Instruct patient not to stop taking atenolol abruptly because angina could worsen and an MI or arrhythmia might occur.
- While patient is being weaned from atenolol, tell him to perform minimal physical activity to prevent chest pain.
- Inform patient that atenolol may alter his blood glucose level and mask symptoms of hypoglycemia.

- Advise patient to report signs of an adverse reaction, such as difficulty breathing, shortness of breath, dizziness, or a rash.

atracurium besylate

Tracrium

Class and Category

Chemical: Biquaternary ammonium ester
Therapeutic: Skeletal muscle relaxant
Pregnancy category: C

Indications and Dosages

▶ *To facilitate endotracheal intubation and induce skeletal muscle relaxation for surgery or mechanical ventilation as adjunct to anesthesia*

I.V. INFUSION OR INJECTION

Adults and children age 2 and over. *Initial:* 0.4 to 0.5 mg/kg by I.V. bolus for nearly complete neuromuscular blockade. *Maintenance:* 0.08 to 0.10 mg/kg 20 to 45 min after initial dose during prolonged surgery. Maintenance doses may be given q 15 to 25 min for patients under balanced anesthesia. For patients undergoing extended surgical procedures, an infusion of 9 to 10 mcg/kg/min may be required after an initial I.V. bolus to counteract the spontaneous return of neuromuscular function, and thereafter 5 to 10 mcg/kg/min is given as a constant infusion.

Children ages 1 month to 2 years receiving halothane anesthesia. *Initial:* 0.3 to 0.4 mg/kg. Frequent maintenance doses may be required.

Route	Onset	Peak	Duration
I.V.	2 to 2.5 min	3 to 5 min	35 to 70 min

Mechanism of Action

Inhibits nerve impulse transmission by competing with acetylcholine for cholinergic receptors on motor end plate.

Incompatibilities

Don't mix atracurium in same syringe or administer it through same I.V. needle as an alkaline solution, such as a barbiturate injection. Don't mix atracurium with lactated Ringer's injection.

Contraindications

Hypersensitivity to atracurium, its components, or benzyl alcohol

Interactions

DRUGS

aminoglycosides, enflurane, furosemide, halothane, isoflurane, lithium, magnesium salts, polymyxin antibiotics, procainamide, quinidine, thiazide diuretics: Possibly enhanced or prolonged atracurium effects

opioid analgesics: Possibly additive histamine release and increased risk and severity of bradycardia and hypotension

Adverse Reactions

CNS: Seizures

CV: Bradycardia, hypertension, hypotension, tachycardia

MS: Inadequate or prolonged neuromuscular blockade

RESP: Apnea, bronchospasm, dyspnea, laryngospasm, wheezing

SKIN: Flushing, rash, urticaria

Other: Anaphylaxis, injection site reaction

Nursing Considerations

- Anticipate using lower doses of atracurium for patients with neuromuscular disease, severe electrolyte disorders, or carcinomatosis because of the risk of enhanced neuromuscular blockade and difficulties with reversal. Lower doses may also be used for patients at risk for adverse reactions related to histamine release.
- Keep atropine nearby to treat atracurium-induced bradycardia.
- For I.V. infusion, dilute atracurium with normnal saline solution, D_5W, or D_5 in normal saline solution. To prepare a solution that yields 200 mcg of atracurium/ml, add 2 ml of atracurium to 98 ml of diluent. To prepare a solution that yields 500 mcg/ml, add 5 ml of atracurium to 95 ml of diluent.
- Store prepared solution in refrigerator or at room temperature for up to 24 hours. Discard unused portion after 24 hours.
- Closely monitor blood pressure of patients with hypotension.
- Monitor patient closely for adverse reactions, especially those associated with histamine release. Be aware that atracurium is more likely than other neuromuscular blockers to cause flushing.
- Before use, store undiluted atracurium at 2° to 8° C (36° to 46° F); don't freeze. Use drug within 14 days if stored at room temperature, even if it's refrigerated later.

PATIENT TEACHING

- Explain purpose of atracurium treatment to patient.

atropine

AtroPen

atropine sulfate

Class and Category

Chemical: Belladonna alkaloid
Therapeutic: Anticholinergic, antimuscarinic
Pregnancy category: C

Indications and Dosages

▶ *To reduce respiratory tract secretions related to anesthesia*

I.V. INJECTION

Adults. 0.4 to 0.6 mg preoperatively.

Children. 0.01 mg/kg up to total of 0.4 mg preoperatively and repeated q 4 to 6 hr, p.r.n.

▶ *To correct bradycardia*

I.V. INJECTION

Adults. 0.4 to 1 mg. If no response to first dose, repeat once after 5 min.

Children. 0.01 to 0.02 mg/kg with a minimum dose of 0.1 mg and a maximum dose of 0.5 mg. If no response to first dose, repeat once after 5 min.

▶ *To treat cholinesterase inhibitor (such as neostigmine, pilocarpine, and methacholine) toxicity*

I.V. INJECTION

Adults. 2 to 4 mg. Then 2 mg q 5 to 10 min until muscarinic signs (bradycardia, vasodilation, and pupil dilation) disappear or signs of atropine intoxication develop.

I.V. INJECTION

Children. 1 mg. Then 0.5 to 1 mg q 5 to 10 min until muscarinic signs disappear or signs of atropine intoxication develop.

▶ *To treat mushroom (muscarine) toxicity*

I.V. INJECTION

Adults. 1 to 2 mg q hr until respiratory signs and symptoms subside.

▶ *To treat pesticide (organophosphate) toxicity*

I.V. INJECTION

Adults. 1 to 2 mg, repeated in 20 to 30 min as soon as cyanosis has cleared. Then dosage continued until definite improvement is maintained, possibly for 2 or more days.

Route	Onset	Peak	Duration
I.V.	Immediate	2 to 4 min	Brief

Mechanism of Action

Inhibits acetylcholine's muscarinic action at the neuroeffector junctions of smooth muscles, cardiac muscles, exocrine glands, SA and AV nodes, and the urinary bladder. In small doses, atropine inhibits salivary and bronchial secretions and diaphoresis. In moderate doses, it increases impulse conduction through the AV node and increases heart rate. In large doses, it decreases GI and urinary tract motility and gastric acid secretion.

Contraindications

Angle-closure glaucoma, asthma, GI obstructive disease (achalasia, pyloric obstruction, pyloroduodenal stenosis), hepatic disease, hypersensitivity to atropine or its components, ileus, intestinal atony, myasthenia gravis, myocardial ischemia, obstructive uropathy, renal disease, severe ulcerative colitis, tachycardia, toxic megacolon, unstable cardiovascular status in acute hemorrhage

Interactions

DRUGS

adsorbent antidiarrheals, antacids: Decreased atropine absorption
amantadine, anticholinergics, antidyskinetics, glutethimide, meperidine, muscle relaxants, phenothiazines, tricyclic antidepressants and other drugs with anticholinergic properties, including antiarrhythmics (disopyramide, procainamide, quinidine), antihistamines, buclizine, meclizine: Increased atropine effects
antimyasthenics: Reduced intestinal motility
cyclopropane: Risk of ventricular arrhythmias
haloperidol: Decreased antipsychotic effect
ketoconazole: Decreased ketoconazole absorption
metoclopramide: Decreased effect on GI motility
opioid analgesics: Increased risk of ileus, severe constipation, and urine retention
potassium chloride, especially wax-matrix forms: Possibly GI ulcers
urinary alkalizers (calcium or magnesium antacids, carbonic anhydrase inhibitors, citrates, sodium bicarbonate): Delayed excretion and increased risk of adverse atropine effects

Adverse Reactions

CNS: Agitation, amnesia, anxiety, ataxia, Babinski's or Chaddock's reflex, behavioral changes, CNS stimulation (with high doses), coma, confusion, decreased concentration, decreased tendon reflexes, delirium, dizziness, drowsiness, fever, hallucinations,

headache, hyperreflexia, insomnia, lethargy, mania, mental disorders, nervousness, paranoia, restlessness, seizures, somnolence, stupor, syncope, vertigo, weakness
CV: Arrhythmias, bradycardia (with low doses), cardiac dilation, chest pain, hypertension, hypotension, left ventricular failure, MI, palpitations, tachycardia (with high doses), weak or impalpable peripheral pulses
EENT: Acute angle-closure glaucoma, altered taste, blepharitis, blindness, blurred vision, conjunctivitis, cyclophoria, cycloplegia, decreased visual acuity or accommodation, dry eyes or conjunctiva, dry mucous membranes, dry mouth, eye irritation, eyelid crusting, heterophoria, increased intraocular pressure, keratoconjunctivitis, lacrimation, laryngitis, laryngospasm, mydriasis, nasal congestion, oral lesions, photophobia, pupils poorly reactive to light, strabismus, tongue chewing
GI: Abdominal distention, abdominal pain, bloating, constipation, decreased bowel sounds or food absorption, delayed gastric emptying, dysphagia, heartburn, ileus, nausea, vomiting
GU: Bladder distention, enuresis, impotence, urinary hesitancy, urinary urgency, urine retention
MS: Dysarthria, hypertonia, muscle twitching
RESP: Bradypnea, dyspnea, inspiratory stridor, pulmonary edema, respiratory failure, shallow breathing, subcostal recession, tachypnea
SKIN: Cold skin, cyanosis, decreased sweating, dermatitis, flushing, rash, urticaria
Other: Anaphylaxis, dehydration, injection site reaction, polydipsia, sensations of warmth

Nursing Considerations

- Avoid using high-dose atropine sulfate therapy in patients with ulcerative colitis because of risk of toxic megacolon or in patients with hiatal hernia and reflux esophagitis because of risk of esophagitis
- **WARNING** Assess for symptoms of toxic doses of atropine, such as excitement, agitation, drowsiness, and confusion, which are likely to affect elderly patients even with low doses. If these symptoms occur, take safety precautions to prevent patient injury.
- Assess bowel and bladder elimination. Notify prescriber if diarrhea, constipation, urinary hesitancy, or urine retention develop.

PATIENT TEACHING

- Advise patient to notify prescriber if he has persistent or severe diarrhea, constipation, or difficulty urinating.

azathioprine sodium

Imuran

azathioprine

Imuran

Class and Category

Chemical: Purine analogue
Therapeutic: Antimetabolite, immunosuppressant
Pregnancy category: D

Indications and Dosages

▶ *To prevent kidney transplant rejection*

I.V. INFUSION, TABLETS

Adults and children. *Initial:* 3 to 5 mg/kg daily I.V. or P.O. as a single dose on or 1 to 3 days before day of transplant, followed by 3 to 5 mg/kg daily I.V. after surgery until P.O. dose is tolerated. *Maintenance:* 1 to 3 mg/kg daily P.O.

DOSAGE ADJUSTMENT Dosage reduced for patients with oliguria (such as from tubular necrosis) after transplantation because their drug or metabolite excretion may be delayed.

Route	Onset	Peak	Duration
I.V., P.O.	4 to 8 wk	Unknown	Several days

Mechanism of Action

May prevent proliferation and differentiation of activated B and T cells by interfering with purine (protein) and nucleic acid (DNA and RNA) synthesis.

Contraindications

Hypersensitivity to azathioprine

Interactions

DRUGS

ACE inhibitors, drugs that affect bone marrow and cell development in bone marrow (such as co-trimoxazole): Possibly severe leukopenia
allopurinol: Possibly increased therapeutic and adverse effects of azathioprine

anticoagulants: Possibly decreased anticoagulant action
cyclosporine: Possibly decreased blood cyclosporine level
methotrexate: Possibly increased blood level of azathioprine metabolite 6-mercaptopurine, which can lead to cell death
neuromuscular blockers: Possibly decreased or reversed action of neuromuscular blocker

Adverse Reactions

CNS: Fever, malaise
GI: Abdominal pain, diarrhea, hepatotoxicity (elevated liver function test results), nausea, pancreatitis, steatorrhea, vomiting
HEME: Leukopenia, macrocytic anemia, pancytopenia, thrombocytopenia
MS: Arthralgia, myalgia
SKIN: Alopecia, rash
Other: Infection, lymphomas and other neoplasms

Nursing Considerations

- Before I.V. administration, add 20 ml of sterile water for injection to azathioprine vial and swirl it until clear solution forms. The resulting drug concentration is 100 mg and can be diluted further, usually in normal saline solutin or D_5W, as prescribed. Calculate infusion rate based on final volume to be infused. Then administer over 30 to 60 minutes or as prescribed (from 5 minutes to 8 hours).
- Obtain results of baseline laboratory tests, including WBC, RBC, and platelet counts. Then expect to monitor results once a week during first month of therapy, twice a month during second and third months of therapy, and once a month or more frequently thereafter.
- Be aware that hematologic reactions typically are dose-related and may occur late in therapy, especially in patients with transplant rejection.
- **WARNING** If WBC count decreases rapidly or remains significantly and consistently low, expect to reduce dosage or discontinue use of azathioprine.
- Periodically monitor liver function test results to detect early signs of hepatotoxicity.
- If patient develops thrombocytopenia, take bleeding precautions, such as avoiding I.M. injections and venipunctures, applying ice to areas of trauma, and checking I.V. infusion sites every 2 hours for bleeding.
- If patient also receives an oral anticoagulant, monitor his PT.

- Know that azathioprine therapy increases the risk of viral, fungal, bacterial, and protozoal infections. Monitor for signs of infection, such as fever, chills, sore throat, and mouth sores. Expect to administer aggressive antibiotic, antiviral, or other drug therapy and to reduce azathioprine dosage.
- Minimize risk of infection. If patient has severe leukopenia, take neutropenic precautions, such as placing him in a private room, limiting visitors, and screening visitors for communicable illnesses.
- If oral azathioprine causes GI upset, administer it in divided doses or with meals.
- Store parenteral form and tablets at 15° to 25° C (59° to 77° F). Keep in a dry place and protect from light.

PATIENT TEACHING

- Advise patient to take oral azathioprine with food or meals to minimize GI upset.
- **WARNING** Teach patient to recognize and report signs of infection, such as sore throat and fever.
- Teach patient how to reduce the risk of bleeding and how to maintain safety so that he doesn't fall.

azithromycin

Zithromax

Class and Category

Chemical: Azalide (subclass of macrolide)
Therapeutic: Antibiotic
Pregnancy category: B

Indications and Dosages

▶ *To treat community-acquired pneumonia*

I.V. INFUSION

Adults and adolescents age 16 or over. 500 mg I.V. as a single dose daily for at least 2 days, followed by 500 mg P.O. as a single dose daily until patient completes 7 to 10 days of therapy.

▶ *To prevent* Mycobacterium avium *complex in patients with advanced HIV infection*

I.V. INFUSION

Adults. 1.2 g once weekly, as indicated.

▶ *To treat pelvic inflammatory disease*

I.V. INFUSION

Adults. 500 mg I.V. as a single dose daily for 1 to 2 days, followed by 250 mg P.O. as a single dose daily until patient completes 7 days of therapy.

Mechanism of Action

Binds to a ribosomal subunit of susceptible bacteria, blocking peptide translocation and inhibiting RNA-dependent protein synthesis. Drug concentrates in phagocytes, macrophages, and fibroblasts, which release it slowly and may help move it to infection sites.

Incompatibilities

Don't add I.V. substances, additives, or drugs to azithromycin I.V. solution, and don't infuse them through the same I.V. line as azithromycin.

Contraindications

Hypersensitivity to azithromycin, erythromycin, or other macrolide antibiotics

Interactions

DRUGS

antacids that contain aluminum or magnesium: Possibly decreased peak blood azithromycin level, but extent of absorption is unchanged
carbamazepine, cyclosporine, phenytoin, terfenadine (drugs metabolized by cytochrome P-450 system): Possibly increased blood levels of these drugs
digoxin: Possibly increased blood digoxin level
dihydroergotamine, ergotamine: Possibly severe peripheral vasospasm and abnormal sensations (acute ergot toxicity)
HMG-CoA reductase inhibitors: Increased risk of severe myopathy or rhabdomyolysis
pimozide: Possibly sudden death
theophylline: Possibly increased blood theophylline level
triazolam: Possibly decreased excretion and increased therapeutic effects of triazolam
warfarin: Possibly increased anticoagulation

FOODS

food: Dramatically increased absorption rate of azithromycin

Adverse Reactions

CNS: Dizziness, fatigue, headache, somnolence, vertigo

CV: Chest pain, elevated serum CK level, palpitations, prolonged QT interval, torsades de pointes
EENT: Hearing loss, mucocutaneous candidiasis, tinnitus
ENDO: Hyperglycemia
GI: Abdominal pain, diarrhea, elevated liver function test results, nausea, pseudomembranous colitis, vomiting
GU: Elevated BUN and serum creatinine levels, nephritis, vaginal candidiasis
HEME: Leukopenia, neutropenia, thrombocytopenia
SKIN: Jaundice, photosensitivity, rash, Stevens-Johnson syndrome, toxic epidermal necrolysis, urticaria
Other: Allergic reaction, angioedema, elevated serum phosphorus level, hyperkalemia, infusion site reaction (such as pain and redness), superinfection

Nursing Considerations

- Obtain culture and sensitivity test results, if possible, before starting therapy.
- Use drug cautiously in patients with hepatic dysfunction (because drug is metabolize in the liver) or renal dysfunction (because effects are unknown in this group).
- **WARNING** Don't give azithromycin by I.V. bolus because it may cause erythema, pain, swelling, tenderness, or other reaction at the site. Infuse it over 60 minutes or longer, as prescribed (typically 1 mg/ml over 3 hours or 2 mg/ml over 1 hour.)
- If hepatic function is impaired, monitor liver function studies because azithromycin is eliminated mainly by the liver.
- Assess patient for bacterial or fungal superinfection, which may occur with prolonged or repeated therapy. If it occurs, expect to give another antibiotic or antifungal.
- Monitor bowel elimination; if needed, obtain stool culture to rule out pseudomembranous colitis. If it occurs, expect to stop azithromycin and give fluid, electrolytes, and antibiotics effective against *Clostridium difficile.*

PATIENT TEACHING

- Tell patient to immediately report evidence of allergic reactions, such as rash, itching, hives, chest tightness, and trouble breathing.
- Warn patient that abdominal pain and loose, watery stools may occur. If diarrhea persists or becomes severe, urge him to contact prescriber and replace fluids.

- Because azithromycin may destroy normal flora, teach patient to watch for and immediately report signs of superinfection, such as white patches in the mouth.

aztreonam

Azactam

Class and Category

Chemical: Monobactam
Therapeutic: Antibiotic
Pregnancy category: B

Indications and Dosages

▶ *To treat infections of the urinary tract, lower respiratory tract, skin, soft tissue, female reproductive tract; intra-abdominal infections; septicemia; and surgical abscesses caused by susceptible strains of gram-negative bacteria*

I.V. INFUSION, I.V. INJECTION

Adults. 0.5 to 2 g q 8 to 12 hr up to a maximum of 8 g daily. For life-threatening systemic infection, 2 g q 6 to 8 hr up to a maximum of 8 g daily.

Children ages 9 months to 16 years. 30 mg/kg q 6 to 8 hr up to 120 mg/kg daily; 50 mg/kg q 4 to 6 hr (for *Pseudomonas aeruginosa*).

DOSAGE ADJUSTMENT If creatinine clearance is 10 to 30 ml/min/1.73 m^2, initial dose is 1 to 2 g; then 50% of usual dose at usual interval. If creatinine clearance less than 10 ml/min/1.73 m^2, initial dose is 500 mg to 2 g; then 25% of the usual dose q 6, 8, or 12 hr.

Route	Onset	Peak	Duration
I.V. infusion, injection	Immediate	Immediate	Unknown

Mechanism of Action

Inhibits bacterial cell wall synthesis in susceptible aerobic gram-negative bacteria. These bacteria assemble rigid, cross-linked cell walls in several steps. Aztreonam affects the final cross-linking stage by inactivating penicillin-binding protein 3 (the enzyme that links cell wall strands), which causes cell lysis and death.

Incompatibilities

Don't mix aztreonam in same I.V. solution as cephradine, metronidazole, or nafcillin sodium. Don't mix it in same I.M. injection solution as local anesthetic.

Contraindications

Hypersensitivity to aztreonam or its components

Interactions

DRUGS

aminoglycosides (prolonged or high-dose therapy): Increased risk of nephrotoxicity and ototoxicity
cefoxitin, imipenem: Possibly antagonized action of aztreonam
furosemide, probenecid: Possibly increased blood aztreonam level

Adverse Reactions

CNS: Confusion, dizziness, fever, headache, insomnia, malaise, paresthesia, seizures, vertigo
CV: Chest pain, hypotension, transient ECG changes
EENT: Altered taste, diplopia, halitosis, mouth ulcers, mucocutaneous candidiasis, nasal congestion, sneezing, tinnitus, tongue numbness
GI: Abdominal cramps, diarrhea, elevated liver function test results, GI bleeding, hepatitis, nausea, pseudomembranous colitis, vomiting
GU: Breast tenderness, elevated serum creatinine level, vaginal candidiasis
HEME: Anemia, eosinophilia, leukocytosis, neutropenia, pancytopenia, positive Coombs' test, prolonged PT and APTT, thrombocytopenia, thrombocytosis
MS: Myalgia
RESP: Bronchospasm, dyspnea, wheezing
SKIN: Diaphoresis, erythema multiforme, exfoliative dermatitis, flushing, jaundice, petechiae, pruritus, purpura, rash, toxic epidermal necrolysis, urticaria
Other: Allergic reaction; injection site pain, phlebitis, swelling, or thrombophlebitis

Nursing Considerations

- Obtain culture and sensitivity test results, if possible, before initiating therapy. If patient is acutely ill, expect to begin therapy before results are available.
- Keep in mind that other antimicrobials may be used with aztreonam in seriously ill patients at risk for gram-positive infection.

- Expect to use I.V. route for patients who need single doses over 1 g and those with life-threatening systemic infections, such as septicemia or peritonitis.
- To reconstitute aztreonam for I.V. bolus injection, use sterile water for injection.
- Immediately after adding diluent to vial, shake it vigorously to mix. After obtaining correct dose, discard unused solution.
- Be aware that reconstituted solution may turn light pink on standing at room temperature. This doesn't affect drug potency.
- Administer I.V. bolus injection directly into I.V. tubing over 3 to 5 minutes.
- **WARNING** When preparing aztreonam for I.V. infusion, use at least 50 ml of appropriate infusion solution per gram of aztreonam. Further dilute drug in I.V. solution, such as normal saline, D_5W, D_5/normal saline, lactated Ringer's, or Ringer's solution.
- Know that I.V. infusion may be administered over 20 to 60 minutes.
- Flush I.V. tubing with solution, such as normal saline solution, before and after administering I.V. infusion to reduce risk of incompatibilities.
- If prescribed, mix aztreonam in same I.V. solution with other antibiotics (such as ampicillin sodium, cefazolin sodium, clindamycin phosphate, gentamicin sulfate, or tobramycin sulfate), or mix it with cloxacillin sodium and vancomycin hydrochloride in peritoneal dialysis solution.
- Prepare solution for I.M. injection using sterile or bacteriostatic water or sodium chloride for injection. Administer injection deep into large muscle, such as in dorsogluteal or ventrogluteal area.
- Assess for signs of bacterial or fungal superinfection, which may occur with prolonged or repeated therapy. If superinfection occurs, treat it as prescribed.
- Monitor bowel elimination; if needed, obtain stool culture to rule out pseudomembranous colitis. If this adverse reaction occurs, expect to discontinue aztreonam and administer fluid, electrolytes, and antibiotics that are effective against Clostridium difficile.
- Evaluate patient's renal and liver function test results, as ordered, if the patient has renal or hepatic impairment.
- Monitor renal function if patient is receiving an aminoglycoside because of the increased risk of nephrotoxicity.

PATIENT TEACHING

- Stress the importance of taking the full course of aztreonam exactly as prescribed, even if the patient feels better before finishing it.
- Teach patient to recognize and immediately report signs and symptoms of allergic reactions, such as chest tightness, difficulty breathing, hives, itching, and rash.
- Warn patient that abdominal pain and loose, watery stools may occur. If diarrhea persists or becomes severe, urge him to contact prescriber and replace fluids.
- Because aztreonam may destroy normal flora, teach patient to watch for and immediately report signs of superinfection, such as white patches in mouth.

B

basiliximab

Simulect

Class and Category

Chemical: Chimeric (murine or human) monoclonal antibody
Therapeutic: Immunosuppressant
Pregnancy category: B

Indications and Dosages

▶ *To prevent acute kidney transplant rejection*

I.V. INFUSION, I.V. INJECTION

Adults and adolescents over age 15. 20 mg within 2 hr before transplant, then 20 mg 4 days after transplant.
Children and adolescents ages 2 to 15. 12 mg/m^2 within 2 hr before transplant, then 12 mg/m^2 4 days after transplant. *Maximum:* 20 mg/dose.

Route	Onset	Peak	Duration
I.V.	Unknown	Unknown	22 to 50 days

Mechanism of Action

Initiates immunosuppression by blocking interleukin-2 receptors located on the surface of activated T cells. Normally, interleukin-2 is released by stimulated T lymphocytes, causing activation and differentiation of other T lymphocytes responsible for cell-mediated immunity.

Incompatibilities

Don't add or infuse any other drugs simultaneously through same I.V. line as basiliximab.

Contraindications

Hypersensitivity to basiliximab or its components

Interactions

None known.

Adverse Reactions

CNS: Asthenia, dizziness, fever, headache, insomnia, tremor
CV: Hypertension, peripheral edema
EENT: Oral candidiasis, pharyngitis, rhinitis
ENDO: Hyperglycemia
GI: Abdominal pain, constipation, diarrhea, indigestion, nausea, vomiting
GU: Dysuria, increased urinary nitrogen level, UTI
HEME: Anemia
MS: Back pain, leg pain
RESP: Cough, dyspnea, upper respiratory tract infection
SKIN: Acne
Other: Hypercholesterolemia, hyperkalemia, hyperuricemia, hypocalcemia, hypokalemia, hypophosphatemia, impaired wound healing, metabolic acidosis, weight gain

Nursing Considerations

- To reconstitute basiliximab, add 5 ml of sterile water for injection to powder and shake vial gently to dissolve. Further dilute with normal saline or D_5W for infusion to a volume of 50 ml. Gently invert infusion bag to avoid foaming; don't shake. Drug should appear clear to opalescent and colorless. Don't use if you detect particles.
- Administer reconstituted drug as a bolus dose directly through a central or peripheral I.V. line, or give the diluted solution I.V. over 20 to 30 minutes. Be aware that bolus dose may cause nausea, vomiting, and a localized injection site reaction, including pain.
- Monitor blood pressure, heart rate, and respiratory status during drug administration and for a brief period thereafter.
- Expect drug to be given as adjunct to cyclosporine and corticosteroids.
- Don't store reconstituted basiliximab at room temperature for longer than 4 hours; don't refrigerate it for longer than 24 hours.
- **WARNING** Be aware that patient may develop hypersensitivity reactions, including anaphylaxis, bronchospasm, dyspnea, hypotension, pruritus, rash, respiratory failure, sneezing, tachycardia, urticaria, and wheezing, on initial exposure or following re-exposure after several months. Notify prescriber immediately if such reactions occur.
- Store unreconstituted drug at 2° to 8° C (36° to 46° F).

PATIENT TEACHING
- Inform patient that second dose of basiliximab will be given 4 days after transplant and that she may also receive cyclosporine and corticosteroid therapy.
- Inform patient that because of drug's immunosuppressant effects, she may experience slower wound healing and be more susceptible to upper respiratory tract infections.

benzquinamide hydrochloride

Emete-Con

Class and Category

Chemical: Benzoquinolizine amide
Therapeutic: Antiemetic
Pregnancy category: Not rated

Indications and Dosages

▶ *To treat nausea and vomiting related to anesthesia or surgery*

I.V. OR I.M. INJECTION

Adults. 25 mg or 0.2 to 0.4 mg/kg by slow infusion (1 ml q 0.5 to 1 min) as a single dose, followed by I.M. doses. Or 50 mg or 0.5 to 1 mg/kg I.M., repeated in 1 hr; then q 3 to 4 hr, p.r.n.

Route	Onset	Peak	Duration
I.V.	15 min	Unknown	Unknown

Mechanism of Action

Exhibits antiemetic, antihistaminic, mild cholinergic, and sedative effects by unknown mechanism.

Contraindications

Hypersensitivity to benzquinamide or its components

Interactions

DRUGS

vasopressors: Increased hypertensive effects

Adverse Reactions

CNS: Chills, dizziness, drowsiness, excitement, fatigue, fever, headache, insomnia, nervousness, restlessness, tremor, weakness
CV: Atrial fibrillation, hypertension, hypotension, premature atrial or ventricular contractions

EENT: Blurred vision, dry mouth, increased salivation
GI: Anorexia, hiccups, nausea
MS: Muscle twitching
SKIN: Diaphoresis, flushing, rash, urticaria

Nursing Considerations

- **WARNING** Avoid I.V. route when administering benzquinamide to patients with cardiovascular disease because sudden blood pressure increases and transient arrhythmias may occur. Use I.V. route only for patients without cardiovascular disease who aren't receiving a preanesthetic or cardiovascular drug.
- Reconstitute drug with 2.2 ml of sterile water or bacteriostatic water for injection containing benzyl alcohol or methylparaben and propylparaben to yield 2 ml of a 25-mg/ml solution.
- Take safety precautions to reduce the risk of injury from CNS depression.
- Store reconstituted drug at room temperature. Solution retains potency for 14 days.

PATIENT TEACHING

- Advise patient to stay in bed after receiving benzquinamide and to call for assistance to reduce the risk of injury.
- Instruct patient to report whether nausea and vomiting have been relieved.

benztropine mesylate

Apo-Benztropine (CAN), Cogentin, PMS Benztropine (CAN)

Class and Category

Chemical: Tertiary amine
Therapeutic: Antidyskinetic, central-acting anticholinergic
Pregnancy category: C

Indications and Dosages

▶ *As adjunct to treat all forms of Parkinson's disease*

I.V. INJECTION, TABLETS

Adults with Parkinson's disease. 1 to 2 mg daily (usual dose) with a range of 0.5 to 6 mg daily.
Adults with idiopathic Parkinson's disease. *Initial:* 0.5 to 1 mg at bedtime. *Maximum:* 4 to 6 mg daily.
Adults with postencephalitic Parkinson's disease. 2 mg daily in one or more doses; may begin with 0.5 mg at bedtime and increase as needed.

▶ *To control extrapyramidal symptoms (except tardive dyskinesia) caused*

by phenothiazines and other neuroleptic drugs
I.V. OR I.M. INJECTION
Adults. 1 to 4 mg once or twice daily.
▶ *To treat acute dystonic reactions*
I.V. OR I.M. INJECTION
Adults. *Initial:* 1 to 2 ml (1 to 2 mg total dose) I.V. or I.M. *Maintenance:* 1 to 2 mg P.O. b.i.d. to prevent recurrence.

Route	Onset	Peak	Duration
I.V., I.M	15 min	Unknown	24 hr
P.O.	1 to 2 hr	Unknown	24 hr

Mechanism of Action
Blocks acetylcholine's action at cholinergic receptor sites. This restores the brain's normal dopamine and acetylcholine balance, which relaxes muscle movement and decreases drooling, rigidity, and tremor. Benztropine also may inhibit dopamine reuptake and storage, which prolongs dopamine's action.

Contraindications
Achalasia, bladder neck obstruction, glaucoma, hypersensitivity to benztropine mesylate or its components, megacolon, myasthenia gravis, prostatic hypertrophy, pyloric or duodenal obstruction, stenosing peptic ulcer

Interactions
DRUGS
amantadine: Possibly increased adverse anticholinergic effects
digoxin: Possibly increased blood digoxin level
haloperidol: Possibly increased schizophrenic symptoms, decreased serum haloperidol level, and development of tardive dyskinesia
levodopa: Possibly decreased levodopa effectiveness
phenothiazines: Possibly reduced phenothiazine effects and increased psychiatric symptoms

Adverse Reactions
CNS: Agitation, confusion, delirium, delusions, depression, disorientation, dizziness, drowsiness, euphoria, excitement, fever, hallucinations, headache, light-headedness, listlessness, memory loss, nervousness, paranoia, psychosis, weakness
CV: Hypotension, mild bradycardia, orthostatic hypotension, palpitations, tachycardia
EENT: Angle-closure glaucoma, blurred vision, diplopia, dry

mouth, increased intraocular pressure, mydriasis, suppurative parotitis
GI: Constipation, duodenal ulcer, epigastric distress, ileus, nausea, vomiting
GU: Dysuria, urinary hesitancy, urine retention
MS: Muscle spasms, muscle weakness
SKIN: Decreased sweating, dermatoses, flushing, rash, urticaria

Nursing Considerations

- Expect to administer I.V. or I.M. benztropine when patient needs more rapid response than oral drug can provide. Be aware that I.M. route is commonly used because it provides effects in about the same time as I.V. route. Watch for improvement a few minutes after administration. If parkinsonian symptoms reappear, expect to repeat dose.
- Know that therapy generally begins with a low dose followed by gradual increases of 0.5 mg every 5 or 6 days because benztropine has a cumulative action.
- Assess muscle rigidity and tremor as a baseline. Then monitor them frequently for improvement, which indicates the effectiveness of benztropine.
- Administer drug before or after meals based on patient's need and response. If patient has increased salivary secretions, expect to administer benztropine after meals. If patient has dry mouth, plan to give drug before meals unless nausea develops.
- **WARNING** When administering benztropine to patient with drug-induced extrapyramidal reactions, be alert for exacerbation of psychiatric symptoms.
- Know that high-dose benztropine therapy may cause weakness and inability to move specific muscle groups. If this occurs, expect to reduce benztropine dosage.
- Store drug at 15° to 30° C (59° to 86° F). Don't freeze.

PATIENT TEACHING

- Warn patient that benztropine has a cumulative effect, increasing her risk of adverse reactions and overdose.
- Caution patient to avoid driving and similar activities until the effects of benztropineare known because drug may cause blurred vision, dizziness, and drowsiness.
- **WARNING** Because benztropine decreases sweating, urge patient to avoid extremely hot or humid conditions to reduce the risk of heatstroke and severe hyperthermia. This is especially important for elderly patients and those who abuse alcohol or have chronic illnesses or CNS disorders.

- Explain to the patient the need to have eye examinations and intraocular pressure measurements periodically because benztropine may cause angle-closure glaucoma and increase intraocular pressure.

betamethasone sodium phosphate

Betnesol (CAN), Celestone Phosphate, Selestoject

Class and Category

Chemical: Synthetic glucocorticoid
Therapeutic: Anti-inflammatory
Pregnancy category: C

Indications and Dosages

▶ *To treat conditions accompanied by severe inflammation and conditions requiring immunosuppression*

I.V. INJECTION (BETAMETHASONE SODIUM PHOSPHATE)

Adults. *Initial:* Variable (given in emergency situations or when oral therapy isn't possible). *Maximum:* 9 mg daily.

▶ *To treat bursitis, gouty arthritis, osteoarthritis, periostitis of cuboid, peritendinitis, rheumatoid arthritis, skin lesions, tenosynovitisintra-articular, intrabursal, or intradermal injection (betamethasone acetate-betamethasone sodium phosphate)*

Adults with bursitis, peritendinitis, or tenosynovitis. 1 ml by intrabursal or intra-articular injection. Three or four injections given q 1 to 2 wk.

Adults with osteoarthritis or rheumatoid arthritis. 0.5 to 2 ml, depending on joint size.

Adults with foot bursitis. 0.25 to 0.5 ml q 3 to 7 days.

Adults with foot tenosynovitis or periostitis of cuboid. 0.5 ml q 3 to 7 days.

Adults with acute gouty arthritis. 0.5 to 1 ml q 3 to 7 days.

Adults with skin lesions. 0.2 ml/cm^2 intradermally, up to 1 ml weekly.

DOSAGE ADJUSTMENT Dosage reduced for elderly patients and accompanied by periodic monitoring of blood pressure and blood glucose and electrolyte levels.

Route	Onset	Peak	Duration
I.V.	Rapid	Unknown	Unknown
Other	Unknown	Unknown	1 to 2 wk*

* For intra-arterial or intrasynovial injection; 1 week for intralesional injection in soft tissue.

Mechanism of Action

Binds to intracellular glucocorticoid receptors and suppresses inflammatory and immune responses by:

- inhibiting neutrophil and monocyte accumulation at inflammation site and suppressing their phagocytic and bactericidal activity
- stabilizing lysosomal membranes
- suppressing antigen response of macrophages and helper T cells
- inhibiting synthesis of inflammatory response mediators, such as cytokines, interleukins, and prostaglandins.

Contraindications

Live virus vaccination, systemic fungal infection

Interactions

DRUGS

anticholinesterase drugs: Possibly antagonized anticholinesterase effects in myasthenia gravis
barbiturates: Possibly decreased effects of betamethasone
cyclosporine: Possibly increased risk of cyclosporine toxicity
digitalis glycosides: Possibly increased risk of digitalis toxicity
estrogens: Possibly decreased excretion of betamethasone
hydantoins, rifampin: Possibly increased excretion and decreased therapeutic effects of betamethasone
insulin, oral antidiabetics: Possibly increased blood glucose level
isoniazid: Possibly decreased blood isoniazid level
ketoconazole: Possibly decreased excretion of betamethasone
oral anticoagulants: Possibly increased or decreased action of anticoagulants, requiring adjusted anticoagulant dosage
oral contraceptives: Possibly increased half-life and concentration and decreased excretion of betamethasone
potassium-wasting diuretics: Increased risk of hypokalemia
salicylates: Possibly decreased blood level and therapeutic effects of salicylates
somatrem: Possibly inhibition of somatrem's growth-promoting effects
theophyllines: Possibly changes in effects of both drugs

Adverse Reactions

CNS: Fatigue, headache, increased ICP with papilledema, insomnia, malaise, neuritis, paresthesia, seizures, steroid psychosis, syncope, vertigo

CV: Arrhythmias, ECG changes, fat embolism, heart failure, hypertension, thromboembolism, thrombophlebitis
EENT: Cataracts, exophthalmos, glaucoma, increased intraocular pressure
ENDO: Cushingoid symptoms (buffalo hump, central obesity, decreased carbohydrate tolerance, fat pad enlargement, moon face), fluid retention, growth suppression in children, hyperglycemia, negative nitrogen balance, secondary adrenocortical and pituitary unresponsiveness (in times of stress)
GI: Abdominal distention, increased appetite, nausea, pancreatitis, peptic ulcer (possibly with perforation), ulcerative esophagitis, vomiting
GU: Amenorrhea, glycosuria, menstrual irregularities
HEME: Leukocytosis
MS: Aseptic necrosis of femoral and humeral heads, loss of muscle mass, muscle weakness, osteoporosis, spontaneous pathologic and vertebral compression fractures, tendon rupture
RESP: Bronchospasm
SKIN: Acneiform lesions, allergic dermatitis, ecchymosis, facial erythema, hirsutism, impaired wound healing, increased sweating, petechiae, lupuslike lesions, purpura, rash, subcutaneous fat atrophy, thin and fragile skin, urticaria
Other: Anaphylaxis, angioedema, hypocalcemia, hypokalemia, sodium retention, suppressed reaction to skin tests, weight gain

Nursing Considerations

- Be aware that betamethasone therapy should be used with great caution in patients with Strongylides (threadworm) infestation because the drug induced immunosuppression may lead to Strongylides hyperinfection and dissemination with widespread larval migration. Severe enterocolitis and life-threatening gram-negative septicemia may follow.
- Expect prescriber to order baseline ophthalmic examination before initiating therapy because prolonged betamethasone use may lead to increased intraocular pressure, glaucoma, and subsequent optic nerve damage. Use betamethasone cautiously in patients with ocular herpes simplex because corneal perforation may occur.
- Assess for signs of infection before administering betamethasone because drug may mask those signs. Because drug may cause immunosuppression, new infection may develop during therapy. If so, expect to administer appropriate antibiotic.

- Review serum electrolyte levels, as ordered, before initiating therapy. Monitor these levels often during therapy to detect imbalances. Sodium and water retention and potassium and calcium depletion may occur with high-dose betamethasone therapy. If so, expect to restrict sodium intake and provide potassium and calcium supplements.
- Because betamethasone is linked to peptic ulcer formation, expect to administer it with an antacid or H_2-receptor blocker.
- **WARNING** Monitor ECG tracings for arrhythmias, and evaluate patient for anaphylactic reactions, such as angioedema and seizures, which have been associated with rapid I.V. administration of high-dose corticosteroids.
- **WARNING** During long-term betamethasone therapy, assess for signs of adrenal suppression and insufficiency (fatigue, hypotension, lassitude, nausea, vomiting, and weakness) when patient is exposed to stress. If she exhibits these signs, notify prescriber at once.
- Watch for signs and symptoms of steroid psychosis, such as delirium, clouded sensorium, euphoria, insomnia, mood swings, personality changes, and severe depression, which may develop 15 to 30 days after therapy begins. Be prepared to discontinue therapy. If this isn't possible, expect to administer psychotropic drugs.
- After intra-articular injection, assess joint for marked increase in pain, local swelling, and more restricted movement. If patient also develops fever and malaise, suspect septic arthritis and notify prescriber immediately. Expect to assist with joint fluid aspiration to confirm septic arthritis.
- Monitor patient for cushingoid signs and symptoms, such as moon face, buffalo hump, central obesity, striae, acne, ecchymosis, and weight gain. Notify prescriber if you detect these symptoms.

PATIENT TEACHING

- Reinforce signs of adrenal insufficiency and possible need for dosage increases during stress. Advise patient to notify prescriber immediately if signs of insufficiency occur or if she's exposed to stress.
- Instruct patient to avoid exposure to infections because drug can cause immunosuppression. Also teach patient to recognize and immediately report signs of infection.
- After intra-articular injection, advise patient not to overuse joint and to continue other treatments such as physical therapy.

biperiden lactate

Akineton Lactate

Class and Category

Chemical: Tertiary amine
Therapeutic: Anticholinergic, antidyskinetic
Pregnancy category: C

Indications and Dosages

▶ *To control extrapyramidal symptoms (except tardive dyskinesia) caused by phenothiazines and other neuroleptic drugs*

I.V. INJECTION

Adults. 2 mg repeated q 30 min until symptoms resolve or maximum of four consecutive doses in 24 hr is reached.

Route	Onset	Peak	Duration
I.V.	15 min	Unknown	1 to 8 hr

Mechanism of Action

Blocks acetylcholine's action at cholinergic receptor sites. This action restores the brain's normal dopamine and acetylcholine balance, which relaxes muscle movement and decreases rigidity and tremors. Biperiden also may inhibit dopamine reuptake and storage, which prolongs dopamine's action.

Contraindications

Achalasia, angle-closure glaucoma, bladder neck obstruction, bowel obstruction, hypersensitivity to biperiden, myasthenia gravis, prostatic hypertrophy, pyloric or duodenal obstruction, stenosing peptic ulcer, toxic megacolon

Interactions

DRUGS

amantadine: Possibly increased adverse anticholinergic effects
digoxin: Possibly increased serum digoxin level
haloperidol: Possibly increased schizophrenic symptoms, decreased serum haloperidol level, and development of tardive dyskinesia
levodopa: Possibly decreased levodopa effectiveness
phenothiazines: Possibly reduced phenothiazine effects and increased psychiatric symptoms

Adverse Reactions

CNS: Agitation, confusion, delirium, delusions, depression, disori-

entation, dizziness, drowsiness, euphoria, excitement, fever, hallucinations, headache, light-headedness, listlessness, memory loss, nervousness, paranoia, psychosis, weakness
CV: Hypotension, mild bradycardia, orthostatic hypotension, palpitations, tachycardia
EENT: Angle-closure glaucoma, blurred vision, diplopia, dry mouth, increased intraocular pressure, mydriasis, photosensitivity, suppurative parotitis
GI: Constipation, ileus, nausea, vomiting
GU: Dysuria, urinary hesitancy, urine retention
MS: Muscle spasms, muscle weakness
SKIN: Decreased sweating, dermatoses, flushing, rash, urticaria

Nursing Considerations

- Expect to give I.V. biperiden when patient needs more rapid response than oral drug can provide. It also may be given I.M.
- Obtain baseline blood pressure and heart rate. Monitor patient for hypotension and other CV effects, and help patient change position as needed.
- Assess muscle rigidity and tremor at baseline, and monitor them often for improvement, which indicates drug effectiveness.
- Inspect solution for particles and discoloration before use.
- Administer I.V. biperiden slowly.
- **WARNING** Be alert for exacerbation of psychiatric symptoms during biperiden therapy.
- Store drug at 15° to 30° C (59° to 86° F) and protect from light. Don't freeze.

PATIENT TEACHING

- Teach patient about possible adverse effects of biperiden, including CNS effects. Advise her to report such symptoms as dizziness, depression, confusion, rash, vision changes, and eye pain.
- Instruct patient to avoid sudden position changes.
- Inform patient that she may experience increased eye sensitivity to light during biperiden therapy.

bivalirudin

Angiomax

Class and Category

Chemical: Hirudin analogue
Therapeutic: Anticoagulant
Pregnancy category: B

Indications and Dosages

▶ *As adjunct to provide anticoagulation and prevent thrombosis in patients with unstable angina who are having percutaneous transluminal coronary angioplasty or percutaneous coronary intervention; to provide anticoagulation and prevent thrombosis in patients with or at risk of heparin-induced thrombocytopenia or heparin-induced thrombocytopenia thrombosis syndrome who are undergoing percutaneous coronary intervention*

I.V. INFUSION

Adults. *Initial:* Immediately before angioplasty, 0.75-mg/kg bolus followed by 1.75 mg/kg/hr as a continuous infusion for duration of procedure. Five minutes after bolus dose and while continuous infusion is running, additional 0.3-mg/kg dose may be given if needed. After procedure, 1.75 mg/kg/hr may be given for 4 hr by continuous infusion, followed by 0.2 mg/kg/hr for up to 20 hr if needed.

DOSAGE ADJUSTMENT Infusion dosage possibly reduced to 1 mg/kg/hr for patients with severe renal impairment (glomerular filtration rate of 10 to 29 ml/min) and to 0.25 mg/kg/hr for dialysis-dependent patients.

Route	Onset	Peak	Duration
I.V.	Immediate	Unknown	1 hr after end of infusion

Mechanism of Action

Selectively binds to thrombin, including thrombin trapped in established clots. Without thrombin, fibrinogen can't convert to fibrin and clots can't form.

Incompatibilities

Don't mix any other drugs in same I.V. line before or during bivalirudin administration. Mixing with alteplase, amiodarone, amphotericin B, chlorpromazine HCL, diazepam, prochlorperazine edisylate, reteplase, streptokinase, and vancomycin HCL can result in haze, particulate formation, or precipitation.

Contraindications

Active major bleeding, hypersensitivity to bivalirudin or its components

Interactions

DRUGS

alteplase, antineoplastic drugs, antithymocyte globulin, heparin, NSAIDs, platelet inhibitors, reteplase, streptokinase, strontium chloride Sr 89, warfarin: Risk of bleeding

porfimer: Possibly decreased efficacy of porfimer photodynamic therapy

salicylates: Increased risk of hypoprothrombinemia and bleeding

Adverse Reactions

CNS: Headache, intracranial hemorrhage
CV: Hypotension, thrombosis
EENT: Bleeding from mouth, epistaxis
GI: Abdominal cramps, diarrhea, GI or retroperitoneal bleeding, nausea, vomiting
GU: Hematuria, vaginal bleeding
HEME: Severe bleeding, thrombocytopenia
MS: Back pain
RESP: Hemoptysis, hemothorax
SKIN: Ecchymosis
Other: Anaphylaxis, injection site bleeding, hematoma, or pain

Nursing Considerations

- To reconstitute bivalirudin, add 5 ml of sterile water for injection to each 250-mg vial and swirl gently until dissolved. For initial infusion, dilute each reconstituted vial in 50 ml of D_5W or normal saline solution to yield 5 mg/ml.
- For subsequent low-rate infusion, further dilute reconstituted drug in 500 ml of D_5W or normal saline solution to a final concentration of 0.5 mg/ml.
- Expect to give patient 300 to 325 mg of aspirin P.O. daily, as prescribed, during bivalirudin therapy.
- **WARNING** Expect to monitor blood coagulation tests before and regularly during therapy because bleeding is a major risk of bivalirudin therapy.
- **WARNING** Monitor patient often for evidence of bleeding because no antidote for bivalirudin is available. If life-threatening bleeding occurs, notify prescriber immediately, stop drug, and prepare to monitor APTT and other coagulation tests as ordered. Be aware that blood transfusions may be needed. Patients with an increased risk of bleeding include females with active menstruation; patients with vascular or organ abnormalities, such as severe uncontrolled hyperten-

sion, advanced renal disease, infective endocarditis, dissecting aortic aneurysm, diverticulitis, hemophilia, hepatic disease (especially from a deficiency in vitamin K–dependent clotting factors), inflammatory bowel disease, or peptic ulcer disease; and those who have recently had a CVA, major surgery (including eye, brain, or spinal cord surgery), large vessel or lumbar puncture, organ biopsy, spinal anesthesia, or major bleeding (including intracranial, GI, intraocular, retroperitoneal, or pulmonary bleeding).

- If patient is receiving gamma brachytherapy, watch closely for evidence of thrombosis (weak or absent pulse, pallor, pain) because drug may increase the risk in these patients.
- If possible, avoid I.M. injections to decrease the risk of bleeding.
- Discard any unused portion of drug.

PATIENT TEACHING

- Inform patient that bivalirudin is a blood thinner used only in the hospital setting.
- Instruct patient to check her skin for bruising or red spots and to immediately report back or stomach pain, difficulty breathing, dizziness or fainting, and unusual bleeding, such as black or tarry stools, blood in urine, coughing up blood, heavy menstrual bleeding, or nosebleeds. Drug may need to be discontinued.
- Urge patient to avoid injury while receiving bivalirudin—for example, by brushing her teeth gently, using a soft-bristled toothbrush.
- Caution patient not to take anti-inflammatory drugs, such as ibuprofen, naproxen, ketoprofen, aspirin, and aspirin-like products, or other blood thinners, such as warfarin, while receiving bivalirudin unless prescriber instructs her to do so.

bleomycin sulfate

Blenoxane

Class and Category

Chemical: Cytotoxic glycopeptide antibiotic mixture
Therapeutic: Antineoplastic antibiotic
Pregnancy category: D

Indications and Dosages

▶ *To treat squamous cell carcinoma of the head and neck (including mouth, tongue, tonsil, sinus, palate, lip, buccal mucosa, gingiva, epiglottis,*

nasopharynx, oropharynx, and larynx), skin, penis, cervix, and vulva; non-Hodgkin's lymphomas; and testicular carcinoma
I.V. INJECTION
Adults and adolescents. 0.25 to 0.5 units/kg or 10 to 20 units/m^2 over at least 10 min once or twice a week.
▶ *To treat Hodgkin's disease*
I.V. INJECTION
Adults and adolescents. *Initial:* 0.25 to 0.5 units/kg or 10 to 20 units/m^2 over at least 10 min once or twice a week. *Maintenance:* 1 unit daily or 5 units weekly if 50% response occurs. Each dose should be administered over at least 10 min.
DOSAGE ADJUSTMENT Patients with Hodgkin's disease or non-Hodgkin's lymphoma are given a test dose of 2 units or less for the first two doses because of possible anaphylactoid reaction. For patients with impaired renal function (regardless of indication), dosage decreased to 50% of normal dose if serum creatinine level is 1.5 to 2 mg/dl; to 25% of normal dose if serum creatinine level is 2.5 to 4 mg/dl; to 20% of normal dose if serum creatinine level is 4 to 6 mg/dl; and to 5% to 10% of normal dose if serum creatinine level is 6 to 10 mg/dl.

Mechanism of Action
May inhibit cell's ability to replicate or reproduce by inhibiting DNA synthesis and, to a lesser extent, RNA and protein synthesis. Bleomycin is effective against both cycling and noncycling cells, but it appears to be most effective in the G_2 phase of cell division.

Incompatibilities
Don't mix bleomycin with D_5W or other solutions containing dextrose to avoid a loss in potency.

Contraindications
Hypersensitivity or a history of idiosyncratic reaction to bleomycin

Interactions
DRUGS
antineoplastics: Increased risk of pulmonary and mucosal toxicity and bone marrow depression
cisplatin: Increased risk of bleomycin toxicity due to bleomycin accumulation

digoxin: Decreased blood digoxin level
general anesthetics: Increased risk of pulmonary deterioration and fibrosis
live virus vaccines: Severe and possibly fatal infections
phenytoin: Decreased blood phenytoin level
vincristine: Increased therapeutic effect of bleomycin

Adverse Reactions

CNS: Chills, fever
CV: Pleuropericarditis, Raynaud's phenomenon, vascular toxicity (cerebral arteritis, CVA, MI, thrombotic microangiopathy), vasospasm (when used in combination with vinblastine for testicular cancer)
EENT: Stomatitis
GI: Anorexia, elevated liver function test results, hepatotoxicity, vomiting
GU: Cystitis, elevated BUN and serum creatinine levels, hematuria
HEME: Decreased hemoglobin level, leukopenia, thrombocytopenia
RESP: Pneumonitis progressing to pulmonary fibrosis, pulmonary toxicity (decreased diffusion capacity, lung volume, and vital capacity; dyspnea; crackles)
SKIN: Alopecia, erythema, hyperkeratosis, hyperpigmentation, mucocutaneous toxicity, nail changes, rash, skin tenderness, striae, vesiculation
Other: Idiosyncratic reaction (chills, fever, hypotension, confusion, faintness, wheezing), injection site phlebitis, tumor site pain, weight loss

Nursing Considerations

- Be aware that bleomycin should be administered only under the supervision of a qualified physician where appropriate diagnostic and treatment facilities are available.
- Follow facility protocols for preparation and handling of antineoplastic drugs and appropriate disposal of used equipment.
- Add 5 or 10 ml of sodium chloride for injection to a 15-unit or 30-unit vial of bleomycin.
- Store reconstituted bleomycin at room temperature and use within 24 hours.
- Be aware that premedication with acetaminophen, steroids, and diphenhydramine may be administered to reduce the risk of anaphylaxis and drug-induced fever.
- Expect pulmonary function tests and chest X-rays to be ordered before initiation of therapy to establish patient's baseline pulmonary status.

- **WARNING** Monitor patient's respiratory status, including auscultation and evaluation of breathing patterns during and after therapy, to assist with early detection of pulmonary toxicity. This complication occurs in about 10% of patients receiving bleomycin, especially elderly patients, those who have received cytotoxic drugs, those who are receiving bleomycin in combination with other antineoplastics, those receiving oxygen therapy during and after surgery, smokers, and patients receiving a total dose greater than 400 units. Expect drug to be discontinued if pulmonary changes are detected. Be aware that pulmonary symptoms can occur up to 1 month after therapy ends.
- Be aware that patients who have been treated with radiation therapy are at increased risk for pulmonary and mucocutaneous toxicity and bone marrow depression.
- **WARNING** Be aware that patients with lymphoma may develop a severe idiosyncratic reaction (chills, fever, hypotension, confusion, faintness, and wheezing) similar to anaphylaxis, especially after first or second dose. This reaction may occur immediately or several hours after dose is given. Notify prescriber immediately if such a reaction occurs. Expect to give antihistamines, corticosteroids, pressor agents, and volume expanders, as prescribed.
- Obtain BUN and serum creatinine levels before starting therapy, and monitor patient for signs and symptoms of declining renal function during therapy, especially if patient has significant renal function impairment.
- Monitor for elevated liver function test results, which may indicate drug-induced hepatotoxicity.
- Monitor patient for signs of adverse skin and mucous membrane effects, which occur in 25% to 50% of patients undergoing bleomycin therapy, usually 2 or 3 weeks after administration of 150 to 200 units.
- Be aware that fraction of inspired oxygen (FIO_2) is maintained at 25%—approximately that of room air—during and after surgery to reduce the risk of pulmonary complications. Expect fluid replacement to be colloid rather than crystalloid.
- Store unreconstituted vials at 2° to 8° C (36° to 46° F).

PATIENT TEACHING

- Teach patient signs and symptoms of adverse reactions associated with bleomycin, and advise her to immediately report any that occur.

- Stress the importance of obtaining periodic chest X-rays, which may be ordered every 1 to 2 weeks, to detect signs of adverse pulmonary reactions.
- Advise patient to inform all health care providers, including dentists, that she is receiving bleomycin.
- Encourage patient to maintain good oral hygiene and adequate nutritional intake. If she develops stomatitis, suggest that she try eating bland, soft foods served cold or at room temperature to decrease irritation.

bretylium tosylate

Bretylate (CAN), Bretylol

Class and Category

Chemical: Bromobenzyl quaternary ammonium compound
Therapeutic: Class III antiarrhythmic
Pregnancy category: C

Indications and Dosages

▶ *To prevent and treat ventricular fibrillation and to treat life-threatening ventricular arrhythmias that don't respond to first-line antiarrhythmics, such as lidocaine*

I.V. INFUSION, I.V. INJECTION

Adults with immediate life-threatening ventricular arrhythmias. *Initial:* 5 mg/kg undiluted by rapid I.V. injection; if ventricular fibrillation persists, 10 mg/kg repeated as often as needed. *Continuous suppression:* 1 to 2 mg/min or 5 to 10 mg/kg of diluted I.V. solution infused over at least 8 min q 6 hr.

Adults with other ventricular arrhythmias. *Initial:* 5 to 10 mg/kg of diluted I.V. solution infused over at least 8 min and repeated q 1 to 2 hr if arrhythmia continues. *Maintenance:* 5 to 10 mg/kg diluted I.V. solution infused over at least 8 min q 6 hr, or 1 to 2 mg/min infused continuously.

DOSAGE ADJUSTMENT Dosing interval increased for patients with impaired renal function because bretylium is excreted primarily by kidneys.

Route	Onset	Peak	Duration
I.V.	5 to 10 min*	6 to 9 hr	6 to 24 hr

* For suppression of ventricular fibrillation; 20 to 120 min for suppression of ventricular tachycardia.

Mechanism of Action

Bretylium prolongs the repolarization phase of the action potential and lengthens the effective refractory period, which helps stop reentry arrhythmias. It also acts on adrenergic nerve terminals. Initially, it causes norepinephrine release, increasing heart rate and blood pressure. Then it blocks norepinephrine release, as shown, decreasing heart rate and blood pressure. It also increases the ventricular threshold, making the ventricular myocardium less responsive to ectopic impulses and preventing ventricular fibrillation.

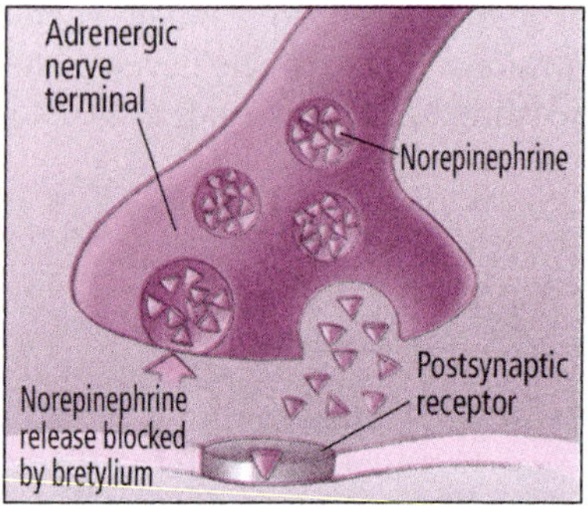

Contraindications

Digitalis toxicity, hypersensitivity to bretylium

Interactions

DRUGS

catecholamines (such as dopamine and norepinephrine): Increased vasopressor effects of catecholamines
digoxin: Possibly worsening of digitalis toxicity

Adverse Reactions

CNS: Anxiety, confusion, dizziness, emotional lability, fever, lethargy, light-headedness, paranoid psychosis, syncope, vertigo
CV: Angina, arrhythmias (including bradycardia and more frequent PVCs), hypotension, orthostatic hypotension, transient hypertension
EENT: Mild conjunctivitis, nasal congestion
GI: Abdominal pain, diarrhea, hiccups, nausea, vomiting
GU: Renal dysfunction
RESP: Dyspnea
SKIN: Diaphoresis, erythematous macular rash, flushing
Other: Injection site pain

Nursing Considerations

- **WARNING** Monitor patients with severe aortic stenosis or pulmonary hypertension for signs of hypotension, a common effect of bretylium therapy.

- Be aware that bretylium is always diluted for I.V. administration *except* when used in life-threatening ventricular fibrillation. In this instance, use *undiluted* bretylium and administer it as quickly as possible.
- Dilute bretylium in a compatible I.V. solution, such as D_5W, D_5/normal saline solution, D_5/lactated Ringer's solution, normal saline solution, 5% sodium bicarbonate, 20% mannitol, 1/6 molar sodium lactate, lactated Ringer's solution, calcium chloride in D_5W, and potassium chloride in D_5W. Dilute to a concentration of at least 500 mg/50 ml.
- Be aware that bretylium is also available in 5% dextrose; this form should be used for I.V. infusion only.
- For I.V. infusion, dilute bretylium and administer at 1 to 2 mg/minute, using an infusion pump or other appropriate rate control device.
- **WARNING** Be aware that patient may experience hypotension while supine. Have patient remain supine until tolerance develops. If her supine systolic blood pressure falls below 75 mm Hg, expect to administer dopamine or norepinephrine and monitor her blood pressure closely because vasopressor effects intensify when these drugs are given together.
- Be alert for transient hypertension and increased frequency of arrhythmias because bretylium initially triggers release of norepinephrine. Monitor patient's ECG tracings and blood pressure continuously, and notify prescriber of changes.
- Monitor serum bretylium level. Notify prescriber if level falls outside therapeutic range of 0.5 to 1.5 mcg/ml.
- Store drug at 15° to 30° C (59° to 86° F). Don't freeze.

PATIENT TEACHING

- Advise patient receiving bretylium to immediately report chest pain or pressure, pain at I.V. site, or rash.
- Warn patient that she may feel dizzy or light-headed even when lying down. Instruct her to remain supine and to ask for assistance when attempting to move or sit up. Tell her that this sensation usually subsides in a few days.

bumetanide

Bumex

Class and Category

Chemical: Sulfonamide derivative
Therapeutic: Loop diuretic

Pregnancy category: C

Indications and Dosages

▶ *To treat edema caused by heart failure, hepatic disease, and renal disease, including nephrotic syndrome*

I.V. INFUSION, I.V. INJECTION

Adults. 0.5 to 1 mg over 1 to 2 min; may repeat q 2 to 3 hr if necessary. *Maximum:* 10 mg daily.

DOSAGE ADJUSTMENT Continuous infusion (12 mg over 12 hr) may be more effective and less toxic than intermittent infusion in patients with severe chronic renal insufficiency.

Route	Onset	Peak	Duration
I.V.	In min	15 to 30 min	3.5 to 4 hr

Mechanism of Action

Inhibits the reabsorption of sodium, chloride, and water in the ascending limb of the loop of Henle, which promotes their excretion and reduces fluid volume.

Contraindications

Anuria, hepatic coma, hypersensitivity to bumetanide or its components, severe electrolyte depletion

Interactions

DRUGS

aminoglycosides: Increased risk of ototoxicity
antihypertensives: Increased antihypertensive effect
indomethacin: Slowed increase in urine and sodium excretion, inhibited plasma renin activity
lithium: Decreased lithium renal clearance, increased risk of lithium toxicity
probenecid: Decreased sodium excretion

Adverse Reactions

CNS: Dizziness, encephalopathy, headache
CV: Chest pain, hypotension
EENT: Ototoxicity
ENDO: Hyperglycemia
GI: Nausea
GU: Azotemia, difficulty maintaining erection, elevated serum creatinine level, premature ejaculation

MS: Muscle spasms
Other: Hyperuricemia, hypocalcemia, hypochloremia, hypokalemia, hyponatremia, hypovolemia

Nursing Considerations

- **WARNING** Be aware that patients who are hypersensitive to sulfonamides may be hypersensitive to bumetanide. Monitor such patients closely when starting therapy.
- Expect to use parenteral route for patients with impaired GI absorption or those for whom oral route isn't practical. Switch to oral route, as prescribed, as soon as possible.
- Discard unused parenteral solution 24 hours after preparation.
- Assess fluid and electrolyte balance closely because bumetanide is a potent diuretic (40 to 60 times more potent than furosemide). Monitor fluid intake and output once every 8 hours, evaluate serum electrolyte levels when ordered, and assess for imbalances.
- **WARNING** Be aware that high-dose or too-frequent administration can cause profound diuresis and water and electrolyte depletion, especially in elderly patients.
- Monitor serum potassium level regularly to check for hypokalemia, especially if patient takes a digitalis glycoside for heart failure or has hepatic cirrhosis, ascites, aldosteronism, potassium-losing nephropathy, diarrhea, or a history of ventricular arrhythmias.
- Assess for signs of ototoxicity, such as tinnitus, daily. Rarely, bumetanide may cause ototoxicity, especially with I.V. administration, high doses, and increased frequency of administration in a patient with renal impairment.
- Monitor results of renal function tests during bumetanide therapy to detect adverse reactions.
- Store drug at 15° to 30° C (59° to 86° F), and protect from light. Don't freeze.

PATIENT TEACHING

- Inform patient that fluid intake and output will be monitored during bumetanide therapy. Advise her to report signs and symptoms of electrolyte imbalance, such as dizziness, headache, and muscle spasms.
- Teach patient about adverse reactions, and tell her to report any that occur.
- Advise patient to avoid potentially hazardous activities until drug's CNS effects are known.

- Review potassium-rich foods, and encourage patient to include them in her daily diet.
- Inform diabetic patient that her blood glucose level will be monitored regularly; urge her to report signs or symptoms of hyperglycemia.

buprenorphine hydrochloride

Buprenex

Class, Category, and Schedule

Chemical: Opioid, thebaine derivative
Therapeutic: Narcotic analgesic
Pregnancy category: C
Controlled substance: Schedule V

Indications and Dosages

▶ *To control moderate to severe pain*

I.V INJECTION

Adults and children age 12 and older. 0.3 mg q 6 hr or more, p.r.n. A second 0.3-mg dose given 30 to 60 min after first dose, if needed.

DOSAGE ADJUSTMENT I.V. dose reduced by half in elderly or debilitated patients and in those who have respiratory disease or also use another CNS depressant.

Children ages 2 to 12. 0.002 to 0.006 mg/kg q 4 to 6 hr, p.r.n.

Route	Onset	Peak	Duration
I.V.	Less than 15 min	Less than 1 hr	6 to 10 hr*

Mechanism of Action

May bind with CNS receptors to alter the perception of and emotional response to pain. Buprenorphine may act by displacing narcotic agonists from their binding sites and competitively inhibiting their actions.

Incompatibilities

Don't administer I.V. buprenorphine through the same I.V. line as diazepam or lorazepam.

Contraindications

Hypersensitivity to buprenorphine or its components

* 4 to 5 hr in children ages 2 to 12.

Interactions

DRUGS

CNS depressants, MAO inhibitors: Additive hypotensive and respiratory and CNS depressant effects of these drugs

narcotic analgesics: Reduced therapeutic effects if buprenorphine is given before another narcotic analgesic

Adverse Reactions

CNS: Dizziness, headache, sedation, vertigo
CV: Bradycardia, hypertension, hypotension
EENT: Miosis
GI: Nausea, vomiting
RESP: Bronchospasm, hypoventilation
SKIN: Diaphoresis, pruritus, rash, urticaria
Other: Anaphylaxis; angioedema; injection site pain, redness, and swelling

Nursing Considerations

- Use buprenorphine cautiously in patients with severe hepatic or renal impairment, myxedema, hypothyroidism, adrenal insufficiency, CNS depression, coma, toxic psychosis, prostatic hypertrophy, urethral stricture, acute alcoholism, alcohol withdrawal syndrome, kyphoscoliosis, or biliary tract dysfunction. Also use cautiously in patients who abuse drugs, have been opioid-dependent, or receive a drug that decreases hepatic clearance.
- Use drug cautiously in patients with head injury, intracranial lesions, or other conditions that could increase CSF pressure.
- WARNING Administer buprenorphine over at least 2 minutes. Be aware that rapid administration of other opioid analgesics has caused anaphylaxis, severe respiratory depression, hypotension, peripheral circulatory collapse, and cardiac arrest. Keep emergency equipment and drugs nearby.
- Inspect injection site for local reactions; don't use the same site twice.
- Monitor vital signs and response to drug often, especially after giving first dose.

PATIENT TEACHING

- Instruct patient to lie down during buprenorphine administration and for a period afterward to lessen drug's hypotensive effects (dizziness, light-headedness) and other adverse effects such as nausea and vomiting.
- Advise patient to change position slowly and to avoid rising quickly from a sitting or lying position.

- Advise patient to avoid potentially hazardous activities until drug's CNS effects are known.

butorphanol tartrate

Stadol

Class, Category, and Schedule

Chemical: Opioid
Therapeutic: Anesthesia adjunct, opioid analgesic
Pregnancy category: C
Controlled substance: Schedule II

Indications and Dosages

▶ *To manage pain*

I.V. INJECTION

Adults. 0.5 to 2 mg (usually 1 mg) q 3 to 4 hr, p.r.n.

▶ *As adjunct to provide preoperative anesthesia*

I.V. INJECTION

Adults. Individualized; average of 2 mg 60 to 90 min before surgery.

▶ *As adjunct to provide anesthesia*

I.V. INJECTION

Adults. Individualized; average of 1 to 4 mg initially and then supplemental doses of 0.5 to 1 mg, p.r.n. Total usually required during surgery is 60 to 180 mcg/kg (0.06 to 0.18 mg/kg).

DOSAGE ADJUSTMENT Dosage reduced by half for elderly patients and those with impaired hepatic or renal function.

Route	Onset	Peak	Duration
I.V.	2 to 3 min	30 min	2 to 4 hr

Mechanism of Action

May bind with and stimulate mu and kappa opiate receptors in the spinal cord and higher levels in the CNS. In this way, butorphanol is believed to alter the perception of and emotional response to pain.

Contraindications

Acute respiratory depression, diarrhea due to poisoning, hypersensitivity to butorphanol or its components (including the preservative benzethonium chloride)

Interactions

DRUGS

CNS depressants: Additive CNS depression

ACTIVITIES

alcohol use: Additive CNS depression

Adverse Reactions

CNS: Anxiety, confusion, difficulty performing purposeful movements, difficulty speaking, dizziness, euphoria, floating feeling, headache, lethargy, nervousness, paresthesia, somnolence, syncope, tremor, vertigo
CV: Chest pain, hypotension, palpitations, tachycardia, vasodilation
EENT: Blurred vision, dry mouth, tinnitus
GI: Anorexia, constipation, epigastric pain, nausea, vomiting
RESP: Apnea, respiratory depression, shallow breathing
SKIN: Clammy skin, pruritus, sensation of warmth

Nursing Considerations

- Give butorphanol slowly, over several minutes. Be aware that rapid administration may cause anaphylaxis, severe respiratory depression, hypotension, peripheral circulatory collapse, and cardiac arrest. Keep emergency equipment and drugs nearby.
- Assess respiratory status closely, especially in patients having an acute asthma attack and those with chronic respiratory disease, hypothyroidism, or conditions that increase CSF pressure, because drug causes respiratory depression. Pediatric, elderly, extremely ill, or debilitated patients and those who have recently taken or are currently taking drugs with respiratory depressant effects are also more sensitive to butorphanol's effects.
- Frequently monitor blood pressure after giving butorphanol. If severe hypertension develops (rare), stop drug at once and notify prescriber. If patient isn't opioid-dependent, expect to administer naloxone to reverse drug's effects.
- Monitor patient for evidence of drug-induced CNS depression or increased CSF pressure, such as altered LOC, restlessness, and irritability, in patients with a head injury, intracranial lesions, or other conditions that could cause these effects. Patients who are taking or have recently taken drugs that depress the CNS are also more susceptible to these effects. Take appropriate safety precautions.
- Because butorphanol can increase cardiac workload, use it with extreme caution in patients with acute MI, ventricular dysfunction, or coronary insufficiency.

- Be aware that butorphanol may induce or exacerbate arrhythmias or seizures in patients with a history of these conditions and may mask symptoms of acute abdominal conditions.
- Monitor patients with renal or hepatic impairment and those receiving a drug that decreases hepatic clearance for signs of increased butorphanol effects because drug is metabolized in the liver and excreted by the kidneys.
- Be aware that patients with a history of drug abuse (including acute alcoholism), emotional instability, or suicidal ideation or attempts are at increased risk for opioid abuse; however, the risk of drug dependence from butorphanol is lower than with some other opioid analgesics.
- Monitor patients with prostatic hypertrophy, renal function impairment, recent urinary tract surgery, or urethral stricture for signs of urine retention, such as difficulty voiding or feeling that the bladder isn't empty after voiding, peripheral edema, or weight gain.
- Store drug at 15° to 30° C (59° to 86° F), and protect from light. Don't freeze.

PATIENT TEACHING

- Instruct patient to lie down during butorphanol administration and for a period afterward to lessen drug's hypotensive effects (dizziness, light-headedness) and other adverse effects, such as nausea and vomiting.
- Advise patient to change position slowly and to avoid rising quickly from a sitting or lying position.
- Advise patient to avoid potentially hazardous activities until drug's CNS effects are known.
- Tell patient to avoid alcohol and other CNS depressants, including OTC drugs, during butorphanol therapy because of possible additive CNS depression.

C

calcitriol (1,25-dihydroxycholecalciferol)

Calcijex

Class and Category

Chemical: Sterol derivative, vitamin D analogue
Therapeutic: Antihypocalcemic, antihypoparathyroid
Pregnancy category: C

Indications and Dosages

▶ *To treat hypoparathyroidism*

I.V. INJECTION

Adults. *Initial:* 1 to 2 mcg 3 times/wk given q other day. Each dose increased 0.5 to 1 mcg at 2- to 4-wk intervals, if needed.

Mechanism of Action

Binds to specific receptors of the intestinal mucosa to increase calcium absorption from the intestines. It also may regulate calcium ion transfer from bone to blood and stimulate calcium reabsorption in the distal renal tubules, making more calcium available in the body.

Contraindications

Hypercalcemia, vitamin D toxicity

Interactions

DRUGS

cholestyramine: Decreased calcitriol absorption
digitalis glycosides: Possibly arrhythmias
ketoconazole: Decreased blood calcitriol level
magnesium-containing antacids (I.V. form): Hypermagnesemia
mineral oil: Decreased blood calcitriol level (with prolonged use of mineral oil)
phenobarbital, phenytoin: Decreased synthesis and blood level of calcitriol
thiazide diuretics: Hypercalcemia

Adverse Reactions
SKIN: Erythema multiforme, lip swelling, pruritus, rash, urticaria

Nursing Considerations
- Make sure patient has adequate calcium intake.
- Store drug at room temperature and protect from heat and direct light.
- In high-dose or long-term calcitriol therapy, be alert for vitamin D toxicity. Early evidence includes abdominal or bone pain, constipation, dry mouth, headache, metallic taste, myalgia, nausea, somnolence, vomiting, and weakness. Late evidence includes albuminuria, anorexia, arrhythmias, azotemia, conjunctivitis (calcific), decreased libido, elevated AST and ALT levels, elevated BUN level, vascular calcification, hypercholesterolemia, hypertension, hyperthermia, irritability, mild acidosis, nephrocalcinosis, nocturia, pancreatitis, photophobia, polydipsia, polyuria, pruritus, rhinorrhea, and weight loss.

PATIENT TEACHING
- Warn patient not to take other forms of vitamin D while taking calcitriol.
- Advise patient to notify prescriber immediately if signs of toxicity, such as headache, irritability, nausea, photophobia, vomiting, weakness, and weight loss, develop.

calcium chloride
Calciject (CAN)

calcium gluceptate
Calcium Stanley (CAN)

calcium gluconate

Class and Category
Chemical: Elemental cation
Therapeutic: Antihypermagnesemic agent, antihypocalcemic agent, calcium replacement, cardiotonic agent
Pregnancy category: C

Indications and Dosages
▶ *To replace calcium in hypocalcemia*
I.V. INFUSION (CALCIUM CHLORIDE)
Adults. 0.5 to 1 g q 1 to 3 days, infused at less than 1 ml/min.
Children. 25 mg/kg given over several minutes.

I.V. INJECTION (CALCIUM GLUCEPTATE)
Adults and children. 1.1 to 4.4 g I.V. at a rate not to exceed 2 ml (36 mg)/min.
I.V. INJECTION (CALCIUM GLUCONATE)
Adults. 970 mg given slowly and repeated if needed until tetany is controlled.
Children. 200 to 500 mg as a single dose given slowly and repeated if needed until tetany is controlled.
▶ *As adjunct to treat magnesium intoxication*
I.V. INJECTION (CALCIUM CHLORIDE)
Adults. 500 mg promptly and repeated p.r.n., based on response.
▶ *As adjunct in cardiac resuscitation*
I.V. INJECTION (CALCIUM CHLORIDE)
Adults. 0.5 to 1 g.
Children. 0.2 ml/kg.
▶ *As adjunct in exchange transfusion*
I.V. INJECTION (CALCIUM GLUCONATE)
Adults. 1.35 mEq after each 100 ml of citrated blood is exchanged.
Neonates. 0.45 mEq after each 100 ml of citrated blood is exchanged.
I.V. INJECTION (CALCIUM GLUCEPTATE)
Neonates. 110 mg after each 100 ml of citrated blood is exchanged.

Mechanism of Action
Increases levels of intracellular and extracellular calcium, which is needed to maintain homeostasis, especially in the nervous and musculoskeletal systems. Also plays a role in normal cardiac and renal function, respiration, coagulation, and cell membrane and capillary permeability. Helps regulate the release and storage of neurotransmitters and hormones.

Incompatibilities
To avoid precipitation, don't administer I.V. calcium chloride, gluceptate, or gluconate through the same I.V. line as bicarbonates, carbonates, phosphates, sulfates, or tartrates. Don't mix with tetracyclines to avoid rendering tetracyclines inactive.

Contraindications
Hypercalcemia, hypersensitivity to calcium salts or their components, hypophosphatemia, renal calculi, ventricular fibrillation

Interactions

DRUGS

atenolol: Decreased blood atenolol level and beta blockade
calcitonin: Possibly antagonized effects of calcitonin in hypercalcemia treatment
calcium supplements, magnesium-containing preparations: Increased serum calcium or magnesium level, especially in patients with impaired renal function
cellulose sodium phosphate: Decreased effectiveness of cellulose sodium phosphate in preventing hypercalciuria
digitalis glycosides: Increased risk of arrhythmias
estrogens, oral contraceptives (estrogen-containing): Increased calcium absorption
etidronate: Decreased etidronate absorption
fluoroquinolones: Reduced fluoroquinolone absorption by calcium carbonate
gallium nitrate: Antagonized effects of gallium nitrate
iron salts: Decreased gastric absorption of iron
magnesium sulfate (parenteral): Neutralized effects of magnesium by parenteral calcium salts
neuromuscular blockers (except succinylcholine): Possibly reversal of neuromuscular blockade by parenteral calcium salts; enhanced or prolonged neuromuscular blockade induced by tubocurarine
norfloxacin: Decreased norfloxacin bioavailability
phenytoin: Decreased bioavailability of phenytoin and calcium
potassium phosphates, potassium and sodium phosphates: Increased risk of calcium deposition in soft tissue
sodium bicarbonate: Possibly milk-alkali syndrome
sodium fluoride: Reduced fluoride and calcium absorption
sodium polystyrene sulfonate: Possibly metabolic alkalosis if patient has renal impairment
tetracyclines: Decreased tetracycline absorption and blood level, leading to decreased anti-infective response
thiazide diuretics: Possibly hypercalcemia
verapamil: Reversed verapamil effects
vitamin A (more than 25,000 units/day): Possibly stimulation of bone loss, decreased effects of calcium supplementation, and hypercalcemia
vitamin D (high doses): Excessively increased calcium absorption

FOODS

caffeine: Possibly decreased calcium absorption

ACTIVITIES
alcohol use (excessive), smoking: Possibly decreased calcium absorption

Adverse Reactions

CNS: Paresthesia
CV: Hypotension, irregular heartbeat
GI: Nausea, vomiting
SKIN: Diaphoresis, flushing, or sensation of warmth
Other: Hypercalcemia; injection site burning, pain, rash, or redness

Nursing Considerations

- **WARNING** Be aware that calcium chloride injection contains three times as much calcium per milliliter as calcium gluconate injection.
- Warm solution to room temperature before administration.
- Don't use calcium gluceptate if you detect crystals.
- If you observe crystals in calcium gluconate, you can dissolve them by warming solution to 30° to 40° C (86° to 104° F).
- Administer I.V. calcium through an infusing I.V. solution, using a small-bore needle inserted into a large vein to minimize irritation. Give calcium slowly to prevent excess calcium from reaching the heart and causing adverse cardiovascular reactions. Adverse reactions often result from too-rapid administration. If ECG tracings are abnormal or patient reports injection site discomfort, expect to temporarily discontinue administration.
- Maintain patient in a recumbent position for 30 minutes after administration to prevent dizziness from hypotension.
- Assess regularly for extravasation because calcium causes necrosis. If infiltration occurs, discontinue I.V. calcium and notify prescriber immediately.
- Regularly monitor serum calcium level and evaluate therapeutic response by verifying the absence of Chvostek's and Trousseau's signs. Be aware that patients with dehydration, electrolyte imbalance, renal function impairment, or sarcoidosis are at increased risk for hypercalcemia. Patients with diarrhea or GI malabsorption may have increased fecal calcium excretion.
- Monitor vital signs and ECG tracings as appropriate. Calcium administration may cause a temporary increase in blood pressure, especially in elderly or hypertensive patients.
- Assess for arrhythmias in patients with cardiac disease, those receiving digitalis glycosides, and those with a history of ventricular fibrillation during cardiac resuscitation.

- Monitor for signs of calculi formation, such as pain radiating from the lumbar region, in patients with a history of renal calculi.
- Store calcium at 15° to 30° C (59° to 86° F), and protect from heat, moisture, and direct light. Don't freeze.

PATIENT TEACHING

- Instruct patient to immediately report pain at calcium injection site.
- Tell patient to avoid excessive use of tobacco and excessive consumption of alcoholic beverages and caffeine-containing products because these substances may decrease calcium absorption.
- Teach patient with hypocalcemia about the need for calcium and vitamin D intake as well as weight-bearing exercise.

capreomycin sulfate

Capastat

Class and Category

Chemical: Polypeptide antibiotic isolated from *Streptomyces capreolus*
Therapeutic: Antitubercular agent
Pregnancy category: C

Indications and Dosages

▶ *As adjunct to treat pulmonary tuberculosis caused by* Mycobacterium tuberculosis *when primary drugs have been ineffective or can't be used because of toxicity*

I.V. INFUSION

Adults. 1 g daily for 60 to 120 days, followed by 1 g two or three times weekly for 12 to 24 mo. *Maximum:* 20 mg/kg daily.

> **Mechanism of Action**
> May interfere with lipid and nucleic acid biosynthesis in actively growing tubercle bacilli.

Contraindications

Hypersensitivity to capreomycin or its components

Interactions

DRUGS

aminoglycosides (parenteral): Increased risk of ototoxicity, nephrotoxicity, and neuromuscular blockade

nephrotoxic drugs (such as amphotericin B): Increased risk of nephrotoxicity
neuromuscular blockers: Enhanced neuromuscular blockade
ototoxic drugs (such as quinidine): Increased risk of ototoxicity
polymyxins (parenteral): Increased risk of nephrotoxicity and neuromuscular blockade

Adverse Reactions

CNS: Dizziness, vertigo
EENT: Ototoxicity
GI: Elevated liver function test results
GU: Nephrotoxicity
HEME: Leukocytosis, leukopenia
SKIN: Maculopapular rash, urticaria
Other: Injection site pain, induration, or bleeding

Nursing Considerations

- Expect capreomycin dosage to be decreased for patients with reduced renal clearance.
- Reconstitute sterile capreomycin powder with 0.9% sodium chloride injection or sterile water for injection. Add 2, 2.15, 2.63, 3.3, or 4.3 ml of diluent to a 1-g vial of capreomycin to yield a concentration of 370, 350, 300, 250, or 200 mg/ml, respectively. Let stand for 2 to 3 minutes to allow for complete dissolution.
- Dilute reconstituted drug for I.V. injection with 100 ml of normal saline solution. Administer over 60 minutes.
- Store reconstituted capreomycin at 2° to 8° C (36° to 46° F) for up to 24 hours. Be aware that a color change to pale straw color with subsequent darkening doesn't indicate loss of potency or development of toxicity.
- Monitor results of renal function tests and assess urine for sediment to detect signs of renal injury or nephrotoxicity.
- Assess patient for changes in hearing. Ensure that he receives audiometric testing and vestibular function assessments regularly.
- Monitor patient closely for signs of a hypersensitivity reaction, such as urticaria and maculopapular rash, especially in patients with a history of hypersensitivity reactions to other drugs.

PATIENT TEACHING

- Advise patient receiving capreomycin to report excessive bleeding at injection site.

- Instruct patient to notify prescriber immediately if he develops hearing loss or ringing in ears.
- Explain the need for frequent laboratory tests to monitor renal function.
- Tell patient that tuberculosis therapy lasts for 12 to 24 months and that another drug will also be prescribed.
- Explain that noncompliance may decrease effectiveness and increase duration of treatment.

caspofungin acetate

Cancidas

Class and Category

Chemical: Echinocandins
Therapeutic: Antifungal
Pregnancy category: C

Indications and Dosages

▶ *To treat invasive aspergillosis in patients refractory to or intolerant of other therapies; to treat candidemia and candidal infections in intra-abdominal abscesses, peritonitis, and pleural space infections*

I.V. INFUSION

Adults. *Initial:* 70 mg on day 1, followed by 50 mg daily. *Maximum:* 70 mg daily.

▶ *To treat presumed fungal infections in febrile, neutropenic patients*

I.V. INFUSION

Adults. *Initial:* 70 mg on day 1, followed by 50 mg daily for at least 14 days, including at least 7 days after neutropenia and symptoms have resolved. Increased to 70 mg daily as needed. *Maximum:* 70 mg daily.

DOSAGE ADJUSTMENT Dosage reduced to 35 mg daily after initial 70-mg loading dose in moderate hepatic insufficiency.

▶ *To treat esophageal candidiasis*

I.V. INFUSION

Adults. 50 mg daily.

DOSAGE ADJUSTMENT Dosage reduced to 35 mg daily in moderate hepatic insufficiency.

Incompatibilities

Don't mix or infuse with other drugs. Don't admix with diluents that contain dextrose.

Contraindications

Hypersensitivity to caspofungin acetate or its components

Mechanism of Action

Caspofungin acetate interferes with fungal cell membrane synthesis by inhibiting the synthesis of b (1,3)-D-glucan. A polypeptide, b (1,3)-D-glucan is the essential component of the fungal cell membrane that makes it rigid and protective. Without it, fungal cells rupture and die. This mechanism of action is most effective against susceptible filamentous fungi, such as *Aspergillus.*

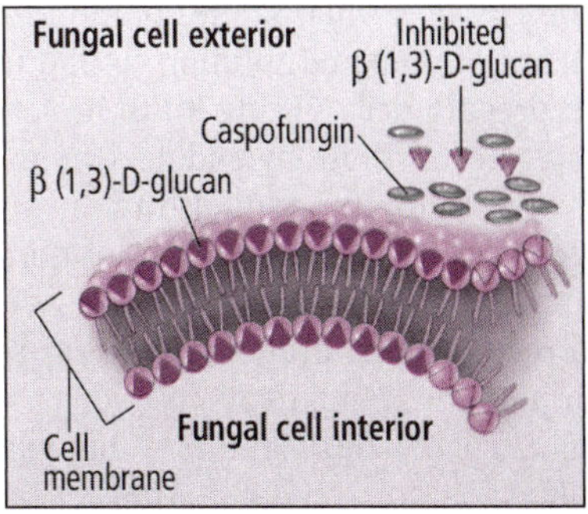

Interactions

DRUGS

carbamazepine, dexamethasone, efavirenz, nelfinavir, nevirapine, phenytoin, rifampin: Possibly decreased blood caspofungin level
cyclosporine: Transient increases in ALT and AST levels
tacrolimus: Possibly decreased blood tacrolimus level

Adverse Reactions

CNS: Chills, dizziness, fever, headache, insomnia, paresthesia, tremor
CV: Edema, hypertension, hypotension, phlebitis, tachycardia, thrombophlebitis
GI: Abdominal pain, diarrhea, elevated liver function test results, hepatic dysfunction, jaundice, nausea, vomiting
GU: Elevated BUN or serum creatinine level, proteinuria, renal insufficiency
HEME: Decreased hemoglobin and hematocrit
MS: Back pain, myalgia
RESP: Bronchospasm, dyspnea, stridor, tachypnea
SKIN: Diaphoresis, erythema, flushing, pruritus, rash, sensation of warmth
Other: Decreased serum bicarbonate level, facial edema, hypercalcemia, hyperkalemia, hyperphosphatemia, hypokalemia, hypomagnesemia, infusion site reaction

Nursing Considerations

- To prepare 70-mg loading dose, let vial reach room temperature. Reconstitute by adding 10.5 ml of normal saline solution

to vial. Dilute for administration by transferring 10 ml of reconstituted drug to 250 ml of normal saline solution.
- To prepare 70-mg loading dose from two 50-mg vials, add 10.5 ml of normal saline solution to each vial; then transfer 14 ml of prepared solution to 250 ml of normal saline solution.
- To prepare daily 50-mg infusion, let vial reach room temperature. Reconstitute by adding 10.5 ml of normal saline solution to vial. Dilute for administration by transferring only 10 ml of reconstituted drug to 250 ml of normal saline solution.
- To prepare daily 50-mg infusion at reduced volume, add 10 ml of reconstituted drug to 100 ml of normal saline solution.
- To prepare 35-mg daily dose for patient with moderate hepatic insufficiency, reconstitute 50-mg vial with 10.5 ml of normal saline solution. To dilute, transfer only 7 ml of reconstituted drug to 250 ml of normal saline solution or, if needed, to 100 ml of normal saline solution.
- When preparing powder for reconstitution, mix gently to obtain a clear solution. Don't use if solution is cloudy or contains precipitate. Discard unused solution after 24 hours.
- Infuse drug slowly over approximately 1 hour.
- Expect to increase daily dose to 70 mg, as prescribed, for patients not responding to carbamazepine, dexamethasone, efavirenz, nelfinavir, nevirapine, phenytoin, or rifampin.
- Watch for flushed skin, and assess patient often for unexplained temperature elevation.
- Assess for airway patency if patient develops excessive facial edema or respiratory stridor. Provide emergency airway management if complete obstruction occurs.
- Monitor patient's liver function test results, as ordered, and report abnormalities.

PATIENT TEACHING
- Urge patient to notify prescriber immediately if he has difficulty talking, swallowing, or breathing during caspofungin administration.

cefazolin sodium

Ancef

Class and Category

Chemical: First-generation cephalosporin, 7-aminocephalosporanic acid
Therapeutic: Antibiotic

Pregnancy category: B

Indications and Dosages

▶ *To treat respiratory tract infections caused by group A beta-hemolytic streptococci,* Haemophilus influenzae, Klebsiella *sp.,* Staphylococcus aureus, *and* Streptococcus pneumoniae; *skin and soft-tissue infections caused by* S. aureus, *group A beta-hemolytic and other strains of streptococci; biliary tract infections caused by* Escherichia coli, Klebsiella *sp.,* Proteus mirabilis, S. aureus, *and various strains of streptococci; bone and joint infections caused by* S. aureus; *genital infections, such as epididymitis and prostatitis, caused by* E. coli, Klebsiella *sp.,* P. mirabilis, *and some strains of enterococci; septicemia caused by* E. coli, Klebsiella *sp.,* P. mirabilis, S. aureus, *and* S. pneumoniae; *and endocarditis caused by group A beta-hemolytic streptococci and* S. aureus

I.V. INFUSION, I.V. INJECTION

Adults. For mild infections, 250 to 500 mg q 8 hr; for moderate to severe infections, 500 to 1,000 mg q 6 to 8 hr; and for severe life-threatening infections, 1,000 to 1,500 mg q 6 hr. *Maximum:* 6 g daily.

Children. For mild to moderate infections, 25 to 50 mg/kg daily divided equally and given t.i.d. or q.i.d.; for severe infections, 100 mg/kg daily divided equally and given t.i.d. or q.i.d.

▶ *To treat pneumococcal pneumonia*

I.V. INFUSION, I.V. INJECTION

Adults. 500 mg q 12 hr.

▶ *To treat acute uncomplicated UTI caused by* E. coli, Klebsiella *sp.,* P. mirabilis, *and some strains of* Enterobacter *and* Enterococcus

I.V. INFUSION, I.V. INJECTION

Adults. 1 g q 12 hr.

▶ *To provide surgical prophylaxis*

I.V. INFUSION, I.V. INJECTION

Adults. 1 g 30 to 60 min before surgery; 0.5 to 1 g during surgery if it lasts 2 hr or longer; 0.5 to 1 g q 6 to 8 hr for 24 hr after surgery.

DOSAGE ADJUSTMENT After initial loading dose appropriate to infection's severity, dosage interval at least 8 hr for adults with creatinine clearance of 35 to 54 ml/min/1.73 m^2; dosage reduced by 50% and given q 12 hr for adults with creatinine clearance of 11 to 34 ml/min/1.73 m^2; and dosage reduced by 50% and given q 18 to 24 hr for adults with creatinine clearance of 10 ml/min/1.73 m^2 or less. Dosage reduced to 60% and given q 12 hr for children with creatinine clearance of

40 to 70 ml/min/1.73 m^2; dosage reduced to 25% and given q 12 hr for children with creatinine clearance of 20 to 40 ml/min/1.73 m^2; and dosage reduced to 10% and given q 24 hr for children with creatinine clearance of 5 to 20 ml/min/1.73 m^2.

Mechanism of Action

Interferes with bacterial cell wall synthesis by inhibiting the final step in the cross-linking of peptidoglycan strands. Peptidoglycan makes cell membranes rigid and protective. Without it, bacterial cells rupture and die.

Incompatibilities

To prevent mutual inactivation, don't mix cefazolin with aminoglycosides. Also avoid mixing cefazolin with other drugs, including pentamidine isethionate.

Contraindications

Hypersensitivity to cephalosporins or their components

Interactions

DRUGS

aminoglycosides, loop diuretics: Additive nephrotoxicity
probenecid: Increased and prolonged blood cefazolin level

Adverse Reactions

CNS: Chills, fever, headache, seizures
CV: Edema
EENT: Hearing loss
GI: Abdominal cramps, diarrhea, elevated liver function test results, hepatic failure, hepatitis, hepatomegaly, nausea, oral candidiasis, pseudomembranous colitis, vomiting
GU: Elevated BUN and serum creatinine levels, nephrotoxicity, renal failure, vaginal candidiasis
HEME: Eosinophilia, hemolytic anemia, hypoprothrombinemia, neutropenia, thrombocytopenia, unusual bleeding
MS: Arthralgia
RESP: Dyspnea
SKIN: Ecchymosis, erythema, erythema multiforme, pruritus, rash, Stevens-Johnson syndrome
Other: Anaphylaxis; injection site pain, redness, and swelling; superinfection

Nursing Considerations

- Use cefazolin cautiously in patients with impaired renal function or a history of GI disease, particularly colitis. Also use drug cautiously in patients who are hypersensitive to penicillin because cross-sensitivity has occurred in 10% of such patients.
- If possible, obtain culture and sensitivity test results, as ordered, before giving drug.
- **WARNING** To prevent unintentional overdose, cefazolin for injection USP and dextrose injection USP shouldn't be used in children who require less than the full adult dose.
- Reconstitute 500-mg vial of drug with 2 ml of sterile water for injection (or 1-g vial with 2.5 ml). Shake well until dissolved.
- For direct I.V. injection, further dilute reconstituted solution with at least 5 ml sterile water for injection. Inject slowly over 3 to 5 minutes in tubing of a flowing compatible I.V. solution.
- For intermittent I.V. infusion, reconstitute 500 to 1,000 mg in 50 to 100 ml of normal saline solution, D_5W, $D_{10}W$, D_5/lactated Ringer's, D_5/0.2 normal saline solution, D_5/0.45 normal saline solution, D_5/normal saline solution, lactated Ringer's injection, 5% or 10% invert sugar in sterile water for injection, 5% sodium bicarbonate (Ancef), or Ringer's injection.
- Store reconstituted cefazolin up to 24 hours at room temperature or 10 days under refrigeration.
- Monitor I.V. site for irritation, phlebitis, and extravasation.
- Monitor BUN and serum creatinine levels for early signs of nephrotoxicity. Also monitor fluid intake and output; decreasing urine output may indicate nephrotoxicity.
- Be aware that an allergic reaction may occur a few days after therapy starts.
- Assess bowel pattern daily; severe diarrhea may indicate pseudomembranous colitis.
- Watch for evidence of superinfection: cough, diarrhea, drainage, fever, malaise, pain, perineal itching, rash, redness, swelling.
- Assess for pharyngitis, ecchymosis, bleeding, and arthralgia; they may indicate a blood dyscrasia.

PATIENT TEACHING

- Instruct patient to complete the prescribed course of therapy.
- Tell patient to immediately report severe diarrhea to prescriber.

cefepime hydrochloride

Maxipime

Class and Category

Chemical: Fourth-generation cephalosporin, 7-aminocephalosporanic acid
Therapeutic: Antibiotic
Pregnancy category: B

Indications and Dosages

▶ *To treat mild to moderate UTI caused by* Escherichia coli, Klebsiella pneumoniae, *or* Proteus mirabilis
I.V. INFUSION
Adults and children age 12 and over. 500 to 1,000 mg q 12 hr for 7 to 10 days.

▶ *To treat severe UTI caused by* E. coli *or* K. pneumoniae, *moderate to severe skin and soft-tissue infections caused by* Staphylococcus aureus *or* Streptococcus pyogenes
I.V. INFUSION
Adults and children age 12 and over. 2 g q 12 hr for 10 days.

▶ *To treat moderate to severe pneumonia caused by* Enterobacter *sp.,* K. pneumoniae, Pseudomonas aeruginosa, *or* Streptococcus pneumoniae
I.V. INFUSION
Adults and children age 12 and over. 1 to 2 g q 12 hr for 10 days.

▶ *To treat febrile neutropenia*
I.V. INFUSION
Adults and children age 12 and over. 2 g q 8 hr for 7 days or until neutropenia resolves.

▶ *To treat complicated intra-abdominal infections (together with metronidazole) caused by alpha-hemolytic streptococci,* Bacteroides fragilis, E. coli, Enterobacter *sp.,* K. pneumoniae, *or* P. aeruginosa
I.V. INFUSION
Adults and children age 12 and over. 2 g q 12 hr for 7 to 10 days.

DOSAGE ADJUSTMENT Dosing interval increased from 12 to 24 hr and from 8 to 12 hr for patients with creatinine clearance of 30 to 60 ml/min/1.73 m^2; dosing interval increased from 8 or 12 hr to 24 hr and dose decreased from 2 g q 12 hr to 1 g q 24 hr (all other doses remain unchanged) for patients with creatinine clearance of 11 to 29 ml/min/1.73 m^2; dosage decreased from 500 mg q 12 hr to 250 mg q 24 hr, from 1,000 mg q 12 hr to 250 mg q 24 hr, from 2,000 mg q 12 hr to 500 mg q 24 hr, and from 2 g q 8 hr to 1 g q 24 hr if creatinine clearance is less than 11 ml/min/1.73 m^2.

Mechanism of Action

Interferes with bacterial cell wall synthesis by inhibiting the final step in the cross-linking of peptidoglycan strands. Peptidoglycan makes cell membranes rigid and protective. Without it, bacterial cells rupture and die.

Incompatibilities

Don't add cefepime to solutions that contain ampicillin in a concentration of more than 40 mg/ml. Don't add drug to solutions that contain aminophylline, gentamycin, metronidazole, netilmicin sulfate, tobramycin, or vancomycin.

Contraindications

Hypersensitivity to cephalosporins or their components

Interactions

DRUGS

aminoglycosides, loop diuretics: Increased risk of renal failure in patients with renal disease

Adverse Reactions

CNS: Chills, fever, headache, seizures
CV: Edema
EENT: Hearing loss
GI: Abdominal cramps, diarrhea, elevated liver function test results, hepatic failure, hepatomegaly, nausea, oral candidiasis, pseudomembranous colitis, vomiting
GU: Elevated BUN level, nephrotoxicity, renal failure, vaginal candidiasis
HEME: Eosinophilia, hemolytic anemia, hypoprothrombinemia, neutropenia, thrombocytopenia, unusual bleeding
MS: Arthralgia
RESP: Dyspnea
SKIN: Ecchymosis, erythema, erythema multiforme, pruritus, rash, Stevens-Johnson syndrome
Other: Anaphylaxis; injection site pain, redness, and swelling; superinfection

Nursing Considerations

- Use cefepime cautiously in patients with impaired renal function or a history of GI disease, particularly colitis. Also use drug cautiously in patients who are hypersensitive to penicillin because cross-sensitivity has occurred in about 10% of such patients.

- If possible, obtain culture and sensitivity test results, as ordered, before giving drug.
- For I.V. infusion, reconstitute according to manufacturer's guidelines. Administer over 30 minutes.
- Be aware that an allergic reaction may occur a few days after therapy starts.
- Monitor BUN and serum creatinine levels for early signs of nephrotoxicity. Also monitor fluid intake and output; decreasing urine output may indicate nephrotoxicity. Be aware that unadjusted dosages of cefepime in renally impaired patients may cause myoclonus and seizures.
- Assess bowel pattern daily; severe diarrhea may indicate pseudomembranous colitis.
- Assess for signs of superinfection, such as perineal itching, fever, malaise, redness, pain, swelling, drainage, rash, diarrhea, and cough or sputum changes.
- Assess for pharyngitis, ecchymosis, bleeding, and arthralgia; they may indicate a blood dyscrasia.

PATIENT TEACHING

- Tell patient to immediately report severe diarrhea to the prescriber.

cefmetazole sodium

Zefazone

Class and Category

Chemical: Second-generation cephalosporin, 7-aminocephalosporanic acid
Therapeutic: Antibiotic
Pregnancy category: B

Indications and Dosages

▶ *To treat UTI caused by* Escherichia coli; *lower respiratory tract infections, such as bronchitis and pneumonia, caused by* E. coli, Haemophilus influenzae, Staphylococcus aureus, *or* Streptococcus pneumoniae; *skin and soft-tissue infections caused by* Bacteroides fragilis, B. melaninogenicus, E. coli, Klebsiella oxytoca, Klebsiella pneumoniae, Morganella morganii, Proteus mirabilis, Proteus vulgaris, S. aureus, Staphylococcus epidermidis, Streptococcus agalactiae, *or* Streptococcus pyogenes; *and intra-abdominal infections caused by* B. fragilis, Clostridium perfringens, E. coli, K. oxytoca, *or* K. pneumoniae

I.V. INFUSION

Adults. 2 g q 6 to 12 hr for 5 to 14 days.

DOSAGE ADJUSTMENT Dosage reduced to 1 to 2 g q 12 hr for patients with creatinine clearance of 50 to 90 ml/min/ 1.73 m^2; 1 to 2 g q 16 hr for patients with creatinine clearance of 30 to 49 ml/min/1.73 m^2; 1 to 2 g q 24 hr for patients with creatinine clearance of 10 to 29 ml/min/1.73 m^2; and 1 to 2 g q 48 hr for patients with creatinine clearance of less than 10 ml/ min/1.73 m^2.

► *To provide surgical prophylaxis for vaginal hysterectomy*

I.V. INFUSION

Adults. 2 g as a single dose given 30 to 90 min before surgery, or 1 g given 30 to 90 min before surgery and repeated 8 and 16 hr later.

► *To provide surgical prophylaxis for abdominal hysterectomy and for high-risk cholecystectomy*

I.V. INFUSION

Adults. 1 g given 30 to 90 min before surgery and repeated 8 and 16 hr later.

► *To provide surgical prophylaxis for cesarean section*

I.V. INFUSION

Adults. 2 g as a single dose after cord is clamped or 1 g after cord is clamped and then repeated 8 and 16 hr later.

► *To provide surgical prophylaxis for colorectal surgery*

I.V. INFUSION

Adults. 2 g as a single dose 30 to 90 min before surgery, or 2 g given 30 to 90 min before surgery and repeated 8 and 16 hr later.

Mechanism of Action

Interferes with bacterial cell wall synthesis by inhibiting the final step in the cross-linking of peptidoglycan strands. Peptidoglycan makes cell membranes rigid and protective. Without it, bacterial cells rupture and die.

Contraindications

Hypersensitivity to cephalosporins or their components

Interactions

DRUGS

aminoglycosides, loop diuretics: Increased risk of nephrotoxicity

anticoagulants: Possibly increased anticoagulant effect

probenecid: Increased and prolonged blood cefmetazole level

ACTIVITIES
alcohol use: Possibly disulfiram-like reaction

Adverse Reactions

CNS: Chills, fever, headache, seizures
CV: Edema
EENT: Hearing loss, oral candidiasis
GI: Abdominal cramps, diarrhea, elevated liver function test results, hepatic failure, hepatomegaly, nausea, pseudomembranous colitis, vomiting
GU: Elevated BUN level, nephrotoxicity, renal failure, vaginal candidiasis
HEME: Eosinophilia, hemolytic anemia, hypoprothrombinemia, neutropenia, thrombocytopenia, unusual bleeding
MS: Arthralgia
RESP: Dyspnea
SKIN: Ecchymosis, erythema, erythema multiforme, pruritus, rash, Stevens-Johnson syndrome
Other: Anaphylaxis, infusion site thrombophlebitis, superinfection

Nursing Considerations

- If possible, obtain culture and sensitivity test results, as ordered, before giving cefmetazole.
- Reconstitute drug with sterile water for injection, bacteriostatic water for injection, or 0.9% sodium chloride for injection.
- Store reconstituted solution for up to 24 hours at room temperature or for up to 7 days when refrigerated. Solution may also be frozen at −20° C (−4° F) or less for up to 6 weeks.
- Dilute primary solution as needed to 1 to 20 mg/ml in D_5W, normal saline solution, lactated Ringer's solution, or 1% lidocaine solution without epinephrine. Diluted solution remains potent for 24 hours if stored at room temperature, for 7 days if refrigerated, and for 6 weeks if frozen.
- Monitor for signs of an allergic reaction, such as difficulty breathing or a rash, especially in patients who are hypersensitive to penicillin, because cross-sensitivity has occurred in about 10% of such patients.
- Monitor BUN and serum creatinine levels to detect early signs of nephrotoxicity, especially in patients with impaired renal function. Also monitor fluid intake and output; decreasing urine output may indicate nephrotoxicity.
- Assess bowel pattern daily; severe diarrhea may indicate pseudomembranous colitis. Patients with a history of GI disease, particularly colitis, are at increased risk.

- Assess for signs of superinfection, such as perineal itching, fever, malaise, redness, pain, swelling, drainage, rash, diarrhea, and cough or sputum changes.
- Assess for pharyngitis, ecchymosis, bleeding, and arthralgia, which may indicate a blood dyscrasia. Monitor PT and bleeding time as ordered.
- Don't refreeze thawed solutions.

PATIENT TEACHING

- Advise patient receiving cefmetazole to immediately report severe diarrheaor signs of blood dyscrasia or superinfection. Inform him that yogurt or buttermilk can help decrease diarrhea.
- Instruct patient to avoid alcohol during therapy and for at least 3 days after taking last dose.
- Review with patient other possibly serious adverse reactions, including difficulty breathing, rash, and chest tightness, and tell him to report any that occur.

cefonicid sodium

Monocid

Class and Category

Chemical: Second-generation cephalosporin, 7-aminocephalosporanic acid
Therapeutic: Antibiotic
Pregnancy category: B

Indications and Dosages

▶ *To treat lower respiratory tract infection caused by* Escherichia coli, Haemophilus influenzae, Klebsiella pneumoniae, *or* Streptococcus pneumoniae; *UTI caused by* E. coli, K. pneumoniae, Morganella morganii, Proteus mirabilis, Proteus vulgaris, *or* Providencia rettgeri; *skin and soft-tissue infections caused by* Staphylococcus aureus, Staphylococcus epidermidis, Streptococcus agalactiae, *or* Streptococcus pyogenes; *septicemia caused by* E. coli *or* S. pneumoniae; *and bone and joint infections caused by* S. aureus

I.V. INFUSION, I.V. INJECTION

Adults. For mild to moderate infection, 1 g q 24 hr; for severe or life-threatening infection, 2 g q 24 hr.

▶ *To treat uncomplicated UTI*

I.V. INFUSION, I.V. INJECTION

Adults. 500 mg q 24 hr.

DOSAGE ADJUSTMENT Initial dose reduced to 75 mg/kg in

patients with impaired renal function. Then dosage reduced to 10 to 25 mg/kg q 24 hr if creatinine clearance ranges from 60 to 79 ml/min/1.73 m^2; 8 to 20 mg/kg q 24 hr if creatinine clearance ranges from 40 to 59 ml/min/1.73 m^2; 4 to 15 mg/kg q 24 hr if creatinine clearance ranges from 20 to 39 ml/min/1.73 m^2; 4 to 15 mg/kg q 48 hr if creatinine clearance ranges from 10 to 19 ml/min/1.73 m^2; 4 to 15 mg/kg q 3 to 5 days if creatinine clearance ranges from 5 to 9 ml/minute/1.73 m^2; and 3 to 4 mg/kg q 3 to 5 days if creatinine clearance is less than 5 ml/min/1.73 m^2.

▶ *To provide surgical prophylaxis*

I.V. INFUSION, I.V. INJECTION

Adults. 1 g 60 min before surgery. Dose repeated once daily, if needed, for 2 days after prosthetic arthroplasty or open-heart surgery.

Mechanism of Action

Interferes with bacterial cell wall synthesis by inhibiting the final step in the cross-linking of peptidoglycan strands. Peptidoglycan makes cell membranes rigid and protective. Without it, bacterial cells rupture and die.

Incompatibilities

To prevent mutual inactivation, don't mix cefonicid with aminoglycosides.

Contraindications

Hypersensitivity to cephalosporins or their components

Interactions

DRUGS

aminoglycosides, loop diuretics: Increased risk of nephrotoxicity
probenecid: Increased and prolonged blood cefonicid level

Adverse Reactions

CNS: Chills, fever, headache, seizures
CV: Edema
EENT: Hearing loss, oral candidiasis
GI: Abdominal cramps, diarrhea, elevated liver function test results, hepatic failure, hepatomegaly, nausea, pseudomembranous colitis, vomiting
GU: Elevated BUN level, nephrotoxicity, renal failure, vaginal candidiasis

HEME: Eosinophilia, hemolytic anemia, hypoprothrombinemia, neutropenia, thrombocytopenia, unusual bleeding
MS: Arthralgia
RESP: Dyspnea
SKIN: Ecchymosis, erythema, erythema multiforme, pruritus, rash, Stevens-Johnson syndrome
Other: Anaphylaxis, infusion site thrombophlebitis, superinfection

Nursing Considerations

- If possible, obtain culture and sensitivity test results, as ordered, before giving cefonicid.
- Reconstitute each 500-mg vial of drug with 2 ml of sterile water for injection (or each 1-g vial with 2.5 ml).
- For I.V. infusion, dilute further in 50 to 100 ml of compatible solution, such as D_5W, $D_{10}W$, D_5/0.2 normnal saline solution, D_5/0.45 normal saline solution, or D_5/normal saline solution.
- Be aware that 1 g of cefonicid/18 ml of sterile water for injection is an isotonic solution.
- Store reconstituted solution at room temperature for up to 24 hours or under refrigeration for up to 72 hours.
- Administer I.V. injection slowly over 3 to 5 minutes through tubing of a flowing compatible I.V. solution.
- Monitor patient for signs of an allergic reaction, such as difficulty breathing or a rash, especially in patients who are hypersensitive to penicillin, because cross-sensitivity has occurred in about 10% of such patients.
- Monitor BUN and serum creatinine levels to detect early signs of nephrotoxicity, especially in patients with impaired renal function. Also monitor fluid intake and output; decreasing urine output may indicate nephrotoxicity.
- Assess bowel pattern daily; severe diarrhea may indicate pseudomembranous colitis. Patients with a history of GI disease, particularly colitis, are at increased risk.
- Assess for signs of superinfection, such as perineal itching, fever, malaise, redness, pain, swelling, drainage, rash, diarrhea, and cough or sputum changes.
- Assess for pharyngitis, ecchymosis, bleeding, and arthralgia, which may indicate a blood dyscrasia. Monitor PT and bleeding time as ordered.
- Before reconstituting drug, store it at 2° to 8° C (36° to 46° F). Protect from light.

PATIENT TEACHING

- Advise patient receiving cefonicid to immediately report severe diarrhea or signs of blood dyscrasia or superinfection. Inform him that yogurt or buttermilk can help decrease diarrhea.
- Review with patient other possibly serious adverse reactions, including difficulty breathing, rash, and chest tightness, and tell him to report any that occur.

cefoperazone sodium

Cefobid

Class and Category

Chemical: Third-generation cephalosporin, 7-aminocephalosporanic acid
Therapeutic: Antibiotic
Pregnancy category: B

Indications and Dosages

▶ *To treat respiratory tract infection caused by* Enterobacter *sp.,* Escherichia coli, Haemophilus influenzae, Klebsiella pneumoniae, Proteus mirabilis, Pseudomonas aeruginosa, Staphylococcus aureus, Streptococcus pneumoniae, Streptococcus pyogenes, *or other streptococci (excluding enterococci); UTI caused by* E. coli *or* P. aeruginosa; *uncomplicated gonorrhea caused by* Neisseria gonorrhoeae; *gynecologic infections caused by anaerobic gram-positive cocci,* Bacteroides *sp.,* Clostridium *sp.,* E. coli, Staphylococcus epidermidis, *or* Streptococcus agalactiae; *bacterial septicemia caused by* E. coli, Klebsiella *sp.,* S. aureus, Serratia marcescens, *or streptococci; skin and soft-tissue infections caused by* P. aeruginosa, S. aureus, *or* S. pyogenes; *and intra-abdominal infections caused by anaerobic gram-negative bacilli,* E. coli, *or* P. aeruginosa

I.V. INFUSION

Adults. 1 to 2 g q 12 hr. For severe infections or those caused by less sensitive organisms, 6 to 12 g daily divided into equal doses and given b.i.d., t.i.d., or q.i.d. *Maximum:* 12 g daily.

Incompatibilities

To prevent mutual inactivation, don't mix cefoperazone with aminoglycosides. Also avoid mixing cefoperazone with other drugs, including pentamidine isethionate.

Contraindications

Hypersensitivity to cephalosporins or their components

Mechanism of Action

Interferes with bacterial cell wall synthesis by inhibiting the final step in the cross-linking of peptidoglycan strands. Peptidoglycan makes cell membranes rigid and protective. Without it, bacterial cells rupture and die.

Interactions

DRUGS

aminoglycosides, loop diuretics: Increased risk of nephrotoxicity
oral anticoagulants, other drugs that affect blood clotting: Increased anticoagulant effect

ACTIVITIES

alcohol use: Disulfiram-like reaction from acetaldehyde accumulation

Adverse Reactions

CNS: Chills, fever, headache, seizures
CV: Edema
EENT: Hearing loss, oral candidiasis
GI: Abdominal cramps, diarrhea, elevated liver function test results, hepatic failure, hepatomegaly, nausea, pseudomembranous colitis, vomiting
GU: Elevated BUN level, nephrotoxicity, renal failure, vaginal candidiasis
HEME: Eosinophilia, hemolytic anemia, hypoprothrombinemia, neutropenia, thrombocytopenia, unusual bleeding
MS: Arthralgia
RESP: Dyspnea
SKIN: Ecchymosis, erythema, erythema multiforme, pruritus, rash, Stevens-Johnson syndrome
Other: Anaphylaxis, infusion site thrombophlebitis, superinfection

Nursing Considerations

- Expect cefoperazone dosage to be reduced for patients with combined renal and hepatic function impairment. Monitor serum drug levels in patients with impaired hepatic function or biliary obstruction who are receiving more than 4 g/day; dosage may need to be reduced.
- If possible, obtain culture and sensitivity test results, as ordered, before giving drug.
- Reconstitute cefoperazone for injection with required amount of diluent; then dilute further in compatible solution, such as D_5W, $D_{10}W$, D_5/lactated Ringer's solution, D_5/0.2 normal saline

solution, D_5/normal saline soluiton, lactated Ringer's solution, normal saline solution, Normosol M and D_5W, or Normosol R. (See manufacturer's guidelines for details.)
- After drug reconstitution, let foam dissipate and inspect solution to ensure complete dissolution.
- Store reconstituted solution of cefoperazone for injection at room temperature for 24 hours.
- Be aware that cefoperazone also comes in a minibag (cefoperazone injection) with a concentration of 1 or 2 g/50 ml. Before use, store minibag at −25° to −10° C (−13° to 14° F). Thaw at room temperature of 25° C (77° F) or under refrigeration at 5° C (41° F). Don't thaw with warm bath or microwave. Make sure that all ice crystals have melted before use.
- After thawing minibag, use it within 48 hours if stored at room temperature or within 14 days if refrigerated. Don't refreeze. Discard solution if it's cloudy or contains precipitate.
- To prevent air embolism, don't administer minibags (cefoperazone injection) using I.V. lines with series connections.
- Give drug as intermittent infusion over 15 to 30 minutes or as continuous infusion. Direct bolus injection isn't recommended.
- Monitor BUN and serum creatinine levels to detect early signs of nephrotoxicity. Also monitor fluid intake and output; decreasing urine output may indicate nephrotoxicity.
- Monitor for signs of an allergic reaction, such as difficulty breathing or a rash, especially in patients who are hypersensitive to penicillin, because cross-sensitivity has occurred in about 10% of such patients.
- Assess bowel pattern daily; severe diarrhea may indicate pseudomembranous colitis. Patients with a history of GI disease, particularly colitis, are at increased risk.
- Assess for pharyngitis, ecchymosis, bleeding, and arthralgia, which may indicate a blood dyscrasia. Monitor PT and bleeding time as ordered. Be prepared to administer vitamin K, if ordered, to treat hypoprothrombinemia.
- Assess for signs of superinfection, such as perineal itching, fever, malaise, redness, pain, swelling, drainage, rash, diarrhea, and cough or sputum changes.
- Before reconstituting cefoperazone for injection, store at 15° to 30° C (59° to 86° F). Protect from light.

PATIENT TEACHING
- Ask patient to avoid alcohol during cefoperazone therapy and for at least 3 days after taking the last dose.

- Instruct patient to immediately report severe diarrhea or signs of blood dyscrasia or superinfection. Inform him that yogurt or buttermilk can help decrease diarrhea.
- Review with patient other possibly serious adverse reactions, including difficulty breathing, rash, and chest tightness, and tell him to report any that occur.

cefotaxime sodium

Claforan

Class and Category

Chemical: Third-generation cephalosporin, 7-aminocephalosporanic acid
Therapeutic: Antibiotic
Pregnancy category: B

Indications and Dosages

▶ *To provide perioperative prophylaxis*

I.V. INFUSION, I.V. INJECTION

Adults and children weighing more than 50 kg (110 lb). 1 g 30 to 90 min before surgery.

▶ *To provide perioperative prophylaxis related to cesarean section*

I.V. INFUSION, I.V. INJECTION

Adults. 1 g as soon as cord is clamped, then 1 g q 6 hr for up to two doses.

▶ *To treat disseminated gonorrhea*

I.V. INFUSION, I.V. INJECTION

Adults and children weighing more than 50 kg. 1 g q 8 hr.

▶ *To treat uncomplicated infections caused by susceptible organisms*

I.V. INFUSION, I.V. INJECTION

Adults and children weighing more than 50 kg. 1 g q 12 hr.
Children ages 1 month to 12 years weighing less than 50 kg. 50 to 180 mg/kg/day in four to six divided doses.
Children ages 1 to 4 weeks. 50 mg/kg I.V. q 8 hr.
Children age 1 week and younger. 50 mg/kg I.V. q 12 hr.

▶ *To treat moderate to severe infections caused by susceptible organisms*

I.V. INFUSION, I.V. INJECTION

Adults and children weighing more than 50 kg. 1 to 2 g q 8 hr.
Children ages 1 month to 12 years weighing less than 50 kg. 50 to 180 mg/kg daily in four to six divided doses. More serious infections, including meningitis, warrant higher dosages.

Children ages 1 to 4 weeks. 50 mg/kg I.V. q 8 hr.
Children age 1 week and younger. 50 mg/kg I.V. q 12 hr.

▶ *To treat septicemia and other infections that commonly require antibiotics in higher doses than those used to treat moderate to severe infections*

I.V. INFUSION, I.V. INJECTION
Adults and children weighing more than 50 kg. 2 g q 6 to 8 hr.

▶ *To treat life-threatening infections caused by susceptible organisms*

I.V. INFUSION, I.V. INJECTION
Adults and children weighing more than 50 kg. 2 g q 4 hr. *Maximum:* 12 g/day.
Children ages 1 month to 12 years weighing less than 50 kg. 50 to 180 mg/kg/day in four to six divided doses.
Children ages 1 to 4 weeks. 50 mg/kg q 8 hr.
Children age 1 week and younger. 50 mg/kg q 12 hr.
DOSAGE ADJUSTMENT Dosage reduced by 50% for patients with estimated creatinine clearance less than 20 ml/min/ 1.73 m^2.

Mechanism of Action

Interferes with bacterial cell wall synthesis by inhibiting the cross-linking of peptidoglycan strands. Peptidoglycan makes cell membranes rigid and protective. Without it, bacterial cells rupture and die.

Incompatibilities

To prevent mutual inactivation, don't mix cefotaxime with aminoglycosides. Also avoid mixing cefotaxime with other drugs, including pentamidine isethionate.

Contraindications

Hypersensitivity to cephalosporins or their components

Interactions

DRUGS
aminoglycosides, loop diuretics: Increased risk of nephrotoxicity
probenecid: Increased and prolonged blood cefotaxime level

Adverse Reactions

CNS: Chills, fever, headache, seizures
CV: Edema
EENT: Hearing loss

GI: Abdominal cramps, diarrhea, elevated liver function test results, hepatic failure, hepatomegaly, nausea, oral candidiasis, pseudomembranous colitis, vomiting
GU: Elevated BUN level, nephrotoxicity, renal failure, vaginal candidiasis
HEME: Eosinophilia, hemolytic anemia, hypoprothrombinemia, neutropenia, thrombocytopenia, unusual bleeding
MS: Arthralgia
RESP: Dyspnea
SKIN: Ecchymosis, erythema, erythema multiforme, pruritus, rash, Stevens-Johnson syndrome, toxic epidermal necrolysis
Other: Anaphylaxis; injection site pain, redness, and swelling; superinfection

Nursing Considerations

- Use cefotaxime cautiously in patients with impaired renal function, a history of GI disease (especially colitis), or hypersensitivity to penicillin; cross-sensitivity has occurred in 10% of such patients.
- If possible, obtain culture and sensitivity test results, as ordered, before giving drug.
- For I.V. use, reconstitute each 0.5-, 1-, or 2-g vial with 10 ml of sterile water for injection. Shake to dissolve.
- For intermittent I.V. infusion, further dilute in 50 to 100 ml of D_5W or normal saline solution.
- **WARNING** When preparing drug for a neonate, don't use diluent that contains benzyl alcohol; it could cause a fatal toxic syndrome.
- Give cefotaxime by I.V. injection over 3 to 5 minutes through tubing of a flowing compatible I.V. solution. Temporarily stop other solutions being given through same I.V. site.
- Discard unused drug after 24 hours if stored at room temperature, 5 days if refrigerated.
- Protect cefotaxime powder and solution from light and heat.
- Monitor I.V. sites for signs of phlebitis or extravasation. Rotate I.V. sites every 72 hours.
- Monitor BUN and serum creatinine levels and fluid intake and output for signs of nephrotoxicity.
- Be aware that an allergic reaction may occur a few days after therapy starts.
- Assess bowel pattern daily; severe diarrhea may indicate pseudomembranous colitis.

- Assess patient for pharyngitis, ecchymosis, bleeding, and arthralgia, which may indicate a blood dyscrasia. Monitor CBC, PT, and bleeding time, as ordered.
- Monitor patient closely for superinfection. If signs appear, notify prescriber and expect to stop drug and give appropriate care.

PATIENT TEACHING

- Instruct patient to immediately report severe diarrhea to prescriber.

cefoxitin sodium

Mefoxin

Class and Category

Chemical: Second-generation cephalosporin, 7-aminocephalosporanic acid
Therapeutic: Antibiotic
Pregnancy category: B

Indications and Dosages

▶ *To provide surgical prophylaxis*

I.V. INFUSION, I.V. INJECTION

Adults. 2 g 30 to 60 min before surgery and then 2 g q 6 hr after first dose for up to 24 hr.

Children age 3 months or over. 30 to 40 mg/kg 30 to 60 min before surgery and then q 6 hr after first dose for up to 24 hr.

▶ *To provide surgical prophylaxis for cesarean section*

I.V. INFUSION, I.V. INJECTION

Adults. 2 g as a single dose as soon as cord is clamped or 2 g as soon as cord is clamped followed by 2 g 4 and 8 hr after initial dose.

▶ *To provide surgical prophylaxis for transurethral prostatectomy*

I.V. INFUSION, I.V. INJECTION

Adults. 1 g 30 to 60 min before surgery and then 1 g q 8 hr for up to 5 days.

▶ *To treat infection, including septicemia, gynecologic infection, intra-abdominal infection, UTI, and infection of the lower respiratory tract, skin, soft tissue, bones, and joints caused by anaerobes (including* Bacteroides *sp.,* Clostridium *sp.,* Fusobacterium *sp.,* Peptococcus niger, *and* Peptostreptococcus *sp.), gram-negative organisms (including* Escherichia coli, Haemophilus influenzae *[and ampicillin-resistant strains],* Klebsiella, *and* Proteus *sp.), and gram-positive organisms (including* Staphylococcus aureus *[penicillinase- and non-penicillinase-producing strains],* Staphylococcus epidermidis, Streptococcus agalactiae, Streptococcus pneumoniae, *and* Streptococcus pyogenes*)*

I.V. INFUSION, I.V. INJECTION

Adults. For uncomplicated infections, 1 g q 6 to 8 hr; for moderate to severe infections, 1 g q 4 hr or 2 g q 6 to 8 hr; for infections that commonly require high-dose antibiotics (such as gas gangrene), 2 g q 4 hr or 3 g q 6 hr.

Children age 3 months or over. 80 to 160 mg/kg/day in equal doses and given q 4 to 6 hr (with higher dosages used for more severe infections). *Maximum:* 12 g/day.

DOSAGE ADJUSTMENT Dosage reduced to 1 to 2 g q 8 to 12 hr if creatinine clearance is 30 to 50 ml/min/1.73 m^2; 1 to 2 g q 12 to 24 hr if clearance is 10 to 29 ml/min/1.73 m^2; 0.5 to 1 g q 12 to 24 hr if clearance is 5 to 9 ml/min/1.73 m^2; and 0.5 to 1 g q 24 to 48 hr if clearance is less than 5 ml/min/1.73 m^2.

Mechanism of Action

Interferes with bacterial cell wall synthesis by inhibiting the final step in the cross-linking of peptidoglycan strands. Peptidoglycan makes cell membranes rigid and protective. Without it, bacterial cells rupture and die.

Incompatibilities

To prevent mutual inactivation, don't mix cefoxitin with aminoglycosides. Also avoid mixing cefoxitin with other drugs, including pentamidine isethionate.

Contraindications

Hypersensitivity to cephalosporins or their components

Interactions

DRUGS

aminoglycosides, loop diuretics: Increased risk of nephrotoxicity

Adverse Reactions

CNS: Chills, fever, headache, seizures

CV: Edema

EENT: Hearing loss

GI: Abdominal cramps, diarrhea, elevated liver function test results, hepatic failure, hepatomegaly, nausea, oral candidiasis, pseudomembranous colitis, vomiting

GU: Elevated BUN level, nephrotoxicity, renal failure, vaginal candidiasis

HEME: Eosinophilia, hemolytic anemia, hypoprothrombinemia, neutropenia, thrombocytopenia, unusual bleeding
MS: Arthralgia
RESP: Dyspnea
SKIN: Ecchymosis, erythema, erythema multiforme, flushing, pruritus, rash, Stevens-Johnson syndrome, urticaria
Other: Anaphylaxis; injection site pain, redness, and swelling; superinfection

Nursing Considerations

- Use cefoxitin cautiously in patients hypersensitive to penicillin; cross-sensitivity has occurred in 10% of such patients. Also use cautiously in patients with a history of GI disease, particularly colitis, because of an increased risk of pseudomembranous colitis.
- If possible, obtain culture and sensitivity test results, as ordered, before giving drug.
- For I.V. use, reconstitute 1 g with 10 ml of sterile water for injection or 2 g with 10 to 20 ml of diluent.
- For I.V. injection, administer slowly over 3 to 5 minutes through tubing of a flowing compatible I.V. solution.
- For intermittent infusion, further dilute with 50 to 100 ml of D_5W or normal saline solution.
- For continuous high-dose infusion, add cefoxitin to I.V. solutions of D_5W, normal saline solution, or D_5/normal saline solution.
- Discard unused drug after 24 hours if stored at room temperature or after 1 week if refrigerated.
- Be aware that powder or solution may darken during storage, a change that doesn't reflect altered potency.
- Be aware that an allergic reaction may occur a few days after therapy starts.
- Monitor BUN and serum creatinine levels for early signs of nephrotoxicity. Also monitor fluid intake and output; decreasing urine output may indicate nephrotoxicity.
- Assess bowel pattern daily; severe diarrhea may indicate pseudomembranous colitis.
- Assess for pharyngitis, ecchymosis, bleeding, and arthralgia; they may indicate a blood dyscrasia.

PATIENT TEACHING

- Tell patient to immediately report severe diarrhea to the prescriber.

ceftazidime

Ceptaz, Fortaz, Tazicef, Tazidime

Class and Category

Chemical: Third-generation cephalosporin, 7-aminocephalosporanic acid
Therapeutic: Antibiotic
Pregnancy category: B

Indications and Dosages

▶ *To treat infection caused by gram-negative organisms (including* Acinetobacter, Citrobacter, Enterobacter, Escherichia coli, Haemophilus influenzae, Klebsiella, Neisseria, Proteus mirabilis, Proteus vulgaris, Pseudomonas aeruginosa, Salmonella, Serratia, *and* Shigella*), gram-positive organisms (including* Streptococcus agalactiae, Streptococcus pneumoniae, *and* Streptococcus pyogenes *[group B streptococci]), as well as* Staphylococcus aureus *(penicillinase- and non–penicillinase-producing strains)*

I.V. INFUSION

Adults and children age 12 and over. 1 g q 8 to 12 hr.

I.V. INFUSION

Children ages 1 month to 12 years. 30 to 50 mg/kg q 8 hr.
Neonates up to age 1 month. 30 mg/kg q 12 hr. *Maximum:* 6 g/day.

▶ *To treat uncomplicated UTI*

I.V. INFUSION

Adults and children age 12 and over. 250 mg q 12 hr.

▶ *To treat complicated UTI*

I.V. INFUSION

Adults and children age 12 and over. 500 mg q 8 to 12 hr.

▶ *To treat uncomplicated pneumonia and mild skin and soft-tissue infection*

I.V. INFUSION

Adults and children age 12 and over. 0.5 to 1 g q 8 hr.

▶ *To treat bone and joint infection*

I.V. INFUSION

Adults and children age 12 and over. 2 g q 12 hr.

▶ *To treat serious gynecologic and intra-abdominal infection, meningitis, and life-threatening infection, especially in immunocompromised patients*

I.V. INFUSION

Adults and children age 12 and over. 2 g q 8 hr.

▶ *To treat pseudomonal lung infection in patients with cystic fibrosis and normal renal function*
I.V. INFUSION
Adults and children age 1 month and over. 30 to 50 mg/kg q 8 hr. *Maximum:* 6 g daily.
Neonates up to age 1 month. 30 mg/kg q 12 hr.
DOSAGE ADJUSTMENT Dosage reduced to 1 g q 12 hr if creatinine clearance is 31 to 50 ml/min/1.73 m^2; to 1 g q 24 hr if clearance is 16 to 30 ml/min/1.73 m^2; to 0.5 g q 24 hr if clearance is 6 to 15 ml/min/1.73 m^2; and to 0.5 g q 48 hr if clearance is less than 6 ml/min/1.73 m^2.

Mechanism of Action

Interferes with bacterial cell wall synthesis by inhibiting the cross-linking of peptidoglycan strands. Peptidoglycan makes the cell membrane rigid and protective. Without it, bacterial cells rupture and die.

Incompatibilities

Don't mix ceftazidime with aminoglycosides to prevent mutual inactivation. Vancomycin is physically incompatible with ceftazidime (precipitate may form); flush I.V. line between these drugs if given through same tubing. Avoid mixing ceftazidime with other drugs, including pentamidine isethionate.

Contraindications

Hypersensitivity to cephalosporins or their components

Interactions

DRUGS
aminoglycosides, loop diuretics: Increased risk of nephrotoxicity

Adverse Reactions

CNS: Chills, fever, headache, seizures
CV: Edema
EENT: Hearing loss
GI: Abdominal cramps, diarrhea, elevated liver function test results, hepatic failure, hepatomegaly, nausea, oral candidiasis, pseudomembranous colitis, vomiting
GU: Elevated BUN level, nephrotoxicity, renal failure, vaginal candidiasis
HEME: Eosinophilia, hemolytic anemia, hypoprothrombinemia, neutropenia, thrombocytopenia, unusual bleeding

MS: Arthralgia
RESP: Dyspnea
SKIN: Ecchymosis, erythema, erythema multiforme, pruritus, rash, Stevens-Johnson syndrome
Other: Anaphylaxis; injection site pain, redness, and swelling; superinfection

Nursing Considerations

- Use ceftazidime cautiously in patients hypersensitive to penicillin because cross-sensitivity occurs in 10% of them. Watch for allergic reactions a few days after therapy starts.
- Use cautiously in patients with a history of GI disease, particularly colitis, because risk of pseudomembranous colitis is increased.
- Know that ceftazidime L-arginine (Ceptaz) is not recommended for children under age 12.
- If possible, obtain culture and sensitivity test results, as ordered, before giving drug.
- Protect ceftazidime powder and reconstituted drug from heat and light; both tend to darken during storage.
- If pharmacy delivers frozen solution, thaw it at room temperature, not in water bath or microwave. Store thawed solution for up to 12 hours at room temperature or 7 days in refrigerator; don't refreeze.
- **WARNING** When preparing drug for neonates or immature infants, don't use diluents containing benzyl alcohol because they are linked to a fatal toxic syndrome.
- For I.V. bolus, reconstitute 1 to 2 g with 10 ml sterile water for injection, D_5W, or sodium chloride for injection. Shake to dissolve. Administer I.V. injection slowly over 3 to 5 minutes through tubing of a flowing compatible I.V. fluid.
- For intermittent infusion, further dilute in 50 to 100 ml of D_5W or normal saline solution. Avoid using sodium bicarbonate injection as a diluent because drug is least stable in it. During ceftazidime administration, temporarily stop other solutions being given at the same I.V. site.
- Rotate I.V. sites every 72 hours. Assess for phlebitis and extravasation.
- Assess bowel pattern daily; severe diarrhea may indicate pseudomembranous colitis.
- Monitor CBC, hematocrit, and serum AST, ALT, bilirubin, LD, and alkaline phosphatase levels during long-term therapy.

- Monitor PT, as ordered, in at-risk patients, such as those with renal or hepatic impairment or poor nutritional state and those receiving anticoagulant or prolonged antibiotic therapy. Notify prescriber if PT decreases, and expect to give vitamin K.
- Assess for perineal itching, fever, malaise, redness, swelling, rash, and change in cough or sputum; they may indicate a superinfection.
- Watch for pharyngitis, ecchymosis, bleeding, and arthralgia (possible blood dyscrasia). Monitor PT and bleeding time.

PATIENT TEACHING

- Urge patient to report severe diarrhea or signs of blood dyscrasia or superinfection.

ceftizoxime sodium

Cefizox

Class and Category

Chemical: Third-generation cephalosporin, 7-aminocephalosporanic acid
Therapeutic: Antibiotic
Pregnancy category: B

Indications and Dosages

▶ *To treat mild to moderate infection of the lower respiratory tract, skin, soft tissue, bones, and joints; septicemia; meningitis; and intra-abdominal infections caused by anaerobes (such as* Bacteroides *sp.,* Peptococcus, *and* Peptostreptococcus*), gram-negative organisms (including* Escherichia coli, Haemophilus influenzae, Klebsiella, *and* Proteus mirabilis*), and gram-positive organisms (including* Enterobacter *sp.,* Serratia *sp.,* Staphylococcus aureus, Staphylococcus epidermidis, Streptococcus agalactiae, Streptococcus pneumoniae, *and* Streptococcus pyogenes*)*

I.V. INFUSION, I.V. INJECTION

Adults and children age 12 and over. 1 to 2 g q 8 to 12 hr.

▶ *To treat severe or refractory infections of the type listed above*

I.V. INFUSION, I.V. INJECTION

Adults and children age 12 and over. 1 g q 8 hr or 2 g q 8 to 12 hr.

▶ *To treat life-threatening infections of the type listed above*

I.V. INFUSION, I.V. INJECTION

Adults and children age 12 and over. 3 to 4 g q 8 hr or, if required, up to 2 g q 4 hr.

▶ *To treat bacterial infection in children*

I.V. INFUSION, I.V. INJECTION

Children age 6 months and over. 50 mg/kg q 6 to 8 hr.

▶ *To treat uncomplicated UTI*

I.V. INFUSION, I.V. INJECTION

Adults. 500 mg q 12 hr.

▶ *To treat pelvic inflammatory disease*

I.V. INFUSION, I.V. INJECTION

Adults. 2 g q 8 hr.

DOSAGE ADJUSTMENT If creatinine clearance is 50 to 79 ml/min/1.73 m^2, dosage reduced to 0.5 g q 8 hr for less severe infections and 0.75 to 1.5 g q 8 hr for life-threatening infections. If creatinine clearance is 5 to 49 ml/min/1.73 m^2, dosage reduced to 0.25 to 0.5 g q 12 hr for less severe infections and 0.5 to 1 g q 12 hr for life-threatening infections. If creatinine clearance is 4 ml/min/1.73 m^2 or less, dosage reduced to 0.5 g q 48 hr or 0.25 g q 24 hr for less severe infections and 0.5 to 1 g q 48 hr or 0.5 g q 24 hr for life-threatening infections.

Mechanism of Action

Interferes with bacterial cell wall synthesis by inhibiting the final step in the cross-linking of peptidoglycan strands. Peptidoglycan makes the cell membrane rigid and protective. Without it, bacterial cells rupture and die.

Incompatibilities

Don't mix ceftizoxime with aminoglycosides to prevent mutual inactivation.

Contraindications

Hypersensitivity to cephalosporins or their components

Interactions

DRUGS

aminoglycosides, loop diuretics: Increased risk of nephrotoxicity
probenecid: Increased and prolonged blood ceftizoxime level

Adverse Reactions

CNS: Chills, fever, headache, seizures
CV: Edema
EENT: Hearing loss
GI: Abdominal cramps, diarrhea, elevated liver function test results, hepatic failure, hepatomegaly, nausea, oral candidiasis, pseudomembranous colitis, vomiting

GU: Elevated BUN level, nephrotoxicity, renal failure, vaginal candidiasis
HEME: Eosinophilia, hemolytic anemia, hypoprothrombinemia, neutropenia, thrombocytopenia, unusual bleeding
MS: Arthralgia
RESP: Dyspnea
SKIN: Ecchymosis, erythema, erythema multiforme, pruritus, rash, Stevens-Johnson syndrome
Other: Anaphylaxis; infusion site pain, redness, and swelling; superinfection

Nursing Considerations

- If possible, obtain culture and sensitivity test results, as ordered, before giving ceftizoxime.
- Reconstitute ceftizoxime for injection with sterile water for injection as follows: for 500-mg vial, add 5 ml; for 1-g vial, add 10 ml; and for 2-g vial, add 20 ml. Shake well. Dilute reconstituted solution further with 50 to 100 ml of a compatible solution, such as normal saline solution or D_5W, before I.V. infusion.
- Be aware that reconstituted drug may be stored for 24 hours at room temperature or 96 hours if refrigerated.
- Administer I.V. injection slowly over 3 to 5 minutes through tubing of a flowing compatible I.V. fluid.
- Be aware that ceftizoxime also comes in a minibag (ceftizoxime injection) with a concentration of 1 or 2 g/50 ml. Before using minibag, store it at –25° to –10° C (–13° to 14° F). Thaw it at room temperature or in refrigerator.
- Discard minibag after 48 hours if stored at room temperature or after 28 days if refrigerated. Don't refreeze. Don't use solution if it contains precipitate or is cloudy.
- To prevent air embolism, don't administer minibag using I.V. lines with series connections.
- Assess I.V. site for extravasation and phlebitis.
- Monitor BUN and serum creatinine levels to detect early signs of nephrotoxicity, especially in patients with impaired renal function. Also monitor fluid intake and output; decreasing urine output may indicate nephrotoxicity.
- Assess bowel elimination pattern daily; severe diarrhea may indicate pseudomembranous colitis. Patients with a history of GI disease, particularly colitis, are at increased risk.
- Monitor for signs of an allergic reaction, such as difficulty breathing or a rash, especially in patients who are hypersensi-

tive to penicillin, because cross-sensitivity has occurred in about 10% of such patients. Be aware that an allergic reaction may occur a few days after therapy starts.

- Assess CBC, hematocrit, and serum AST, ALT, bilirubin, LD, and alkaline phosphatase levels during long-term therapy.
- Assess for pharyngitis, ecchymosis, bleeding, and arthralgia, which may indicate a blood dyscrasia. Monitor PT and bleeding time as ordered.
- Assess patient for evidence of superinfection, such as perineal itching, fever, redness, swelling, rash, and change in cough or sputum.
- Before reconstituting drug, store it at 15° to 30° C (59° to 86° F).

PATIENT TEACHING

- Advise patient receiving ceftizoxime to immediately report severe diarrhea or signs of blood dyscrasias or superinfection. Inform him that yogurt and buttermilk can help maintain intestinal flora and decrease diarrhea.
- Review with patient other possibly serious adverse reactions, such as difficulty breathing, rash, and chest tightness, and tell him to report any that occur.

ceftriaxone sodium

Rocephin

Class and Category

Chemical: Third-generation cephalosporin, 7-aminocephalosporanic acid
Therapeutic: Antibiotic
Pregnancy category: B

Indications and Dosages

▶ *To treat infection of the lower respiratory tract, skin, soft tissue, urinary tract, bones, and joints; sinusitis; intra-abdominal infections; and septicemia caused by anaerobes (including* Bacteroides bivius, Bacteroides fragilis, Bacteroides melaninogenicus, *and* Peptostreptococcus *sp.), gram-negative organisms (including* Citrobacter *sp.,* Enterobacter aerogenes, Escherichia coli, Haemophilus influenzae, Klebsiella *sp.,* Neisseria *sp.,* Proteus mirabilis, Proteus vulgaris, Providencia *sp.,* Salmonella *sp.,* Serratia marcescens, Shigella, *and some strains of* Pseudomonas aeruginosa*), and gram-positive organisms (including* Staphylococcus aureus, Streptococcus pneumoniae, *and* Streptococcus pyogenes*)*

I.V. INFUSION

Adults. 1 to 2 g once daily or in equally divided doses b.i.d. *Maximum:* 4 g daily.

Children. 50 to 75 mg/kg daily in divided doses q 12 hr. *Maximum:* 2 g daily.

▶ *To treat meningitis*

I.V. INFUSION

Children. *Initial:* 100 mg/kg on first day; then 100 mg/kg once daily or in divided doses q 12 hr for 7 to 14 days. *Maximum:* 4 g daily.

▶ *To treat disseminated gonoccocal infection and pelvic inflammatory disease*

I.V. INFUSION

Adults: 1 g q 24 hr.

▶ *To treat gonococcal meningitis and endocarditis*

I.V. INFUSION

Adults. 1 to 2 g q 12 hr for 10 to 14 days (meningitis) or for 4 wk or longer (endocarditis).

▶ *To provide surgical prophylaxis*

I.V. INFUSION

Adults. 1 g 30 min to 2 hr before surgery.

Mechanism of Action

Interferes with bacterial cell wall synthesis by inhibiting the final step in the cross-linking of peptidoglycan strands. Peptidoglycan makes the cell membrane rigid and protective. Without it, bacterial cells rupture and die.

Incompatibilities

Don't admix ceftriaxone with pentamidine isethionate, labetalol, or other antibiotics, such as aminoglycosides, because of potential for incompatibility, such as substantial mutual inactivation.

Contraindications

Hypersensitivity to cephalosporins or their components

Interactions

DRUGS

aminoglycosides, loop diuretics: Increased risk of nephrotoxicity

Adverse Reactions

CNS: Chills, fever, headache, seizures

CV: Edema

EENT: Hearing loss

GI: Abdominal cramps, diarrhea, elevated liver function test results, hepatic failure, hepatomegaly, nausea, oral candidiasis, pseudolithiasis, pseudomembranous colitis, vomiting
GU: Elevated BUN level, nephrotoxicity, renal failure, vaginal candidiasis
HEME: Eosinophilia, hemolytic anemia, hypoprothrombinemia, neutropenia, thrombocytopenia, unusual bleeding
MS: Arthralgia
RESP: Allergic pneumonitis, dyspnea
SKIN: Ecchymosis, erythema, erythema multiforme, pruritus, rash, Stevens-Johnson syndrome
Other: Anaphylaxis; injection site pain, redness, and swelling; superinfection

Nursing Considerations

- Use ceftriaxone cautiously in patients who are hypersensitive to penicillins because cross-sensitivity has occurred in about 10% of such patients.
- If possible, obtain culture and sensitivity results, as ordered, before giving drug.
- Protect powder from light.
- For I.V. use, reconstitute with an appropriate diluent, such as sterile water for injection or sodium chloride for injection, as follows: 250-mg vial, add 2.4 ml; 500-mg vial, add 4.8 ml; 1-g vial, add 9.6 ml; and 2-g vial, add 19.2 ml to yield 100 mg/ml. For piggyback bottles, reconstitute with 10 ml of diluent indicated above for 1-g bottle and 20 ml for 2-g bottle. After reconstitution, further dilute to 50 to 100 ml with diluent indicated above and infuse over 30 minutes.
- Monitor BUN and serum creatinine levels to detect early signs of nephrotoxicity. Also, monitor fluid intake and output; decreasing urine output may indicate nephrotoxicity.
- Monitor patient for allergic reactions a few days after therapy starts.
- Assess CBC, hematocrit, and serum AST, ALT, bilirubin, LD, and alkaline phosphatase levels during long-term therapy.
- Assess bowel pattern daily; severe diarrhea may indicate pseudomembranous colitis.
- Assess for perineal itching, fever, malaise, redness, swelling, rash, and change in cough or sputum; they may indicate a superinfection.
- Assess for pharyngitis, ecchymosis, bleeding, and arthralgia; they may indicate a blood dyscrasia.

PATIENT TEACHING

- Tell patient to immediately report severe diarrhea or evidence of blood dyscrasia or superinfection to prescriber.

cefuroxime sodium

Zinacef

Class and Category

Chemical: Second-generation cephalosporin, 7-aminocephalosporanic acid
Therapeutic: Antibiotic
Pregnancy category: B

Indications and Dosages

▶ *To treat disseminated gonococcal infection and uncomplicated pneumonia*

I.V. INFUSION, I.V. INJECTION

Adults. 750 mg q 8 hr.

▶ *To treat bone and joint infection*

I.V. INFUSION, I.V. INJECTION

Adults. 1.5 g q 8 hr.
Children over age 3 months. 50 to 150 mg/kg/day in divided doses q 8 hr. *Maximum:* Adult dose.

▶ *To treat bacterial meningitis*

I.V. INFUSION

Adults. 1.5 to 3 g q 8 hr.
Children over age 1 month. 50 to 80 mg/kg q 6 to 8 hr.
Neonates up to age 1 month. 33.3 to 50 mg/kg q 8 to 12 hr.

▶ *To treat moderate infection other than those listed above*

I.V. INFUSION, I.V. INJECTION

Adults. 750 mg q 8 hr for 5 to 10 days.

I.V. INFUSION, I.V. INJECTION

Children over age 3 months. 50 mg/kg daily in equally divided doses q 6 to 8 hr.

▶ *To treat severe or complicated infection other than those listed above*

I.V. INFUSION, I.V. INJECTION

Adults. 1.5 g q 8 hr.
Children over age 3 months. 100 mg/kg daily in equally divided doses q 6 to 8 hr.

▶ *To treat life-threatening infections other than those listed above*

I.V. INFUSION, I.V. INJECTION

Adults. 1.5 g q 6 hr.

▶ *To provide perioperative prophylaxis*

I.V. INFUSION, I.V. INJECTION

Adults. 1.5 g 30 to 60 min before surgery (at induction of anesthesia for open-heart surgery), and then 0.75 g q 8 hr thereafter (1.5 g q 12 hr for total of 6 g with open-heart surgery).

DOSAGE ADJUSTMENT Parenteral dosage reduced to 0.75 g q 12 hr if creatinine clearance is 10 to 20 ml/min/1.73 m^2 or to 0.75 g q 24 hr if less than 10 ml/min/1.73 m^2.

Mechanism of Action

Interferes with bacterial cell wall synthesis by inhibiting the final step in the cross-linking of peptidoglycan strands. Peptidoglycan makes the cell membrane rigid and protective. Without it, bacterial cells rupture and die.

Incompatibilities

Don't admix parenteral cefuroxime with other antibiotics, such as aminoglycosides, because of potential for incompatibility, such as substantial mutual inactivation. If they're administered concurrently, don't mix them in the same I.V. bag or bottle.

Contraindications

Hypersensitivity to cephalosporins or their components

Interactions

DRUGS

aminoglycosides, loop diuretics: Increased risk of nephrotoxicity
antacids, H_2-receptor antagonists, omeprazole: Decreased cefuroxime axetil absorption
probenecid: Increased and prolonged blood cefuroxime level

Adverse Reactions

CNS: Chills, fever, headache, seizures
CV: Edema
EENT: Hearing loss, oral candidiasis
GI: Abdominal cramps, diarrhea, elevated liver function test results, hepatic failure, hepatomegaly, nausea, pseudomembranous colitis, vomiting
GU: Elevated BUN level, nephrotoxicity, renal failure, vaginal candidiasis
HEME: Eosinophilia, hemolytic anemia, hypoprothrombinemia, neutropenia, thrombocytopenia, unusual bleeding
MS: Arthralgia
RESP: Dyspnea

SKIN: Ecchymosis, erythema, erythema multiforme, pruritus, rash, Stevens-Johnson syndrome
Other: Anaphylaxis; injection site edema, pain, and redness; superinfection

Nursing Considerations

- Use cefuroxime cautiously in patients hypersensitive to penicillin because cross-sensitivity has occurred in 10% of such patients.
- If possible, obtain culture and sensitivity results, as ordered, before giving drug.
- For I.V. use, reconstitute following manufacturer's instructions according to type of preparation available. Solution ranges in color from light yellow to amber.
- If using a container of frozen parenteral solution, thaw at room temperature or under refrigeration before administration; make sure all ice crystals have melted. Don't force thawing by microwave irradiation.
- Store reconstituted parenteral drug for up to 24 hours at room temperature or 96 hours in refrigerator. (Thawed solutions may be stable for 24 hours at room temperature or 28 days if refrigerated.)
- Administer I.V. injection over 3 to 5 minutes through tubing of a flowing compatible I.V. fluid.
- Monitor I.V. site for extravasation and phlebitis.
- Monitor patient's BUN and serum creatinine levels and fluid intake and output to detect signs of nephrotoxicity. Monitor patients with renal impairment closely because they may have greater toxic reactions to cefuroxime.
- Monitor patient for allergic reactions continuing up to a few days after therapy starts. Patients with a history of some form of allergy, especially to drugs, are at increased risk for an allergic reaction.
- Assess bowel pattern daily; severe diarrhea may indicate pseudomembranous colitis. If it's suspected, stop drug, as ordered, and provide treatment as prescribed.
- Assess patient for pharyngitis, ecchymosis, bleeding, and arthralgia, which may indicate a blood dyscrasia.
- Monitor PT and bleeding time, as ordered. Be prepared to administer vitamin K, if ordered, to treat hypothrombinemia.

PATIENT TEACHING

- Instruct patient to shake oral suspension well before measuring each dose and to use an accurate liquid-measuring device for each dose.

- Advise patient using single-dose packets of oral suspension to empty the contents of one packet into a glass and add at least 10 ml (2 tsp) of cold water; apple, grape, or orange juice; or lemonade. Tell him to stir well and consume entire mixture at once.
- Inform patient that yogurt and buttermilk help maintain intestinal flora and can decrease diarrhea during therapy.
- Instruct patient to immediately report to prescriber severe diarrhea or evidence of blood dyscrasia.

cephapirin sodium

Cefadyl

Class and Category

Chemical: First-generation cephalosporin, 7-aminocephalosporanic acid
Therapeutic: Antibiotic
Pregnancy category: B

Indications and Dosages

▶ *To treat respiratory tract infection, skin and soft-tissue infections, UTI, septicemia, endocarditis, and osteomyelitis caused by gram-negative organisms (including* Escherichia coli, Haemophilus influenzae, Klebsiella *sp., and* Proteus mirabilis*) and gram-positive organisms (including group A beta-hemolytic streptococci,* Streptococcus pneumoniae, *and staphylococci, including coagulase-positive, coagulase-negative, and penicillinase-producing—but not methicillin-resistant—strains of* Staphylococcus aureus*)*

I.V. INFUSION, I.V. INJECTION

Adults. 0.5 to 1 g q 4 to 6 hr. *Maximum:* 12 g daily.
Children over age 3 months. 40 to 80 mg/kg/day divided into four equal doses and given q 6 hr. *Maximum:* 12 g daily.

▶ *To provide surgical prophylaxis*

I.V. INFUSION, I.V. INJECTION

Adults. 1 to 2 g 30 to 60 min before surgery, 1 to 2 g during long procedure, and 1 to 2 g q 6 hr after surgery for 24 hr.
DOSAGE ADJUSTMENT For open-heart surgery or prosthetic arthroplasty, prophylaxis continued for 3 to 5 days after procedure, if needed.

Contraindications

Hypersensitivity to cephalosporins or their components

Mechanism of Action

Interferes with bacterial cell wall synthesis by inhibiting the final step in the cross-linking of peptidoglycan strands. Peptidoglycan makes the cell membrane rigid and protective. Without it, bacterial cells rupture and die.

Interactions

DRUGS

aminoglycosides, loop diuretics: Increased risk of nephrotoxicity
probenecid: Increased and prolonged blood cephapirin level

Adverse Reactions

CNS: Chills, fever, headache, seizures
CV: Edema
EENT: Hearing loss
GI: Abdominal cramps, diarrhea, elevated liver function test results, hepatic failure, hepatomegaly, nausea, oral candidiasis, pseudomembranous colitis, vomiting
GU: Elevated BUN level, nephrotoxicity, renal failure, vaginal candidiasis
HEME: Eosinophilia, hemolytic anemia, hypoprothrombinemia, neutropenia, thrombocytopenia, unusual bleeding
MS: Arthralgia
RESP: Dyspnea
SKIN: Ecchymosis, erythema, erythema multiforme, pruritus, rash, Stevens-Johnson syndrome
Other: Anaphylaxis; infusion site pain, redness, and swelling; superinfection

Nursing Considerations

- If possible, obtain culture and sensitivity test results, as ordered, before giving cephapirin.
- For I.V. injection, reconstitute 1 g with 10 ml or more of appropriate diluent, such as sterile water for injection. Administer I.V. injection slowly over 3 to 5 minutes through tubing of a flowing compatible I.V. fluid.
- For I.V. infusion, dilute further in 50 ml of D_5W or normal saline solution and infuse over 15 to 30 minutes. Stop primary I.V. solution during cephapirin administration.
- Store reconstituted drug for 12 to 48 hours (depending on diluent used) at room temperature or for 10 days in refrigerator.
- Don't administer a cloudy solution.
- Assess I.V. site for extravasation and phlebitis.

- Monitor BUN and serum creatinine levels to detect early signs of nephrotoxicity, especially in patients with impaired renal function. Also monitor fluid intake and output; decreasing urine output may indicate nephrotoxicity.
- Monitor for signs of an allergic reaction, such as difficulty breathing or a rash, especially in patients who are hypersensitive to penicillin, because cross-sensitivity has occurred in about 10% of such patients. Be aware that an allergic reaction may occur a few days after therapy starts.
- Assess CBC, hematocrit, and serum AST, ALT, bilirubin, LD, and alkaline phosphatase levels during long-term therapy.
- Assess bowel elimination pattern daily; severe diarrhea may indicate pseudomembranous colitis. Patients with a history of GI disease, particularly colitis, are at increased risk.
- Assess for pharyngitis, ecchymosis, bleeding, and arthralgia, which may indicate a blood dyscrasia. Monitor PT and bleeding time, as ordered.
- Assess for furry tongue, perineal itching, and loose, foul-smelling stools, any of which may indicate superinfection.
- Before reconstituting cephapirin for injection, store it at 15° to 30° C (59° to 86° F).

PATIENT TEACHING

- Instruct patient receiving cephapirin to immediately report severe diarrhea or signs of blood dyscrasias or superinfection. Inform him that yogurt and buttermilk can help maintain intestinal flora and decrease diarrhea during therapy.
- Review with patient other possibly serious adverse reactions, such as difficulty breathing, rash, and chest tightness, and tell him to report any that occur.

chloramphenicol sodium succinate

Chloromycetin

Class and Category

Chemical: Dichloroacetic acid derivative
Therapeutic: Antibiotic
Pregnancy category: Not rated

Indications and Dosages

▶ *To treat serious infection for which less potentially dangerous drugs are ineffective or contraindicated*

I.V. INFUSION

Adults. 12.5 mg/kg q 6 hr. *Maximum:* 4 g daily.

Children. 12.5 mg/kg q 6 hr.
Full-term infants age 2 weeks and over. 12.5 mg/kg q 6 hr or 25 mg/kg q 12 hr.
Preterm and full-term infants up to age 2 weeks. 6.25 mg/kg q 6 hr.

▶ *To treat bacteremia or meningitis*

I.V. INFUSION

Children. 50 to 100 mg/kg daily in divided doses q 6 hr.

DOSAGE ADJUSTMENT Dosage limited to 25 mg/kg daily for infants and children with immature metabolic processes.

Mechanism of Action

Produces a bacteriostatic effect on susceptible organisms by inhibiting protein synthesis, thereby preventing amino acids from being transferred to growing polypeptide chains.

Contraindications

Hypersensitivity to chloramphenicol or its components

Interactions

DRUGS

alfentanil: Prolonged alfentanil effect
barbiturates: Increased blood barbiturate level; decreased blood chloramphenicol level
blood-dyscrasia–causing drugs (such as captropil and cephalosporins), bone marrow depressants (including colchicine and methotrexate): Increased bone marrow depression
chlorpropamide, tolbutamide: Increased hypoglycemic effects of these drugs
clindamycin, erythromycin, lincomycin: Decreased antibacterial effects of these drugs
cyclophosphamide: Decreased or delayed activation of cyclophosphamide, increased bone marrow depression
hepatic enzyme inducers (including rifampin): Decreased blood chloramphenicol level
hydantoins: Increased blood hydantoin level, possibly resulting in toxicity, including increased bone marrow depression; decreased blood chloramphenicol level
iron salts: Increased serum iron level
oral anticoagulants: Enhanced anticoagulant effect
oral contraceptives containing estrogen: Decreased contraceptive effect with prolonged chloramphenicol use

penicillins: Decreased penicillin activity, synergistic effects with treatment of certain microorganisms
vitamin B_{12}: Antagonized hematopoietic response to vitamin B_{12}

Adverse Reactions

CNS: Confusion, delirium, depression, fever, headache, peripheral neuropathy
CV: Gray syndrome in neonates
EENT: Glossitis, optic neuritis, stomatitis
GI: Diarrhea, nausea, vomiting
HEME: Aplastic anemia, bone marrow depression, granulocytopenia, hypoplastic anemia, leukopenia, reticulocytopenia, thrombocytopenia
SKIN: Macular or vesicular rash, urticaria
Other: Anaphylaxis, angioedema

Nursing Considerations

- **WARNING** Keep in mind that chloramphenicol should never be used to treat minor infections or for prophylaxis because of the many serious toxicities associated with its use.
- Be aware that patients with impaired or immature renal function (especially neonates and infants) may require reduced dosage. Monitor chloramphenicol concentrations, as ordered.
- Prepare a 10% solution by adding 10 ml of sterile water for injection or D_5W to each 1-g vial of chloramphenicol. Administer over at least 1 minute.
- Know that diluted I.V. solution is stable for 24 to 48 hours when stored at room temperature or refrigerated (depending on manufacturer's recommendation). Don't use if it's cloudy.
- Monitor CBC as ordered for signs of blood dyscrasias, including leukopenia and thrombocytopenia.
- Assess for fever, sore throat, tiredness, unusual bleeding, or ecchymosis, which may indicate a blood dyscrasia.
- Perform neurologic assessments regularly, looking for signs and symptoms of peripheral neuropathy.
- **WARNING** If early signs of gray syndrome (failure to feed, pallor, cyanosis, abdominal distention, irregular respirations, and vasomotor collapse) appear, notify prescriber and be prepared to stop drug immediately.
- Be aware that chloramphenicol may increase bone marrow depression in patients receiving radiation therapy.
- Be aware that administering chloramphenicol at term or during labor puts neonate at risk for gray syndrome and administering drug to breast-feeding woman may have toxic effects on infant.

- Before reconstituting chloramphenicol, store it at 15° to 25° C (59° to 77° F).

PATIENT TEACHING

- Instruct patient receiving chloramphenicol to immediately report signs of blood dyscrasias.
- **WARNING** Advise patient to be alert for signs of potentially fatal, irreversible bone marrow depression, which leads to aplastic anemia and is characterized by fever, pallor, pharyngitis, severe fatigue and weakness, and unusual bleeding or bruising. Bone marrow depression may occur weeks to months after therapy and seems unrelated to administration route. Stress the importance of follow-up care.
- Urge patient to use a soft-bristled toothbrush and to avoid using toothpicks or dental floss because of increased risk of infection and gingival bleeding due to drug's effects on blood counts.

chlordiazepoxide hydrochloride

Librium

Class, Category, and Schedule

Chemical: Benzodiazepine
Therapeutic: Antianxiety agent
Pregnancy category: Not rated
Controlled substance: Schedule IV

Indications and Dosages

▶ *To provide short-term management of severe anxiety*

I.V. INJECTION

Adults. *Initial:* 50 to 100 mg. Then 25 to 50 mg t.i.d. or q.i.d., p.r.n. *Maximum:* 300 mg daily.

▶ *To provide short-term treatment of acute alcohol withdrawal*

I.V. INJECTION

Adults. *Initial:* 50 to 100 mg. Repeated in 2 to 4 hr, followed by individualized oral dosage if needed to control symptoms. *Maximum:* 300 mg daily.

DOSAGE ADJUSTMENT Dosage reduced to 25 to 50 mg for elderly or debilitated patients and for children age 12 and older.

Contraindications

Hypersensitivity to chlordiazepoxide or its components

Interactions

DRUGS

cimetidine, disulfiram, fluoxetine, isoniazid, ketoconazole, metoprolol, oral

contraceptives, propoxyphene, propranolol, valproic acid: Increased blood chlordiazepoxide level
CNS depressants: Increased CNS effects
digoxin: Increased blood digoxin level and risk of digitalis toxicity
levodopa: Decreased efficacy of levodopa's antiparkinsonian effects
neuromuscular blockers: Potentiated, counteracted, or diminished effects of neuromuscular blockers
phenytoin: Possibly increased phenytoin toxicity
probenecid: Shortened onset of action or prolonged effect of chlordiazepoxide
rifampin: Decreased chlordiazepoxide effects
theophyllines: Antagonized sedative effects of chlordiazepoxide
ACTIVITIES
alcohol use: Increased CNS effects

Mechanism of Action

May potentiate the effects of gamma-aminobutyric acid (GABA) and other inhibitory neurotransmitters by binding to specific benzodiazepine receptors in the limbic and cortical areas of the CNS. By binding to these receptors, chlordiazepoxide increases GABA's inhibitory effects and blocks cortical and limbic arousal, which helps control emotional behavior. It also helps relieve symptoms of alcohol withdrawal by causing CNS depression.

Adverse Reactions

CNS: Ataxia, confusion, depression, drowsiness
CV: ECG changes, hypotension, tachycardia
GI: Hepatic dysfunction
HEME: Agranulocytosis
SKIN: Jaundice
Other: Infusion site pain, redness, and swelling

Nursing Considerations

- **WARNING** Be aware that prolonged use of therapeutic doses of chlordiazepoxide can lead to dependence.
- Reconstitute ampule contents with 5 ml of sterile water for injection or sodium chloride for injection. Agitate gently until completely dissolved. Administer slowly over 1 minute immediately after reconstitution. Discard unused portions.
- **WARNING** Don't use supplied diluent (provided for I.M. use) to prepare drug for I.V. use because air bubbles form on the surface.

- Be aware that rapid I.V. administration may cause apnea, hypotension, bradycardia, and cardiac arrest. Keep emergency equipment and drugs nearby. Observe patient for 5 hours or longer, as needed.
- Monitor patients with porphyria for signs of an exacerbation, such as fever, photosensitivity, abdominal pain, and neuropathy.
- Monitor patient for adverse reactions, especially if he has hypoalbuminemia, which increases drug's sedative effects.
- Observe for signs of phlebitis or thrombophlebitis after I.V. administration.
- Monitor patients with impaired hepatic or renal function for signs of increased CNS effects due to slowed chlordiazepoxide metabolism or excretion because drug is metabolized by liver and excreted by kidneys.
- Monitor a hyperactive, aggressive child or any patient with a history of psychiatric disorders for paradoxical reactions, such as excitement, stimulation, and acute rage, during first 2 weeks of therapy.
- Before reconstituting chlordiazepoxide, store it at 15° to 30° C (59° to 86° F).

PATIENT TEACHING

- Caution patient about possible drowsiness, and advise him to avoid activities requiring alertness until chlordiazepoxide's full CNS effects are known.

chlorothiazide

Diuril

chlorothiazide sodium

Diuril

Class and Category

Chemical: Sulfonamide derivative
Therapeutic: Antihypertensive, diuretic
Pregnancy category: B

Indications and Dosages

▶ *To produce diuresis*

I.V. INFUSION, I.V. INJECTION

Adults. 250 mg q 6 to 12 hr.

Route	Onset	Peak	Duration
I.V.	15 min	4 hr	6 to 12 hr

Mechanism of Action

A thiazide diuretic, chlorothiazide inhibits sodium (Na^+) reabsorption and promotes movement of Na^+, chloride (Cl^-), and water (H_2O) from blood in peritubular capillaries into the nephron's distal convoluted tubule, as shown. Initially, chlorothiazide may reduce blood pressure by decreasing extracellular fluid volume, plasma volume, and cardiac output. It also directly dilates arteries. After several weeks, extracellular fluid volume, plasma volume, and cardiac output return to normal. Peripheral vascular resistance remains decreased.

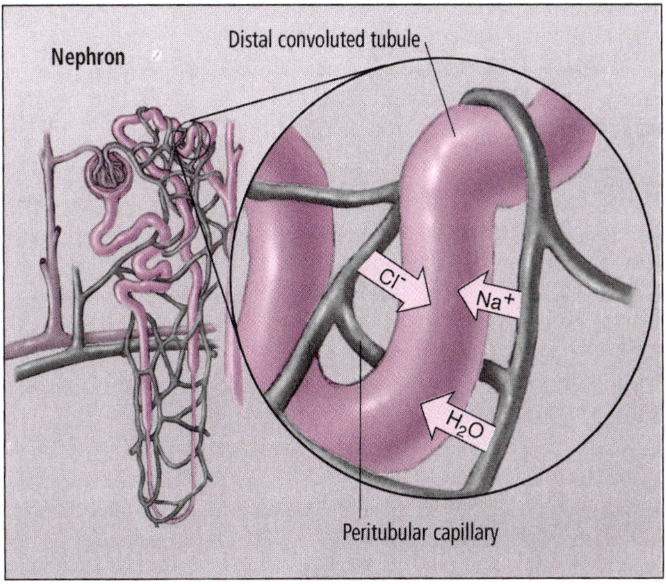

Contraindications

Anuria; hepatic coma; hypersensitivity to chlorothiazide, its components, sulfonamides, or related thiazide diuretics; renal failure

Interactions

DRUGS

allopurinol: Increased risk of allopurinol hypersensitivity
amiodarone: Increased risk of arrhythmias from hypokalemia
amphotericin B, glucocorticoids: Intensified electrolyte depletion
anesthetics: Potentiated effects of anesthetics
anticholinergics: Increased chlorothiazide absorption
anticoagulants, methenamines, sulfonylureas: Decreased effects of these drugs

antihypertensives: Increased antihypertensive effect
antineoplastics: Prolonged antineoplastic-induced leukopenia
calcium: Possibly increased blood calcium level
cholestyramine, colestipol: Decreased chlorothiazide absorption
diazoxide: Hyperglycemia, hypotension
digitalis glycosides: Increased risk of digitalis-induced arrhythmias
dopamine: Increased diuretic effect of both drugs
lithium: Increased risk of lithium toxicity
loop diuretics: Synergistic effects, resulting in profound diuresis and serious electrolyte imbalances
methyldopa: Potential development of hemolytic anemia
neuromuscular blockers: Increased neuromuscular blockade
NSAIDs: Possibly reduced diuretic effect of chlorothiazide
sympathomimetics: Possibly inhibited antihypertensive effect of chlorothiazide
vitamin D: Enhanced vitamin D action

Adverse Reactions

CNS: Dizziness, headache, paresthesia, restlessness, vertigo, weakness
CV: Orthostatic hypotension
ENDO: Hyperglycemia
GI: Abdominal cramps, anorexia, constipation, diarrhea, gastric irritation, nausea, pancreatitis, vomiting
GU: Glycosuria, hematuria, impotence, interstitial nephritis, renal dysfunction or failure
HEME: Agranulocytosis, aplastic anemia, hemolytic anemia, leukopenia, thrombocytopenia
MS: Muscle spasms
SKIN: Jaundice, photosensitivity, purpura, rash, urticaria
Other: Anaphylactic reactions, hypercalcemia, hyperuricemia, hypochloremic alkalosis, hypokalemia, hypomagnesemia, hyponatremia, hypovolemia

Nursing Considerations

- Don't give parenteral form of chlorothiazide by I.M. or subcutaneous route.
- For I.V. use, reconstitute with at least 18 ml of sterile water for injection. Discard unused solution after 24 hours. Reconstituted solution is compatible with dextrose solution or normal saline solution for infusion.
- Watch I.V. site closely. If extravasation occurs, stop infusion and tell prescriber at once.

- Weigh patient daily to assess fluid loss and drug effectiveness. Also, check blood pressure often if used to treat hypertension; antihypertensive effect may not appear for days.
- Assess patient for electrolyte imbalances.
- Monitor renal function closely, especially in elderly patients, because the risk of toxicity increases with renal impairment.

PATIENT TEACHING

- Encourage patient to eat a high-potassium diet.
- Instruct patient to rise slowly to minimize effects of orthostatic hypotension.
- Tell patient to immediately notify prescriber about weakness, cramps, nausea, vomiting, restlessness, excessive thirst, drowsiness, tiredness, increased heart rate, diarrhea, sudden joint pain, or dizziness.
- Inform patient with diabetes mellitus that his blood glucose will be monitored and that his oral antidiabetic dosage may need to be increased.

chlorpromazine hydrochloride

Largactil (CAN), Thorazine

Class and Category

Chemical: Propylamine derivative of phenothiazine
Therapeutic: Antiemetic, antipsychotic, tranquilizer
Pregnancy category: Not rated

Indications and Dosages

▶ *To provide intraoperative control of nausea and vomiting*

I.V. INJECTION

Adults. 25 mg diluted to 1 mg/ml with sodium chloride for injection and given at a rate not to exceed 2 mg q 2 min. *Maximum:* 25 mg.

Children age 6 months and over. 0.275 mg/kg diluted to at least 1 mg/ml with sodium chloride for injection and given at a rate not to exceed 1 mg q 2 min. *Maximum:* 75 mg/day for children ages 5 to 12 years or weighing 50 to 100 lb; 40 mg daily for children up to age 5 years or weighing up to 50 lb.

▶ *To treat intractable hiccups*

I.V. INFUSION

Adults. 25 to 50 mg diluted in 500 to 1,000 ml of normal saline solution and administered at 1 mg/min with patient in supine position.

▶ *To treat tetanus (usually as adjunct to barbiturates)*
I.V. INFUSION
Adults. 25 to 50 mg diluted to at least 1 mg/ml and given at no more than 1 mg/min.
Children age 6 months and over. 0.55 mg/kg q 6 to 8 hr, diluted to at least 1 mg/ml and given at no more than 1 mg/2 min. *Maximum:* 75 mg daily for children ages 5 to 12 or weighing 50 to 100 lb; 40 mg daily for children up to age 5 or weighing up to 50 lb.
DOSAGE ADJUSTMENT Dosage possibly reduced for patients with hepatic dysfunction. Dosage reduced to one-third to one-half the normal adult dosage for elderly or debilitated patients.

Mechanism of Action

Depresses areas of the brain that control activity and aggression, including the cerebral cortex, hypothalamus, and limbic system, by an unknown mechanism. Chlorpromazine prevents nausea and vomiting by inhibiting or blocking dopamine receptors in the medullary chemoreceptor trigger zone and peripherally by blocking the vagus nerve in the GI tract. It may relieve anxiety by causing indirect reduction in arousal and increased filtering of internal stimuli to the reticular activating system in the brain stem.

Incompatibilities

Don't mix chlorpromazine with thiopental, atropine, or solutions that don't have a pH of 4 to 5 because a precipitate will form. Don't mix chlorpromazine injection in same syringe with other drugs.

Contraindications

Comatose states; hypersensitivity to chlorpromazine, phenothiazines, or their components; use of large amounts of CNS depressants

Interactions

DRUGS
amphetamines: Decreased amphetamine effectiveness, decreased antipsychotic effectiveness of chlorpromazine
barbiturates: Decreased plasma level and, possibly, effectiveness of chlorpromazine
CNS depressants: Prolonged and intensified CNS depression
metrizamide: Possibly lowered seizure threshold
oral anticoagulants: Decreased anticoagulant effect

phenytoin: Interference with phenytoin metabolism, increased risk of phenytoin toxicity
propranolol: Increased plasma levels of both drugs
thiazide diuretics: Possibly increased orthostatic hypotension
ACTIVITIES
alcohol use: Prolonged and intensified CNS depression

Adverse Reactions

CNS: Drowsiness, extrapyramidal reactions (dystonia, fever, motor restlessness, pseudoparkinsonism, and tardive dyskinesia), neuroleptic malignant syndrome, seizures
CV: ECG changes, such as nonspecific, usually reversible Q- and T-wave changes; orthostatic hypotension; tachycardia
EENT: Blurred vision, dry mouth, nasal congestion, ocular changes (fine particle deposits in lens and cornea) with long-term therapy
ENDO: Gynecomastia, hyperglycemia, hypoglycemia, lactation, moderate breast engorgement
GI: Constipation, ileus, nausea
GU: Amenorrhea, ejaculation disorders, impotence, priapism, urine retention
HEME: Agranulocytosis, aplastic anemia, eosinophilia, hemolytic anemia, leukopenia, pancytopenia, thrombocytopenic purpura
SKIN: Exfoliative dermatitis, jaundice, photosensitivity, tissue necrosis, urticaria

Nursing Considerations

- Protect chlorpromazine solution from light. Solution should be clear and colorless to pale yellow. Discard markedly discolored solution.
- Don't inject drug subcutaneously because it can cause severe tissue necrosis.
- Wear gloves when working with liquid or injectable form because parenteral solution may cause contact dermatitis.
- For I.V. injection, dilute chlorpromazine with sodium chloride for injection to a concentration that yields 1 mg/ml before administration.
- **WARNING** Be aware that chlorpromazine contains benzyl alcohol, which can cause a fatal toxic syndrome in neonates or immature infants, characterized by CNS, respiratory, circulatory, and renal impairment and metabolic acidosis. Dosage has not been established for infants younger than age 6 months.
- **WARNING** Be alert for possible suppressed cough reflex, which increases patient's risk of aspirating vomitus.

- **WARNING** If neuroleptic malignant syndrome (hyperpyrexia, muscle rigidity, altered mental status, autonomic instability) develops, notify prescriber immediately and expect to discontinue drug and begin intensive medical treatment. Monitor carefully for recurrence if patient resumes antipsychotic therapy.
- Monitor patients (especially children) with chronic respiratory disorders (such as severe asthma or emphysema) or acute respiratory tract infections for exacerbations of these conditions caused by chlorpromazine's CNS depressant effects. Be aware that patients with cardiovascular, hepatic, or renal disease are at increased risk for developing hypotension, heart failure, and arrhythmias.
- Monitor patients with a history of hepatic encephalopathy from cirrhosis for increased sensitivity to drug's CNS effects.
- Because of chlorpromazine's anticholinergic effects, monitor patients with a history of or predisposition to glaucoma for evidence of this disorder, such as eye pain, vision changes, or nausea and vomiting from increased intraocular pressure.
- Be aware that drug should be used cautiously in those who are exposed to organophosphorus insecticides.
- Monitor patients who have been exposed to extreme heat for heatstroke due to drug-induced suppression of temperature regulation. Symptoms include tachycardia, fever, and confusion.
- Be aware that pediatric and elderly patients are at increased risk for developing hypotension amd extrapyramidal reactions, especially if they're acutely ill or debilitated.
- Before reconstituting chlorpromazine, store it at 15° to 30° C (59° to 86° F).

PATIENT TEACHING

- Because chlorpromazine may cause drowsiness, dizziness, and blurred vision (especially during the first few days of therapy), advise patient to avoid potentially hazardous activities until drug's CNS effects are known.
- Advise patient, especially if elderly, to rise slowly from a supine or seated position to avoid dizziness, light-headedness, and fainting.
- Urge patient to avoid alcohol because of possible additive effects and hypotension.
- Inform patient that drug may reduce body's response to heat and cold; advise him to avoid temperature extremes, as in very cold or hot showers.

- If patient reports dry mouth, suggest sugarless chewing gum, hard candy, and fluids.
- Urge patient to report sudden sore throat or other signs of infection.

cidofovir

Vistide

Class and Category

Chemical: Synthetic purine nucleotide analogue
Therapeutic: Antiviral
Pregnancy category: C

Indications and Dosages

I.V. INFUSION

▶ *To treat cytomegalovirus (CMV) retinitis in patients with AIDS*

Adults. Induction dose of 5 mg/kg infused over 1 hr once q wk for 2 wk. *Maintenance:* 5 mg/kg infused over 1 hr once q 2 wk. Probenecid should be given before and after each cidofovir dose.
DOSAGE ADJUSTMENT Maintenance dosage reduced to 3 mg/kg if serum creatinine level increases by 0.3 or 0.4 mg/dl above baseline.

Mechanism of Action

Ultimately converted by pyrimidine nucleoside monophosphate kinase and other cellular enzymes to cidofovir diphosphate. Cidofovir diphosphate suppresses cytomegalovirus (CMV) replication by incorporation into and termination of the growing DNA chain, and by selective inhibition and inactivation of viral DNA polymerase, an enzyme used in the viral DNA replication process.

Incompatibilities

Don't add other drugs or supplements to cidofovir solutions.

Contraindications

Concurrent administration within 7 days of other nephrotoxic drugs; direct intraocular injection; hypersensitivity to cidofovir or severe hypersensitivity to probenecid or other sulfa-containing drugs; serum creatinine level greater than 1.5 mg/dl, calculated creatinine clearance less than or equal to 55 ml/min/1.73 m^2, or urine protein level greater than or equal to 100 mg/dl (proteinuria greater than or equal to 2+)

Interactions

DRUGS

nephrotoxic drugs (such as aminoglycosides, amphotericin B, foscarnet, NSAIDs, and pentamidine): Increased risk of nephrotoxicity

Adverse Reactions

CNS: Asthenia, fever, headache
EENT: Iritis, ocular hypotony, uveitis, vision changes
GI: Anorexia, diarrhea, nausea, vomiting
GU: Elevated serum creatinine level, nephrotoxicity, proteinuria
HEME: Neutropenia
Other: Decreased serum sodium bicarbonate levels, metabolic acidosis

Nursing Considerations

- **WARNING Be aware that cidofovir is for I.V. infusion only and is not for direct intraocular injection.**
- Monitor serum creatinine and urine protein levels within 48 hours of an upcoming cidofovir dose, as ordered. Expect maintenance dosage to be decreased if serum creatinine level increases by 0.3 or 0.4 mg/dl above baseline. Expect therapy to be discontinued if serum creatinine level increases by at least 0.5 mg/dl above baseline or if patient develops proteinuria of 3+ or more.
- Monitor WBC count with differential before cidofovir dose to detect drug-induced neutropenia. Also, assess patient for signs of neutropenia, including fever, chills, and sore throat.
- Expect to administer 2 g of probenecid 3 hours before each dose of cidofovir and 1 g 2 hours and 8 hours after each dose—for a total of 4 g—to minimize the risk of nephrotoxicity.
- Give at least 1 L of normal saline solution over 1 to 2 hours immediately before giving cidofovir. Another infusion of 1 L of normal saline solution over 1 to 3 hours may be prescribed for patients who can tolerate the extra fluid, to be started when cidofovir infusion starts or immediately afterward.
- Be aware that adverse reactions can vary when cidofovir is given in combination therapy. Review information for all drugs given as part of a specific regimen, including drug interactions and adverse effects.
- Be aware that an antiemetic may be prescribed to help reduce nausea from probenecid. Also, be prepared to administer prophylactic or therapeutic antihistamines or acetaminophen if patient develops an allergic or hypersensitivity reaction.

- Be aware that cidofovir has mutagenic properties. Follow facility protocol for preparation and handling of such drugs and for appropriate disposal of used equipment. Thoroughly wash any skin exposed to cidofovir with soap and water.
- Inspect each vial of cidofovir before administration; discard it if you detect particles or discoloration. Dilute each dose of cidofovir with 100 ml of normal saline solution. Give within 24 hours. Diluted solutions not used immediately may be stored at 2° to 8° C (36° to 46° F) but must be used within the original 24-hour period. Allow refrigerated solution to return to room temperature before giving it.
- Administer cidofovir at a constant rate over a 1-hour period, using an infusion pump.
- Assess patient for changes in vision, such as decreased vision, which may indicate decreased intraocular pressure. Ensure that patient's intraocular pressure is measured periodically.

PATIENT TEACHING

- Instruct patient to eat some food before each dose of probenecid to help reduce drug-related nausea and vomiting.
- Stress the importance of taking the full course of probenecid with each dose of cidofovir to decrease the risk of adverse reactions.
- Advise patient to comply with follow-up ophthalmic exams to assess drug effectiveness and monitor for adverse reactions. Inform patient that CMV retinitis may continue to progress during and following treatment.
- Inform patient who is also receiving zidovudine that a dosage adjustment or temporary discontinuation of zidovudine may be needed on the day of cidofovir therapy.
- If patient develops neutropenia, urge him to avoid sports and other activities that increase the risk of accidental injury. Also advise him to take measures to avoid infection, such as maintaining good oral hygiene (for example, by using a soft-bristled toothbrush) and washing hands before touching eyes or nose.

cimetidine hydrochloride

Novo-Cimetine (CAN), Tagamet

Class and Category

Chemical: Imidazole derivative
Therapeutic: Antiulcer agent, gastric acid secretion inhibitor, H_2-receptor antagonist

Pregnancy category: B

Indications and Dosages

▶ *To treat and prevent recurrence of duodenal ulcer*

I.V. INJECTION

Adults. *Initial:* 300 mg q 6 to 8 hr. Dosage increased, if needed, by increasing frequency. *Maximum:* 2,400 mg daily.

▶ *To treat active, benign gastric ulcer*

I.V. INJECTION

Adults and adolescents. *Initial:* 300 mg q 6 to 8 hr. Dosage increased, if needed, by increasing frequency. *Maximum:* 2,400 mg/day.

▶ *To treat pathologic hypersecretory conditions, such as Zollinger-Ellison syndrome*

I.V. INJECTION

Adults and adolescents. *Initial:* 300 mg q 6 to 8 hr. Dosage increased, if needed, by increasing frequency. *Maximum:* 2,400 mg daily.

▶ *To prevent stress-related upper GI bleeding during hospitalization*

I.V. INFUSION

Adults. 50 mg/hr by continuous infusion for 7 days.

Route	Onset	Peak	Duration
I.V.	Unknown	Unknown	4 to 5 hr

Mechanism of Action

Blocks histamine's action at H_2-receptor sites on the stomach's parietal cells. This action reduces gastric fluid volume and acidity. Cimetidine also decreases the amount of gastric acid that's secreted in response to food, caffeine, insulin, betazole, or pentagastrin.

Incompatibilities

Don't mix cimetidine in same I.V. solution with aminophylline or barbiturates. Don't mix drug in same syringe with pentobarbital sodium.

Contraindications

Hypersensitivity to cimetidine or its components

Interactions

DRUGS

antacids, anticholinergics, metoclopramide: Decreased cimetidine absorption

benzodiazepines, calcium channel blockers, carbamazepine, chloroquine, labetalol, lidocaine, metoprolol, metronidazole, moricizine, pentoxifylline, phenytoin, propafenone, propranolol, quinidine, quinine, sulfonylureas, tacrine, theophyllines, triamterene, tricyclic antidepressants, valproic acid, warfarin: Reduced metabolism and increased blood levels and effects of these drugs, possibly toxicity from these drugs
carmustine: Increased carmustine myelotoxicity
digoxin, fluconazole: Possibly decreased blood levels of these drugs
ferrous salts, indomethacin, ketoconazole, tetracyclines: Decreased effects of these drugs
flecainide: Increased flecainide effects
fluorouracil: Increased blood fluorouracil level after long-term cimetidine use
ketoconazole: Decreased blood ketoconazole level
opioid analgesics: Increased toxic effects of opioid analgesics
oral anticoagulants: Increased anticoagulant effect
procainamide: Increased blood procainamide level
succinylcholine: Increased neuromuscular blockade
tocainide: Decreased tocainide effects
FOODS
caffeine: Reduced metabolism and increased blood level and effects of caffeine
ACTIVITIES
alcohol use: Possibly increased blood alcohol level

Adverse Reactions

CNS: Confusion, dizziness, hallucinations, headache, peripheral neuropathy, somnolence
ENDO: Mild gynecomastia if used longer than 1 month
GI: Mild and transient diarrhea
GU: Impotence, transiently elevated serum creatinine level
SKIN: Rash

Nursing Considerations

- Don't use cimetidine if solution is discolored or contains precipitate.
- For I.V. injection, dilute cimetidine in normal saline solution to a total volume of 20 ml. Inject drug over 5 minutes or more.
- Use diluted solution within 48 hours when stored at room temperature.
- **WARNING** Be aware that rapid administration of cimetidine can increase patient's risk of developing arrhythmias and hypotension.

- For intermittent I.V. infusion, dilute drug in at least 50 ml of D_5W or other compatible I.V. solution. Infuse over 15 to 20 minutes.
- Be especially alert for confusion in elderly or debilitated patients who receive cimetidine.
- Before using cimetidine, store it at 15° to 30° C (59° to 86° F).

PATIENT TEACHING

- Advise patient to avoid alcohol during cimetidine therapy to prevent interactions.
- Caution patient that cigarette smoking increases gastric acid secretion and can worsen gastric disease.

ciprofloxacin

Cipro I.V.

Class and Category

Chemical: Fluoroquinolone derivative
Therapeutic: Antibiotic
Pregnancy category: C

Indications and Dosages

▶ *To prevent inhalation anthrax after exposure or to treat inhalation anthrax*

I.V. INFUSION

Adults and adolescents. 400 mg q 12 hr for 60 days.
Children. 10 mg/kg q 12 hr for 60 days. *Maximum:* 400 mg/dose or 800 mg daily.

▶ *To treat acute sinusitis caused by gram-negative organisms (including* Campylobacter jejuni, Citrobacter diversus, Citrobacter freundii, Enterobacter cloacae, Escherichia coli, Haemophilus influenzae, Haemophilus parainfluenzae, Klebsiella pneumoniae, Morganella morganii, Neisseria gonorrhoeae, Proteus mirabilis, Proteus vulgaris, Providencia rettgeri, Providencia stuartii, Pseudomonas aeruginosa, Serratia marcescens, Shigella flexneri, *and* Shigella sonnei*) and gram-positive organisms (including* Enterococcus faecalis, Staphylococcus aureus, Staphylococcus epidermidis, *and* Streptococcus pneumoniae*)*

I.V. INFUSION

Adults. For mild to moderate infection, 400 mg q 12 hr.

▶ *To treat bone and joint infections caused by susceptible organisms listed above*

I.V. INFUSION

Adults. For mild to moderate infection, 400 mg q 12 hr for 4 to 6 wk. For severe or complicated infection, 400 mg q 8 hr.

▶ *To treat skin and soft-tissue infection caused by susceptible organisms listed above*

I.V. INFUSION

Adults. For mild to moderate infection, 400 mg q 12 hr. For severe or complicated infections, 400 mg q 8 hr.

▶ *To treat chronic bacterial prostatitis caused by susceptible organisms listed above*

I.V. INFUSION

Adults. 400 mg q 12 hr.

▶ *To treat UTIs caused by susceptible organisms listed above*

I.V. INFUSION

Adults. For mild to moderate infection, 200 mg q 12 hr. For severe or complicated infection, 400 mg q 12 hr.

▶ *To treat lower respiratory tract infections caused by susceptible organisms listed above*

I.V. INFUSION

Adults. For mild to moderate infection, 400 mg q 12 hr. For severe or complicated infection, 400 mg q 8 hr.

▶ *To treat intra-abdominal infections caused by susceptible organisms listed above*

I.V. INFUSION

Adults. 400 mg q 8 hr along with parenteral metronidazole.

▶ *To treat mild to severe nosocomial pneumonia caused by susceptible organisms listed above*

I.V. INFUSION

Adults. 400 mg q 8 hr.

▶ *To treat typhoid fever caused by* Salmonella typhi *or infectious diarrhea caused by* C. jejuni, E. coli, S. flexneri, *or* S. sonnei

DOSAGE ADJUSTMENT Dosage reduced to 250 to 500 mg q 12 hr in patients with creatinine clearance of 30 to 50 ml/min/1.73 m^2; and to 250 to 500 mg P.O. or 200 to 400 mg I.V. q 18 hr in patients with creatinine clearance of 5 to 29 ml/min/1.73 m^2.

Incompatibilities

Don't administer parenteral ciprofloxacin with aminophylline, amoxicillin, cefepime, clindamycin, dexamethasone, floxacillin, furosemide, heparin, or phenytoin.

Mechanism of Action
Inhibits the enzyme DNA gyrase, which is responsible for the unwinding and supercoiling of bacterial DNA before it replicates, and causes bacterial cells to die.

Contraindications
Hypersensitivity to ciprofloxacin, quinolones, or their components; concurrent therapy with tizanidine

Interactions
DRUGS
antacids, didanosine, iron supplements, sucralfate, zinc- or iron-containing multivitamins: Decreased ciprofloxacin absorption
cyclosporine: Elevated serum creatinine and cyclosporine levels
glyburide: Severe hypoglycemia
methylxanthines, theophylline, tizanidine: Increased blood levels of these drugs leading possibly to increased toxicity
NSAIDs (except acetylsalicylic acid): Increased risk of seizures with high doses of ciprofloxacin
oral anticoagulants: Enhanced anticoagulant effects
phenytoin: Increased or decreased blood phenytoin level
probenecid: Increased blood level of ciprofloxacin and, possibly, toxicity
FOODS
caffeine: Increased caffeine effects
dairy products: Delayed drug absorption

Adverse Reactions
CNS: Agitation, anxiety, cerebral thrombosis, confusion, dizziness, headache, insomnia, light-headedness, migraine, nightmares, paranoia, peripheral neuropathy, restlessness, seizures, syncope, toxic psychosis
CV: Angina, atrial flutter, cardiopulmonary arrest, cardiovascular collapse, hypertension, MI, orthostatic hypotension, palpitations, phlebitis, tachycardia, torsades de pointes, vasculitis, ventricular ectopy
EENT: Oral candidiasis
GI: Abdominal pain, constipation, diarrhea, elevated liver function test results, flatulence, GI bleeding, hepatic failure or necrosis, hepatitis, indigestion, intestinal perforation, jaundice, nausea, necrosis pancreatitis, pseudomembranous colitis, vomiting
GU: Crystalluria, hematuria, increased serum creatinine level, in-

terstitial nephritis, nephrotoxicity, renal calculi, renal failure, urine retention, vaginal candidiasis
HEME: Agranulocytosis, bone marrow depression, hemolytic anemia, lymphadenopathy, pancytopenia
MS: Tendon rupture
RESP: Bronchospasm, pulmonary embolism, respiratory arrest
SKIN: Erythema multiforme, exfoliative dermatitis, photosensitivity, rash, Stevens-Johnson syndrome, toxic epidermal necrolysis, urticaria
Other: Acidosis, anaphylaxis, angioedema, serum sickness–like reaction

Nursing Considerations

- Obtain culture and sensitivity test results, as ordered, before giving ciprofloxacin.
- Use drug cautiously in patients with CNS disorders.
- Dilute I.V. ciprofloxacin concentrate to 1 to 2 mg/ml using D_5W or sodium chloride for injection. Don't dilute solutions that come from the manufacturer in D_5W before I.V. infusion. Infuse slowly over 1 hour.
- Store reconstituted solution for up to 14 days at room temperature or refrigerated.
- Be aware that patient should be well hydrated during therapy to help prevent alkaline urine, which may lead to crystalluria and nephrotoxicity.
- Assess patient's hepatic, renal, and hematologic functions periodically, as ordered, for patients receiving prolonged therapy.
- Monitor patient closely for diarrhea, which may reflect pseudomembranous colitis. If it occurs, notify prescriber and expect to withhold ciprofloxacin and treat diarrhea.
- Assess patient for evidence of peripheral neuropathy. Notify prescriber and expect to stop drug if patient complains of pain, burning, tingling, numbness, or weakness in extremities or if physical examination reveals deficits in light touch, pain, temperature, position sense, vibratory sensation, or motor strength.
- Monitor patients (especially children, elderly patients, and patients receiving corticosteroids) for evidence of tendon rupture, such as pain, inflammation, and swelling at the site. Be aware that tendon rupture may occur during or after ciprofloxacin therapy. Notify prescriber about suspected tendon rupture, and have patient rest and refrain from exercise until tendon rupture has been ruled out. If present, expect to provide supportive care as ordered.

- Assess patient's skin routinely for signs of rash or other hypersensitivity reactions because ciprofloxacin may cause serious skin reactions. Stop drug at first sign of reaction and notify prescriber.

PATIENT TEACHING

- Encourage patient to drink plenty of fluids during therapy to help prevent crystalluria.
- Urge patient to avoid caffeinated products because caffeine may accumulate in the body during ciprofloxacin therapy and cause excessive stimulation.
- Instruct patient to notify prescriber at first sign of allergy, such as rash.
- Urge patient to avoid hazardous activities until CNS effects of drug are known.
- Advise patient to notify prescriber about severe or prolonged diarrhea, changes in limb sensation or movement, and pain, inflammation, or swelling over a joint.
- Tell patient to notify prescriber at first sign of rash or other hypersensitivity reaction.

cisplatin

Platinol (CAN), Platinol-AQ

Class and Category

Chemical: Inorganic metal complex
Therapeutic: Alkylating-like antineoplastic
Pregnancy category: D

Indications and Dosages

▶ *To treat metastatic testicular tumors*

I.V. INFUSION

Adults. 20 mg/m^2 daily for 5 days q 21-day cycle. *Maximum:* 120 mg/m^2 for each course.

▶ *To treat metastatic ovarian tumors*

I.V. INFUSION

Adults also receiving cyclophosphamide sequentially. 75 to 100 mg/m^2 per cycle q 4 wk. *Maximum:* 120 mg/m^2 for each course.

Adults not receiving cyclophosphamide. 100 mg/m^2 per cycle q 4 wk. *Maximum:* 120 mg/m^2 for each course.

Adults also receiving paclitaxel. 75 mg/m^2 q 3 wk for six courses. *Maximum:* 120 mg/m^2 for each course.

▶ *To treat advanced bladder cancer*
I.V. INFUSION
Adults: 50 to 70 mg/m^2 per cycle q 3 or 4 wk. *Maximum:* 120 mg/m^2 for each course.

> **Mechanism of Action**
> May bind to DNA within the cell, thus interfering with DNA function and synthesis. May also have a smaller effect on RNA synthesis. Cisplatin's actions are cell-cycle-phase–nonspecific.

Incompatibilities
Don't use needles or I.V. sets containing aluminum to administer cisplatin because a precipitate could form and potency could be decreased.

Contraindications
Hearing impairment, hypersensitivity to cisplatin or other platinum-containing drugs, myelosuppression

Interactions
DRUGS
antihistamines, buclizine, cyclizine, loxapine, meclizine, phenothiazines, thioxanthenes, trimethobenzamide: Possibly masked ototoxicity effects
bleomycin: Increased risk of bleomycin toxicity
blood-dyscrasia–causing drugs (including ACE inhibitors, cephalosporins, and NSAIDs): Increased leukopenic and thrombocytopenic effects of cisplatin
bone marrow depressants (such as amphotericin B, colchicine, and paclitaxel): Increased effects of these drugs
nephrotoxic drugs (such as acyclovir, aminoglycosides, and penicillamine): Potentiated risk of nephrotoxicity
ototoxic drugs (such as capreomycin, furosemide, and NSAIDs): Increased risk of ototoxicity
vaccines, killed virus: Possibly decreased antibody response to vaccine
vaccines, live virus: Possibly increased adverse effects of vaccine virus, life-threatening infection, and decreased antibody response to vaccine

Adverse Reactions
CNS: Neurotoxicity
EENT: Optic neuritis, ototoxicity, papilledema, stomatitis, vision changes

ENDO: Syndrome of inappropriate ADH secretion
GI: Anorexia, nausea, vomiting
GU: Nephrotoxicity, uric acid nephropathy
HEME: Anemia, hemolytic anemia, leukopenia, thrombocytopenia
SKIN: Extravasation
Other: Anaphylaxis, hyperuricemia, hypocalcemia, hypomagnesemia

Nursing Considerations

- Be aware that cisplatin should be administered only under the supervision of a qualified physician or nurse in settings where appropriate diagnostic and treatment facilities are available.
- **WARNING** Make sure that emergency equipment and drugs, such as antihistamines, epinephrine, and I.V. corticosteroids, are available in case of anaphylaxis.
- Follow facility protocols for preparation and handling of antineoplastic drugs and appropriate disposal of used equipment.
- **WARNING** To decrease the risk of inadvertent overdose, contact prescriber if cumulative cisplatin dose for each cycle exceeds 100 mg/m^2.
- Monitor creatinine clearance, serum uric acid, and BUN levels, as ordered, before initiating cisplatin therapy and before each subsequent course to detect early signs of nephrotoxicity. Expect dosage to be reduced for patients with impaired renal function.
- Monitor CBC, including hematocrit, platelet count, and WBC count with differential, before and periodically during therapy.
- Monitor serum electrolyte levels, including magnesium, sodium, potassium, and calcium levels, before initiating therapy and before each subsequent course. Be aware that tetany associated with hypocalcemia and hypomagnesemia has been reported.
- Hydrate patient, as ordered, with 1 to 2 L of fluid 8 to 12 hours before cisplatin administration.
- **WARNING** Wear gloves when handling cisplatin. If cisplatin comes in contact with skin or mucosa, immediately and thoroughly wash skin with soap and water and flush mucosa with water.
- Dilute prescribed dose of cisplatin with 2 L of D_5/0.45 normal saline solution or D_5/0.3 normal saline solution that contains 37.5 g of mannitol.
- **WARNING** Don't expose cisplatin to needles or administration sets containing aluminum because a precipitate will form and drug potency will be decreased.

- Anticipate dosage reduction if patient is also receiving radiation therapy or a drug that depresses bone marrow.
- Reconstitute cisplatin for injection (available in Canada only) by adding 10 or 50 ml of sterile water for injection to 10- or 50-mg vial, respectively. Further dilute using D_5/0.45 normal saline solution or D_5/0.3 normal saline solution. Diluted solution is stable for 20 hours at 27° C (80° F). Protect from light if not used within 6 hours of removal from vial.
- Administer an antiemetic, as prescribed, before initiation of cisplatin therapy. Infuse cisplatin as prescribed. Protect from light if diluted cisplatin is not administered within 6 hours.
- Be prepared to hydrate patient for 24 hours after cisplatin administration, and assess for adequate urine output.
- Observe patient for signs of leukopenia or infection, including fever, chills, pharyngitis, tiredness or weakness, and unusual bleeding or ecchymosis.
- Perform neurologic assessment to check for signs of neurotoxicity, such as paresthesia of the hands and feet, loss of taste or motor function, seizures, muscle spasms, and areflexia. Expect to discontinue cisplatin therapy if neurotoxicity occurs.
- Monitor serum uric acid level, especially in patients with a history of gout or urate calculi. Be aware that allopurinol may be prescribed to help prevent uric acid nephropathy. Expect antigout drug dosage to be adjusted if blood uric acid level is elevated from cisplatin therapy.
- Assess for signs of extravasation at I.V. infusion site, such as redness, swelling, or pain. Be aware that concentrations greater than 0.5 mg/ml put the patient at increased risk for tissue cellulitis, fibrosis, and necrosis.
- Be aware that effects of radiation therapy or bone marrow depressants may be increased when these treatments are administered concurrently with cisplatin. Patients with a history of bone marrow depression, chickenpox (including recent exposure), or herpes zoster are at increased risk for severe generalized disease.
- Monitor patient for signs and symptoms of syndrome of inappropriate ADH secretion, including dizziness, confusion, agitation, and tiredness or weakness.
- Expect subsequent courses of cisplatin therapy to be initiated after an appropriate time interval when serum creatinine level is below 1.5 mg/dl or BUN level is below 25 mg/dl (or both); platelet count is above or equal to 100,000/mm^3; WBC count is

greater than or equal to 4,000/mm^3; and audiometric testing indicates hearing is within normal limits.

- Store cisplatin injection at 15° to 25° C (59° to 77° F); don't refrigerate.
- Store cisplatin for injection (available in Canada only) at 15° to 30° C (59° to 86° F), and protect from light.

PATIENT TEACHING

- Instruct patient receiving cisplatin to immediately report unusual bruising or bleeding; black, tarry stools; blood in urine or stools; pinpoint red spots on skin; numbness or tingling in fingers or toes; and ringing in ears or hearing loss.
- Urge patient not to receive live or killed virus vaccines during cisplatin therapy and for 3 months to 1 year after completion of therapy, unless approved by prescriber. Instruct him to avoid people who have received such vaccines or to wear a protective mask when he's around them.
- Caution patient to avoid sports and other activities that increase the risk of accidental injury. Also advise him to take measures to avoid infection, such as maintaining good oral hygiene (for example, by using soft-bristled toothbrush) and washing hands before touching eyes or nose.
- Stress the importance of keeping scheduled follow-up appointments and undergoing prescribed diagnostic tests, such as neurologic function studies and audiometric testing, before each course of cisplatin to monitor for adverse drug effects.
- Suggest that patient with stomatitis eat soft, bland foods served cold or at room temperature to decrease irritation.

clindamycin phosphate

Cleocin, Dalacin C Phosphate (CAN)

Class and Category

Chemical: Lincosamide
Therapeutic: Antibacterial and antiprotozoal antibiotic
Pregnancy category: B

Indications and Dosages

▶ *To treat serious respiratory tract infection caused by anaerobes such as occur with anaerobic pneumonitis, empyema, and lung abscess and those caused by pneumococci, staphylococci, and streptococci; serious skin and soft-tissue infections caused by anaerobes, staphylococci, and streptococci; septicemia caused by anaerobes; intra-abdominal infections caused by anaerobes such as occur with intra-abdominal abscess and peritonitis; infections of the female pelvis and genital tract caused by anaerobes such as occur with endometritis, nongonococcal tubo-ovarian abscess, pelvic cellulitis, and postsurgical vaginal cuff infection; bone and joint infections caused by* Staphylococcus aureus; *as adjunct therapy in chronic bone and joint infections*

I.V. INFUSION

Adults and adolescents age 16 and over. For serious infections, 600 to 1,200 mg daily in equally divided doses b.i.d. to q.i.d.; for severe infections, 1,200 to 2,700 mg daily in equally divided doses b.i.d. to q.i.d.; for life-threatening infections, 4,800 mg daily in equally divided doses b.i.d. to q.i.d.

Children ages 1 month to 16 years. 20 to 40 mg/kg/day in equally divided doses t.i.d. or q.i.d., depending on severity of infection.

Neonates younger than age 1 month. 15 to 20 mg/kg daily in equally divided doses t.i.d. or q.i.d., depending on severity of infection.

Mechanism of Action

Inhibits protein synthesis in susceptible bacteria by binding to the 50S subunits of bacterial ribosomes and preventing peptide bond formation, which causes bacterial cells to die.

Incompatibilities

Don't administer clindamycin with aminophylline, ampicillin, barbiturates, calcium gluconate, magnesium sulfate, or phenytoin because these drugs are physically incompatible.

Contraindications

Hypersensitivity to clindamycin or lincomycin

Interactions

DRUGS

chloramphenicol, erythromycin: Possibly antagonized effects of clindamycin

neuromuscular blockers: Increased neuromuscular blockade

Adverse Reactions

CNS: Fatigue, headache

CV: Hypotension

EENT: Glossitis, metallic or unpleasant taste, stomatitis

GI: Abdominal pain, diarrhea, esophagitis, nausea, pseudomembranous colitis, vomiting
HEME: Agranulocytosis, eosinophilia, leukopenia, neutropenia, thrombocytopenic purpura
SKIN: Pruritus, rash, urticaria
Other: Anaphylaxis, infusion site thrombophlebitis, superinfection

Nursing Considerations

- Expect to obtain a specimen for culture and sensitivity testing before giving first dose of clindamycin.
- Give I.V. dose by infusion only; don't give bolus dose. Dilute 300 mg of clindamycin in 50 ml of diluent and give over 10 minutes. Dilute 600 mg of clindamycin in 100 ml of diluent and give over 20 minutes. Dilute 900 mg of clindamycin in 100 ml of diluent and give over 30 minutes.
- Store diluted parenteral solution for up to 24 hours at room temperature.
- **WARNING** When preparing clindamycin for administration to neonates or premature infants, don't use drug that contains benzyl alcohol because it may cause a fatal toxic syndrome characterized by CNS, respiratory, circulatory, and renal impairment and metabolic acidosis.
- Be aware that drug should be used cautiously in patients with atopy, significant allergies, or a history of asthma.
- Check I.V. site frequently for phlebitis and irritation.
- Monitor results of liver function tests, CBC, and platelet counts during prolonged therapy.
- Monitor serum drug levels, as ordered, in patients with impaired hepatic or renal function who are receiving high doses. A dosage adjustment may be necessary.
- Observe patient for evidence of superinfection, such as vaginal itching and sore mouth, and for signs of pseudomembranous colitis, which may occur 2 to 9 days after therapy begins. Patients with a history of GI disease, particularly colitis or regional enteritis, are at increased risk for colitis. Be aware that antibiotic-related diarrhea and colitis are more common and may be more severe and less well tolerated in elderly patients.
- Before diluting drug, store it at 15° to 30° C (59° to 86° F).

PATIENT TEACHING

- Advise patient receiving clindamycin to immediately report signs or symptoms of colitis (severe diarrhea and abdominal cramps) or superinfection (an inflamed mouth or vagina), as well as rash or lesions.

coagulation Factor VIIa (recombinant)

NovoSeven

Class and Category

Chemical: Vitamin K–dependent glycoprotein
Therapeutic: Antihemophilic, hemostatic
Pregnancy category: C

Indications and Dosages

▶ *To treat bleeding episodes in pagtients with hemophilia A or B or with inhibitors to Factor VIII or Factor IX*

I.V. INJECTION

Adults. 90 mcg/kg injected over 2 to 5 minutes q 2 hr until hemostasis achieved; then q 3 to 6 hr, as needed.

▶ *To prevent bleeding in surgical intervention or invasive procedure in hemophilia A or B patients with inhibitors to Factor VIII or Factor IX*

I.V. INJECTION

Adults. 90 mcg/kg injected over 2 to 5 minutes immediately before surgery or procedure; then q 2 hr throughout surgery or procedure. After minor surgery, 90 mcg/kg injected over 2 to 5 minutes q 2 hr for 48 hr; then 90 mcg/kg injected over 2 to 5 minutes q 2 to 6 hr until healing has occurred. After major surgery, 90 mcg/kg over 2 to 5 minutes q 2 hr for 5 days; then 90 mcg/kg over 2 to 5 minutes q 4 hr until healing has occurred.

▶ *To treat or prevent bleeding episodes in patients with congenital Factor VII deficiency*

I.V. INFUSION

Adults. 15 to 30 mcg/kg over 2 to 5 minutes q 4 to 6 hr until hemostasis occurs.

▶ *To treat patients with acquired hemophilia*

I.V. INFUSION

Adults. 70 to 90 mcg/kg over 2 to 5 minutes q 2 to 3 hr until hemostasis occurs.

Mechanism of Action

Factor VIIa actuvates the extrinsic pathway of coagulation by forming complexes with tissue factor to activate factors IX and X. Activated Factor X complexes with other factors to convert prothrombin to thrombin. Thrombin then converts fibrinogen to fibrin which leads to the formation of a hemostatic plug to produce local hemostais. This process may also occur on the surface of activated platelets.

Contraindications

Hypersensitivity to recombinant coagulation Factor VIIa; its components; or to mouse, hamster or bovine proteins.

Interactions

DRUGS

activated and nonactivated prothrombin complex concentrates: Increased risk of thrombosis

Adverse Reactions

CNS: Fever, headache
CV: Acute MI, bradyarrhythmia, chest tightness or pain, edema, hypertension, hypotension, supraventricular tachycardia, thrombosis
EENT: Epistaxis
GI: Nausea, vomiting
HEMA: Disseminated intravascular coagulation, hemorrhage
MS: Arthralgia
RESP: Wheezing
SKIN: Pruritis, purpura, rash, urticaria
Other: Anaphylaxis, injection site reaction

Nursing Considerations

- Be aware that patients with disseminated intravascular coagulation, advanced atherosclerotic disease, crush injury, septicemia, or receiving concomitant treatment with activated or nonactivated prothrombin complex concentrate are at increased risk for a thrombotic event such as myocardial ischemia or infarction and cerebral ischemia or infarction.
- Monitor Factor VII–deficient patients' PT and Factor VII coagulant activity before and after administration of drug. If Factor VIIa activity fails to reach the expected level, the PT is not corrected or bleeding is not controlled, notify prescriber. The patient may have developed antibodies to the drug. Be prepared to obtain specimen for antibody analysis.
- Reconstitute drug with the correct amount of sterile water (2.2 ml for 1.2-mg vial, 4.3 ml for 2.4-mg vial, and 8.5 ml for 4.8-mg vial). Clean rubber stopper with alcohol and insert the syringe needle into the center of the stopper, aiming the needle against the side of the vial so the stream of sterile water runs down the vial wall. Do not inject the diluent directly onto the powder. Gently swirl vial until powder is dissolved. Do not shake reconstituted solution. If solution is foamy, let solution settle before giving it. Once reconstituted, use within 3 hours.

- Monitor patient's clotting status closely. If intravascular coagulation is confirmed by test results or signs and symptoms occur, notify prescriber and expect to reduce dosage or stop drug.

PATIENT TEACHING

- Tell patient to immediately report any signs and symptoms of an allergic reaction, such as hives, rash, chest tightness, or difficulty breathing.
- Inform patient that he will need regular laboratory tests to determine effectiveness of drug.

codeine phosphate

Class, Category, and Schedule

Chemical: Phenanthrene derivative
Therapeutic: Opioid analgesic
Pregnancy category: C
Controlled substance: Schedule II

Indications and Dosages

▶ *To treat mild to moderate pain*

I.V. INJECTION

Adults. 15 to 60 mg q 4 hr. *Usual:* 30 mg/dose.

Mechanism of Action

May produce analgesia through partial metabolism to morphine. Codeine binds with mu, delta, and kappa receptors in the spinal cord and with mu_1 and $kappa_3$ receptors at higher levels in the CNS, altering the perception of—and emotional response to—pain. By binding with these receptors, the drug decreases levels of intracellular cAMP, which inhibits adenylate cyclase activity. This action prevents the release of pain neurotransmitters, such as substance P and dopamine.

Contraindications

Hypersensitivity to codeine, other opioids, or their components; significant respiratory depression

Interactions

DRUGS

anticholinergics, paregoric: Increased risk of severe constipation
antihypertensives, diuretics: Potentiated hypotensive effects
buprenorphine: Decreased effectiveness of codeine
CNS depressants: Additive CNS effects

hydroxyzine: Increased codeine analgesic effect, increased CNS depressant and hypotensive effects
MAO inhibitors: Increased risk of unpredictable, severe, and sometimes fatal reactions
metoclopramide: Antagonized effect of metoclopramide on GI motility
naloxone: Antagonized codeine analgesic effect
naltrexone: Precipitated withdrawal symptoms in codeine-dependent patients
neuromuscular blockers: Additive respiratory depressant effects
other opioid analgesics: Additive CNS and respiratory depressant effects and hypotensive effects
ACTIVITIES
alcohol use: Additive CNS effects

Adverse Reactions

CNS: Coma, delirium, depression, disorientation, dizziness, drowsiness, euphoria, hallucinations, headache, lack of coordination, lethargy, light-headedness, mental and physical impairment, mood changes, restlessness, sedation, seizures, tremor
CV: Bradycardia, heart block, orthostatic hypotension, palpitations, tachycardia
EENT: Altered taste, blurred vision, diplopia, dry mouth, laryngeal edema, laryngospasm, miosis
GI: Abdominal cramps and pain, anorexia, constipation, flatulence, ileus, nausea, vomiting
GU: Decreased libido, difficult ejaculation, dysuria, impotence, oliguria, ureteral spasm, urinary incontinence, urine retention
MS: Muscle rigidity
RESP: Apnea, bronchoconstriction, bronchospasm, depressed cough reflex, respiratory depression
SKIN: Diaphoresis, flushing, pallor, pruritus, rash, urticaria
Other: Anaphylaxis, facial edema, physical and psychological dependence

Nursing Considerations

- Instruct patient to lie down during codeine administration and for a period afterward to lessen dizziness, light-headedness, nausea, and vomiting.
- **WARNING** Administer diluted codeine solution slowly over several minutes. Rapid administration may cause serious adverse reactions, including anaphylaxis, severe respiratory depression, hypotension, peripheral circulatory collapse, and

cardiac arrest. Make sure emergency equipment and drugs are available.
- Evaluate for therapeutic response, including decreased pain and facial grimacing.
- Monitor respiratory depth, effort, and rate. Notify prescriber immediately if respiratory rate drops below 10 breaths/minute; patients having an acute asthma attack and those with chronic respiratory disease are at increased risk. Pediatric, elderly, debilitated, or extremely ill patients are at increased risk for drug's respiratory depressant effects.
- Monitor patient for evidence of drug-induced CNS depression or increased CSF pressure, such as altered LOC, restlessness, and irritability, in patients with a head injury, intracranial lesions, or other conditions that could cause these effects. Patients who are taking or have recently taken drugs that cause CNS depression are also more susceptible to these effects. Take appropriate safety precautions.
- Be aware that codeine may induce or exacerbate arrhythmias or seizures in patients with a history of these conditions and may mask symptoms of acute abdominal conditions.
- **WARNING** Assess patient for signs of physical and psychological dependence.
- Be aware that patients with a history of drug abuse (including acute alcoholism), emotional instability, or suicidal ideation or attempts are at increased risk for opioid abuse; however, the risk of drug dependence is lower with codeine than with some other opioid analgesics.
- Assess urine output; a decrease may signal urine retention.
- Store drug at 15° to 30° C (59° to 86° F). Protect from freezing and light.

PATIENT TEACHING
- Advise patient to avoid alcohol and other CNS depressants, including OTC preparations, during codeine therapy because of possible additive CNS effects.
- Advise patient to avoid potentially hazardous activities until drug's CNS effects are known.
- Caution patient to get up slowly from a sitting or lying position.
- To prevent constipation, encourage patient to consume plenty of fluids and high-fiber foods, if not contraindicated by another condition.
- Advise patient to notify prescriber if he becomes short of breath or has difficulty breathing.

colchicine

Class and Category

Chemical: Colchicum alkaloid derivative
Therapeutic: Antigout agent, anti-inflammatory
Pregnancy category: D

Indications and Dosages

▶ *To prevent gouty arthritis attacks*

I.V. INFUSION, I.V. INJECTION

Adults. 0.5 to 1 mg once or twice daily. *Maximum:* 4 mg daily.

▶ *To treat acute gouty arthritis*

I.V. INFUSION, I.V. INJECTION

Adults. 2 mg over 2 to 5 min; then 0.5 mg q 6 hr or 1 mg q 6 to 12 hr until pain decreases. *Maximum:* 4 mg daily.

DOSAGE ADJUSTMENT For elderly patients, maximum dosage reduced to 2 mg/24 hr. After initial course of therapy, patient should receive no further colchicine in any form for 21 days.

Route	Onset	Peak	Duration
I.V.	In 6 to 12 hr	Unknown	Unknown

Mechanism of Action

In gouty arthritis, leukocytes release chemotactic factors, degradation enzymes, and other inflammatory substances through phagocytosis of urate crystals in affected joints. Colchicine helps stop this process, probably by disrupting microtubules within leukocytes.

Normally, microtubules contribute to cell structure and movement. When colchicine binds to tubulin (the protein from which microtubules are made), the microtubule falls apart, as shown. This process disrupts cell function and keeps leukocytes from invading joints and causing inflammation.

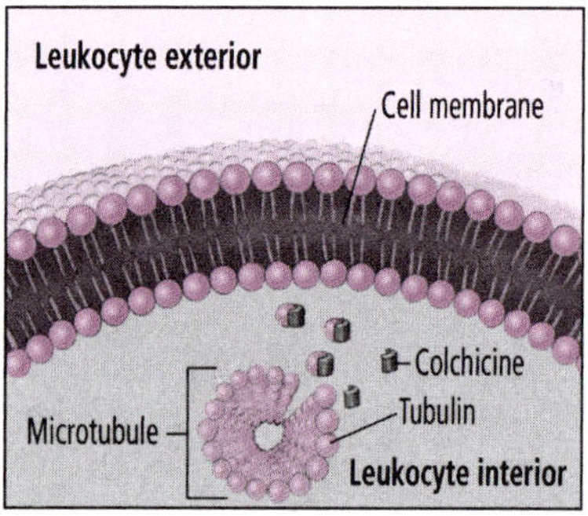

Contraindications

Blood dyscrasias; hypersensitivity to colchicine or its components; serious cardiac, GI, hepatic, or renal disorders

Incompatibilities

Don't combine colchicine with bacteriostatic agents, any solution or injection that contains D_5W, or any other solution that may change colchicine's pH because precipitation may occur.

Interactions

DRUGS

anticoagulants (such as heparin), platelet aggregation inhibitors (such as aspirin), thrombolytics (such as alteplase): Possibly significantly increased risk of GI ulceration or hemorrhage

antineoplastics: Possibly increased serum uric acid level and decreased therapeutic effectiveness of colchicine

cyclosporine: Increased blood cyclosporine level

NSAIDs (such as phenylbutazone): Possibly increased risk of bone marrow depression, GI bleeding, leukopenia, or thrombocytopenia

vitamin B_{12}: Possibly impaired absorption of and increased dosage requirements for vitamin B_{12}

ACTIVITIES

alcohol use: Increased risk of adverse GI effects

Adverse Reactions

CNS: Peripheral neuropathy

CV: Arrhythmias

GI: Abdominal pain, diarrhea, nausea, vomiting

HEME: Agranulocytosis, aplastic anemia, thrombocytopenia

MS: Myopathy

SKIN: Alopecia, rash

Other: Injection site pain and tenderness, median nerve neuritis in affected arm, and skin and soft-tissue necrosis if extravasation occurs

Nursing Considerations

- **WARNING** To prevent extravasation, ensure that the I.V. catheter is patent and correctly positioned before administering colchicine. Throughout therapy, check I.V. injection site frequently for pain, tenderness, and skin peeling. Consult prescriber about switching to oral form as soon as possible. Avoid S.C. or I.M. administration of colchicine because these routes may cause tissue necrosis and sloughing.

- **WARNING** Don't give colchicine by any route within 7 days after a full I.V. course (4 mg) because of the risk of toxicity. Be aware that elderly or debilitated patients and those with a history of cardiac disease or impaired renal or hepatic function are at increased risk for cumulative toxicity.
- Expect to monitor CBC and platelet and reticulocyte counts at baseline and every 3 months after therapy starts.
- Dilute drug with 10 to 20 ml of normal saline solution. Don't use a diluent that contains a bacteriostatic agent. Alternatively, administer colchicine through a free-flowing I.V. line with normal saline solution into a large vein. Don't use colchicine if solution is cloudy or contains sediment.
- Administer I.V. form over 2 to 5 minutes.
- Notify prescriber immediately and expect to stop therapy if patient develops signs or symptoms of colchicine toxicity, such as abdominal pain, diarrhea, nausea, or vomiting.
- Store drug at 15° to 30° C (59° to 86° F); protect from freezing and light.

PATIENT TEACHING

- Instruct patient to return for blood tests every 3 months, as ordered, during colchicine therapy.
- Explain that gouty arthritis pain and swelling typically subside in 24 to 48 hours after therapy begins.
- Advise patient to immediately report abdominal pain, diarrhea, nausea, or vomiting.

conivaptan hydrochloride

Vaprisol

Class and Category

Chemical: Arginine vasopressin antagonist (antidiuretic hormone)
Therapeutic: Aquaretic (sodium/water stabilizer)
Pregnancy category: C

Indications and Dosages

▶ *To treat euvolemic hyponatremia in hospitalized patients, such as those with syndrome of inappropriate antidiuretic hormone, hypothyroidism, adrenal insufficiency, or pulmonary disorders*

I.V. INFUSION

Adults. *Loading dose:* 20 mg over 30 min, followed by 20 mg as a continuous infusion over 24 hr. An additional 20 mg daily may be given by continuous infusion for 1 to 3 days, as needed. *Maxi-*

mum: 40 mg daily with total duration of therapy, including loading dose, not to exceed 4 days.

Route	Onset	Peak	Duration
I.V.	Unknown	24 hr	Unknown

Mechanism of Action

Conivaptan binds with arginine vasopressin V2 receptor sites in the collecting ducts of the kidneys. By doing so, it blocks the action of arginine vasopressin on the V2 receptor, decreasing water resorption in the collecting ducts. This increases excretion of free water (urine output) and increases serum sodium concentration, thereby correcting the water and sodium imbalance.

Incompatibilities

Don't mix conivaptan with lactated Ringer's solution, normal saline solution, or other drugs.

Contraindications

Hypersensitivity to conivaptan or its components; patients with hypovolemic hyponatremia; use with potent CYP3A4 inhibitors, such as clarithromycin, indinavir, itraconazole, ketoconazole, and ritonavir

Interactions

DRUGS

amphotericin B, cisplatin, corticosteroids: Possibly additive hypokalemic effects
clarithromycin, indinavir, itraconazole, ketoconazole, ritonavir, and other strong CYP3A4 inhibitors: Increased blood conivaptan level
digoxin: Possibly increased digoxin level and risk of digioxin toxicity
drugs metabolized by CYP3A4, such as HMG-CoA reductase inhibitors: Possibly increased risk of rhabdomyolysis

Adverse Reactions

CNS: Confusion, fever, headache, insomnia
CV: Atrial fibrillation, hypertension, hypotension, orthostatic hypotension, peripheral edema
EENT: Dry mouth, oral candidiasis
ENDO: Hyperglycemia, hypoglycemia
GI: Constipation, diarrhea, nausea, thirst, vomiting
GU: Hematuria, pollakiuria, polyuria, UTI
HEME: Anemia

RESP: Pneumonia
SKIN: Erythema
Other: Dehydration, hypokalemia, hypomagnesemia, hyponatremia, infusion site reactions (erythema, pain, phlebitis, swelling)

Nursing Considerations

- Be aware that conivaptan shouldn't be used to treat patients with heart failure.
- Use conivaptan cautiously in patients with hepatic or renal dysfunction because conivaptan levels remain elevated longer in these patients, increasing exposure to the drug.
- Administer conivaptan only through large veins, and change the infusion site every 24 hours. This drug may cause serious infusion site reactions even when diluted and infused correctly. Inspect the site regularly; change it immediately if reactions occur, such as erythema, pain, phlebitis, or swelling.
- Dilute 20-mg (4-ml) loading dose with 100 ml of 5% dextrose injection before administration. Gently invert the bag several times to mix thoroughly. Use mixture within 24 hours, infusing over 30 minutes.
- Dilute 20-mg (4-ml) or 40-mg (8-ml) continuous infusion dose with 250 ml of D_5W before administration. Gently invert the bag several times to mix thoroughly. Infuse immediately over 24 hours. If infusion is interrupted for any reason, discard any remaining solution 24 hours after mixing.
- Monitor patient's neurologic status and serum sodium level closely during conivaptan therapy because a rapid increase in serum sodium level (more than 12 mEq/L/24 hr) may cause serious neurologic impairment. If serum sodium level rises faster than expected, stop infusion temporarily and notify prescriber. If it continues to rise, expect to stop conivaptan. If hyponatremia persists or recurs and the patient has no neurologic abnormalities, conivaptan may be resumed at a reduced rate.
- Monitor patient's vital signs, and assess patient regularly for evidence of hypovolemia. If patient develops hypovolemia or hypotension while receiving conivaptan, stop infusion, notify prescriber, and provide supportive care, as prescribed. After hypovolemia and hypotension have been corrected, drug may be resumed at a reduced rate.
- Store ampules in cardboard container, protected from light, until ready for use.

PATIENT TEACHING

- Instruct patient to report infusion site discomfort immediately.

- Tell patient that frequent laboratory tests will be needed to monitor his serum sodium level and volume status.

co-trimoxazole
(sulfamethoxazole and trimethoprim)

Bactrim, Septra

Class and Category

Chemical: Sulfonamide derivative (sulfamethoxazole), dihydrofolic acid analogue (trimethoprim)
Therapeutic: Antibiotic
Pregnancy category: C

Indications and Dosages

▶ *To treat acute otitis media, shigellosis, UTI, and other infections caused by gram-negative organisms (including* Enterobacter *sp.,* Escherichia coli, Haemophilus ducreyi, Haemophilus influenzae, *indole-positive* Proteus *sp.,* Klebsiella pneumoniae, Neisseria gonorrhoeae, Proteus mirabilis, Providencia *sp.,* Salmonella *sp.,* Serratia *sp., and* Shigella *sp.) and gram-positive organisms (including group A beta-hemolytic streptococci,* Nocardia *sp.,* Staphylococcus aureus, *and* Streptococcus pneumoniae*)*

I.V. INFUSION

Adults and children over age 2 months. 40 to 50 mg/kg of sulfamethoxazole (SMZ) and 8 to 10 mg/kg of trimethoprim (TMP) daily in divided doses q 6, 8, or 12 hr for up to 5 days for shigellosis, 14 days for UTI.

▶ *To treat* Pneumocystis jiroveci (carinii) *pneumonia*

I.V. INFUSION

Adults and children over age 2 months. 75 to 100 mg/kg of SMZ and 15 to 20 mg/kg of TMP daily in three or four divided doses q 6 to 8 hr for up to 14 days.

Mechanism of Action

Blocks two consecutive steps in the formation of essential nucleic acids and proteins in susceptible organisms. Sulfamethoxazole inhibits synthesis of dehydrofolic acid (a nucleic acid) by competing with para-aminobenzoic acid. Trimethoprim inhibits the action of the enzyme dihydrofolate reductase, thus blocking production of tetrahydrofolic acid.

Incompatibilities

Don't mix co-trimoxazole with other drugs or solutions.

Contraindications

Age younger than 2 months; hypersensitivity to sulfamethoxazole, sulfonamides, trimethoprim, or their components; megaloblastic anemia caused by folate deficiency

Interactions

DRUGS

ACE inhibitors: Possibly increased risk of hyperkalemia (elderly patients)
cyclosporine: Decreased blood level and therapeutic effectiveness of cyclosporine, increased risk of nephrotoxicity
digoxin: Possibly increased blood digoxin level resulting in increased risk of digoxin toxicity
diuretics: Increased risk of thrombocytopenic purpura (elderly patients)
indomethacin: Possibly increased blood co-trimoxazole level
methotrexate: Increased blood methotrexate level and risk of methotrexate toxicity
phenytoin: Possibly decreased hepatic clearance and prolonged half-life of phenytoin
pyrimethamine (dosage greater than 25 mg/wk): Increased risk of megaloblastic anemia
sulfonylureas: Possibly increased hypoglycemic effects of sulfonylureas
tricyclic antidepressants: Decreased effectiveness of tricyclic antidepressant
warfarin: Increased anticoagulant effects

Adverse Reactions

CNS: Anxiety, aseptic meningitis, ataxia, chills, depression, fatigue, hallucinations, headache, insomnia, seizures, vertigo
EENT: Glossitis, stomatitis
GI: Abdominal pain, anorexia, diarrhea, hepatitis, nausea, pancreatitis, pseudomembranous enterocolitis, vomiting
GU: Crystalluria, renal failure, toxic nephrosis
HEME: Agranulocytosis, eosinophilia, hemolytic anemia, leukopenia, methemoglobinemia, neutropenia, thrombocytopenia
RESP: Cough, dyspnea
SKIN: Dermatitis, erythema, photosensitivity, rash, Stevens-Johnson syndrome, toxic epidermal necrolysis, urticaria
Other: Anaphylaxis, hyperkalemia, injection site inflammation and pain

Nursing Considerations

- Use cautiously in patients with impaired hepatic or renal function, severe allergy or bronchial asthma, or possible folate deficiency (patient who are elderly, long-term alcoholic, taking anticonvulsants, or malnourished or have malabsorption).
- Expect to obtain culture and sensitivity test results before beginning co-trimoxazole.
- For I.V. infusion, dilute each 5 ml of cotrimoxazole with 75 to 125 ml of D_5W before administration.
- When giving drug to neonates, don't mix with solutions that contain benzyl alcohol because this preservative has been linked to a fatal toxic syndrome involving circulatory, CNS, renal, and respiratory impairment and metabolic acidosis.
- Infuse slowly over 60 to 90 minutes.
- Assess for evidence of blood dyscrasia, including bleeding, ecchymosis, and joint pain, especially in elderly patients who are also taking a thiazide diuretic.
- Monitor older patients closely because of increased risk of bone marrow suppression, hyperkalemia, and severe skin reactions.

PATIENT TEACHING

- Instruct patient to notify prescriber immediately if rash, severe diarrhea, or other serious adverse reactions occur.

cyclophosphamide

Cytoxan, Neosar, Procytox (CAN)

Class and Category

Chemical: Nitrogen mustard derivative
Therapeutic: Alkylating antineoplastic
Pregnancy category: D

Indications and Dosages

▶ *To treat acute lymphocytic or nonlymphocytic leukemia, chronic myelocytic or lymphocytic leukemia, neuroblastoma, retinoblastoma, and Hodgkin's disease or non-Hodgkin's lymphoma*

I.V. INFUSION, I.V. INJECTION

Adults. *Initial:* 40 to 50 mg/kg in divided doses over 2 to 5 days, or 10 to 15 mg/kg q 7 to 10 days, or 3 to 5 mg/kg twice weekly. *Maintenance:* Varies with diagnosis and patient's clinical and hematologic response to, and tolerance of, therapy.

Children. *Initial:* 2 to 8 mg/kg or 60 to 250 mg/m^2 q wk or in divided doses for 6 or more days. *Maintenance:* 10 to 15 mg/kg q

7 to 10 days, or 30 mg/kg q 3 to 4 wk or when bone marrow recovers.

▶ *To treat breast, epithelial, or ovarian cancer; multiple myeloma; and mycosis fungoides*

I.V. INFUSION, I.V. INJECTION

Adults. *Initial:* 40 to 50 mg/kg in divided doses over 2 to 5 days, or 10 to 15 mg/kg q 7 to 10 days, or 3 to 5 mg/kg twice weekly. *Maintenance:* Varies with diagnosis and patient's clinical and hematologic response and tolerance to therapy.

DOSAGE ADJUSTMENT Dosage varies, depending on regimen used. Dosage may be reduced when cyclophosphamide is used with other cytotoxic drugs.

Mechanism of Action

After biotransformation in the liver, crosslinks with strands of DNA and RNA to interfere with the growth of susceptible, rapidly proliferating malignant cells. Cyclophosphamide inhibits protein synthesis within the cell and also has immunosuppressive qualities. Its actions are cell-cycle-phase–nonspecific.

Contraindications

Hypersensitivity to cyclophosphamide, severely depressed bone marrow

Interactions

DRUGS

allopurinol: Increased toxic effects of cyclophosphamide on bone marrow

blood-dyscrasia–causing drugs (cephalosporins, cisplatin): Increased leukopenic and thrombocytopenic effects of cyclophosphamide

bone marrow depressants (such as colchicine and methotrexate): Increased bone marrow depression

busulfan: Decreased cyclophosphamide clearance, possibly leading to cyclophosphamide toxicity

chloramphenicol: Decreased cyclophosphamide effectiveness

cocaine: Increased risk of prolonged cocaine effects and toxicity

cytarabine: Cardiomyopathy and risk of death

daunorubicin, doxorubicin: Risk of increased cardiotoxicity

hepatic enzyme inducers (such as allopurinol and erythromycin): Decreased half-life and increased activity of cyclophosphamide

immunosuppressants (such as azathioprine, chlorambucil, corticosteroids, and cyclosporine): Increased risk of infection and development of neoplasms

lovastatin: Increased risk of rhabdomyolysis and acute renal failure in heart transplant patients
oral anticoagulants: Decreased or increased anticoagulant activity
pentostatin, trastuzumab: Increased risk of cardiotoxicity
phenobarbital: Increased metabolism and leukopenic activity of cyclophosphamide
succinylcholine: Enhanced neuromuscular blockade effects of succinylcholine
tamoxifen: Increased risk of thromboembolism
thiazide diuretics: Increased risk of granulocytopenia
vaccines, killed virus: Possibly decreased antibody response to vaccine
vaccines, live virus: Possibly increased adverse effects of vaccine, severe infection, and decreased antibody response to vaccine

Adverse Reactions

CNS: Dizziness, headache
CV: Cardiotoxicity (including acute myopericarditis and cardiomyopathy)
EENT: Stomatitis
ENDO: Condition resembling syndrome of inappropriate ADH secretion (SIADH), hyperglycemia
GI: Anorexia, diarrhea, epigastric pain, hemorrhagic colitis, hepatitis, nausea, vomiting
GU: Amenorrhea, azoospermia, hemorrhagic and nonhemorrhagic cystitis, infertility, nephrotoxicity, oligospermia, uric acid nephropathy
HEME: Anemia, leukopenia, thrombocytopenia
RESP: Interstitial pulmonary fibrosis, pneumonitis
SKIN: Alopecia, darkened nails, diaphoresis, flushing or erythema of face, hyperpigmentation, pruritus, rash, urticaria
Other: Anaphylaxis, hyperkalemia, hyperuricemia, hyponatremia, impaired wound healing, infection, injection site edema, pain, or redness

Nursing Considerations

- Follow facility protocol for preparation and handling of antineoplastic drugs and for appropriate disposal of used equipment.
- Anticipate dosage reduction if patient is also receiving radiation therapy or a drug that depresses bone marrow.
- Monitor liver and renal function test results before and periodically during therapy because drug is metabolized in the liver and excreted by the kidneys.
- Monitor CBC, including hematocrit, platelet count, and WBC count with differential, before and periodically during therapy.

- Be prepared to hydrate patient before and after therapy to minimize the risk of hemorrhagic cystitis and to help eliminate drug-induced uric acid accumulation.
- Prepare a solution with a concentration of 20 mg/ml by adding appropriate amount of sterile water for injection or bacteriostatic water for injection (paraben-preserved only) if specified by manufacturer. Shake until dissolved. Be aware that nonlyophilized form of cyclophosphamide for injection may take up to 6 minutes to dissolve; lyophilized form takes about 45 seconds.
- **WARNING When preparing drug for administration to neonates or premature infants, don't use diluents that contain benzyl alcohol because they have been linked to a fatal toxic syndrome characterized by CNS, respiratory, circulatory, and renal impairment and metabolic acidosis.**
- Solution may be diluted further for I.V. infusion with D_5W, D_5/normal saline solution, D_5/lactated Ringer's solution, lactated Ringer's solution, 0.45 normal saline solution, or sodium lactate injection. Use within 24 hours if stored at room temperature or within 6 days if refrigerated.
- Be aware that adverse reactions can vary when cyclophosphamide is used in combination therapy. Review all drugs given in the regimen, including drug interactions and adverse effects.
- Assess patient for signs of hemorrhagic cystitis, including hematuria and dysuria, and expect to discontinue cyclophosphamide therapy if you detect them.
- Monitor serum uric acid level, especially in patients with a history of gout or urate calculi. Expect a dosage adjustment of antigout drugs if blood uric acid level is elevated from cyclophosphamide therapy. Be aware that uricosuric antigout drugs may increase the risk of uric acid nephropathy.
- Observe patient for signs of leukopenia or infection, including fever, chills, pharyngitis, tiredness or weakness, and unusual bleeding or ecchymosis.
- Monitor patients who have undergone an adrenalectomy for increased toxic effects of cyclophosphamide. Expect dosages of replacement steroids and cyclophosphamide to be adjusted.
- Be aware that effects of radiation therapy or bone marrow depressants may be increased when these therapies are administered concurrently with cyclophosphamide. Patients with a history of bone marrow depression, chickenpox (including recent exposure), or herpes zoster are at increased risk for severe generalized disease.

- Assess urine output and urinary specific gravity to assess for a syndrome resembling SIADH. Obtain urine specimen, as ordered, for microscopic examination for hematuria periodically during therapy and for several hours after a large dose.
- Monitor patient for signs of dizziness, confusion, and agitation, which could indicate a syndrome similar to SIADH. Tiredness and weakness are also symptoms.
- Be aware that some patients receiving cyclophosphamide have developed a second malignancy, such as leukemia or bladder or renal cancer; a causal relationship hasn't been established.
- Store unopened cyclophosphamide below 25° C (77° F).

PATIENT TEACHING

- Tell patient receiving cyclophosphamide to immediately report unusual bruising or bleeding; black, tarry stools; blood in urine or stools; or pinpoint red spots on the skin.
- Review with patient the need for adequate fluid intake and frequent urination (including at least once at night) to help prevent hemorrhagic cystitis and to aid in elimination of excess uric acid, which may result from cyclophosphamide treatment.
- Instruct patient to consult prescriber if he requires dental surgery or emergency treatment with general anesthesia within 10 days of cyclophosphamide treatment.
- Advise patient not to receive live or killed virus vaccines during therapy and for 3 months to 1 year after completion of cyclophosphamide therapy, unless approved by prescriber. Urge patient to avoid people who have received such vaccines or to wear a protective mask when he's around them.
- Caution patient to avoid sports and other activities that increase the risk of accidental injury. Also advise him to take measures to avoid infection, such as maintaining good oral hygiene (for example, by using soft-bristled toothbrush) and washing hands before touching eyes or nose.
- Advise patient with thrombocytopenia to avoid alcohol and aspirin to reduce the risk of GI bleeding.
- Suggest that patient with stomatitis eat soft, bland foods served cold or at room temperature to decrease irritation.
- Inform patient that his hair should grow back following treatment but that color and texture may be different.
- Inform patient that although cyclophosphamide may reduce sperm count and function and ovarian function, he should use a barrier method of birth control during therapy.

cyclosporine (cyclosporin A)

Neoral, Sandimmune, SangCya

Class and Category

Chemical: Tolypocladium inflatum Gams- or *Cylindrocarpon lucidum* Booth–derived polypeptide
Therapeutic: Antipsoriatic, antirheumatic, immunosuppressant
Pregnancy category: C

Indications and Dosages

▶ *To prevent or treat organ rejection in kidney, liver, and heart allogenic transplantation*

I.V. INFUSION

Adults. 2 to 6 mg/kg daily starting 4 to 12 hr before surgery and continuing postoperatively until patient can tolerate oral form.

Mechanism of Action

Causes immunosuppression by inhibiting the proliferation of T lymphocytes, the production and release of lymphokines, and the release of interleukin-2.

Contraindications

Abnormal renal function, neoplastic diseases, and uncontrolled hypertension in patients with psoriasis or rheumatoid arthritis (modified capsules and oral solution); hypersensitivity to cyclosporine, its components, or polyoxyethylated castor oil (I.V. infusion)

Interactions

DRUGS

ACE inhibitors, angiotensin II receptor antagonists, potassium-sparing diuretics, potassium supplements: Increased risk of hyperkalemia
amiodarone, azithromycin, bromocriptine, clarithromycin, colchicine, danazol, diltiazem, erythromycin, fluconazole, hormonal contraceptives, imatinib, itraconazole, ketoconazole, methylprednisolone, metoclopromide, nicardipine, quinupristin and dalfopristin, verapamil: Increased blood cyclosporine level
amphotericin B, azapropazon, cimetidine, ciprofloxacin, colchicine, co-trimoxazole, fibric acid derivatives (such as bezafibrate and fenofibrate), gentamicin, ketoconazole, melphalan, NSAIDs, ranitidine, tacrolimus, tobramycin, vancomycin: Increased risk of nephrotoxicity

atorvastatin, fluvastatin, lovastatin, pravastatin, simvastatin: Increased risk of myotoxicity
carbamazepine, nafcillin, octreotide, orlistat, phenobarbital, phenytoin, rifampin, St. John's wort, sulfinpyrazone, terbinafine, ticlopidine: Decreased blood cyclosporine level and therapeutic response
digoxin: Increased blood digoxin level and risk of digitalis toxicity
indinavir, nelfinavir, ritonavir, saquinavir: Possibly increased blood cyclosporine level
methotrexate: Increased blood methotrexate level
methylprednisolone (high dose): Increased risk of seizures
other immunosuppressants: Possibly excessive immunosuppression
prednisolone: Increased blood prednisolone level
sirolimus: Increased blood sirolimus level
vaccines (killed or live virus): Possibly suppressed immune response and increased adverse effects of vaccine
FOODS
Grapefruit, grapefruit juice: Increased risk of nephrotoxicity
Potassium-rich foods: Increased risk of hyperkalemia

Adverse Reactions

CNS: Altered level of consciousness, confusion, headache, intracranial hypertension, loss of motor function, paresthesia, psychiatric disturbances, seizures, tremor
CV: Chest pain, hypertension
EENT: Gingival hyperplasia, optic disc edema, oral candidiasis, visual impairment
ENDO: Gynecomastia
GI: Diarrhea, nausea, pancreatitis, vomiting
GU: Albuminuria, hematuria, proteinuria, renal failure
HEME: Anemia, leukopenia, thrombocytopenia
SKIN: Acne, flushing, hirsutism, rash
Other: Anaphylaxis, hyperkalemia, hypomagnesemia, lymphoma

Nursing Considerations

- Prepare I.V. infusion by diluting each milliliter of concentrate in 20 to 100 ml of normal saline solution or D_5W. Use glass containers because of possible leaching of diethylhexyphthalate from polyvinyl chloride bags into cyclosporine solution.
- Give infusion over 2 to 6 hours or, if needed, over 24 hours.
- **WARNING** Closely monitor for anaphylaxis at least during first 30 minutes of I.V. administration. Make sure emergency equipment and drugs are immediately available.
- **WARNING** Be aware that rapid I.V. infusion may cause acute nephrotoxicity.

- Don't draw blood to measure cyclosporine level through same I.V. tubing used to administer drug, even if line was flushed after administration. Blood level may be falsely elevated.
- Discard diluted solution after 24 hours.
- Monitor blood pressure, especially in patients with a history of hypertension, because drug can worsen this condition. Expect to decrease cyclosporine dosage if hypertension develops.
- Monitor results of liver and renal function tests, as ordered, to detect signs of decreased function.
- Although uncommon, cyclosporine may cause neurotoxicity, especially after liver transplantation. Watch for evidence of encephalopathy: impaired consciousness, loss of motor function, psychiatric disurbance, seizures, and visual disturbance.
- Be aware that cyclosporine may increase serum cholesterol level and St. John's wort may decrease blood cyclosporine level.

PATIENT TEACHING

- Instruct patient not to receive virus vaccines during therapy. Urge him to avoid people who have received such vaccines or to wear a protective mask when he's around them.
- Caution patient to avoid exposure to infection during therapy because cyclosporine causes immunosuppression.
- Urge patient to maintain good dental hygiene because of risk of gingival hyperplasia.

D

daclizumab (dacliximab)

Zenapax

Class and Category

Chemical: Monoclonal antibody
Therapeutic: Immunosuppressant
Pregnancy category: C

Indications and Dosages

▶ *To prevent acute organ rejection after kidney transplantation*

I.V. INFUSION

Adults and children. 1 mg/kg given in five doses: dose 1 given no more than 24 hr before transplantation; doses 2 through 5 at 14-day intervals.

> **Mechanism of Action**
> Inhibits interleukin-2–mediated activation of lymphocytes, which prevents WBCs from attacking the transplanted kidney. Daclizumab also reduces the body's infection-fighting ability.

Contraindications

Hypersensitivity to daclizumab or its components

Interactions

None known.

Adverse Reactions

CNS: Anxiety, chills, depression, dizziness, fatigue, fever, headache, insomnia, paresthesia, tremor, weakness
CV: Chest pain, edema, hypertension, hypotension, tachycardia, thrombosis
EENT: Blurred vision, pharyngitis, rhinitis
ENDO: Hyperglycemia
GI: Abdominal distention and pain, constipation, diarrhea, flatu-

lence, gastritis, heartburn, hemorrhoids, indigestion, nausea, vomiting
GU: Dysuria, hematuria, hydronephrosis, oliguria, renal insufficiency, renal tubular necrosis, urine retention
HEME: Bleeding
MS: Arthralgia, back pain, leg cramps, myalgia
RESP: Atelectasis, cough, crackles, dyspnea, hypoxia, lung congestion, pleural effusion, pulmonary edema
SKIN: Acne, diaphoresis, hirsutism, impaired wound healing, night sweats, pruritus, rash
Other: Dehydration, fluid overload, injection site pain and redness, lymphocele

Nursing Considerations

- Avoid shaking daclizumab vial before use. Dilute calculated dose of daclizumab in 50 ml of normal saline solution. Gently invert bag to mix; to prevent foaming, don't shake it.
- Don't use solution if it contains particles or is discolored.
- Use room temperature solution within 4 hours or refrigerated solution within 24 hours; discard unused solution.
- Because daclizumab's compatibility with other drugs isn't known, don't add or simultaneously infuse other drugs through same I.V. line.
- Administer drug through a peripheral or central vein over 15 minutes.
- Monitor blood glucose level for increases during therapy.
- **WARNING** Although daclizumab seldom causes severe hypersensitivity reactions, keep drugs that treat such reactions readily available.
- Before using drug, store it at 2° to 8° C (36° to 46° F). Don't freeze or shake; protect from direct light.

PATIENT TEACHING

- Urge patient to complete full course of daclizumab therapy and to return for scheduled follow-up visits.

dantrolene sodium

Dantrium, Dantrium Intravenous

Class and Category

Chemical: Hydantoin derivative, imidazolidinedione sodium salt
Therapeutic: Malignant hyperthermia therapy adjunct
Pregnancy category: C (parenteral), not rated (oral)

Indications and Dosages

▶ *To prevent malignant hyperthermia before surgery*

I.V. INFUSION

Adults and children. *Initial:* 2.5 mg/kg infused over 1 hr 60 to 75 min before anesthesia. Additional individualized doses given as needed during surgery.

CAPSULES

Adults and children. 4 to 8 mg/kg daily in divided doses t.i.d. or q.i.d. 1 or 2 days before surgery, with last dose given 3 to 4 hr before surgery.

▶ *To treat malignant hyperthermia*

I.V. INJECTION

Adults and adolescents. *Initial:* 1 mg/kg by rapid bolus, repeated as needed until symptoms subside or cumulative dose of 10 mg/kg has been reached. Dose is repeated if symptoms reappear.

▶ *To treat postmalignant hyperthermic crisis*

I.V. INJECTION

Adults and children. *Initial:* Individualized dosage beginning with 1 mg/kg or more as needed if oral therapy can't be used. *Maximum:* 10 mg/kg total dose.

CAPSULES

Adults and children. 4 to 8 mg/kg daily in divided doses q.i.d. for 1 to 3 days.

Mechanism of Action

Prevents calcium release from the sarcoplasmic reticulum of skeletal muscle cells. Blocked calcium release inhibits the activation of acute catabolism associated with malignant hyperthermia.

Incompatibilities

Don't administer dantrolene with acidic solutions, including D_5W and normal saline solution.

Contraindications

For oral drug only: Active hepatic disease (such as cirrhosis and hepatitis), conditions in which spasticity helps maintain upright posture and improve balance or function, skeletal muscle spasms caused by rheumatic disorders

Interactions

DRUGS

calcium channel blockers (especially verapamil): Possibly hyperkalemia, life-threatening arrhythmias, and shock

sedatives: Possibly profound sedation

ACTIVITIES

alcohol use: Possibly increased CNS depression

Adverse Reactions

CNS: Dizziness, drowsiness, fatigue, light-headedness, malaise, slurred speech or other speech problems, weakness

CV: Heart failure, pericarditis

GI: Abdominal cramps, diarrhea, dysphagia, hepatitis, hepatotoxicity, nausea, vomiting

GU: Enuresis

MS: Decreased grip strength, myalgia

RESP: Dyspnea, feeling of suffocation, pleural effusion

SKIN: Erythema, extravasation with tissue damage, urticaria

Other: Thrombophlebitis

Nursing Considerations

- Reconstitute each vial of dantrolene with 60 ml of sterile water for injection (without a bacteriostatic agent). Shake vial until clear. Store reconstituted solution at room temperature, protected from direct sunlight. Discard after 6 hours.
- To prevent precipitation of reconstituted drug, transfer it to a plastic I.V. bag, rather than a glass bottle, for infusion. Don't use solution if it contains precipitate or is cloudy.
- Because drug has a high pH, infuse into a central vein, if possible, to avoid tissue damage from extravasation.
- Monitor blood pressure and heart rate often during drug administration to detect tachycardia and blood pressure changes.
- Monitor results of liver function tests—especially ALT, AST, alkaline phosphatase, and total bilirubin levels—for hepatotoxicity.
- Be aware that oral form of dantrolene is also used to treat chronic spastic conditions. Consult manufacturer's insert for additional dosage guidelines, nursing considerations, and adverse reactions associated with long-term oral use.
- Before reconstituting dantrolene, store it at 15° to 30° C (59° to 86° F), and avoid prolonged exposure to light.

PATIENT TEACHING

- Inform patient that dantrolene may weaken her grip strength as well as muscles used for walking and climbing stairs. Advise her

to be careful when eating to avoid problems due to difficulty swallowing.
- Caution patient about drug's sedating effects. Instruct her to avoid sedatives, unless prescribed, and other sedating substances, such as alcohol.
- Advise patient to report yellow skin or sclerae, itching, or fatigue.

daptomycin

Cubicin

Class and Category

Chemical: Cyclic lipopetide
Therapeutic: Antibacterial
Pregnancy category: B

Indications and Dosages

▶ *To treat complicated skin and skin-structure infections caused by* Staphylococcus aureus *(including methicillin-resistant microorganisms);* Staphylococcus pyogenes, Streptococcus agalactiae, Streptococcus dysgalactiae *subsp.* equisimilis, *and* Enterococcus faecalis *(vancomycin-susceptible isolates only).*

I.V. INFUSION

Adults. 4 mg/kg over 30 min once daily q 24 hr for 7 to 14 days.

▶ *To treat* S. aureus *bacteremia including those with right-sided infective endocarditis, caused by methicillin-susceptible and methicillin-resistant isolates*

I.V. INFUSION

Adults. 6 mg/kg over 30 min once daily for 2 to 6 weeks

DOSAGE ADJUSTMENT For patients with a creatinine clearance less than 30 ml/min, dosage interval increased to once every 48 hours

Route	Onset	Peak	Duration
I.V.	Unknown	72 hr	Unknown

Mechanism of Action

Binds to bacterial membranes, allowing efflux of potassium to cause depolarization of the membrane potential. With the loss of the membrane potential, inhibition of protein, DNA, and RNA synthesis occur, which causes bacterial cell death.

Incompatibilities

Daptomycin is incompatible with dextrose-containing diluents and should not be given with other I.V. substances, additives, or other medications

Contraindications

Hypersensitivity to daptomycin or its components

Interactions

DRUGS

HMG-CoA reductase inhibitors: Increased risk of myopathy

Adverse Reactions

CNS: Anxiety, asthenia, confusion, dizziness, fever, headache, insomnia, neuropathy
CV: Chest pain, edema, heart failure, hypertension, hypotension
EENT: Throat pain
ENDO: Hyperglycemia, hypoglycemia
GI: Abdominal pain, abnormal liver function tests, constipation, decreased appetite, diarrhea, dyspepsia, elevated CK level, GI hemorrhage, nausea, vomiting
GU: Renal failure, UTI
HEME: Anemia
MS: Arthralgia, back pain, limb pain, muscle pain or weakness, myopathy, osteomyelitis, rhabdomyolysis
RESP: Cough, dyspnea, pleural effusion, pneumonia
SKIN: Cellulitis, diaphoresis, erythema, rash, pruritis, truncal erythema, urticaria
Other: Anaphylaxis, bacteremia, *Candida* infection, fungal infection, hyperkalemia, hypokalemia, injection site reactions, sepsis

Nursing Considerations

- Expect to obtain samples for culture and sensitivity tests before daptomycin treatment begins.
- Reconstitute daptomycin powder with 10 ml normal saline solution and then further dilute with normal saline solution. If kept at room temperature, use within 12 hours; if refrigerated, use within 48 hours.
- Administer as an I.V. infusion over 30 minutes.
- Be aware that daptomycin is compatible with normal saline and lactated Ringer's solutions. It is not compatible with dextrose-containing solutions.
- Monitor patient's bowel elimination. If diarrhea develops, obtain stool culture to check for pseudomembranous colitis. If

confirmed, expect to stop drug and give fluid, electrolytes, and antibiotics effective against *Clostridium difficile.*

- Obtain repeated blood cultures, as ordered, if patient has persistent or relapsing *S. aureus* infection or has a poor response to daptomycin therapy. Surgical intervention at the site of the infection (such as debridement, removal of prosthetic device, or valve replacement) may be needed.
- Assess patient regularly for muscle pain or weakness, particularly affecting the arms or legs. If present, notify prescriber.
- Montior patient's CK level weekly or more often if the patient has recently or is currently receiving therapy with an HMG-CoA reductase inhibitor or has renal insufficiency. If CK level is elevated, increase monitoring frequency. Expect to discontinue drug if patient develops unexplained signs and symptoms of myopathy with CK level of 1,000 to 2,000 units/L. If CK level exceeds 2,000 units/L, expect to stop giving drug if patient is symptom-free.
- Monitor patient closely for signs and symptoms of neuropathy. If present, notify prescriber.

PATIENT TEACHING

- Tell patient to report unexplained muscle or limb pain or weakness to prescriber.
- Instruct patient to alert prescriber if signs and symptoms of an allergic reaction occur, such as a rash, itching, hives, or difficulty breathing.
- Inform patient that regular blood tests will be needed throughout daptomycin therapy.
- Tell patient with bacteremia that daptomycin therapy may be needed for up to 6 weeks.

darbepoetin alfa

Aranesp

Class and Category

Chemical: 165-amino acid glycoprotein identical to human erythropoietin
Therapeutic: Antianemic
Pregnancy category: C

Indications and Dosages

▶ *To treat anemia from chronic renal failure*

I.V. INJECTION

Adults. *Initial:* 0.45 mcg/kg as a single dose q wk. *Maintenance:*

Dosage individualized and increased once a month to maintain a hemoglobin level of 12 g/dl or less.

DOSAGE ADJUSTMENT Dosage reduced by about 25% if hemoglobin level increases and approaches 12 g/dl. If hemoglobin level continues to increase, doses temporarily withheld until hemoglobin level begins to decrease; then therapy is restarted at a dose about 25% below previous dose. Dosage reduced by about 25% if hemoglobin level increases by more than 1.0 g/dl in a 2-week period. Dosage increased by about 25% of previous dose if hemoglobin level increases less than 1 g/dl over 4 weeks but only if serum ferritin level is 100 mcg/L or greater and serum transferrin saturation is 20% or greater. Further increases made at 4-week intervals until specified hemoglobin level is obtained.

DOSAGE ADJUSTMENT For conversion from epoetin alfa to darbepoetin alfa, drug given q wk for patient who previously received epoetin alfa two to three times/wk and once every 2 wk for patient who previously received epoetin alfa once/wk. For patients being converted from epoetin alfa, 6.25 mcg/wk darbepoetin alfa given q wk for patients who received less than 2,500 units/wk of epoetin alfa; 12.5 mcg/wk darbepoetin alfa given q wk for patients who received 2,500 to 4,999 units/wk of epoetin alfa; 25 mcg/wk darbepoetin alfa given q wk for patients who received 5,000 to 10,999 units/wk of epoetin alfa; 40 mcg/wk darbepoetin alfa given q wk for patients who received 11,000 to 17,999 units/wk of epoetin alfa; 60 mcg/wk darbepoetin alfa given q wk for patients who received 18,000 to 33,999 units/wk of epoetin alfa; 100 mcg/wk darbepoetin alfa given q wk for patients who received 34,000 to 89,999 units/wk of epoetin alfa; 200 mcg/wk darbepoetin alfa given q wk for patients who received 90,000 or more units/wk of epoetin alfa.

Route	Onset	Peak	Duration
I.V.	2 to 6 wk	Unknown	Unknown

Mechanism of Action

Stimulates the release of reticulocytes from the bone marrow into the bloodstream, where they develop into mature RBCs.

Incompatibilities

Don't mix darbepoetin alfa with any other drug.

Contraindications

Hypersensitivity to human albumin or products made from mammal cells; uncontrolled hypertension

Interactions

DRUGS

None known

Adverse Reactions

CNS: Asthenia, dizziness, fatigue, fever, headache, seizures
CV: Arrhythmias, cardiac arrest, chest pain, congestive heart failure, hypertension, hypotension, peripheral edema, vascular access hemorrhage, vascular access thrombosis
GI: Abdominal pain, constipation, diarrhea, nausea, vomiting
MS: Arthralgia, back pain, limb pain, myalgia
RESP: Bronchitis, cough, dyspnea, upper respiratory tract infection
SKIN: Rash, urticaria
Other: Antibody formation against darbepoetin alfa, fluid overload, infection, flulike symptoms, injection site pain, sepsis

Nursing Considerations

- Before starting therapy, expect to correct folic acid or vitamin B_{12} deficiencies because these conditions may interfere with drug's effectiveness.
- To ensure effective drug response, expect to obtain serum ferritin level and serum transferrin saturation before beginning and during therapy, as ordered. If serum ferritin level is less than 100 mcg/l or serum transferrin saturation is less than 20%, expect to begin supplemental iron therapy.
- Don't shake vial during preparation to avoid denaturing drug and rendering it biologically inactive.
- Discard drug if you see particulate matter or discoloration.
- Don't dilute drug before giving it.
- Discard unused portion of drug because it contains no preservatives.
- Monitor blood pressure frequently during therapy for hypertension. Expect to reduce dosage or withhold drug if blood pressure is poorly controlled with antihypertensive and dietary measures.

- Monitor hemoglobin level weekly, as ordered, until hemoglobin stabilizes and maintenance dosage has been achieved. Thereafter, monitor hemoglobin level regularly, as ordered. After each dosage adjustment, expect to monitor hemoglobin level weekly for 4 weeks until hemoglobin level stabilizes in response to dosage change.
- **WARNING** Assess patient for a sudden but rare change in condition that may reflect a severe anemia as a result of loss of response to darbepoetin alfa. If this occurs, be prepared for patient to undergo tests as ordered to rule out infections, inflammatory or malignant processes, osteofibrosis cystica, occult blood loss, hemolysis, severe aluminum toxicity, or bone marrow fibrosis, any of which may compromise an erythropoietic response.
- **WARNING** Be aware that the risk of cardiac arrest, seizures, CVA, exacerbations of hypertension, congestive heart failure, vascular thrombosis, vascular ischemia, vascular infarction, acute MI, and fluid overload with peripheral edema increases if hemoglobin level increases more than about 1 g/dl during any 2-week period. Expect to decrease darbepoetin dosage if this occurs.
- Institute seizure precautions according to facility policy.
- For patients with chronic renal failure who aren't receiving dialysis, expect to administer doses lower than those given to patients receiving dialysis. Also, monitor renal function test results and fluid and electrolyte balance in these patients for signs of deteriorating renal function.
- Store drug at 2° to 8° C (36° to 46° F). Don't freeze, and protect from light.

PATIENT TEACHING

- Advise patient that the risk of seizures is highest during the first 90 days of drug therapy. Discourage her from engaging in hazardous activities during this time.
- Stress the importance of complying with the dosage regimen and keeping follow-up medical and laboratory appointments.
- Advise patient to follow up with her prescriber for blood pressure monitoring.
- Encourage patient to eat adequate quantities of iron-rich foods.
- Review possible adverse reactions, and urge patient to notify prescriber if she experiences chest pain, headache, rash, seizures, shortness of breath, or swelling.

decitabine

Dacogen

Class and Category

Chemical: Analogue of natural nucleoside 2′-deoxycytidine
Therapeutic: Antineoplastic
Pregnancy category: D

Indications and Dosages

▶ *To treat myelodysplastic syndromes (MDS), including secondary MDS of all French-American-British subtypes and intermediate 1 and 2 and high-risk International Prognostic Scoring System groups*

I.V. INFUSION

Adults. 15 mg/m^2 over 3 hr; then repeated q 8 hr for 3 days, with cycle repeated q 6 wk for a minimum of four cycles.

DOSAGE ADJUSTMENT For hematologic recovery that requires more than 6 wk but less than 8 wk, treatment delayed for up to 2 wk and dose temporarily reduced to 11 mg/m^2 q 8 hr. For hematologic recovery that requires more than 8 wk but less than 10 wk, treatment delayed up to 2 more wk and dose reduced to 11 mg/m^2 q 8 hr with dosage maintained or increased in subsequent cycles as clinically indicated.

Mechanism of Action

After phosphorylation and incorporation into DNA, inhibits DNA methyltransferase, resulting in hypomethylation of DNA and cellular differentiation. In neoplastic cells, hypomethylation may restore normal function to genes essential for control of cellular differentiation and proliferation. Decitabine also may kill rapidly dividing cells by forming covalent adducts between DNA methyltransferase and decitabine-saturated DNA.

Contraindications

Hypersensitivity to decitabine or its components

Interactions

DRUGS

live-virus vaccines: increased risk of infection resulting from vaccine

Adverse Reactions

CNS: Anxiety, cerebral edema, confusion, dizziness, fatigue, fever, headache, hypoesthesia, insomnia, intracranial hemorrhage, lethargy, malaise, rigors

CV: Atrial fibrillation, cardiac arrest, chest discomfort or pain, heart failure, hypotension, MI, peripheral edema
EENT: Bleeding gums, blurred vision, lip or tongue ulceration, oral mucous petechiae, oral candidasis, pharyngitis, postnasal drip, sinusitis, stomatitis
ENDO: Hyperglycemia
GI: Abdominal distention or pain, anorexia, ascities, abdominal pain, constipation, decreased appetite, diarrhea, dysphagia, dyspepsia, gastroesophageal reflux disease, hyperbilirubinemia, nausea, vomiting
GU: Dysuria, urinary frequency, UTI
HEME: Anemia, leukopenia, neutropenia, thrombocytopenia, thrombocythemia
MS: Arthralgia, back or limb pain, myalgia
RESP: Decreased breath sounds, cough, crackles, hypoxia, pneumonia, pulmonary edema
SKIN: Alopecia, cellulites, ecchymosis, erythema, hematoma, pallor, petechiae, pruritis, rash, urticaria
Other: Bacteremia, candidal infection, dehydration, facial edema, hyperkalemia, hypoalbuminemia, hypokalemia, hypomagnesemia, hyponatremia, injection site swelling, pain and redness; lymphodenpathy

Nursing Considerations

- Use cautiously in patients with liver or renal impairment.
- Follow facility protocols for preparation and handling of antineoplastic drugs and for appropriate disposal of used equipment.
- Reconstitute with 10 ml sterile water using aseptic technique. Upon reconstitution know that each ml contains approximately 5 mg of decitabine. Immediately after reconstitution, further dilute with normal saline solution, dextrose 5%, or lactated Ringer's solution to a final drug concentration of 0.1 to 1 mg/ml. Use within 15 minutes or if delay is anticipated, reconstitute drug using cold dilution solution and store in refrigerator for up to 7 hr.
- Monitor CBC, including hematocrit, platelet count, and WBC with differential as well as electrolytes, liver enzymes and serum creatinine before and intermittently during decitabine therapy, as ordered.
- Assess for signs of infection, such as fever, if patient develops leukopenia. Expect to obtain appropriate specimens for culture and sensitivity testing.

• **WARNING** Monitor patient closely for non-hematological toxicities such as active or uncontrolled infections, a serum creatinine level greater than 2 mg/dl, or serum glutamic pyruvic transaminase or total bilirubin levels 2 times or more the upper normal limits. If present, notify prescriber and expect decitabine therapy to be withheld until resolved.

PATIENT TEACHING

• Advise male patients not to father a child during decitabine therapy and for 2 months after. Also urge female patients to use contraception to avoid pregnancy during therapy and to notify prescriber immediately if pregnancy occurs.
• Advise patient to have dental work completed before beginning decitabine therapy, if possible, or to defer such work until blood counts return to normal because drug can delay healing and cause gingival bleeding. Teach patient proper oral hygiene, and advise him to use a soft-bristled toothbrush.
• Instruct patient who develops bone marrow depression to avoid persons with infections. Advise him to report fever, cough, or lower back or side pain as these signs and symptoms may indicate infection.
• Stress the importance of avoiding accidental cuts from sharp objects, such as razor blades or fingernail clippers, because excessive bleeding or infection may occur.
• Advise patient with stomatitis to eat bland, soft foods served cold or at room temperature to decrease irritation.
• Stress the importance of complying with the dosage regimen and of keeping follow-up medical appointments and appointments for laboratory tests.

desmopressin acetate

DDAVP Injection, Octostim (CAN)

Class and Category

Chemical: Synthetic ADH analogue
Therapeutic: Antidiuretic, antihemorrhagic
Pregnancy category: B

Indications and Dosages

▶ *To control symptoms of central diabetes insipidus*

I.V. INFUSION

Adults. 2 to 4 mcg daily in divided doses b.i.d. Dosage adjusted as needed.

▶ *To prevent or manage bleeding episodes in hemophilia A or mild to*

moderate type I von Willebrand's disease
I.V. INFUSION
Adults and children weighing more than 10 kg (22 lb). 0.3 mcg/kg diluted in 50 ml of normal saline solution and infused over 15 to 30 min. If used preoperatively, give 30 min before procedure.
Children who weigh 10 kg or less. 0.3 mcg/kg diluted in 10 ml of normal saline solution and infused over 15 to 30 min. If used preoperatively, dose is given 30 min before procedure.

Route	Onset	Peak	Duration
I.V.	15 to 30 min*	30 to 60 min*	3 hr†

Mechanism of Action
Exerts an antidiuretic effect similar to that of vasopressin by increasing cellular permeability of renal collecting ducts and distal tubules, thus enhancing water reabsorption, reducing urine flow, and increasing osmolality. As an antihemorrhagic, drug increases blood level of clotting Factor VIII (antihemophilic factor) and activity of von Willebrand's Factor (factor VII_{VWF}). It also may increase platelet aggregation and adhesion at injury sites by directly affecting blood vessel walls.

Contraindications
Hypersensitivity to desmopressin or its components

Interactions
DRUGS
carbamazepine, chlorpropamide, clofibrate: Possibly potentiated antidiuretic effect of desmopressin
demeclocycline, lithium: Possibly decreased antidiuretic effect of desmopressin
vasopressor drugs: Possibly potentiated vasopressor effect of desmopressin

Adverse Reactions
CNS: Asthenia, chills, dizziness, headache
CV: Hypertension (with high doses), transient hypotension
EENT: Conjunctivitis, epistaxis, lacrimation, nasal congestion (nasal form), ocular edema, pharyngitis, rhinitis
GI: Nausea

* For antihemorrhagic effect.
† For von Willebrand's disease; 4 to 20 hr for mild hemophilia A.

GU: Vulvar pain (parenteral form)
SKIN: Flushing
Other: Anaphylaxis, injection site pain and redness; water intoxication

Nursing Considerations

- Use desmopressin cautiously in patients with conditions associated with fluid and electrolyte imbalance, such as cystic fibrosis; such patients are prone to hyponatremia.
- Monitor blood pressure frequently during therapy.

PATIENT TEACHING

- To prevent hyponatremia and water intoxication in a child or an elderly patient, instruct family to restrict fluids as prescribed.
- Urge patient to notify prescriber if adverse reactions occur.

dexamethasone sodium phosphate

Cortastat, Dalalone, Decadrol, Decaject, Dexacorten, Dexasone, Dexone, Hexadrol Phosphate, Primethasone, Solurex

Class and Category

Chemical: Synthetic adrenocortical steroid
Therapeutic: Anti-inflammatory, diagnostic aid, immunosuppressant
Pregnancy category: C

Indications and Dosages

▶ *To treat endocrine disorders, such as congenital adrenal hyperplasia, hypercalcemia with cancer, and nonsuppurative thyroiditis; acute episodes or exacerbations of rheumatic disorders; collagen diseases, such as systemic lupus erythematosus and acute rheumatic carditis; severe dermatologic diseases; severe allergic conditions, such as seasonal or perennial allergic rhinitis, bronchial asthma, serum sickness, and drug hypersensitivity reactions; respiratory diseases, such as symptomatic sarcoidosis, Löffler's syndrome, berylliosis, fulminating or disseminated pulmonary tuberculosis, and aspiration pneumonitis; hematologic disorders, such as idiopathic thrombocytopenic purpura and secondary thrombocytopenia in adults, autoimmune hemolytic anemia, aplastic crisis, and congenital hypoplastic anemia; tuberculous meningitis and trichinosis with neurologic or myocardial involvement*

▶ *To manage leukemias and lymphomas in adults and acute leukemia in children; to induce diuresis or remission of proteinuria in idiopathic nephrotic syndrome without uremia or nephrotic syndrome caused by systemic lupus erythematosus*

▶ *To provide palliative therapy during acute exacerbations of GI diseases, such as ulcerative colitis and regional enteritis*
I.V. INJECTION
Adults. Highly individualized dosage based on severity of disorder. *Usual:* 0.75 to 9 mg daily as a single dose or in divided doses.
▶ *To manage adrenocortical insufficiency*
I.V. INJECTION
Adults. 0.5 to 9 mg daily as a single dose or in divided doses.
▶ *To decrease cerebral edema*
I.V. INJECTION
Adults. 10 mg I.V. followed by 4 mg I.M. q 6 hr. Decreased after 2 to 4 days, if needed, gradually tapering off over 5 to 7 days unless inoperable or recurring brain tumor is present. If such a tumor is present, dosage gradually decreased after 2 to 4 days to maintenance dosage of 2 mg I.M. q 8 to 12 hr and switched to P.O. regimen as soon as possible.
▶ *To treat unresponsive shock*
I.V. INFUSION AND INJECTION
Adults. 20 mg as a single dose followed by 3 mg/kg over 24 hr as a continuous infusion; 40 mg as a single dose followed by 40 mg q 2 to 6 hr, as needed; or 1 mg/kg as a single dose. All regimens used for no more than 3 days.

Mechanism of Action

Binds to intracellular glucocorticoid receptors and suppresses inflammatory and immune responses by:
- inhibiting neutrophil and monocyte accumulation at inflammation site and suppressing their phagocytic and bactericidal activity
- stabilizing lysosomal membranes
- suppressing antigen response of macrophages and helper T cells
- inhibiting synthesis of inflammatory response mediators, such as cytokines, interleukins, and prostaglandins.

Contraindications

Administration of live virus vaccine to patient or family member, hypersensitivity to dexamethasone or its components (including sulfites), idiopathic thrombocytopenic purpura (I.M. use), systemic fungal infections

Interactions

DRUGS

aminoglutethimide, antacids, barbiturates, carbamazepine, hydantoins, mitotane, rifampin: Decreased dexamethasone effectiveness
amphotericin B (parenteral), carbonic anhydrase inhibitors: Risk of hypokalemia
anticholinesterases: Decreased anticholinesterase effectiveness in myasthenia gravis
aspirin, NSAIDs: Increased risk of adverse GI effects
cholestyramine: Increased dexamethasone clearance
cyclosporine: Increased activity of both drugs, possibly resulting in seizures
digoxin: Increased risk of digitalis toxicity related to hypokalemia
ephedrine: Decreased half-life and increased clearance of dexamethasone
erythromycin, indinavir: Increased clearance and decreased plasma concentrations of these drugs
estrogens, ketoconazole, macrolide antibiotics: Decreased dexamethasone clearance
isoniazid: Decreased blood isoniazid level
neuromuscular blockers: Possibly potentiated or counteracted neuromuscular blockade
oral anticoagulants: Altered coagulation times, requiring reduced anticoagulant dosage
oral contraceptives: Increased half-life and concentration of dexamethasone
phenytoin: Increased risk of seizures
potassium-wasting diuretics: Increased potassium loss and risk of hypokalemia
salicylates: Decreased blood level and effectiveness of salicylates
somatrem: Possibly inhibition of somatrem's growth-promoting effect
thalidomide: Increased risk of toxic epidermal necrolysis
theophyllines: Altered effects of either drug
toxoids, vaccines: Decreased antibody response

ACTIVITIES

alcohol use: Increased risk of GI bleeding

Adverse Reactions

CNS: Depression, emotional lability, euphoria, fever, headache, increased ICP with papilledema, insomnia, light-headedness, malaise, neuritis, neuropathy, paresthesia, psychosis, seizures, syncope, tiredness, vertigo, weakness

CV: Arrhythmias, bradycardia, edema, fat embolism, heart failure, hypercholesterolemia, hyperlipidemia, hypertension, myocardial rupture, tachycardia, thromboembolism, thrombophlebitis, vasculitis
EENT: Cataracts, glaucoma, vision changes (all forms); epistaxis, loss of smell and taste, nasal burning and dryness, oral candidiasis, perforated nasal septum, pharyngitis, rebound nasal congestion, rhinorrhea, sneezing (nasal aerosol)
ENDO: Cushingoid symptoms, decreased iodine uptake, growth suppression in children, hyperglycemia, menstrual irregularities, secondary adrenocortical and pituitary unresponsiveness
GI: Abdominal distention, bloody stools, elevated liver function test results, heartburn, hepatomegaly, increased appetite, indigestion, intestinal perforation, melena, nausea, pancreatitis, peptic ulcer with possible perforation, ulcerative esophagitis, vomiting
GU: Glycosuria, increased or decreased number and motility of spermatozoa, perineal irritation, urinary frequency
HEME: Leukocytosis, leukopenia
MS: Aseptic necrosis of femoral and humeral heads; muscle atrophy, spasms, or weakness; myalgia; osteoporosis; pathologic fracture of long bones; tendon rupture (intra-articular injection); vertebral compression fracture
RESP: Bronchospasm
SKIN: Acne, allergic dermatitis, diaphoresis, ecchymosis, erythema, hirsutism, necrotizing vasculitis, petechiae, subcutaneous fat atrophy, striae, thin and fragile skin, urticaria
Other: Aggravated or masked signs of infection, anaphylaxis, angioedema, hypernatremia, hypocalcemia, hypokalemia, hypokalemic alkalosis, impaired wound healing, metabolic acidosis, sodium and fluid retention, suppressed skin test reaction, weight gain

Nursing Considerations

- Use dexamethasone cautiously in patients with congestive heart failure, hypertension, or renal insufficiency because drug can cause sodium retention, which may lead to edema and hypokalemia.
- Also use cautiously in patients who have had intestinal sugery and in those with peptic ulcer, diverticulitis, or ulcerative colitis because of the risk of perforation.
- Give once-daily dose of dexamethasone in the morning to coincide with the body's natural cortisol secretion.

- Be aware that dosage forms with a concentration of 24 mg/ml are for I.V. use only.
- **WARNING** Avoid subcutaneous injection; it may cause atrophy and sterile abscess.
- Inject undiluted I.V. dose directly into I.V. tubing of infusing compatible solution over 30 seconds or less, as prescribed.
- **WARNING** Don't give acetate form by I.V. injection.
- Expect to taper drug rather than stopping it abruptly; prolonged use can cause adrenal suppression.
- Monitor fluid intake and output and daily weight, and assess patient for crackles, dyspnea, peripheral edema, and steady weight gain.
- Periodically evaluate growth if patient is a child.
- Test stool for occult blood.
- Monitor results of hematology studies as well as blood glucose and serum electrolyte, cholesterol, and lipid levels. Dexamethasone may cause hyperglycemia, hypernatremia, hypocalcemia, hypokalemia, or leukopenia. It also may increase serum cholesterol and lipid levels, and it may decrease iodine uptake by the thyroid.
- Assess for evidence of osteoporosis, Cushing's syndrome, and other systemic effects during long-term use.
- Monitor neonate for signs of hypoadrenocorticism if mother received dexamethasone during pregnancy. Be aware that some preparations also contain benzyl alcohol, which may cause a fatal toxic syndrome in neonates and immature infants.
- Assess for hypersensitivity reactions after giving acetate or sodium phosphate form; both may contain bisulfites or parabens, inactive ingredients to which some people are allergic.

PATIENT TEACHING

- Caution patient to avoid alcoholic beverages during therapy because they increase the risk of GI bleeding.
- Advise patient to follow a low-sodium, high-potassium, high-protein diet, if prescribed, to help minimize weight gain (common with this drug). Instruct her to inform prescriber if she's on a special diet.
- Instruct patient not to stop using drug abruptly.
- Advise patient to notify prescriber if condition recurs or worsens after dosage is reduced or therapy stops.
- Urge patient to have regular eye examinations during long-term use.

- Advise patient receiving long-term therapy to carry medical identification and to notify all health care providers that she takes dexamethasone.
- Instruct patient (especially a child) to avoid close contact with anyone who has chickenpox or measles and to notify prescriber immediately if exposure occurs.
- Advise patient and family members to avoid live virus vaccinations, such as oral polio vaccine, during therapy unless prescriber approves.
- Inform diabetic patient that drug may affect her blood glucose level.
- Advise patient to notify prescriber about anorexia, depression, light-headedness, malaise, muscle pain, nausea, vomiting, and signs of early hyperadrenocorticism (abdominal distention, amenorrhea, easy bruising, extreme weakness, facial hair, increased appetite, moon face, weight gain). Inform patient and family about possible changes in appearance.
- Encourage patient to notify prescriber about illness, surgery, or changes in stress level.

dexrazoxane

Zinecard

Class and Category

Chemical: Piperazinedione
Therapeutic: Cardioprotective agent, chelating agent
Pregnancy category: C

Indications and Dosages

▶ *To prevent or reduce severity of cardiomyopathy associated with doxorubicin therapy in women with metastatic breast cancer*

I.V. INJECTION

Adults. *Initial:* 500 mg/m^2 for every 50 mg/m^2 of doxorubicin q 3 wk.

DOSAGE ADJUSTMENT In patients with hyperbilirubinemia, dosage proportionately reduced (depending on severity) to maintain a dexrazoxane-to-doxorubicin ratio of 10:1. In patients with creatinine clearance of less than 40 ml/min, dosage decreased 50%.

Incompatibilities

Don't mix dexrazoxane in same I.V. line with other drugs.

Mechanism of Action

Rapidly enters cardiac cells and acts as an intracellular heavy metal chelator. In cardiac tissues, anthracyclines, such as doxorubicin, form complexes with iron or copper, resulting in damage to cardiac cell membranes and mitochondria. Dexrazoxane combines with intracellular iron and protects against anthracycline-induced free radical damage to the myocardium. It also prevents the conversion of ferrous ions back to ferric ions for use by free radicals.

Contraindications

Hypersensitivity to dexrazoxane or its components; use with chemotherapy regimens that do not contain an anthracycline, such as daunorubicin, doxorubicin, epirubicin, idarubicin, or mitoxantrone

Interactions

bone marrow depressants: Possibly enhanced bone marrow depression

Adverse Reactions

HEME: Myelosuppression including granulocytopenia, leukopenia, or thrombocytopenia
Other: Injection site pain

Nursing Considerations

- **WARNING** Use gloves when preparing reconstituted solution. If dexrazoxane powder or solution comes in contact with your skin or mucosa, immediately and thoroughly wash with soap and water.
- Reconstitute drug by mixing with 25 or 50 ml of 0.167 molar sodium lactate, supplied by the manufacturer, to produce a final concentration of 10 mg/ml. Administer reconstituted solution by slow I.V. push, or further dilute with either normal saline solution or D_5W to a concentration of 1.3 to 5 mg/ml, as prescribed, for rapid I.V. infusion.
- Be aware that dexrazoxane may interfere with tumor response to doxorubicin, especially in patients receiving drug at start of fluorouracil-doxorubicin-cyclophosphamide therapy.
- Monitor patient with immunosuppression or decreased bone marrow reserves resulting from prior chemotherapy or radiation therapy to prevent worsening of her condition. Notify prescriber if condition deteriorates.

PATIENT TEACHING

- Inform patient that dexrazoxane is used to protect the heart from damage caused by myelosuppression and that she'll be given the drug by a health care professional in the hospital or clinic before receiving chemotherapy.
- Inform patient that dexrazoxane and chemotherapy may make her feel generally unwell, but urge her to continue treatment unless prescriber tells her to stop.
- Instruct patient to report chills, fever, mouth sores, pain at injection site, sore throat, unusual bleeding or bruising, unusual tiredness or weakness, and vomiting. Dosage may need to be changed or therapy stopped.
- Inform patient that drug may exacerbate symptoms of bone marrow suppression caused by anthracycline chemotherapy, including increased risk of infection.
- Teach patient importance of avoiding injury and infection during dexrazoxane therapy. For example, advise her to use a soft-bristled toothbrush to prevent damage to teeth and gums; to avoid people with colds, the flu, or bronchitis; and to avoid anyone who has recently had oral polio vaccine because of the increased risk of infection from live virus.

dextrose
(D-glucose)

2.5% Dextrose Injection, 5% Dextrose Injection, 10% Dextrose Injection, 20% Dextrose Injection, 25% Dextrose Injection, 50% Dextrose Injection, 60% Dextrose Injection, 70% Dextrose Injection

Class and Category

Chemical: Monosaccharide
Therapeutic: Antidiabetic, nutritional supplement
Pregnancy category: C

Indications and Dosages

▶ *To treat insulin-induced hypoglycemia*

I.V. INFUSION OR INJECTION

Adults and children. *Initial:* 20 to 50 ml of 50% solution given at 3 ml/min. *Maintenance:* 10% to 15% solution by continuous infusion until blood glucose level reaches therapeutic range.
Infants and neonates. 2 ml/kg of 10% to 25% solution until blood glucose level reaches therapeutic range.

▶ *To replace calories*

I.V. INFUSION

Adults and children. Individualized dosage of 2.5%, 5%, or 10% solution, based on need for fluids or calories and given through peripheral I.V. line. Or a 10% to 70% solution given through a large central vein, if needed, typically mixed with amino acids or other solutions.

Route	Onset	Peak	Duration
I.V.	2 to 3 min	Unknown	Unknown

Mechanism of Action

Prevents protein and nitrogen loss, promotes glycogen deposition, prevents or decreases ketosis, and, in large amounts, acts as an osmotic diuretic. Dextrose is readily metabolized and undergoes oxidation to carbon dioxide and water. The oral form—glucose—is absorbed directly into the bloodstream from the intestines and is distributed, used, or stored in the liver.

Incompatibilities

Don't give dextrose through same infusion set as blood or blood products because pseudoagglutination of RBCs may occur.

Contraindications

For all solutions: Diabetic coma with excessively elevated blood glucose level

For concentrated solutions: Anuria, alcohol withdrawal syndrome in dehydrated patient, glucose-galactose malabsorption syndrome, hepatic coma, intracranial or intraspinal hemorrhage, overhydration

Interactions

DRUGS

corticosteroids, corticotropin: Increased risk of fluid and electrolyte imbalance if dextrose solution contains sodium ions

Adverse Reactions

CNS: Confusion, fever

GU: Glycosuria

Other: Dehydration; hyperosmolar coma; hypervolemia; hypovolemia; injection site extravasation with tissue necrosis, infection, phlebitis, and venous thrombosis

Nursing Considerations

- Use dextrose cautiously in patients with renal impairment because dextrose solutions contain aluminum, which may reach toxic levels when these patients receive prolonged parenteral therapy.
- Give highly concentrated dextrose solution by central venous catheter—not by subcutaneous or I.M. route.
- **WARNING** Avoid rapid or excessive administration of dextrose solution in a very low–birth-weight infant because it can increase serum osmolality and possibly cause intracerebral hemorrhage.
- Assess infusion site regularly for signs of infiltration, such as pain or swelling.
- Assess for glucosuria by using a urine reagent strip or collecting a urine sample and reviewing urinalysis results.
- When discontinuing a concentrated solution, expect to give a 5% to 10% dextrose infusion to avoid rebound hypoglycemia.
- Monitor patient for signs of hypervolemia, such as jugular vein distention and crackles.

PATIENT TEACHING

- Instruct patient to monitor her blood glucose level as directed.
- Stress the importance of reporting discomfort, pain, or signs of infection at I.V. site.

dezocine

Dalgan

Class and Category

Chemical: Aminotetralin, synthetic opioid
Therapeutic: Opioid analgesic
Pregnancy category: C

Indications and Dosages

▶ *To relieve pain*

I.V. INJECTION

Adult. *Initial:* 5 mg, followed by 2.5 to 10 mg q 2 to 4 hr, p.r.n. *Maximum:* 120 mg daily.

Route	Onset	Peak	Duration
I.V.	15 min	30 min	2 to 4 hr

Contraindications

Hypersensitivity to dezocine or its components

Mechanism of Action
Binds with opioid receptors at many CNS sites, which alters the perception of and emotional response to pain.

Interactions
DRUGS

CNS depressants, general anesthetics, hypnotics, sedatives, tranquilizers: Increased CNS depression

other opioid analgesics: Possibly decreased therapeutic effects of other opioid and withdrawal symptoms in patient receiving long-term opioid therapy

ACTIVITIES

alcohol use: Increased CNS depression

Adverse Reactions
CNS: CNS toxicity (delirium, delusions, mental depression), dizziness, sedation, vertigo
CV: Chest pain, hypertension, hypotension, irregular heartbeat
GI: Nausea, vomiting
GU: Decreased urine output, dysuria, urinary frequency
RESP: Atelectasis, cough, dyspnea, respiratory depression
Other: Injection site redness and swelling

Nursing Considerations
- Have patient lie down during dezocine administration and for a period afterward to lessen drug's hypotensive effects (dizziness, light-headedness) and other adverse effects, such as nausea and vomiting.
- **WARNING Administer dezocine slowly. Rapid administration of other opioid analgesics has caused anaphylaxis, severe respiratory depression, hypotension, peripheral circulatory collapse, and cardiac arrest. Keep emergency equipment and drugs nearby.**
- Be aware that dosage reduction may be required for patients with respiratory disease (to avoid decreased respiratory drive and increased airway resistance); impaired hepatic function, including cirrhosis (because elimination half-life may be prolonged); or impaired renal function as well as for elderly, debilitated, or severely ill patients (who may be more sensitive to drug's effects).
- Discard solution if it contains precipitate.

- Frequently monitor blood pressure and pulse and respiratory rates after giving first dose.
- **WARNING** Avoid administering dezocine to a patient who is opioid-dependent. Doing so may precipitate withdrawal symptoms because drug can antagonize opioid effects. Patients with a history of drug abuse (including acute alcoholism), emotional instability, or suicidal ideation or attempts are at increased risk for abuse.
- Assess patient for pain relief, and document your findings frequently.
- Assess respiratory status in patients with acute respiratory depression because dezocine can worsen this condition. Patients having an acute asthma attack and those with chronic disease are at increased risk for respiratory depression.
- Monitor patients with a history of common bile duct disorders for signs of increased biliary pressure, such as pain in upper midline area that may radiate to back and right shoulder.
- Monitor for worsening condition in patients with diarrhea caused by poisoning or pseudomembranous colitis.
- Assess patient's urine output; decreasing output may signal urine retention.
- Monitor for signs of drug-induced CNS depression or increased CSF pressure, such as altered LOC, restlessness, and irritability, in patients with a head injury, intracranial lesions, or other conditions that could cause these effects. Patients who are taking or have recently taken drugs that cause CNS depression are also more susceptible to these effects. Take appropriate safety precautions.
- Be aware that patients with hypothyroidism are at increased risk for respiratory depression and prolonged CNS depression.
- Be aware that dezocine may affect GI motility or mask symptoms of acute abdominal conditions.

PATIENT TEACHING

- Instruct patient to report if dezocine doesn't relieve pain within 1 hour.
- Advise patient to avoid potentially hazardous activities until drug's CNS effects are known.
- Advise patient to change position slowly to minimize dizziness and light-headedness.
- Urge patient to avoid alcohol and other drugs that cause CNS depression during dezocine therapy.

diazepam

Diazemuls, Dizac, Valium

Class, Category, and Schedule

Chemical: Benzodiazepine
Therapeutic: Anticonvulsant, anxiolytic, sedative-hypnotic, skeletal muscle relaxant
Pregnancy category: D
Controlled substance: Schedule IV

Indications and Dosages

▶ *To relieve anxiety*

I.V. INJECTION

Adults. 2 to 5 mg q 3 to 4 hr, p.r.n., for moderate anxiety; 5 to 10 mg q 3 to 4 hr, p.r.n., for severe anxiety.
Children. Individualized dosage. *Maximum:* 0.25 mg/kg given over 3 min and repeated after 15 to 30 min if needed and after another 15 to 30 min if needed.

▶ *To treat symptoms of acute alcohol withdrawal*

I.V. INJECTION

Adults. 10 mg and then 5 to 10 mg in 3 to 4 hr, if needed.

▶ *To provide muscle relaxation, sedation*

I.V. INJECTION

Adults. 5 to 10 mg and then 5 to 10 mg in 3 to 4 hr, if needed.
DOSAGE ADJUSTMENT Dosage reduced to 2 to 5 mg/dose and increased as needed and tolerated for debilitated patients.

▶ *To treat status epilepticus and severe recurrent seizures*

I.V. INJECTION

Adults. 5 to 10 mg repeated q 10 to 15 min, as needed, up to a cumulative dose of 30 mg. Regimen repeated, if needed, in 2 to 4 hr. (Use I.M. route if I.V. access is impossible.)
Children age 5 and over. 1 mg repeated q 2 to 5 min, as needed, up to a cumulative dose of 10 mg. Regimen repeated, if needed, in 2 to 4 hr.
Children ages 1 month to 5 years. 0.2 to 0.5 mg repeated q 2 to 5 min, as needed, up to a cumulative dose of 5 mg. Regimen repeated, if needed, in 2 to 4 hr.

▶ *To provide preoperative sedation*

I.V. INJECTION

Adults. 5 to 10 mg 30 min before surgery.

▶ *To reduce anxiety before cardioversion*

I.V. INJECTION

Adults. 5 to 15 mg 5 to 10 min before procedure.

▶ *To reduce anxiety before endoscopic procedures*
I.V. INJECTION
Adults. Up to 20 mg titrated to desired sedation and administered immediately before procedure.
▶ *To treat tetanus*
I.V. INJECTION
Adults and children age 5 and over. *Initial:* 5 to 10 mg repeated q 3 to 4 hr, if needed. Sometimes larger doses are needed for adults.
DOSAGE ADJUSTMENT For debilitated patients, initial dose reduced to 2 to 5 mg and increased gradually as needed and tolerated.
Children ages 1 month to 5 years. 1 to 2 mg repeated q 3 to 4 hr, as needed.

Mechanism of Action

May potentiate the effects of gamma-aminobutyric acid (GABA) and other inhibitory neurotransmitters by binding to specific benzodiazepine receptors in the limbic and cortical areas of the CNS. GABA inhibits excitatory stimulation, which helps control emotional behavior. The limbic system contains a highly dense area of benzodiazepine receptors, which may explain the drug's antianxiety effects. Diazepam also suppresses the spread of seizure activity caused by seizure-producing foci in the cortex, thalamus, and limbic structures.

Incompatibilities

Don't mix diazepam injection with aqueous solutions. Don't mix diazepam emulsion with morphine or glycopyrrolate or administer it through an infusion set that contains polyvinyl chloride.

Contraindications

Acute angle-closure glaucoma, hypersensitivity to diazepam or its components, untreated open-angle glaucoma

Interactions

DRUGS
cimetidine, disulfiram, fluoxetine, isoniazid, itraconazole, ketoconazole, metoprolol, oral contraceptives, propoxyphene, propranolol, valproic acid: Decreased diazepam metabolism, increased blood level and risk of adverse effects of diazepam
CNS depressants: Increased CNS depression
digoxin: Increased serum digoxin level and risk of digitalis toxicity
levodopa: Decreased antidyskinetic effect of levodopa

probenecid: Faster onset or more prolonged effects of diazepam
ranitidine: Delayed elimination and increased blood level of diazepam
rifampin: Decreased blood diazepam level
theophyllines: Antagonized sedative effect of diazepam
ACTIVITIES
alcohol use: Increased CNS depression

Adverse Reactions

CNS: Anterograde amnesia, anxiety, ataxia, confusion, depression, dizziness, drowsiness, fatigue, headache, insomnia, lethargy, light-headedness, sedation, sleepiness, slurred speech, tremor, vertigo
CV: Hypotension, palpitations, phlebitis, tachycardia, thrombophlebitis
EENT: Blurred vision, diplopia, increased salivation
GI: Anorexia, constipation, diarrhea, nausea, vomiting
GU: Libido changes, urinary incontinence, urine retention
RESP: Respiratory depression
SKIN: Dermatitis
Other: Physical and psychological dependence

Nursing Considerations

- Protect diazepam injection from light. Don't use solution if it is more than slightly yellow or contains precipitate.
- Don't mix emulsion form with anything other than its emulsion base. Otherwise, it may become unstable and increase the risk of serious adverse reactions.
- Before administering emulsion form, ask if patient is allergic to soybeans because this form contains soybean oil.
- Administer diazepam directly into an I.V. line inserted in a large vein or through I.V. tubing as close to insertion site as possible at a rate of at least 5 mg/minute. For an infant or a child, administer I.V. injection slowly over 3 minutes.
- Administer emulsion form within 6 hours of opening ampule because this form contains no preservatives and allows rapid microbial growth. Use polyethylene-lined or glass infusion sets and polyethylene or polypropylene plastic syringes for administration. Don't use a filter with a pore size of less than 5 microns because it may break down the emulsion.
- **WARNING** Be aware that patients with a history of seizure disorders may have seizures when diazepam is started or suddenly withdrawn. Monitor patients with Lennox-Gastaut syndrome or absence seizures for tonic status epilepticus.

- Monitor for increased sedation, especially in patients with hypoalbuminemia.
- Monitor hepatic and renal function blood test results in patients with impaired renal or hepatic function because diazepam is metabolized in the liver and excreted by the kidneys.
- **WARNING** Observe for signs of physical and psychological dependence: a strong desire or need to continue taking diazepam, a need to increase dosage to maintain drug effects, and posttherapy withdrawal symptoms, such as abdominal cramps, insomnia, irritability, nervousness, and tremor.
- Observe for signs of phlebitis or thrombophlebitis after administration.
- Store diazepam injection at 15° to 30° C (59° to 86° F). Store diazepam emulsion below 25° C (77° F). Protect from freezing and light.

PATIENT TEACHING

- Inform patient that diazepam may cause drowsiness, and advise her to avoid activities requiring alertness until drug's CNS effects are known.
- Urge patient to avoid CNS depressants and alcohol during therapy.
- Instruct patient not to take drug more often, in greater quantities, or for a longer time than prescribed. Inform her that physical and psychological dependence can occur, and teach her to recognize signs of dependence.
- Instruct patient not to abruptly stop taking drug without prescriber supervision. Caution patient with a history of seizures that abrupt drug withdrawal may trigger them.

diazoxide

Hyperstat

Class and Category

Chemical: Benzothiadiazine derivative
Therapeutic: Antihypertensive, antihypoglycemic
Pregnancy category: C

Indications and Dosages

▶ *To treat severe hypertension in hospitalized patients*

I.V. INJECTION

Adults and children. *Initial:* 1 to 3 mg/kg by rapid bolus, repeated q 5 to 15 min until diastolic pressure falls below 100 mm Hg. Repeated in 4 hr and again in 24 hr, if needed, until oral antihypertensive therapy begins. *Maximum:* 150 mg/dose, 1.2 g daily.

Route	Onset	Peak	Duration
I.V.	1 min	2 to 5 min	2 to 12 hr

Mechanism of Action

Directly affects smooth muscle cells of peripheral arteries and arterioles, causing them to dilate. This action decreases peripheral resistance, which helps reduce blood pressure. Diazoxide also inhibits insulin release from the pancreas, stimulates catecholamine release, and increases hepatic glucose release.

Contraindications

Acute aortic dissection; hypersensitivity to diazoxide, thiazides, other sulfonamide derivatives, or their components; treatment of compensatory hypertension (as occurs with aortic coarctation)

Interactions

DRUGS

allopurinol, colchicine, probenecid, sulfinpyrazone: Increased serum uric acid level

antihypertensives: Additive hypotensive effects

beta blockers: Increased hypotensive effects of diazoxide

diuretics (especially thiazides): Potentiated hyperglycemic, hyperuricemic, and antihypertensive effects of diazoxide

estrogens, NSAIDs, sympathomimetics: Antagonized hypotensive effects of diazoxide

insulin, oral antidiabetic drugs: Possibly decreased effectiveness of these drugs

oral anticoagulants: Increased anticoagulant effects

peripheral vasodilators, ritodrine: Additive, possibly severe, hypotensive effects

Adverse Reactions

CNS: Anxiety, apprehension, cerebral ischemia, confusion, dizziness, euphoria, headache, insomnia, light-headedness, malaise, somnolence, weakness

CV: Bradycardia, chest pain, hypotension, orthostatic hypotension, palpitations, peripheral edema, tachycardia, transient hypertension

EENT: Blurred vision, dry mouth, increased salivation, taste perversion, tinnitus, transient hearing loss

ENDO: Transient hyperglycemia

GI: Abdominal pain, anorexia, constipation, diarrhea, ileus, nausea, vomiting
HEME: Thrombocytopenia
MS: Gout
SKIN: Diaphoresis, flushing, pruritus, rash, sensation of warmth
Other: Allergic reaction, extravasation with injection site cellulitis and pain; fluid and sodium retention

Nursing Considerations

- Administer diazoxide undiluted over 10 to 30 seconds. Don't give drug by I.M. or subcutaneous route.
- Keep patient supine during I.V. injection and for 1 hour afterward.
- Monitor blood pressure throughout treatment to check for hypertension. Before ending surveillance, measure patient's standing blood pressure if she's ambulatory.
- Monitor patients with uncompensated heart failure for signs of fluid retention and worsening heart failure due to diazoxide's effects.
- Monitor patients with impaired cardiac or cerebral circulation for exacerbations caused by drug-related abrupt blood pressure reduction, mild tachycardia, and decreased blood perfusion.
- Frequently assess I.V. site for extravasation because the alkaline drug can irritate tissue.
- If diabetic patient receives diazoxide to treat hypertension, monitor for signs and symptoms of hyperglycemia because parenteral form commonly causes transient hyperglycemia.
- Be aware that patients with impaired renal function may require reduced dosage because drug effects may be prolonged.
- Monitor patients with a history of gout for signs of exacerbation, such as joint redness or swelling and hyperuricemia.
- Monitor blood glucose level of all patients who receive diazoxide to determine if drug has raised blood glucose level to normal.
- Store drug at 15° to 30° C (59° to 86° F); protect from freezing and light.

PATIENT TEACHING

- Inform patient that she'll be on bed rest until oral diazoxide therapy starts.
- Caution patient not to take antidiabetic drugs unless prescribed.
- Advise patient to report signs of hyperglycemia, such as increased urinary frequency, increased thirst, and fruity breath.

digoxin

Lanoxin Injection, Lanoxin Injection Pediatric

Class and Category

Chemical: Digitalis glycoside
Therapeutic: Antiarrhythmic, cardiotonic
Pregnancy category: C

Indications and Dosages

▶ *To treat heart failure, atrial flutter, atrial fibrillation, and paroxysmal atrial tachycardia with rapid digitalization*

I.V. INJECTION

Adults. *Loading:* 10 to 15 mcg/kg in 3 divided doses q 6 to 8 hr, with first dose equal to 50% of total dose. *Maintenance:* 125 to 350 mcg daily, given once or twice daily.

Children over age 10. *Loading:* 8 to 12 mcg/kg in 3 or more divided doses, with first dose equal to 50% of total dose. Subsequent doses given q 6 to 8 hr. *Maintenance:* 2 to 3 mcg/kg once daily.

Children ages 6 to 10. *Loading:* 15 to 30 mcg/kg in 3 or more divided doses, with first dose equal to 50% of total dose. Subsequent doses given q 6 to 8 hr. *Maintenance:* 4 to 8 mcg/kg daily in two divided doses.

Children ages 2 to 5. *Loading:* 25 to 35 mcg/kg in 3 or more divided doses, with first dose equal to 50% of total dose. Subsequent doses given q 6 to 8 hr. *Maintenance:* 6 to 9 mcg/kg daily in two divided doses.

Infants ages 1 to 24 months. *Loading:* 30 to 50 mcg/kg in 3 or more divided doses, with first dose equal to 50% of total dose. Subsequent doses given q 6 to 8 hr. *Maintenance:* 7.5 to 12 mcg/kg daily in two divided doses.

Full-term neonates. *Loading:* 20 to 30 mcg/kg in 3 or more divided doses, with first dose equal to 50% of total dose. Subsequent doses given q 6 to 8 hr. *Maintenance:* 5 to 8 mcg/kg daily in two divided doses.

Premature neonates. *Loading:* 15 to 25 mcg/kg in 3 or more divided doses, with first dose equal to 50% of total dose. Subsequent doses given q 6 to 8 hr. *Maintenance:* 4 to 6 mcg/kg/ daily in two divided doses.

DOSAGE ADJUSTMENT Dosage carefully adjusted for elderly or debilitated patients and those who have implanted pacemakers because they may develop toxicity at doses tolerated by most patients.

Route	Onset	Peak	Duration
I.V.	5 to 30 min	1 to 5 hr	3 to 4 days

Mechanism of Action

Increases the force and velocity of myocardial contraction, resulting in positive inotropic effects. Digoxin produces antiarrhythmic effects by decreasing the conduction rate and increasing the effective refractory period of the AV node.

Incompatibilities

Don't mix digoxin in the same container or I.V. line as other other drugs.

Contraindications

Hypersensitive carotid sinus syndrome, hypersensitivity to digoxin, presence or history of digitalis toxicity or idiosyncratic reaction to digoxin, ventricular fibrillation, ventricular tachycardia unless heart failure unrelated to digoxin therapy occurs

Interactions

DRUGS

amiodarone, propafenone: Elevated blood digoxin level, possibly to toxic level
antacids: Inhibited digoxin absorption
antiarrhythmics, pancuronium, parenteral calcium salts, rauwolfia alkaloids, sympathomimetics: Possibly increased risk of arrhythmias
diltiazem, verapamil: Increased blood digoxin level, possibly excessive bradycardia
edrophonium: Excessive slowing of heart rate
erythromycin, neomycin, tetracycline: Possibly increased blood digoxin level
hypokalemia-causing drugs, potassium-wasting diuretics: Increased risk of digitalis toxicity from hypokalemia
indomethacin: Decreased renal clearance and increased blood level of digoxin
magnesium sulfate (parenteral): Possibly cardiac conduction changes and heart block
quinidine, quinine: Increased blood digoxin level
spironolactone: Increased half-life and risk of adverse effects of digoxin
succinylcholine: Increased risk of digoxin-induced arrhythmias

sucralfate: Decreased digoxin absorption

Adverse Reactions

CNS: Anxiety, confusion, depression, drowsiness, extreme weakness, hallucinations, headache, syncope
CV: Arrhythmias, heart block
EENT: Blurred vision, colored halos around objects
GI: Abdominal discomfort or pain, anorexia, diarrhea, nausea, vomiting
SKIN: Rash
Other: Electrolyte imbalances

Nursing Considerations

- Before giving each dose of digoxin, take patient's apical pulse and notify prescriber if pulse is below 60 beats/minute (or other specified level).
- Administer drug undiluted, or dilute with a fourfold or greater volume of sterile water for injection, normal saline solution, or D_5W for I.V. administration. Once diluted, administer immediately over at least 5 minutes. Discard if solution is markedly discolored or contains precipitate.
- Monitor closely for signs of digitalis toxicity: altered mental status, arrhythmias, heart block, nausea, vision disturbances, and vomiting. If they appear, notify prescriber, check serum digoxin level as ordered, and expect to withhold drug until level is known. Monitor ECG tracing continuously.
- If patient has acute or unstable chronic atrial fibrillation, assess for drug effectiveness. Ventricular rate may not normalize even when serum drug level falls within therapeutic range; raising the dosage probably won't produce a therapeutic effect and may lead to toxicity.
- Frequently obtain ECG tracings as ordered in elderly patients because of their smaller body mass and reduced renal clearance. Elderly patients, especially those with coronary insufficiency, are more susceptible to arrhythmias—particularly ventricular fibrillation—if digitalis toxicity occurs.
- Monitor serum electrolyte—especially potassium—levels regularly because hypokalemia predisposes patient to digitalis toxicity and serious arrhythmias. Also monitor potassium levels frequently if patient is receiving potassium salts in addition to digoxin because hyperkalemia in such a patient can be fatal.
- Store drug at 15° to 25° C (59° to 77° F); protect from freezing and light.

PATIENT TEACHING
- Urge patient to report adverse reactions, such as GI distress, palpitations, or pulse changes.

digoxin immune Fab (ovine)
Digibind

Class and Category
Chemical: Digoxin-specific antigen-binding fragments
Therapeutic: Digitalis glycoside antidote
Pregnancy category: C

Indications and Dosages
▶ *To treat acute toxicity from a known amount of digoxin elixir or tablets*
I.V. INJECTION
Adults and children. Individualized dosage based on amount ingested. Dose (mg) = dose ingested (mg) multiplied by 0.8 and then divided by 0.5, multiplied by 38, and rounded up to next whole vial.
▶ *To treat acute toxicity from a known quantity of digoxin capsules, digitoxin tablets, or I.V. injection of digoxin or digitoxin*
I.V. INJECTION
Adults and children. Individualized dosage based on amount ingested. Dose (mg) = dose ingested (mg) divided by 0.5, then multiplied by 38 and rounded up to next whole vial.
▶ *To treat acute toxicity from an unknown amount of digoxin or digitoxin during long-term therapy*
I.V. INJECTION
Adults and children. Individualized dosage for digoxin toxicity: Dose (mg) = serum digoxin level (ng/ml) multiplied by body weight (kg), then divided by 100, and then multiplied by 38. Individualized dosage for digitoxin toxicity: Dose (mg) = serum digitoxin level (ng/ml) multiplied by body weight (kg) and then divided by 1,000, multiplied by 38, and rounded up to next whole vial.
DOSAGE ADJUSTMENT Higher dose administered, as prescribed, if the dose based on ingested amount differs substantially from the dose based on serum digoxin or digitoxin level. Dose repeated after several hours, if needed.

Route	Onset	Peak	Duration
I.V.	15 to 30 min	Unknown	8 to 12 hr

Mechanism of Action

Binds with digoxin or digitoxin molecules. The resulting complex is excreted through the kidneys. As the free serum digoxin level declines, tissue-bound digoxin enters the serum and also is bound and excreted.

Contraindications

Hypersensitivity to digoxin immune Fab

Interactions

None known.

Adverse Reactions

CV: Increased ventricular rate (in atrial fibrillation), worsening of heart failure or low cardiac output
Other: Allergic reaction (difficulty breathing, urticaria), febrile reaction, hypokalemia

Nursing Considerations

- Expect each 38-mg vial of purified digoxin immune Fab to bind with about 0.5 mg of digoxin or digitoxin.
- Reconstitute by dissolving 38 mg of drug in 4 ml of sterile water for injection to yield 9.5 mg/ml. Mix gently. Further dilute with normal saline solution to a convenient volume for I.V. infusion. For very small doses, reconstituted 38-mg vial may be diluted with 34 ml of normal saline solution to yield 1 mg/ml. Use reconstituted solution promptly or, if necessary, store it for up to 4 hours at 2° to 8° C (36° to 46° F).
- **WARNING** Before administering digoxin immune Fab to high-risk patient, test for allergic reaction as prescribed by diluting 0.1 ml of reconstituted drug in 9.9 ml of sodium chloride for injection and then injecting 0.1 ml (9.5 mcg/0.1 ml) intradermally. After 20 minutes, observe for an urticarial wheal surrounded by erythema. Alternatively, perform a scratch test by placing one drop of 9.5 mcg/0.1 ml dilution on patient's skin and making a ¼″ scratch through drop with a sterile needle. Inspect site in 20 minutes. Test is considered positive if it produces a wheal surrounded by erythema. If test causes a systemic reaction, apply tourniquet above test site, notify prescriber, and prepare to respond to anaphylaxis. Be aware that if a skin or systemic reaction occurs, additional drug shouldn't be given unless essential; if more of the drug must be given, expect prescriber to pretreat patient with cor-

ticosteroids and diphenhydramine. Prescriber should be on standby to treat anaphylaxis.

- When preparing digoxin immune Fab for an infant, reconstitute drug as ordered and administer with a tuberculin syringe.
- When administering drug to a child, monitor for fluid volume overload.
- When giving a large dose, expect a faster onset but watch closely for febrile reaction. Monitor body temperature and ECG tracing during treatment. Make sure emergency equipment and drugs are readily available.
- Administer I.V. infusion through a 0.22-micron membrane filter over 30 minutes. Keep in mind that drug may be given by rapid I.V. injection if cardiac arrest is imminent.
- Monitor serum potassium level frequently, especially during first few hours of therapy, because potassium level may drop rapidly.
- Be aware that patient may not be redigitalized for several days or even longer, until fragments of digoxin immune Fab have been eliminated from body. This process may be delayed in patients with impaired renal function because drug is eliminated by kidneys.

PATIENT TEACHING

- Teach patient the purpose of digoxin immune Fab and how it will be administered.
- Advise patient to notify you immediately if she experiences adverse reactions, especially difficulty breathing and urticaria.

dihydroergotamine mesylate

D.H.E. 45, Dihydroergotamine-Sandoz (CAN), Migranal

Class and Category

Chemical: Semisynthetic ergot alkaloid
Therapeutic: Antimigraine
Pregnancy category: X

Indications and Dosages

▶ *To treat acute migraine with or without aura*

I.V. INJECTION

Adults. 1 mg, repeated in 1 hr, if needed. *Maximum:* 6 mg/wk.

Route	Onset	Peak	Duration
I.V.	5 min	15 min to 2 hr	About 8 hr

Mechanism of Action

Produces intracranial and peripheral vasoconstriction by binding to all known 5-hydroxytryptamine$_1$ (5-HT$_1$) receptors, alpha$_1$- and alpha$_2$-adrenergic receptors, and dopaminergic receptors. Activation of 5-HT$_1$ receptors on intracranial blood vessels probably constricts large intracranial arteries and closes arteriovenous anastomoses to relieve migraine headache. Activation of 5-HT$_1$ receptors on sensory nerves in the trigeminal system also may inhibit the release of pro-inflammatory neuropeptides.

Peripherally, dihydroergotamine causes vasoconstriction by stimulating alpha-adrenergic receptors. At therapeutic doses, it inhibits norepinephrine reuptake, increasing vasoconstriction. The drug constricts veins more than arteries, increasing venous return while decreasing venous stasis and pooling.

Contraindications

Coronary artery disease, including vasospasm; hemiplegic or basilar migraine; hypersensitivity to dihydroergotamine or other ergot alkaloids; malnutrition; peripheral vascular disease or after vascular surgery; pregnancy; sepsis; severe hepatic or renal impairment; severe pruritus; uncontrolled hypertension; use of macrolide antibiotics or protease inhibitors; use within 24 hours of 5-hydroxytryptamine$_1$ (5-HT$_1$) agonist, ergotamine-containing or ergot-type drug, or methysergide

Interactions

DRUGS

beta blockers: Possibly peripheral vasoconstriction and peripheral ischemia, increased risk of gangrene

macrolides, protease inhibitors: Possibly increased risk of vasospasm, acute ergotism with peripheral ischemia

nitrates: Decreased antianginal effects of nitrates

other ergot drugs, including ergoloid mesylates, ergonovine, methylergonovine, methysergide, and sumatriptan: Increased risk of serious adverse effects from nasal dihydroergotamine

systemic vasoconstrictors: Risk of severe hypertension

ACTIVITIES

smoking: Possibly increased ischemic response to ergot therapy

Adverse Reactions

CNS: Anxiety, confusion, dizziness, fatigue, headache, paresthesia, somnolence, weakness

CV: Bradycardia, chest pain, peripheral vasospasm (calf or heel

pain with exertion, cool and cyanotic hands and feet, leg weakness, weak or absent pulses), tachycardia
EENT: Abnormal vision; dry mouth; epistaxis, nasal congestion or rhinitis, and sore nose (nasal spray); miosis; pharyngitis; sinusitis; taste perversion
GI: Diarrhea, nausea, vomiting
MS: Muscle stiffness
SKIN: Localized edema of face, feet, fingers, and lower legs; sensation of heat or warmth; sudden diaphoresis

Nursing Considerations

- **WARNING Monitor patient for signs of dihydroergotamine overdose, such as abdominal pain, confusion, delirium, dizziness, dyspnea, headache, nausea, pain in legs or arms, paresthesia, seizures, and vomiting.**
- Assess peripheral pulses, skin sensation, warmth, and capillary refill. After giving nasal dihydroergotamine, monitor for signs of widespread blood vessel constriction and adverse reactions caused by decreased circulation to many body areas.

PATIENT TEACHING

- If patient experiences a headache different from her usual migraines, caution her not to use dihydroergotamine and to notify prescriber.
- Advise patient to avoid alcohol, which can exacerbate or cause headaches, and to avoid smoking, which may cause an ischemic response.
- Warn patient about possible dizziness during or after a migraine for which she took dihydroergotamine.

diltiazem hydrochloride

Cardizem

Class and Category

Chemical: Benzothiazepine derivative
Therapeutic: Antianginal, antiarrhythmic, antihypertensive
Pregnancy category: C

Indications and Dosages

▶ *To treat atrial fibrillation, atrial flutter, and paroxysmal supraventricular tachycardia*

I.V. INFUSION OR INJECTION

Adults and adolescents. 0.25 mg/kg given by bolus over 2 min. If response is inadequate after 15 min, 0.35 mg/kg given by bolus over 2 min. Then 10 mg/hr for continued reduction of heart rate after bolus, increased by 5 mg/hr, as needed. *Maximum:* 15 mg/hr for up to 24 hr.

Route	Onset	Peak	Duration
I.V.	3 min	2 to 7 min	30 min to 10 hr*

Mechanism of Action

Diltiazem inhibits calcium movement into coronary and vascular smooth-muscle cells by blocking slow calcium channels in cell membranes, as shown. This action decreases intracellular calcium, which:

- inhibits smooth-muscle cell contractions
- decreases myocardial oxygen demand by relaxing coronary and vascular smooth muscle, reducing peripheral vascular resistance and systolic and diastolic blood pressures
- slows AV conduction time and prolongs AV nodal refractoriness
- interrupts the reentry circuit in AV nodal reentrant tachycardias.

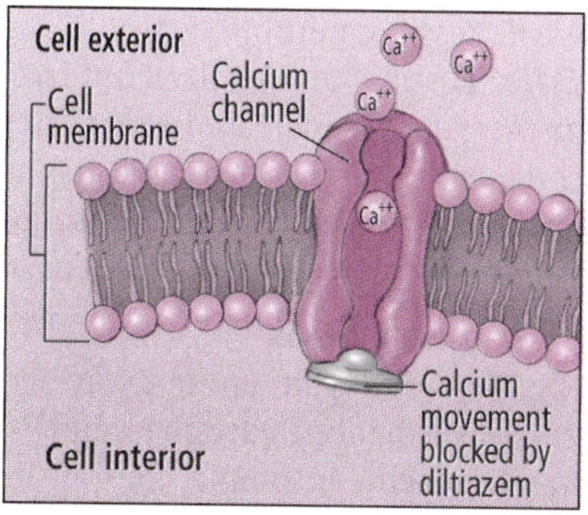

Incompatibilities

Don't give diltiazem through same I.V. line as acetazolamide, acyclovir, aminophylline, ampicillin sodium/sulbactam sodium, cefamandole, cefoperazone, diazepam, furosemide, heparin, hydrocortisone sodium succinate, methylprednisolone sodium succinate, mezlocillin, nafcillin, phenytoin, rifampin, or sodium bicarbonate.

Contraindications

Acute MI; cardiogenic shock; Lown-Ganong-Levine or Wolff-Parkinson-White syndrome, second- or third-degree AV block, and sick sinus syndrome, unless artificial pacemaker is in place; pulmonary edema; systolic blood pressure below 90 mm Hg; ventricular tachycardia (wide complex)

* For infusion; 1 to 3 hr for injection.

Interactions

DRUGS

anesthetics: Additive hypotension; possibly decreased cardiac contractility, conductivity, and automaticity
benzodiazepines: Increased risk of prolonged sedation
beta blockers: Possibly increased risk of adverse cardiovascular effects
buspirone: Increased effects and risk of buspirone toxicity
carbamazepine, cyclosporine, lovastatin, quinidine, theophyllines: Decreased hepatic clearance and increased serum levels of these drugs, leading to toxicity
cimetidine: Decreased diltiazem metabolism, increased blood diltiazem level
digoxin: Increased blood digoxin level
lithium: Possibly neurotoxicity
NSAIDs: Possibly antagonized antihypertensive effect of diltiazem
prazocin: Possibly increased risk of hypotension
procainamide: Possibly increased risk of prolonged QT interval
quinidine: Increased risk of adverse quinidine effects
rifampin: Decreased blood diltiazem level to undetectable amounts

Adverse Reactions

CNS: Abnormal gait, amnesia, asthenia, depression, dizziness, dream disturbances, extrapyramidal reactions, fatigue, hallucinations, headache, insomnia, nervousness, paresthesia, personality change, somnolence, syncope, tremor, weakness
CV: Angina, atrial flutter, AV block (first-, second-, and third-degree), bradycardia, bundle-branch block, heart failure, hypotension, palpitations, peripheral edema, PVCs, sinus arrest, sinus tachycardia, 12-lead ECG abnormalities, ventricular fibrillation, ventricular tachycardia
EENT: Amblyopia, dry mouth, epistaxis, eye irritation, gingival bleeding and hyperplasia, gingivitis, nasal congestion, retinopathy, taste perversion, tinnitus
ENDO: Hyperglycemia
GI: Anorexia, constipation, diarrhea, elevated liver function test results, indigestion, nausea, thirst, vomiting
GU: Acute renal failure, impotence, nocturia, polyuria, sexual dysfunction
HEME: Hemolytic anemia, leukopenia, prolonged bleeding time, thrombocytopenia
MS: Arthralgia, muscle spasms, myalgia
RESP: Cough, dyspnea

SKIN: Alopecia, diaphoresis, erythema multiforme, exfoliative dermatitis, flushing, leukocytoclastic vasculitis, petechiae, photosensitivity, pruritus, purpura, rash, Stevens-Johnson syndrome, toxic epidermal necrolysis, urticaria
Other: Angioedema, hyperuricemia, weight gain

Nursing Considerations

- Use diltiazem cautiously in patients with impaired hepatic or renal function, and monitor liver and renal function test results, as appropriate; diltiazem is metabolized mainly in the liver and excreted by the kidneys.
- **WARNING** Monitor blood pressure, pulse rate, and heart rate and rhythm by continuous ECG as appropriate during therapy. Keep emergency equipment and drugs available.
- Assess patient for signs of heart failure.
- If patient takes digoxin, watch for signs of digitalis toxicity, such as nausea, vomiting, halo vision, and elevated serum digoxin level.
- Administer sublingual nitroglycerin, as prescribed, during diltiazem therapy.
- Expect to discontinue drug if adverse skin reactions, usually transient, persist.

PATIENT TEACHING

- Urge patient to report chest pain, difficulty breathing, dizziness, fainting, irregular heartbeat, rash, or swollen ankles.

dimenhydrinate

Dinate, Dramanate, Gravol (CAN), Hydrate

Class and Category

Chemical: Ethanolamine derivative
Therapeutic: Antiemetic, antihistamine, antivertigo agent
Pregnancy category: B

Indications and Dosages

▶ *To treat nausea, vomiting, dizziness, or vertigo with motion sickness*

I.V. INFUSION, I.V. INJECTION

Adults and adolescents. 50 mg in 10 ml of normal saline solution given slowly, over at least 2 min, q 4 hr p.r.n.
Children. 1.25 mg/kg or 37.5 mg/m^2 in 10 ml of normal saline solution given slowly, over at least 2 min, q 6 hr p.r.n. *Maximum:* 300 mg daily.

Route	Onset	Peak	Duration
I.V.	Immediate	Unknown	3 to 6 hr

Mechanism of Action
May inhibit vestibular stimulation and labyrinthine stimulation and function by acting on the otolith system and, with larger doses, on the semicircular canals.

Contraindications
Hypersensitivity to dimenhydrinate or its components, premature and full-term neonates

Interactions
DRUGS
aminoglycosides and other ototoxic drugs: Masked symptoms of ototoxicity
anticholinergics and drugs with anticholinergic activity: Potentiated anticholinergic effects of dimenhydrinate
apomorphine: Possibly decreased emetic response to apomorphine in treatment of poisoning
barbiturates and other CNS depressants: Possibly increased CNS depression
MAO inhibitors: Increased anticholinergic and CNS depressant effects of dimenhydrinate
ACTIVITIES
alcohol use: Possibly increased CNS depression

Adverse Reactions
CNS: Confusion, drowsiness, hallucinations, nervousness, paradoxical stimulation
CV: Hypotension, palpitations, tachycardia
EENT: Blurred vision, diplopia, dry eyes, dry mouth, nasal congestion
GI: Anorexia, constipation, diarrhea, epigastric discomfort, nausea, vomiting
GU: Dysuria
HEME: Hemolytic anemia
RESP: Thickening of bronchial secretions, wheezing
SKIN: Photosensitivity, rash, urticaria
Other: Anaphylaxis

Nursing Considerations

- **WARNING** Don't administer dimenhydrinate to premature or full-term neonates. Some I.V. preparations may contain benzyl alcohol, which can cause a fatal toxic syndrome characterized by CNS, respiratory, circulatory, and renal impairment and metabolic acidosis.
- **WARNING** Be aware that 50-mg/ml concentration of dimenhydrinate is intended for I.M. use. For I.V. administration, the solution *must* be diluted further with at least 10 ml of diluent, such as D_5W or normal saline solution, for each milliliter of dimenhydrinate.
- Monitor patients with prostatic hypertrophy, stenosing peptic ulcer, pyloroduodenal obstruction, bladder neck obstruction, narrow angle glaucoma, bronchial asthma, or cardiac arrhythmias for signs and symptoms of exacerbation of these conditions resulting from drug's anticholinergic effects.
- Monitor elderly patients for signs of increased sensitivity to dimenhydrinate, such as excessive drowsiness, confusion, and restlessness.
- Assess for signs of paradoxical stimulation, such as nightmares, unusual excitement, nervousness, restlessness, or irritability, especially in children and elderly patients.
- Store drug at 15° to 30° C (59° to 86° F); don't freeze.

PATIENT TEACHING

- Because drug may cause drowsiness, instruct patient to avoid hazardous activities until its CNS effects are known.
- Advise patient to inform health care providers of dimenhydrinate therapy, especially if she's being evaluated for medical conditions that are affected by this drug, such as appendicitis.
- Instruct patient to avoid alcohol, sedatives, and tranquilizers while receiving this drug.
- Encourage patient to use sunscreen to prevent photosensitivity reactions.

diphenhydramine hydrochloride

Benadryl, Hyrexin

Class and Category

Chemical: Ethanolamine derivative
Therapeutic: Antianaphylactic adjunct, antidyskinetic, antiemetic, antihistamine, antivertigo agent
Pregnancy category: B

Indications and Dosages

▶ *To treat hypersensitivity reactions, such as perennial and seasonal allergic rhinitis, vasomotor rhinitis, allergic conjunctivitis, uncomplicated allergic skin eruptions, and transfusion reactions*

I.V. INJECTION

Adults and adolescents. 10 to 50 mg q 4 to 6 hr up to 100 mg/dose, if needed. *Maximum:* 400 mg daily.

Children. 1.25 mg/kg q 4 to 6 hr. *Maximum:* 300 mg daily.

▶ *To prevent motion sickness or treat vertigo*

I.V. INJECTION

Adults and adolescents. *Initial:* 10 mg; increased to 20 to 50 mg q 2 to 3 hr, if needed. *Maximum:* 100 mg/dose, 400 mg daily.

Children. 1 to 1.5 mg/kg I.M. q 4 to 6 hr, p.r.n. *Maximum:* 300 mg daily.

▶ *To treat symptoms of Parkinson's disease and drug-induced extrapyramidal reactions in elderly patients who can't tolerate more potent antidyskinetic drugs*

I.V. INJECTION

Adults and adolescents. 10 to 50 mg q.i.d., as needed. *Maximum:* 100 mg/dose, 400 mg daily.

Route	Onset	Peak	Duration
I.V.	Immediate	1 to 3 hr	6 to 8 hr

Mechanism of Action

Binds to central and peripheral H_1 receptors, competing with histamine for these sites and preventing it from reaching its site of action. By blocking histamine, diphenhydramine produces antihistamine effects: inhibiting respiratory, vascular, and GI smooth-muscle contraction; decreasing capillary permeability, which reduces wheals, flares, and itching; and decreasing salivary and lacrimal gland secretions.

Diphenhydramine also produces antidyskinetic effects, possibly by inhibiting acetylcholine in the CNS. The drug's antiemetic and antivertigo effects may be related to its ability to bind to CNS muscarinic receptors and depress vestibular stimulation and labyrinthine function.

Contraindications

Bladder neck obstruction, hypersensitivity to diphenhydramine or its components, lower respiratory tract symptoms (including asthma), narrow-angle glaucoma, pyloroduodenal obstruction, stenosing peptic ulcer, symptomatic benign prostatic hyperplasia, use within 14 days of MAO inhibitor therapy

Interactions

DRUGS

anticholinergics and drugs with anticholinergic activity: Potentiated anticholinergic effects of diphenhydramine
apomorphine: Possibly decreased emetic response to apomorphine in treatment of poisoning
barbiturates, other CNS depressants: Possibly increased CNS depression
MAO inhibitors: Increased anticholinergic and CNS depressant effects of diphenhydramine

ACTIVITIES

alcohol use: Possibly increased CNS depression

Adverse Reactions

CNS: Confusion, dizziness, drowsiness
CV: Arrhythmias, palpitations, tachycardia
EENT: Blurred vision, diplopia
GI: Epigastric distress, nausea
HEME: Agranulocytosis, hemolytic anemia, thrombocytopenia
RESP: Thickened bronchial secretions
SKIN: Photosensitivity

Nursing Considerations

- Expect to give parenteral form of diphenhydramine only when oral ingestion isn't possible.
- Don't exceed a rate of 25 mg/minute when administering diphenhydramine.
- Expect to discontinue drug at least 72 hours before skin tests for allergies because drug may inhibit cutaneous histamine response, thus producing false-negative results.
- Store drug at 15° to 30° C (59° to 86° F); protect from freezing and light.

PATIENT TEACHING

- Because diphenhydramine may cause drowsiness, advise patient to avoid potentially hazardous activities until its CNS effects are known.
- Urge patient to avoid alcohol and other CNS depressants, such as sedatives and tranquilizers, while receiving diphenhydramine.
- Instruct her to use sunscreen to prevent photosensitivity reactions.

dipyridamole

Persantine

Class and Category

Chemical: Pyrimidine
Therapeutic: Coronary vasodilator, diagnostic aid, platelet aggregation inhibitor
Pregnancy category: B

Indications and Dosages

▶ *To aid diagnosis during thallium perfusion imaging of myocardium*

I.V. INFUSION

Adults. 0.57 mg/kg in 50 ml of D_5W infused over 4 min. *Maximum:* 60 mg.

Route	Onset	Peak	Duration
I.V.	Unknown	3.8 to 8.7 min*	Unknown

Mechanism of Action

May increase the intraplatelet level of adenosine, which causes coronary vasodilation and inhibits platelet aggregation. Dipyridamole also may increase the intraplatelet level of cAMP and may inhibit formation of the potent platelet activator stimulant thromboxane A2, which decreases platelet activation. Vasodilation and increased blood flow occur preferentially in nondiseased coronary vessels, which results in redistribution of blood away from significantly diseased vessels. These changes in perfusion are observed during thallium imaging studies.

Contraindications

Asthma, hypersensitivity to dipyridamole or its components, hypotension, unstable angina pectoris

Interactions

DRUGS

adenosine: Potentiated effects of adenosine
cefamandole, cefoperazone, cefotetan, plicamycin, valproic acid: Possibly hypoprothrombinemia and increased risk of bleeding
heparin, NSAIDs, thrombolytics: Possibly increased risk of bleeding
theophylline: Reversal of coronary vasodilation caused by dipyridamole, possibly false-negative thallium imaging result

* After start of infusion, for increased velocity of coronary artery blood flow.

warfarin: Increased risk of dizziness, abdominal distress, headache and rash

Adverse Reactions

CNS: Dizziness, headache
CV: Angina, arrhythmias, ECG changes (specifically ST-segment and T-wave changes)
GI: Abdominal pain, diarrhea, nausea, vomiting
RESP: Dyspnea
SKIN: Flushing, pruritus, rash

Nursing Considerations

- Protect I.V. form of dipyridamole from direct light and from freezing.
- Monitor blood pressure, pulse rate and rhythm, and breath sounds every 10 to 15 minutes during I.V. infusion.
- Keep parenteral aminophylline available to relieve adverse reactions to dipyridamole infusion.
- At therapeutic doses, expect adverse reactions to be minimal and transient. They typically resolve with long-term use.

PATIENT TEACHING

- Tell patient that dipyridamole usually is given with other anticoagulants.
- Urge her to keep appointments for coagulation tests.
- Instruct patient to seek immediate emergency treatment if chest pain occurs.
- Caution patient to consult prescriber before taking aspirin and other OTC NSAIDs because of increased risk of bleeding.

dobutamine hydrochloride

Dobutrex

Class and Category

Chemical: Synthetic catecholamine
Therapeutic: Cardiac stimulant
Pregnancy category: Not rated

Indications and Dosages

▶ *To treat low cardiac output and heart failure*

I.V. INFUSION

Adults. 2.5 to 10 mcg/kg/min as continuous infusion, adjusted according to hemodynamic response.
Children. 5 to 20 mcg/kg/min as continuous infusion, adjusted according to hemodynamic response.

Route	Onset	Peak	Duration
I.V.	1 to 2 min	Unknown	Less than 5 min

Mechanism of Action

Primarily stimulates $beta_1$-adrenergic receptors and mildly stimulates $beta_2$- and $alpha_1$-adrenergic receptors. $Beta_1$-receptor stimulation produces a positive inotropic effect on the myocardium. This increases cardiac output by boosting myocardial contractility and stroke volume. Increased myocardial contractility raises coronary blood flow and myocardial oxygen consumption. Systolic blood pressure typically rises as a result of increased stroke volume. Other hemodynamic effects include decreased systemic vascular resistance, which reduces afterload, and decreased ventricular filling pressure, which reduces preload.

Incompatibilities

Don't combine dobutamine with cefamandole, cefazolin, cephalothin, ethacrynate sodium, heparin sodium, hydrocortisone sodium succinate, or penicillin because these drugs are incompatible. Don't mix dobutamine with alkaline solutions, such as sodium bicarbonate, because of possible incompatibility. Don't use diluents that contain sodium bisulfite or ethanol. Don't mix dobutamine in same solution with other drugs.

Contraindications

Hypersensitivity to dobutamine or its components, idiopathic hypertrophic subaortic stenosis

Interactions

DRUGS

beta blockers: Possibly increased alpha-adrenergic activity and peripheral resistance
bretylium: Potentiated vasopressor activity, possibly arrhythmias
cyclopropane, halothane: Possibly serious arrhythmias
guanethidine: Decreased hypotensive effect of guanethidine, possibly resulting in severe hypertension
thyroid hormones: Increased cardiovascular effects of thyroid hormones or dobutamine
tricyclic antidepressants: Possibly potentiated cardiovascular and vasopressor effects of dobutamine, resulting in arrhythmias, hyperpyrexia, or severe hypertension

Adverse Reactions

CNS: Fever, headache, nervousness, restlessness
CV: Angina, bradycardia, hypertension, hypotension, palpitations, PVCs, tachycardia
GI: Nausea, vomiting
RESP: Dyspnea
SKIN: Extravasation with tissue necrosis and sloughing, rash
Other: Allergic reaction, hypokalemia

Nursing Considerations

- Avoid giving dobutamine to patients with uncorrected hypovolemia. Expect prescriber to order whole blood or plasma volume expanders to correct hypovolemia. Also avoid giving dobutamine to patients with acute MI because it can intensify or extend myocardial ischemia.
- Dilute concentrate with at least 50 ml of compatible I.V. solution. A common dilution is 500 mg (40 ml from 250-ml bag) in 210 ml of D_5W or normal saline solution to yield 2,000 mcg/ml. Or dilute 1,000 mg (80 ml from 250-ml bag) in 170 ml of D_5W or normal saline solution to yield 4,000 mcg/ml. Adjust maximum concentration according to patient's fluid requirements, as prescribed. Don't exceed 5,000 mcg/ml. Discard solution after 24 hours.
- Inspect parenteral solution for particles and discoloration before administering it.
- Administer drug using an infusion pump.
- Monitor patients who are allergic to sulfites because commercially available dobutamine injections contain sodium bisulfite and may cause anaphylaxis-like signs and symptoms.
- Keep in mind that patients with atrial fibrillation should be adequately digitalized before administration. Monitor such patients for signs of increased AV conduction, such as increased heart rate.
- Monitor blood pressure frequently during therapy, preferably by continuous intra-arterial monitoring; a systolic pressure increase of 10 to 20 mm Hg may indicate a dobutamine-induced increase in cardiac output.
- If hypotension develops, expect to reduce dosage or discontinue drug.
- Monitor heart rate and rhythm continuously for PVCs, which may result from drug's stimulatory effect on the heart's conduction system, and sinus tachycardia, which results from positive

chronotropic effect of beta stimulation and may increase the heart rate by 5 to 15 beats/minute.
- Monitor hemodynamic parameters, such as central venous pressure, pulmonary artery wedge pressure, and cardiac output, as indicated, to assess drug's effectiveness.
- **WARNING** Monitor serum potassium level to check for hypokalemia, a rare result of $beta_2$ stimulation that causes electrolyte imbalances.
- Monitor urine output hourly, as appropriate, to assess for improved renal blood flow.
- Be aware that dobutamine isn't indicated for long-term treatment of heart failure because it may not be effective and may increase the risk of hospitalization and death.
- Before diluting drug, store it at 15° to 30° C (59° to 86° F).

PATIENT TEACHING
- Explain the need for frequent hemodynamic monitoring during dobutamine therapy.

dolasetron mesylate

Anzemet

Class and Category

Chemical: Carboxylate monomethanesulfonate
Therapeutic: Antiemetic
Pregnancy category: B

Indications and Dosages

▶ *To prevent nausea and vomiting from chemotherapy*

I.V. INJECTION

Adults and children over age 16. 1.8 mg/kg or 100 mg as a single dose within 30 min before chemotherapy.

Children ages 2 to 16. 1.8 mg/kg as a single dose within 30 min before chemotherapy. *Maximum:* 100 mg.

ORAL SOLUTION

Adults and children over age 16. 100 mg within 1 hr before chemotherapy.

Children ages 2 to 16. 1.8 mg/kg within 1 hr before chemotherapy. *Maximum:* 100 mg.

▶ *To prevent postoperative nausea and vomiting*

I.V. INJECTION

Adults and children over age 16. 12.5 mg 15 min before end of anesthesia.

Children ages 2 to 16. 0.35 mg/kg 15 min before end of anesthesia. *Maximum:* 12.5 mg/dose.

ORAL SOLUTION

Adults and children over age 16. 100 mg within 2 hr before surgery.

Children ages 2 to 16. 1.2 mg/kg within 2 hr before surgery. *Maximum:* 100 mg.

▶ *To treat postoperative nausea and vomiting*

I.V. INJECTION

Adults and children over age 16. 12.5 mg as a single dose as soon as symptoms develop.

Children ages 2 to 16. 0.35 mg/kg as a single dose as soon as symptoms develop. *Maximum:* 12.5 mg/dose.

Mechanism of Action

With its active metabolite hydrodolasetron, prevents activation of the serotonin 5-hydroxytryptamine$_3$ (5-HT$_3$) receptors located peripherally on the vagal nerve terminals and centrally in the chemoreceptor trigger zone, thereby decreasing the vomiting reflex.

Contraindications

Hypersensitivity to dolasetron or its components

Interactions

DRUGS

atenolol: Possibly decreased clearance of dolasetron
cimetidine: Possibly increased blood dolasetron level
rifampin: Possibly decreased blood dolasetron level

Adverse Reactions

CNS: Headache
CV: Bradycardia, ECG changes, hypertension, hypotension, tachycardia
GI: Diarrhea
SKIN: Rash
Other: Anaphylaxis, injection site pain

Nursing Considerations

- Administer up to 100 mg of dolasetron I.V. in 30 seconds or dilute drug in normal saline solution, D_5W, D_5/0.45 normal saline solution, or lactated Ringer's solution and infuse for up to 15 minutes, as prescribed.

- Flush I.V. line with compatible solution before and after drug administration.
- Expect to prepare an oral solution of dolasetron for patients unable to swallow tablets by diluting injection solution with apple or apple-grape juice.
- **WARNING** Monitor patients receiving dolasetron for ECG changes, including prolonged PR, QTc, and JT intervals and widened QRS complex.
- Store drug at 20° to 25° C (68° to 77° F) and protect from light.

PATIENT TEACHING

- Advise parents of pediatric patients and patients who have difficulty swallowing that oral solution can be prepared by diluting injection form of dolasetron with apple or apple-grape juice.
- Inform patient that oral solution may be refrigerated for up to 48 hours but should be discarded after 2 hours at room temperature.

dopamine hydrochloride

Intropin, Revimine (CAN)

Class and Category

Chemical: Catecholamine
Therapeutic: Cardiac stimulant, vasopressor
Pregnancy category: C

Indications and Dosages

▶ *To correct hypotension that is unresponsive to adequate fluid volume replacement or occurs as part of shock syndrome caused by bacteremia, chronic cardiac decompensation, drug overdose, MI, open-heart surgery, renal failure, trauma, or other major systemic illnesses; to improve low cardiac output*

I.V. INFUSION

Adults. 0.5 to 3 mcg/kg/min for vasodilation of renal arteries; 2 to 10 mcg/kg/min for positive inotropic effects and increased cardiac output; 10 mcg/kg/min, increased gradually according to patient's response, for increased systolic and diastolic blood pressures.

Children. 0.5 to 3 mcg/kg/min for vasodilation of renal arteries; 5 to 20 mcg/kg/min for increased cardiac output and systolic and diastolic blood pressures.

DOSAGE ADJUSTMENT Initial dosage reduced to 10% of usual amount if patient has received an MAO inhibitor in previous 2 to 3 wk.

Route	Onset	Peak	Duration
I.V.	In 5 min	Unknown	Up to 10 min

Mechanism of Action

Stimulates dopamine$_1$ (D_1) and dopamine$_2$ (D_2) postsynaptic receptors. D_1 receptors mediate vasodilation in renal, mesenteric, coronary, and cerebral blood vessels. D_2 receptors, when stimulated, inhibit norepinephrine release. In higher doses, dopamine also stimulates alpha$_1$ and alpha$_2$ receptors, causing vascular smooth-muscle contraction.

At doses of 0.5 to 3 mcg/kg/minute, this naturally occurring catecholamine mainly affects dopaminergic receptors in renal, mesenteric, coronary, and cerebral vessels, resulting in vasodilation, increased renal blood flow, improved GFR, and increased urine output. At doses of 2 to 10 mcg/kg/minute, dopamine stimulates beta$_1$-adrenergic receptors, increasing cardiac output while maintaining dopaminergic-induced vasodilation. At doses of 10 mcg/kg/minute or more, alpha-adrenergic agonism takes over, causing increased peripheral vascular resistance and renal vasoconstriction.

Incompatibilities

Don't add dopamine to 5% sodium bicarbonate, alkaline I.V. solutions, oxidizing agents, or iron salts.

Contraindications

Pheochromocytoma, uncorrected ventricular fibrillation, ventricular tachycardia and other tachyarrhythmias

Interactions

DRUGS

alpha blockers, haloperidol, loxapine, phenothiazines, thioxanthenes: Antagonized peripheral vasoconstriction with high doses of dopamine

anesthetics (such as chloroform, enflurane, halothane, isoflurane, and methoxyflurane): Increased risk of severe atrial and ventricular arrhythmias

antihypertensives, diuretics used as antihypertensives: Possibly decreased antihypertensive effects of these drugs

beta blockers: Antagonized beta receptor–mediated inotropic effects of dopamine

digitalis glycosides: Possibly increased risk of arrhythmias and additive inotropic effects

diuretics: Possibly increased diuretic effects of dopamine or diuretic

doxapram: Possibly increased vasopressor effects
ergot alkaloids: Enhanced peripheral vasoconstriction
guanadrel, guanethidine: Possibly decreased antihypertensive effects of these drugs and potentiated vasopressor response to dopamine, resulting in hypertension and arrhythmias
levodopa: Possibly increased risk of arrhythmias
MAO inhibitors: Prolonged and intensified cardiac stimulation and vasopressor effect of dopamine
maprotiline, tricyclic antidepressants: Possibly potentiated cardiovascular and vasopressor effects of dopamine, resulting in arrhythmias, hyperpyrexia, or severe hypertension
mecamylamine, methyldopa: Possibly decreased hypotensive effects of these drugs and enhanced vasopressor effect of dopamine
methylphenidate: Possibly potentiated vasopressor effect of dopamine
nitrates: Possibly decreased antianginal effect of nitrates; possibly decreased vasopressor effect of dopamine, resulting in hypotension
oxytoxic drugs: Possibly severe hypertension
phenoxybenzamine: Possibly antagonized peripheral vasoconstriction of dopamine, causing hypotension and tachycardia
phenytoin: Possibly sudden bradycardia and hypotension
rauwolfia alkaloids: Possibly decreased hypotensive effects of these drugs
sympathomimetics: Possibly increased adverse cardiovascular and other effects
thyroid hormones: Increased risk of coronary insufficiency

Adverse Reactions

CNS: Headache
CV: Angina, bradycardia, hypertension, hypotension, palpitations, peripheral vasoconstriction, sinus tachycardia, ventricular arrhythmias
GI: Nausea, vomiting
RESP: Dyspnea
SKIN: Extravasation with tissue necrosis
Other: Allergic reaction

Nursing Considerations

- If possible, avoid giving dopamine to patients with occlusive vascular disease, such as atherosclerosis, Buerger's disease, diabetic endarteritis, or Raynaud's disease, because of the risk of decreased peripheral circulation.
- Inspect parenteral solution for particles and discoloration before administration.

- Dilute dopamine concentrate with a compatible I.V. solution before administering. Typical dilution is 400 mg in 250 ml to yield 1.6 mg/ml. Don't exceed 3.2 mg/ml.
- Be aware that drug also comes premixed with D_5W in concentrations of 800 mcg, 1.6 mg, and 3.2 mg. Monitor for elevated glucose levels, as ordered, in patients with subclinical or overt diabetes mellitus because this finding may signal an exacerbation.
- If patient has hypovolemia, ensure adequate fluid resuscitation before giving drug.
- Give drug by I.V. infusion using an infusion pump.
- **WARNING** When the infusion rate exceeds 20 mcg/kg/minute, monitor for excessive vasoconstriction and loss of renal vasodilating effects. Don't exceed an infusion rate of 50 mcg/kg/minute.
- If you must infuse more than 20 mcg/kg/minute of dopamine to maintain blood pressure, expect to infuse norepinephrine as prescribed.
- Administer infusion through a central catheter to avoid extravasation and tissue necrosis. If you must administer drug through a peripheral line, inspect site frequently for signs of extravasation and necrosis. If you detect such signs, start a new I.V. line for dopamine infusion, discontinue previous I.V. line, and notify prescriber immediately.
- If drug extravasates, expect prescriber to give 5 to 10 mg of phentolamine diluted in 10 to 15 ml of normal saline solution, as prescribed. Phentolamine infiltrates directly into area to antagonize vasoconstriction and minimize sloughing and tissue necrosis.
- Titrate dopamine gradually to minimize hypotension, especially after a high infusion rate.
- Monitor blood pressure continuously with an intra-arterial line, as indicated.
- Place patient on continuous ECG monitoring, and assess heart rate and rhythm for arrhythmias.
- Assess patients with cardiac disease, particularly coronary artery disease, for signs of exacerbation or adverse cardiac reactions because dopamine increases myocardial oxygen demand.
- Monitor hemodynamic parameters, such as central venous pressure, pulmonary artery wedge pressure, and cardiac output, as indicated, to assess drug's effectiveness.
- Monitor urine output hourly as appropriate to assess for improved renal blood flow.

- Monitor patients who are allergic to sulfites for signs and symptoms of an allergic reaction because some forms of dopamine contain sulfites.
- Store dopamine at 15° to 30° C (59° to 86° F); don't freeze this drug.

PATIENT TEACHING

- Explain the need for frequent hemodynamic monitoring during dopamine therapy.

doxapram hydrochloride

Dopram

Class and Category

Chemical: Pyrrolidinone derivative
Therapeutic: Respiratory stimulant
Pregnancy category: B

Indications and Dosages

▶ *To stimulate respiration in COPD-related acute respiratory insufficiency*

I.V. INFUSION

Adults and adolescents. 1 to 2 mg/min titrated according to respiratory response. *Maximum:* 3 mg/min for up to 2 hr.

▶ *To treat respiratory depression after anesthesia*

I.V. INFUSION

Adults and adolescents. 5 mg/min until desired response occurs and then reduced to 1 to 3 mg/min. *Maximum:* Cumulative dose of 4 mg/kg or 300 mg.

I.V. INJECTION

Adults and adolescents. 0.5 to 1 mg/kg, repeated q 5 min, if needed. *Maximum:* 1.5 mg/kg as a single dose or 2 mg/kg q 5 min.

Route	Onset	Peak	Duration
I.V.	20 to 40 sec	1 to 2 min	5 to 12 min

Mechanism of Action

Activates peripheral carotid, aortic, and other chemoreceptors to stimulate respiration, resulting in increased tidal volume and respiratory rate. Doxapram also may increase respiratory rate and tidal volume by directly stimulating the respiratory center in the medulla oblongata.

Incompatibilities

To avoid precipitation and gas formation, don't mix doxapram with alkaline solutions, such as aminophylline, sodium bicarbonate, or 2.5% thiopental.

Contraindications

Age less than 1 month; cerebral edema; CVA; head injury; hypersensitivity to doxapram or its components; mechanical disorders of ventilation, including acute bronchial asthma, flail chest, muscle paresis, obstruction, pneumothorax, and pulmonary fibrosis; pulmonary embolism; seizure disorder; severe cardiovascular disorder; severe hypertension; uncompensated heart failure

Interactions

DRUGS

chloroform, cyclopropane, enflurane, halothane, isoflurane, methoxyflurane, trichloroethylene: Possibly adverse myocardial effects if doxapram given within 10 minutes of these drugs
CNS stimulants: Possibly excessive CNS stimulation, resulting in arrhythmias, insomnia, irritability, nervousness, or seizures
MAO inhibitors, sympathomimetics: Additive vasopressor effects
skeletal muscle relaxants: Masked residual effects of muscle relaxants

Adverse Reactions

CNS: Disorientation, dizziness, headache
CV: Arrhythmias, including sinus tachycardia; hypertension
GI: Diarrhea, hiccups, nausea, vomiting
GU: Urine retention
RESP: Bronchospasm, cough, dyspnea
SKIN: Diaphoresis
Other: Injection site pain, redness, swelling, and thrombophlebitis

Nursing Considerations

- Avoid giving doxapram to patients receiving mechanical ventilation.
- Maintain a patent airway, and assess for optimal oxygenation before administering drug.
- Monitor I.V. insertion site for extravasation and signs of thrombophlebitis or local skin irritation.
- If hypertension or dyspnea develops suddenly, stop infusion as directed.
- Assess for early signs of overdose, including enhanced deep tendon reflexes, skeletal muscle hyperactivity, and tachycardia.

PATIENT TEACHING
- Explain the need for frequent pulse and blood pressure monitoring.

doxorubicin hydrochloride

Adriamycin PFS, Adriamycin RDF, Rubex

Class and Category

Chemical: Anthracycline glycoside
Therapeutic: Antibiotic antineoplastic
Pregnancy category: D

Indications and Dosages

▶ *To treat disseminated neoplastic conditions, such as acute lymphoblastic or acute myeloblastic leukemia; Wilms' tumor; neuroblastoma; soft-tissue and bone sarcomas; breast, bronchogenic, gastric, ovarian, transitional cell bladder, or thyroid cancer; Hodgkin's disease; or malignant lymphoma*

I.V. INFUSION OR INJECTION

Adults. 60 to 75 mg/m^2 administered over at least 3 to 5 min q 21 days when given as a single agent, or 40 to 60 mg/m^2 administered over at least 3 to 5 min q 21 to 28 days when given in combination therapy.

Children. 30 mg/m^2 for 3 days q 4 wk.

DOSAGE ADJUSTMENT Dosage varies, depending on regimen used. Dosage may be reduced when doxorubicin is used in combination with other cytotoxic drugs. Dosage reduced by 50% when plasma bilirubin level is 1.2 to 3 mg/ml and by 75% when plasma bilirubin level is 3.1 to 5 mg/ml.

Mechanism of Action

Binds directly to DNA by inserting (intercalating) itself between two DNA bases, which inhibits the synthesis of DNA and RNA and produces single-strand breaks in DNA. In addition, doxorubicin undergoes an enzymatic reduction, resulting in the multi-step production of a hydroxyl radical, which may lead to cell death by reacting with DNA, RNA, cell membranes, and proteins. Doxorubicin is active in all phases of the cell cycle, though cell cycle phase S is most sensitive.

Incompatibilities

Don't mix doxorubicin with heparin or fluorouracil because a precipitate will form. Don't mix doxorubicin with other drugs or with bacteriostatic agents.

Contraindications

Patients who've received maximum acceptable doses of doxorubicin, daunorubicin, idarubicin, or other anthracyclines and anthracenes; marked myelosuppression from prior antitumor therapy or radiation therapy

Interactions

DRUGS

actinomycin D: Acute "recall" pneumonitis after local radiation therapy in children
blood-dyscrasia–causing drugs (such as cephalosporins and cisplatin): Increased leukopenic and thrombocytopenic effects of doxorubicin
bone marrow depressants (such as colchicine and methotrexate): Increased bone marrow depression
carbamazepine: Decreased blood carbamazepine level
cisplatin: Risk of leukemia
cyclophosphamide: Potentiated cyclophosphamide-induced hemorrhagic cystitis, increased risk of doxorubicin-induced cardiotoxicity
cyclosporine: Possibly decreased doxorubicin metabolism; increased risk of severe and prolonged hematologic toxicity, coma, and seizures
cytarabine: Possibly necrotizing colitis
dactinomycin, mitomycin, nifedipine, and other calcium channel blockers: Increased risk of doxorubicin-induced cardiotoxicity
digoxin: Decreased absorption of digoxin
fosphenytoin, phenytoin: Possibly decreased blood phenytoin level
methotrexate and other hepatotoxic drugs: Possibly impaired hepatic function, increased risk of doxorubicin toxicity
paclitaxel: Decreased doxorubicin clearance
phenobarbital: Possibly increased doxorubicin excretion
progesterone: Possibly enhanced doxorubicin-induced neutropenia and thrombocytopenia
streptozocin: Possibly inhibited hepatic metabolism of doxorubicin
trastuzumab: Possibly increased incidence and severity of cardiac dysfunction
vaccines, killed virus: Possibly decreased antibody response to vaccine
vaccines, live virus: Possibly increased adverse effects of vaccine, severe infection, and decreased antibody response to vaccine

Adverse Reactions

CNS: Chills, fever

CV: Arrhythmias, cardiomyopathy, cardiotoxicity
EENT: Conjunctivitis, esophagitis, stomatitis
GI: Diarrhea, GI ulceration or necrosis, nausea, vomiting
GU: Uric acid nephropathy, reddish urine
HEME: Anemia, leukopenia, myelosuppression, thrombocytopenia
SKIN: Alopecia; cellulitis; extravasation; hyperpigmentation of soles, palms, or nails; erythematous streaking along vein used for insertion; infusion site pain; recall postirradiation erythema; urticaria
Other: Hyperuricemia

Nursing Considerations

- **WARNING** Be aware that doxorubicin hydrochloride liposome should not be substituted for doxorubicin hydrochloride. These drugs are not interchangeable; severe adverse reactions may result.
- Be aware that doxorubicin should be administered only under the supervision of a qualified physician and that initial treatment usually takes place in a hospital.
- Follow facility protocols for preparation and handling of antineoplastic drugs and appropriate disposal of used equipment.
- Monitor patient's liver and renal function tests and CBC, including hematocrit, platelet count, and WBC count with differential, before and periodically during therapy. Be aware that cardiac evaluation, including ECG, radionuclide angiography to determine ejection fraction, and echocardiography, will be performed before, during, and sometimes after doxorubicin therapy.
- Be aware that doxorubicin is available in various concentrations. Reconstitute doxorubicin with 0.9% sodium chloride injection to a final concentration of 2 mg/ml. Withdraw appropriate amount of air from vial when preparing drug to prevent pressure build-up. Shake vial to allow contents to dissolve. Inspect solution for particles or discoloration before administration.
- Use most reconstituted solutions within 7 days if stored at room temperature and in normal room light, or within 15 days if refrigerated at 2° to 8° C (36° to 46° F) and protected from sunlight. However, consult manufacturer's recommendations because some preparations may be stable for a shorter period.
- Administer doxorubicin into a large vein by a free-flowing I.V. infusion of D_5W or normal saline solution over at least 3 minutes. Watch for red streaking along vein or facial flushing, which may indicate too-rapid administration.

- Wash your skin thoroughly with soap and water and irrigate your eyes if exposed to doxorubicin.
- Avoid contact with patient's urine or other body fluids—for example, by wearing latex gloves when caring for pediatric patients—for at least 5 days after each treatment.
- **WARNING** Monitor patient for signs of doxorubicin-induced cardiotoxicity, including cardiomyopathy and life-threatening heart failure, which may occur during therapy or months to years afterward. Patients with a history of prior mediastinal irradiation and young or elderly patients receiving concurrent cyclophosphamide therapy are at increased risk for developing cardiotoxicity at lower doses. Be prepared to administer digitalis preparations, diuretics, and afterload reducers such as ACE inhibitors if heart failure occurs.
- Monitor serum uric acid level before and during therapy, especially in patients with a history of gout or urate calculi. Expect antigout drug dosage to be adjusted if blood uric acid level is elevated from doxorubicin therapy. Oral hydration and allopurinol may be administered to prevent uric acid nephropathy.
- Monitor patients with a history of bone marrow depression, chickenpox (including recent exposure), and herpes zoster because they're at increased risk for severe generalized disease. Assess patients with leukopenia for signs of infection, including fever, chills, and cough.
- Be aware that adverse reactions can vary when doxorubicin is administered in combination therapy. Review information for all drugs administered as part of a specific regimen, including drug interactions and adverse effects.
- Assess I.V. insertion site for signs of extravasation, such as redness or pain. Tissue necrosis can occur because drug is a vesicant. (However, extravasation can be painless or can occur even with blood return in I.V. line.) If extravasation occurs, immediately stop injection or infusion and apply ice. Then restart injection or infusion in another vein.
- Before reconstituting doxorubicin, store it at 15° to 30° C (59° to 86° F) and protect from light.

PATIENT TEACHING

- Instruct patient receiving doxorubicin to immediately report adverse reactions, such as unusual bruising or bleeding; black, tarry stools; blood in urine or stools; or pinpoint red spots on skin.
- Inform patient that urine may be red-tinged for 1 or 2 days after treatment.

- Stress the importance of keeping scheduled follow-up appointments and undergoing prescribed diagnostic tests, such as cardiac evaluation, especially to parents of pediatric patients, who are at increased risk for delayed cardiotoxicity, delayed growth, and temporary gonadal impairment.
- Caution patient to avoid sports and other activities that increase the risk of accidental injury. Also advise her to take measures to avoid infection, such as maintaining good oral hygiene (for example, by using soft-bristled toothbrush) and washing hands before touching eyes or nose.
- Advise patient with thrombocytopenia to avoid alcohol and aspirin to reduce the risk of GI bleeding.
- Advise patient not receive live or killed virus vaccines during therapy and for 3 months to 1 year after therapy is completed, unless approved by prescriber. Urge her to avoid people who have received such vaccines or to wear a protective mask when she's around them.
- Suggest that patient with stomatitis eat soft, bland foods served cold or at room temperature to decrease irritation.
- Inform patient that her hair should grow back after therapy but that the color and texture may be different.
- Advise female patient not to breast-feed during therapy.
- Urge both male and female patients to use two methods of birth control during therapy.

doxorubicin hydrochloride liposome

Caelyx (CAN), Doxil

Class and Category

Chemical: Anthracycline
Therapeutic: Antibiotic antineoplastic
Pregnancy category: D

Indications and Dosages

▶ *To treat Kaposi's sarcoma associated with AIDS*

I.V. INFUSION

Adults. 20 mg/m^2 over 30 min q 3 wk.

▶ *To treat refractory ovarian cancer*

I.V. INFUSION

Adults. 40 to 50 mg/m^2 infused at 1 mg/min initially to minimize risk of infusion reaction; then drug infused over 1 to 2 hr. Repeated q 4 wk.

DOSAGE ADJUSTMENT Dosage reduced by 50% when

serum bilirubin level is 1.2 to 3 mg/dl and by 75% when serum bilirubin level is 3 mg/dl.

Mechanism of Action

May induce fragmentation of tumor cell DNA by inhibiting topo-isomerase II, an enzyme that usually acts to catalyze the breakage and reformation of DNA linkages. Antitumor activity and toxicity may be related to the formation of intracellular oxygen free radicals, which may lead to cell death after reaction with DNA, RNA, cell membranes, and proteins. Liposomal encapsulation may enhance doxorubicin accumulation in Kaposi's sarcoma (KS) lesions and allow passage through endothelial cell gaps present in lesions similar to those of KS.

Incompatibilities

Don't mix liposomal doxorubicin with diluents other than D_5W or with other drugs or bacteriostatic agents.

Contraindications

Breast-feeding women, hypersensitivity to doxorubicin hydrochloride or to liposomal components

Interactions

DRUGS

actinomycin D: Acute "recall" pneumonitis after local radiation therapy in children
blood-dyscrasia–causing drugs (such as cephalosporins and cisplatin): Increased leukopenic and thrombocytopenic effects of doxorubicin
bone marrow depressants (such as colchicine and methotrexate): Increased bone marrow depression
carbamazepine: Decreased blood carbamazepine level
cisplatin: Risk of leukemia
cyclophosphamide: Potentiated cyclophosphamide-induced hemorrhagic cystitis, increased risk of doxorubicin-induced cardiotoxicity
cyclosporine: Possibly decreased doxorubicin metabolism; increased risk of severe and prolonged hematologic toxicity, coma, and seizures
cytarabine: Possibly necrotizing colitis
dactinomycin, mitomycin, nifedipine, and other calcium channel blockers: Increased risk of doxorubicin-induced cardiotoxicity
digoxin: Decreased blood digoxin level
fosphenytoin, phenytoin: Possibly decreased blood phenytoin level

methotrexate and other hepatoxic drugs: Possibly impaired hepatic function, increased risk of doxorubicin toxicity
paclitaxel: Decreased doxorubicin clearance
phenobarbital: Possibly increased doxorubicin excretion
progesterone: Possibly enhanced doxorubicin-induced neutropenia and thrombocytopenia
streptozocin: Possibly inhibited hepatic metabolism of doxorubicin
trastuzumab: Possibly increased incidence and severity of cardiac dysfunction
vaccines, killed virus: Possibly decreased antibody response to vaccine
vaccines, live virus: Possibly increased adverse effects of vaccine, severe infection, and decreased antibody response to vaccine

Adverse Reactions

CNS: Anxiety, asthenia, chills, dizziness, fever, headache, insomnia
CV: Cardiotoxicity (dose-related or cumulative effect), chest pain
EENT: Conjunctivitis, mucous membrane disorder (changes in mouth or nose lining), oral candidiasis, pharyngitis, stomatitis, taste perversion
GI: Abdominal pain, anorexia, constipation, diarrhea, dysphagia, ileus, nausea, vomiting
GU: Reddish urine
HEME: Anemia, leukopenia, neutropenia, thrombocytopenia
MS: Back pain
RESP: Dyspnea, pneumonia
SKIN: Alopecia, injection site pain, jaundice, palmar-plantar erythrodysesthesia, rash, recall postirradiation erythema, pruritus
Other: Allergic reaction, infection, infusion reaction

Nursing Considerations

- **WARNING** Be aware that doxorubicin hydrochloride should not be substituted for doxorubicin hydrochloride liposome. These drugs are not interchangeable; severe adverse reactions may result.
- Be aware that liposomal doxorubicin should be administered only under the supervision of a qualified physician.
- Follow facility protocols for preparation and handling of antineoplastic drugs and appropriate disposal of used equipment.
- Monitor hepatic and renal function tests and CBC, including hematocrit, platelet count, and WBC count with differential, before and periodically during therapy. Be aware that cardiac evaluation, including ECG, radionuclide angiography to determine ejection fraction, and echocardiography, will be performed

before, during, and sometimes after doxorubicin hydrochloride liposome therapy.

- Wear gloves and other protective garments (according to facility protocol) when working with this drug. Wash skin thoroughly with soap and water to remove drug if exposed.
- Dilute up to 90 mg of liposomal doxorubicin in 250 ml of D_5W. Inspect solution for particles before administration and discard if particles are present. Be aware that liposomal doxorubicin is a red, translucent solution.
- Use diluted solution within 24 hours if stored at 2° to 8° C (36° to 46° F). Administer without an in-line filter.
- Monitor patient for signs of an infusion reaction, such as flushing, dyspnea, facial edema, headache, chills, back pain, chest or throat tightness, and hypotension. Such a reaction may resolve if infusion rate is decreased; however, in most patients, it will resolve within several hours or a day after infusion is terminated.
- **WARNING** Monitor patient for drug-induced cardiotoxicity, including cardiomyopathy and life-threatening heart failure, which may occur during therapy or months to years afterward. Patients with a history of prior mediastinal irradiation, those who are receiving concurrent cyclophosphamide therapy, and those who have previously received anthracyclines or anthracenediones are at increased risk for developing cardiotoxicity at lower doses. Be prepared to administer digitalis preparations, diuretics, and afterload reducers such as ACE inhibitors if heart failure occurs.
- Monitor patient for stomatitis, signs of bone marrow depression, or palmar-plantar erythrodysesthesia (swelling, pain, erythema, and skin peeling of hands and feet); these adverse reactions may require dosage reduction or drug discontinuation.
- Monitor patients with a history of bone marrow depression, chickenpox (including recent exposure), and herpes zoster because they're at increased risk for severe generalized disease. Assess patients with leukopenia for signs of infection, including fever, chills, and cough.
- Assess I.V. insertion site for signs of extravasation, such as redness or pain. (However, extravasation can be painless.) If extravasation occurs, immediately stop injection or infusion and apply ice. Follow facility protocol, if available, for management of extravasation. Then restart injection or infusion in another vein.
- Before diluting liposomal doxorubicin, store it at 2° to 8° C (36° to 46° F). Drug may be frozen for up to 1 month.

PATIENT TEACHING

- Instruct patient receiving liposomal doxorubicin to immediately report adverse reactions, such as swelling, blisters, or burning of hands or feet; unusual bruising or bleeding; black, tarry stools; blood in urine or stools; or red pinpoint spots on the skin.
- Inform patient that urine may be red-tinged for 1 or 2 days after treatment.
- Stress the importance of keeping scheduled follow-up appointments and undergoing prescribed diagnostic tests, such as cardiac evaluation.
- Caution patient to avoid sports and other activities that increase the risk of accidental injury. Also advise her to take measures to avoid infection, such as maintaining good oral hygiene (for example, by using soft-bristled toothbrush) and washing hands before touching eyes or nose.
- Advise patient with thrombocytopenia to avoid alcohol and aspirin to reduce the risk of GI bleeding.
- Advise patient not to receive live or killed virus vaccines during therapy and for a period afterward, unless approved by prescriber. Urge her to avoid people who have received such vaccines or to wear a protective mask when she's around them.
- Advise patient with stomatitis to try eating soft, bland foods served cold or at room temperature to decrease irritation.
- Inform patient that her hair should grow back after treatment but that the color and texture may be different.
- Advise female patient not to breast-feed during therapy.
- Urge both male and female patients to use two methods of birth control during therapy.

doxycycline hyclate

(contains 100 or 200 mg of base per injection vial)
Vibramycin

Class and Category

Chemical: Oxytetracycline derivative
Therapeutic: Antibiotic
Pregnancy category: D

Indications and Dosages

▶ *To treat cutaneous, GI, or inhalation anthrax*

I.V. INFUSION

Adults, adolescents, and children weighing more than 45 kg (99 lb). 100 mg (base) q 12 hr for 60 days.

Children weighing less than 45 kg. 2.2 mg/kg (base) q 12 hr for 60 days.

I.V. INFUSION

Adults and children over age 8 weighing more than 45 kg. 200 mg (base) daily or 100 mg (base) q 12 hr on day 1 and then 100 to 200 mg (base) daily or 50 to 100 mg (base) q 12 hr. *Maximum:* 300 mg (base) daily.

Children weighing 45 kg or less. 4.4 mg (base)/kg daily or 2.2 mg (base)/kg q 12 hr on day 1 and then 2.2 to 4.4 mg (base)/kg daily or 1.1 to 2.2 mg (base)/kg q 12 hr.

▶ *To treat epididymo-orchitis caused by* Chlamydia trachomatis *or* Neisseria gonorrhoeae *or nongonococcal urethritis caused by* C. trachomatis *or* Ureaplasma urealyticum

I.V. INFUSION

Adults and children over age 8 weighing more than 45 kg. 200 mg (base) daily or 100 mg (base) q 12 hr on day 1 and then 100 to 200 mg (base) daily or 50 to 100 mg (base) q 12 hr. *Maximum:* 300 mg (base) daily.

Children weighing 45 kg or less. 4.4 mg (base)/kg daily or 2.2 mg (base)/kg q 12 hr on day 1 and then 2.2 to 4.4 mg (base)/kg daily or 1.1 to 2.2 mg (base)/kg q 12 hr.

▶ *To treat early syphilis in penicillin-allergic patients*

I.V. INFUSION

Adults and children over age 8 weighing more than 45 kg. 150 mg (base) q 12 hr for at least 10 days. *Maximum:* 300 mg (base) daily.

Children weighing 45 kg or less. 4.4 mg (base)/kg daily or 2.2 mg (base)/kg q 12 hr on day 1 and then 2.2 to 4.4 mg (base)/kg daily or 1.1 to 2.2 mg (base)/kg q 12 hr.

▶ *To treat syphilis of more than 1 year's duration in patients allergic to penicillin*

I.V. INFUSION

Adults and children over age 8 weighing more than 45 kg. 150 mg (base) q 12 hr for at least 10 days. *Maximum:* 300 mg (base) daily.

Children weighing 45 kg or less. 4.4 mg (base)/kg daily or 2.2 mg (base)/kg q 12 hr on day 1 and then 2.2 to 4.4 mg (base)/kg daily or 1.1 to 2.2 mg (base)/kg q 12 hr.

▶ *To treat all other infections caused by susceptible organisms*

I.V. INFUSION

Adults and children over age 8 weighing more than 45 kg. 200 mg (base) daily or 100 mg (base) q 12 hr on day 1 and then

100 to 200 mg (base) daily or 50 to 100 mg (base) q 12 hr. *Maximum:* 300 mg (base) daily.
Children weighing 45 kg or less. 4.4 mg (base)/kg daily or 2.2 mg (base)/kg q 12 hr on day 1 and then 2.2 to 4.4 mg (base)/kg daily or 1.1 to 2.2 mg (base)/kg q 12 hr.

Mechanism of Action

Exerts a bacteriostatic effect against a wide variety of gram-positive and gram-negative organisms. Doxycycline is more lipophilic than other tetracyclines, which allows it to pass more easily through the bacterial lipid bilayer, where it binds reversibly to 30S ribosomal subunits. Bound doxycycline blocks the binding of aminoacyl transfer RNA to messenger RNA, thus inhibiting bacterial protein synthesis.

Contraindications

Hypersensitivity to any tetracycline

Interactions

DRUGS

antacids that contain aluminum, calcium, magnesium, or zinc; calcium supplements; choline and magnesium salicylates; iron salts; laxatives that contain magnesium: Decreased doxycycline absorption and therapeutic effects
barbiturates, carbamazepine, phenytoin: Increased clearance and decreased effects of doxycycline
cholestyramine, colestipol: Decreased doxycycline absorption
digoxin: Increased bioavailability of digoxin, possibly leading to digitalis toxicity
oral anticoagulants: Possibly increased hypo-prothrombinemic effects of these drugs
oral contraceptives: Decreased effectiveness of estrogen-containing oral contraceptives, increased risk of breakthrough bleeding
penicillins: Inhibited bactericidal action
sodium bicarbonate: Altered doxycycline absorption from increased gastric pH

FOODS

dairy products, other foods high in calcium or iron: Decreased doxycycline absorption

Adverse Reactions

CNS: Paresthesia
CV: Phlebitis

EENT: Black "hairy" tongue, glossitis, hoarseness, oral candidiasis, pharyngitis, stomatitis, tooth discoloration
GI: Anorexia; bulky, loose stools; diarrhea; dysphagia; enterocolitis; epigastric distress; esophageal ulceration; hepatotoxicity; nausea; rectal candidiasis; vomiting
GU: Anogenital lesions, dark yellow or brown urine, elevated BUN level, vaginal candidiasis
HEME: Eosinophilia, hemolytic anemia, neutropenia, thrombocytopenia, thrombocytopenic purpura
SKIN: Dermatitis, photosensitivity, rash, urticaria
Other: Anaphylaxis, injection site phlebitis

Nursing Considerations

- Avoid giving doxycycline to breast-feeding women because of the risk of enamel hypoplasia, inhibited linear skeletal growth, oral and vaginal candidiasis, photosensitivity reactions, and tooth discoloration in breast-feeding infant.
- Avoid giving drug to children younger than age 8; it may cause permanent discoloration and enamel hypoplasia of developing teeth.
- Expect to adjust dosage for patients who have hepatic disease to avoid drug accumulation.
- **WARNING** Don't give doxycycline by I.M. or subcutaneous route.
- Observe patient frequently for injection site phlebitis, a common adverse reaction to I.V. administration.
- Monitor liver function test results as appropriate to detect hepatotoxicity.
- Expect doxycycline to increase risk of oral, rectal, or vaginal candidiasis—especially in elderly or debilitated patients and those on prolonged therapy—by changing the normal balance of microbial flora.
- Monitor patient closely for diarrhea, which may indicate pseudomembranous colitis. If diarrhea occurs, notify prescriber and expect to withhold doxycycline. Expect to treat pseudomembranous colitis with fluids, electrolytes, protein, and an antibiotic effective against Clostridium difficile.

PATIENT TEACHING

- Instruct patient to drink plenty of fluids while taking doxycycline to reduce the risk of esophageal burning and ulceration.
- Advise patients who take an oral contraceptive to use an additional contraceptive method during therapy.

- If patient is being treated for a sexually transmitted disease, explain that her partner may need treatment as well.
- Instruct patient to notify prescriber immediately if she experiences anorexia, diarrhea, epigastric distress, nausea, and vomiting during therapy.
- Alert female patients that doxycycline may raise the risk of vaginal candidiasis. Tell them to report vaginal itching or discharge.

droperidol

Inapsine

Class and Category

Chemical: Butyrophenone derivative
Therapeutic: Anesthesia adjunct, antiemetic, sedative-hypnotic
Pregnancy category: C

Indications and Dosages

▶ *To provide anesthesia premedication*

I.V. INJECTION

Children. 0.075 to 0.15 mg/kg I.V. 30 to 60 min before surgery. (For adults and adolescents, drug is given by I.M. injection, 2.5 to 5 mg I.M. 30 to 60 min before surgery.)

▶ *To induce anesthesia*

I.V. INJECTION

Adults and adolescents. *Initial:* 1.25 to 2.5 mg/9 to 11 kg (20 to 25 lb) or 0.1 to 0.14 mg/kg given with general anesthesia. *Maintenance*: Additional 1.25 to 2.5 mg, as needed.

Children. 0.075 to 0.15 mg/kg given with general anesthesia.

▶ *As adjunct to regional anesthesia*

I.V. INJECTION

Adults and adolescents. 2.5 to 5 mg.

▶ *To provide sedative-hypnotic effects for diagnostic procedures performed without anesthesia (conscious sedation)*

I.V. INJECTION

Adults and adolescents. 1.25 to 5 mg 30 to 60 min before procedure, followed by another 1.25 to 2.5 mg I.V., if indicated.

▶ *To prevent postoperative nausea and vomiting*

I.V. INJECTION

Adults and adolescents. 7 to 20 mcg/kg after procedure.

Children. 0.02 to 0.075 mg/kg after procedure.

DOSAGE ADJUSTMENT Initial dosage reduced for elderly patients because of increased risk of hypotension and excessive sedation.

Route	Onset	Peak	Duration
I.V.	3 to 10 min	30 min	2 to 4 hr

Mechanism of Action
Produces sedation by blocking postsynaptic dopamine receptors in the limbic system. Droperidol may reduce nausea by blocking dopamine receptors in the chemoreceptor trigger zone in the reticular formation of the medulla oblongata. It also may produce antiemetic effects by attaching to postsynaptic gamma-aminobutyric acid receptors in the chemoreceptor trigger zone.

Contraindications
Hypersensitivity to droperidol or its components

Interactions
DRUGS
amoxapine, haloperidol, loxapine, metoclopramide, metyrosine, molindone, olanzapine, phenothiazines, pimozide, rauwolfia alkaloids, risperidone, tacrine, thioxanthenes: Possibly increased risk of severe extrapyramidal reactions
anesthetics: Possibly hypotension and peripheral vasodilation
antihypertensives: Possibly orthostatic hypotension
bromocriptine, levodopa: Possibly inhibited actions of these drugs
CNS depressants: Additive CNS depression
epinephrine: Possibly paradoxical reduction of blood pressure
propofol: Possibly decreased antiemetic effect of both drugs
ACTIVITIES
alcohol use: Additive CNS depression

Adverse Reactions
CNS: Anxiety, drowsiness, dystonia, restlessness
CV: Hypertension, hypotension, sinus tachycardia
EENT: Fixed upward position of eyeballs, laryngospasm
MS: Spasms of tongue, face, neck, and back muscles
RESP: Bronchospasm

Nursing Considerations
- Monitor blood pressure frequently in patients with cardiac disease, who may not be able to compensate for droperidol's hypotensive effect.
- Assess patients with parkinsonism for worsening of condition, which may be an adverse effect of droperidol use.

- Monitor heart rate and ECG in patients with hypokalemia, hypomagnesemia, or preexisitng QT interval prolongation and in those with acute alcoholism because they're at increased risk for arrhythmias and, rarely, sudden death.
- Assess patients with pheochromocytoma for hypertension and tachycardia.
- Monitor patients with epilepsy, severe depression, parkinsonism, or impaired cardiovascular function for signs of exacerbation.
- Expect altered LOC to last for up to 12 hours after drug is given.
- If drug causes extrapyramidal reactions, such as restlessness, dystonia, and oculogyric crisis, expect to administer an anticholinergic, such as benztropine or diphenhydramine. Be sure to maintain a patent airway and oxygenation.
- If severe hypotension develops, expect to administer phenylephrine. If hypotension is related to hypovolemia, expect to administer fluids.
- Store drug at 15° to 30° C (59° to 86° F) and protect from light.

PATIENT TEACHING

- Instruct patient to ask for help with ambulation on first postoperative day because LOC may be altered for up to 12 hours.
- Caution patient to avoid drinking alcohol, taking CNS depressants, driving, and operating machinery for 24 hours after receiving droperidol.

E•F

eflornithine hydrochloride (alpha-difluoromethylornithine, DFMO)

Ornidyl

Class and Category

Chemical: Difluoromethylornithine
Therapeutic: Antiprotozoal
Pregnancy category: C

Indications and Dosages

▶ *To treat the meningoencephalitic stage of* Trypanosoma brucei gambiense *infection (sleeping sickness)*

I.V. INFUSION

Adults. 100 mg/kg given over at least 45 min q 6 hr for 14 days.

Route	Onset	Peak	Duration
I.V.	Unknown	4 to 6 hr	Unknown

Mechanism of Action

Inhibits the enzyme ornithine decarboxylase, which is needed for decarboxylation of ornithine. This process is the first step in polyamine synthesis, which is needed for protozoal cell division and differentiation.

Incompatibilities

Don't administer eflornithine with any other drug.

Contraindications

Hypersensitivity to eflornithine or its components

Interactions

DRUGS

other bone marrow depressants (such as chloramphenicol and doxorubicin): Possibly increased bone marrow depression
ototoxic drugs (such as aminoglycosides and NSAIDs): Increased risk of ototoxicity with long-term eflornithine therapy

Adverse Reactions

CNS: Asthenia, dizziness, headache, seizures
EENT: Hearing loss
GI: Abdominal pain, anorexia, diarrhea, vomiting
HEME: Anemia, eosinophilia, leukopenia, myelosuppression, thrombocytopenia
Other: Alopecia, facial edema

Nursing Considerations

- Monitor creatinine clearance of patients with impaired renal function, and plan to reduce eflornithine dosage, as prescribed, based on results.
- Before drug infusion, dilute eflornithine concentrate with sterile water for injection. Using strict aseptic technique, withdraw the contents of a 100-ml vial and inject 25 ml into each of four I.V. diluent bags that contain 100 ml of sterile water. The resulting solution contains 40 mg/ml of eflornithine (5,000 mg of eflornithine in 125 ml total volume).
- Store bags of diluted eflornithine at 4° C (39° F) to reduce the risk of contamination. Use diluted drug within 24 hours.
- Expect to monitor CBC, including platelet count, before treatment, twice weekly during treatment, and weekly after therapy stops until hematologic values return to baseline.
- Don't give other I.V. drugs while infusing eflornithine.
- Take infection-control and bleeding precautions because drug may cause myelosuppression. Adjust dosage or stop therapy as prescribed, based on severity.
- Take seizure precautions during therapy.
- Consult prescriber about the need for serial audiography, if appropriate, to detect hearing loss.
- Store undiluted vials at room temperature, and protect from freezing and light.

PATIENT TEACHING

- Stress the importance of keeping follow-up medical appointments because relapse may occur for up to 24 months after eflornithine treatment ends.
- Teach patient how to follow infection-control and bleeding precautions if myelosuppression occurs.
- Instruct patient to report adverse reactions to prescriber.
- Caution patient about the risk of seizures; advise him not to perform potentially hazardous activities during therapy.

enalaprilat

Vasotec I.V.

Class and Category

Chemical: Dicarbocyl-containing angiotensin-converting enzyme (ACE) inhibitor
Therapeutic: Antihypertensive
Pregnancy category: C (first trimester), D (later trimesters)

Indications and Dosages

▶ *To control hypertension*

I.V. INJECTION

Adults. 1.25 mg q 6 hr.

DOSAGE ADJUSTMENT Initial dose reduced to 0.625 mg for patients who have sodium and water depletion from diuretic therapy, are receiving diuretics, or have a creatinine clearance below 30 ml/min/1.73 m^2. If response is inadequate after 1 hr, 0.625 mg is repeated and therapy continued at 1.25 mg q 6 hr.

Route	Onset	Peak	Duration
I.V.	15 min	1 to 4 hr	About 6 hr

Mechanism of Action

May reduce blood pressure by affecting the renin-angiotensin-aldosterone system. By inhibiting ACE, enalaprilat:

- prevents conversion of angiotensin I to angiotensin II, a potent vasoconstrictor that also stimulates the adrenal cortex to secrete aldosterone
- may inhibit renal and vascular production of angiotensin II
- decreases the serum angiotensin II level and increases serum renin activity, thereby decreasing aldosterone secretion and slightly increasing the serum potassium level and fluid loss
- decreases vascular tone and blood pressure
- inhibits aldosterone release, which reduces sodium and water reabsorption and increases their excretion, further reducing blood pressure.

Contraindications

History of angioedema from previous ACE inhibitor therapy; hypersensitivity to enalapril, enalaprilat, or their components

Interactions

DRUGS

allopurinol, bone marrow depressants (such as amphotericin B and

methotrexate), procainamide, systemic corticosteroids: Possibly increased risk of fatal neutropenia or agranulocytosis
cyclosporine, potassium-sparing diuretics, potassium supplements: Increased risk of hyperkalemia
diuretics, other antihypertensives: Additive hypotensive effects
lithium: Increased blood lithium level and lithium toxicity
NSAIDs: Possibly reduced antihypertensive effects of enalapril and enalaprilat
sympathomimetics: Possibly reduced therapeutic effects of enalapril and enalaprilat
FOODS
potassium-containing salt substitutes: Increased risk of hyperkalemia
ACTIVITIES
alcohol use: Possibly additive hypotensive effect

Adverse Reactions

CNS: Ataxia, confusion, CVA, depression, dizziness, dream disturbances, fatigue, headache, insomnia, nervousness, peripheral neuropathy, somnolence, syncope, vertigo, weakness
CV: Angina, arrhythmias, cardiac arrest, hypotension, MI, orthostatic hypotension, palpitations, pulmonary embolism and infarction, Raynaud's phenomenon
EENT: Blurred vision, conjunctivitis, dry eyes and mouth, glossitis, hoarseness, lacrimation, loss of smell, pharyngitis, rhinorrhea, stomatitis, taste perversion, tinnitus
ENDO: Gynecomastia
GI: Abdominal pain, anorexia, constipation, diarrhea, hepatic failure, hepatitis, ileus, indigestion, melena, nausea, pancreatitis, vomiting
GU: Flank pain, impotence, oliguria, renal failure, UTI
MS: Muscle spasms
RESP: Asthma, bronchitis, bronchospasm, cough, dyspnea, pneumonia, pulmonary edema, pulmonary infiltrates, upper respiratory tract infection
SKIN: Alopecia, diaphoresis, erythema multiforme, exfoliative dermatitis, flushing, pemphigus, photosensitivity, pruritus, rash, Stevens-Johnson syndrome, toxic epidermal necrolysis, urticaria
Other: Anaphylaxis, angioedema, herpes zoster, hyperkalemia

Nursing Considerations

- Be aware that patients with impaired renal function may require a decreased dosage or less frequent doses of enalaprilat because of the risk of increased blood enalaprilat level and hyperkalemia. Monitor urinary protein level before and periodically during enalaprilat therapy.

- Administer enalaprilat undiluted, or dilute with up to 50 ml of D_5W, normal saline solution, dextrose 5% in normal saline solution, or dextrose 5% in lactated Ringer's solution. Use diluted enalaprilat within 24 hours if stored at room temperature. Administer each dose over at least 5 minutes.
- Measure blood pressure immediately after first dose and frequently for at least 2 hours thereafter. If hypotension requires a dosage reduction, monitor blood pressure frequently for 2 hours after reduced dose is administered and frequently for another hour after blood pressure has stabilized.
- Monitor blood pressure regularly during therapy. If patient develops hypotension, place him in supine position and expect to give I.V. normal saline solution or another volume expander, as prescribed.
- Monitor heart rate and rhythm. Expect to obtain repeated 12-lead ECG tracings.
- Monitor laboratory test results to check hepatic and renal function, leukocyte count, and serum potassium level.
- Monitor closely for angioedema of the face, lips, tongue, glottis, larynx, and limbs. If patient develops angioedema of the face and lips, stop drug and give an antihistamine, as prescribed, for symptoms. If tongue, glottis, or larynx is involved, assess for airway obstruction and prepare to give epinephrine 1:1,000 (0.3 to 0.5 ml) S.C. and maintain a patent airway.
- Closely assess for anaphylaxis in patients who receive dialysis with high-flux membranes, treatment with Hymenoptera venom, or LDL apheresis with dextran sulfate.
- Store drug between 15° and 30° C (59° and 86° F).

PATIENT TEACHING

- Inform patient that he may experience light-headedness and fainting, especially during first few days of enalaprilat therapy. Advise him to change position slowly and to avoid potentially hazardous activities until drug's CNS effects are known.
- Inform patient that diarrhea, excessive sweating, vomiting, and other conditions may cause dehydration, which can lead to dizziness, fainting, and very low blood pressure during therapy. Urge sufficient fluid intake to prevent dehydration and related adverse reactions. Instruct patient to report severe or prolonged diarrhea or vomiting.

- Urge patient to immediately report angioedema and other adverse reactions, including persistent dry cough.
- Advise patient to consult prescriber before using salt substitutes, potassium supplements, or other drugs (including OTC drugs) while receiving enalaprilat.

epinephrine (adrenaline)

Adrenalin, Ana-Guard

epinephrine hydrochloride

Adrenalin

Class and Category

Chemical: Catecholamine
Therapeutic: Antianaphylactic, bronchodilator, cardiac stimulant, vasopressor
Pregnancy category: C

Indications and Dosages

▶ *To treat anaphylaxis*

I.V. INFUSION

Adults and adolescents. 100 to 250 mcg given slowly.

▶ *To treat severe anaphylactic shock*

I.V. INFUSION

Adults. 1 mcg/min titrated to 2 to 10 mcg/min for desired hemodynamic response.

▶ *To treat cardiac arrest*

I.V. INJECTION

Adults. 0.5 to 1 mg q 3 to 5 min during resuscitation.
Children. 10 mcg/kg followed by 100 mcg/kg q 3 to 5 min, if needed. If two doses produce no response, subsequent doses are increased to 200 mcg/kg q 5 min.
Neonates. 10 to 30 mcg/kg q 3 to 5 min.

Route	Onset	Peak	Duration
I.V.	Rapid	Unknown	1 to 2 min

Incompatibilities

Don't mix epinephrine with alkalies or oxidizing agents, including bromine, chlorine, chromates, iodine, metal salts (as from iron), nitrites, oxygen, and permanganates, because these substances can destroy epinephrine.

Mechanism of Action

Acts on alpha and beta receptors. This nonselective adrenergic agonist stimulates:

- $alpha_1$ receptors, which constricts arteries and may decrease bronchial secretions.
- presynaptic $alpha_2$ receptors, which inhibits norepinephrine release by way of negative feedback.
- postsynaptic $alpha_2$ receptors, which constricts arteries.
- $beta_1$ receptors, which induces positive chronotropic and inotropic responses.
- $beta_2$ receptors, which dilates arteries, relaxes bronchial smooth muscles, increases glycogenolysis, and prevents mast cells from secreting histamine and other substances, thus reversing bronchoconstriction and edema.

Contraindications

Cerebral arteriosclerosis, coronary insufficiency, counteraction of phenothiazine-induced hypotension, dilated cardiomyopathy, general anesthesia with halogenated hydrocarbons or cyclopropane, hypersensitivity to epinephrine or its components, labor, angle-closure glaucoma, organic brain damage, shock (nonanaphylactic)

Interactions

DRUGS

alpha-adrenergic blockers, drugs with alpha-adrenergic action, rapid-acting vasodilators: Blockage of epinephrine's alpha-adrenergic effect, possibly causing severe hypotension and tachycardia
amyl nitrite, nitrates: Decreased antianginal effects
antihypertensives, diuretics used to treat hypertension: Decreased antihypertensive effects
beta blockers: Mutual inhibition of therapeutic effects, possibly severe hypertension and cerebral hemorrhage
digoxin, quinidine: Increased risk of arrhythmias
dihydroergotamine, ergoloid mesylates, ergonovine, ergotamine, methylergonovine, methysergide, oxytocin: Increased risk of vasoconstriction, causing gangrene, peripheral vascular ischemia, or severe hypertension
hydrocarbon inhalation anesthetics: Increased risk of severe atrial and ventricular arrhythmias
insulin, oral antidiabetic drugs: Decreased effects of these drugs
MAO inhibitors: Possibly increased vasopressor effect of epinephrine and hypertensive crisis

maprotiline, tricyclic antidepressants: Potentiated cardiovascular effects of epinephrine, possibly causing arrhythmias, hyperpyrexia, severe hypertension, or tachycardia
sympathomimetics: Additive CNS stimulation, increased cardiovascular effects of either drug
thyroid hormones: Increased effects of either drug
xanthines: Increased CNS stimulation, additive toxic effects

Adverse Reactions

CNS: Anxiety, chills, fever, dizziness, drowsiness, hallucinations, headache, insomnia, light-headedness, nervousness, restlessness, seizures, tremor, weakness
CV: Chest discomfort or pain; fast, irregular, or slow heartbeat; palpitations; severe hypertension
EENT: Blurred vision, dry mouth or throat, miosis
GI: Anorexia, heartburn, nausea, vomiting
GU: Dysuria
MS: Muscle twitching, severe muscle spasms
RESP: Dyspnea
SKIN: Cold skin, diaphoresis, ecchymosis, flushed or red face or skin, pallor, tissue necrosis
Other: Hyperkalemia, hypokalemia, injection site pain or stinging

Nursing Considerations

- Use epinephrine with extreme caution in patients with angina, arrhythmias, asthma, degenerative heart disease, or emphysema. Epinephrine's inotropic effect equals that of dopamine and dobutamine; its chronotropic effect exceeds that of both.
- Use drug cautiously in elderly patients and those with cardiovascular disease (other than listed above), diabetes mellitus, hypertension, hyperthyroidism, prostatic hypertrophy, and psychoneurologic disorders.
- Be aware that some preparations contain sulfites, which may cause allergic-type reactions. However, the presence of sulfites in epinephrine should not deter its use in a patient with anaphylaxis, even if patient is sensitive to sulfites. Monitor patient closely for adverse effects.
- Dilute the 1:1,000 (1-mg/ml) solution of parenteral epinephrine before I.V. administration.
- Shake suspension thoroughly before withdrawing dose; refrigerate it between uses.
- Inspect epinephrine solution or suspension before use. If it's pink or brown, air has entered a multidose vial. If it's discolored

or contains particles, discard it. Also discard unused portions of parenteral epinephrine.
- When injecting drug, rotate sites because repeated injections in the same site may cause vasoconstriction and localized necrosis.
- Be aware that drug shouldn't be given by intra-arterial injection because marked vasoconstriction may cause gangrene.
- Monitor for potassium imbalances. Initially, hyperkalemia occurs when hepatocytes release potassium. Hypokalemia may quickly follow as skeletal muscles take up potassium.
- To minimize insomnia, give last dose a few hours before bedtime.
- **WARNING** To treat cardiac arrest, at least twice the peripheral I.V. dose of epinephrine may be given by endotracheal instillation. Two dilutions are needed for this regimen; use great caution to avoid medication errors.

PATIENT TEACHING
- Advise patient to notify prescriber if symptoms don't improve or if they improve but then worsen.
- Advise patient to notify prescriber immediately if he experiences blurred vision, chest pain, difficulty breathing, a fast or irregular heartbeat, or increased sweating.

epoetin alfa
(EPO, erythropoietin alfa, recombinant erythropoietin, r-HuEPO)

Epogen, Eprex (CAN), Procrit

Class and Category

Chemical: 165–amino acid glycoprotein identical to human erythropoietin
Therapeutic: Antianemic
Pregnancy category: C

Indications and Dosages

▶ *To treat anemia from renal failure*

I.V. INJECTION

Adults and adolescents. *Initial:* 50 to 100 units/kg 3 times/wk, increased by 25 units/kg after 8 wk if hematocrit hasn't risen by 5 or 6 points or is below desired range (30% to 36%). *Maintenance:* Dosage gradually decreased by 25 units/kg q 4 wk or more to lowest dose that keeps hematocrit at 30% to 36%. *Maximum:* 300 units/kg 3 times/wk.

Children on dialysis. 50 units/kg 3 times/wk; increased after 8 wk if hematocrit hasn't risen by 5 or 6 points and is still below desired range of 30% to 36%. *Maintenance:* Dosage gradually decreased to lowest dose that keeps hematocrit at 30% to 36%.

▶ *To treat anemia in HIV-infected patients who take zidovudine*

I.V. INJECTION

Adults with serum erythropoietin level of 500 mU/ml or less who receive 4,200 mg or less of zidovudine/wk. *Initial:* 100 units/kg 3 times/wk, increased by 50 to 100 units/kg q 4 to 8 wk after 8 wk of therapy. *Maintenance:* Dosage gradually titrated to maintain desired response, based on such factors as variations in zidovudine dosage and occurrence of infection or inflammation. *Maximum:* 300 units/kg 3 times/wk.

Route	Onset	Peak	Duration
I.V., S.C.	In 2 to 6 wk	In 2 mo	About 2 wk

Mechanism of Action

Stimulates the release of reticulocytes from the bone marrow into the bloodstream, where they develop into mature RBCs.

Incompatibilities

Don't mix epoetin alfa with any other drug.

Contraindications

Hypersensitivity to human albumin or products made from mammal cells, uncontrolled hypertension

Interactions

DRUGS

antihypertensives: Increased blood pressure (to hypertensive level), especially when hematocrit rises rapidly
heparin: Increased heparin requirement in hemodialysis patients
iron supplements: Increased iron requirement and need for increased dose

Adverse Reactions

CNS: Anxiety, asthenia, CVA, dizziness, fatigue, fever, headache, insomnia, paresthesia, seizures
CV: Chest pain, deep vein thrombosis, edema, hypertension, MI, tachycardia
GI: Constipation, diarrhea, indigestion, nausea, vomiting
GU: UTI

HEME: Polycythemia
MS: Arthralgia, bone pain, muscle weakness
RESP: Cough, dyspnea, pulmonary congestion, upper respiratory tract infection
SKIN: Rash, pruritus, urticaria
Other: Flulike symptoms, hyperkalemia, injection site reaction, trunk pain

Nursing Considerations

- Use epoetin alfa cautiously in patients who have conditions that could decrease or delay response to drug, such as aluminum intoxication, folic acid deficiency, hemolysis, infection, inflammation, iron deficiency, malignant neoplasm, osteitis (fibrosa cystica), or vitamin B_{12} deficiency.
- Also use drug cautiously in patients with cardiovascular disorders caused by hypertension, a history of seizures, vascular disease, or a hematologic disorder, such as hypercoagulation, myelodysplastic syndrome, or sickle cell disease.
- **WARNING** Be aware that the multidose vial of epoetin contains benzyl alcohol, which can cause a fatal toxic syndrome in neonates and immature infants characterized by CNS, respiratory, circulatory, and renal impairment and metabolic acidosis.
- Don't shake vial during preparation to avoid denaturing glycoprotein and inactivating epoetin alfa.
- Discard unused portion of single-dose vial because it contains no preservatives. Discard unused portion of multidose vial after 21 days.
- Be aware that baseline hemoglobin level should be above 10 but below 13 g/dl if drug is given to patient scheduled for surgery.
- Expect to increase heparin dose if patient receives hemodialysis because epoetin alfa can increase the RBC volume, which could cause clots to form in the dialyzer, hemodialysis vascular access, or both.
- Expect to give an iron supplement (I.V. iron dextran, if needed) because iron requirements rise when erythropoiesis consumes existing iron stores.
- Monitor drug effectiveness by checking hematocrit, typically twice weekly until it stabilizes at 30% to 36%. After that, monitoring can be less frequent.
- Take seizure precautions.

- Be aware that the risk of hypertensive or thrombotic complications increases if the hematocrit rises more than 4 points in 2 weeks.

PATIENT TEACHING

- Advise patient that the risk of seizures is highest during the first 90 days of epoetin alfa therapy. Urge him not to engage in hazardous activities during this time.
- Stress the need to comply with dosage regimen and keep follow-up medical and laboratory appointments.
- Encourage patient to eat iron-rich foods.
- Review possible adverse reactions, and urge patient to notify prescriber if he experiences chest pain, headache, hives, rapid heartbeat, rash, seizures, shortness of breath, or swelling.

epoprostenol sodium (PGI$_2$, PGX, prostacyclin)

Flolan

Class and Category

Chemical: Natural prostaglandin
Therapeutic: Antihypertensive, vasodilator
Pregnancy category: B

Indications and Dosages

▶ *To provide long-term treatment of primary pulmonary hypertension and pulmonary hypertension secondary to scleroderma spectrum of diseases*

I.V. INFUSION

Adults. *Initial:* 2 nanograms/kg/min, increased by 2 nanograms/kg/min q 15 min or longer until dose-limiting adverse reactions (such as abdominal, chest, or musculoskeletal pain; anxiety; bradycardia; dizziness; dyspnea; flushing; headache; hypotension; nausea; tachycardia; and vomiting) occur. *Maintenance:* Dosage started at 4 nanograms/kg/min less than maximum rate tolerated during initial titration. If maximum rate tolerated was less than 5 nanograms/kg/min, long-term infusion rate is started at 50% of maximum rate.

DOSAGE ADJUSTMENT Continuous infusion rate adjusted based on persistence, recurrence, or worsening of primary pulmonary hypertension and dose-related adverse reactions.

Incompatibilities

Don't mix epoprostenol with other parenteral solutions or drugs.

Mechanism of Action

Acts as a natural prostaglandin to directly relax vascular smooth muscles, resulting in arterial dilation and inhibition of platelet aggregation. These actions decrease pulmonary vascular resistance, increase cardiac index and oxygen delivery, and limit thrombus formation.

Contraindications

Hypersensitivity to epoprostenol or its components; long-term use in patients with heart failure caused by severe left ventricular systolic dysfunction; pulmonary edema that developed while establishing epoprostenol dosage

Interactions

DRUGS

anticoagulants, antiplatelet drugs, NSAIDs: Increased risk of bleeding
antihypertensives, diuretics, vasodilators: Decreased blood pressure
digoxin: Possibly increased digoxin bioavailability

Adverse Reactions

CNS: Anxiety, chills, confusion, dizziness, fever, headache, nervousness, paresthesia, syncope, weakness
CV: Bradycardia, chest pain, hypotension, tachycardia
GI: Abdominal pain, diarrhea, nausea, vomiting
HEME: Thrombocytopenia
MS: Arthralgia, jaw pain, myalgia
RESP: Dyspnea, hypoxia
SKIN: Flushing
Other: Flulike symptoms, injection site infection and pain, sepsis, weight gain or loss

Nursing Considerations

- Reconstitute epoprostenol only with sterile diluent that comes in package. Don't dilute reconstituted epoprostenol.
- To make 100 ml of reconstituted solution at 3,000 nanograms/ml, dissolve contents of 0.5-mg vial with 5 ml of diluent; withdraw 3 ml and add enough diluent to make 100 ml. To make 100 ml of solution at 5,000 nanograms/ml, dissolve contents of 0.5-mg vial with 5 ml of diluent; withdraw contents and add enough diluent to make 100 ml. To make 100 ml of solution at 10,000 nanograms/ml, dissolve contents of two 0.5-mg vials each with 5 ml of diluent; withdraw contents and add enough diluent to make 100 ml. To make 100 ml of solution at

15,000 nanograms/ml, dissolve contents of 1.5-mg vial with 5 ml of diluent; withdraw contents and add enough diluent to make 100 ml.

- Give continuous infusion through a central venous catheter. Use peripheral I.V. route only until central access is established.
- Use an ambulatory infusion pump that is small, lightweight, and able to deliver 2 nanograms/kg/minute. It should have alarms for occlusion, end of infusion, and low battery. Use a polyvinyl chloride, polypropylene, or glass reservoir. Keep a backup pump and infusion set nearby to minimize disruptions in delivery.
- Administer a single container of reconstituted solution at room temperature over 8 hours. For extended use at temperatures above 25° C (77° F), use a cold pouch with frozen gel packs to keep drug at 2° to 8°C (36° to 46° F) for 12 hours. Don't expose to direct sunlight.
- After a new infusion rate has been established, monitor closely for adverse reactions. Measure blood pressure each time with patient standing and supine. Also, monitor heart rate for several hours after dosage adjustment. Assess for signs of pulmonary edema, such as dyspnea, anxiety, and hemoptysis, which may be associated with veno-occlusive disease.
- During prolonged infusion, watch for dose-related adverse reactions. If they occur, expect to decrease infusion rate by 2 nanograms/kg/minute every 15 minutes, as prescribed, until adverse reactions resolve.
- **WARNING** Avoid abrupt withdrawal or a sudden large reduction in infusion rate, which could cause rebound pulmonary hypertension (asthenia, dizziness, dyspnea) or death.
- Expect lower dosage to be ordered for elderly patients, especially those with hepatic, renal, or cardiac impairment or other diseases and those who may receive other drugs that can interact with epoprostenol.
- Protect reconstituted drug from light, and refrigerate for no longer than 48 hours. Discard solution that has been frozen or that has been refrigerated for longer than 48 hours.
- Before reconstituting epoprostenol, store it and diluent at 15° to 25° C (59° to 77° F); protect from freezing and light.

PATIENT TEACHING

- Inform patient that epoprostenol is infused continuously through a permanent indwelling central venous catheter by a small infusion pump.

- Stress that patient must commit to long-term therapy, possibly for years.
- Teach patient or caregiver how to reconstitute drug, administer it, and care for the permanent central venous catheter.
- Urge patient to maintain prescribed infusion rate and to consult prescriber before altering it.
- Caution patient that even brief interruptions in drug delivery may cause rapid worsening of symptoms.
- Instruct patient to notify prescriber if adverse reactions occur. Stress the importance of keeping follow-up appointments to assess for adverse reactions and evaluate his response to therapy.
- Make sure patient or caregiver has ready access to emergency phone numbers. Advise patient to carry medical identification documenting his use of epoprostenol and its purpose.
- Caution patient to avoid saunas, hot baths, and sunbathing, which can increase the risk of hypertension.

eptifibatide

Integrilin

Class and Category

Chemical: Cyclic heptapeptide
Therapeutic: Platelet aggregation inhibitor
Pregnancy category: B

Indications and Dosages

▶ *To treat unstable angina and non–Q-wave MI*

I.V. INFUSION

Adults. *Initial:* 180 mcg/kg over 1 to 2 min as soon as possible after diagnosis. *Maintenance:* 2 mcg/kg/min by continuous infusion beginning immediately after initial dose and continuing until discharge or coronary artery bypass grafting, up to 72 hr.

DOSAGE ADJUSTMENT For patients with serum creatinine level of 2 to 4 mg/dl, initial dosage reduced to 135 mcg/kg over 1 to 2 min and maintenance dosage to 0.5 mcg/kg/min by continuous infusion. Drug discontinued before coronary artery bypass graft surgery or if platelet count falls below 100,000/mm^3.

▶ *To prevent thrombosis related to percutaneous transluminal coronary angioplasty (PTCA)*

I.V. INFUSION

Adults. *Initial:* 135 mcg/kg over 1 to 2 min immediately before procedure. *Maintenance:* 0.5 mcg/kg/min by continuous infusion beginning immediately after initial dose and continuing for 20 to 24 hr. *Maximum:* 96 hr of therapy.

Route	Onset	Peak	Duration
I.V.	Immediate	In 15 min	4 to 8 hr

Mechanism of Action

Reversibly inhibits platelet aggregation by preventing the binding of fibrinogen, von Willebrand factor, and other adhesive ligands to the platelet receptor glycoprotein IIb/IIIa on activated platelets. Thus, eptifibatide disrupts the final cross-linking stage of platelet aggregation—and thrombus formation.

Incompatibilities

Don't administer eptifibatide through the same I.V. line as furosemide.

Contraindications

Active bleeding or CVA during previous 30 days, bleeding diathesis, dependence on dialysis, history of hemorrhagic CVA, hypersensitivity to eptifibatide, major surgery during previous 4 weeks, serum creatinine level of 2 mg/dl or higher for 180-mcg/kg dose or 2-mcg/kg/min infusion, serum creatinine level of 4 mg/dl or higher for 135-mcg/kg dose or 0.5-mcg/kg/min infusion, severe uncontrolled hypertension (systolic pressure above 200 mm Hg, diastolic pressure above 110 mm Hg), thrombocytopenia (platelet count below 100,000/mm^3)

Interactions

DRUGS

anticoagulants, clopidogrel, dipyridamole, NSAIDs, thrombolytics, ticlopidine: Additive pharmacologic effects, increased risk of bleeding
other platelet aggregation inhibitors (especially inhibitors of platelet receptor glycoprotein IIb/IIIa, such as abciximab): Increased risk of additive pharmacologic effects

Adverse Reactions

CNS: Intracranial hemorrhage
CV: Hypotension
GI: Hematemesis
GU: Hematuria
HEME: Bleeding, decreased hemoglobin level, thrombocytopenia
Other: Anaphylaxis

Nursing Considerations

- Expect to obtain hematocrit, platelet count, and hemoglobin and serum creatinine levels before starting eptifibatide therapy to detect abnormalities. Also expect to obtain baseline APTT and PT.
- Withdraw bolus dose of eptifibatide from a 10-ml (2-mg/ml) vial into a syringe.
- Using a vented I.V. infusion set, administer a continuous infusion directly from the 100-ml (0.75 mg/ml) vial. Be sure to center the spike in the circle on top of the vial stopper.
- Be aware that eptifibatide may be administered in same I.V. line as normal saline solution or dextrose 5% in normal saline solution containing potassium at a concentration of 60 mEq/L. It also may be administered in same I.V. line as alteplase, atropine, dobutamine, heparin, lidocaine, meperidine, metoprolol, midazolam, morphine, nitroglycerin, or verapamil.
- Expect to keep APTT at 50 to 70 seconds or according to facility protocol during therapy unless patient undergoes PTCA.
- If patient undergoes PTCA, expect to maintain his activated clotting time between 300 and 350 seconds during the procedure.
- During therapy, avoid arterial and venous punctures, I.M. injections, urinary catheter use, nasotracheal or nasogastric intubation, and use of noncompressible I.V. sites, such as subclavian and jugular veins.
- Expect to discontinue eptifibatide and heparin and monitor patient closely if platelet count falls below 100,000/mm^3.
- Plan to discontinue drug, as prescribed, if patient undergoes coronary artery bypass surgery.

PATIENT TEACHING

- Instruct patient to immediately report bleeding during eptifibatide therapy.
- Reassure patient that he'll be monitored closely during therapy.
- Advise patient to avoid activities that may lead to bruising and bleeding.

erythromycin gluceptate

(contains 500 or 1,000 mg of base per vial)

Ilotycin

erythromycin lactobionate

(contains 500 or 1,000 mg of base per vial)

Erythrocin

Class and Category

Chemical: Macrolide
Therapeutic: Antiacne agent, antibiotic
Pregnancy category: B

Indications and Dosages

▶ *To treat mild to moderate upper respiratory tract infections caused by* Haemophilus influenzae, Streptococcus pneumoniae, *or* Streptococcus pyogenes *(group A beta-hemolytic streptococcus)*

I.V. INFUSION

Adults. 250 to 500 mg (base) q 6 hr for 10 days.

Children. 250 to 500 mg (base) q.i.d. or 20 to 50 mg (base)/kg daily in divided doses for 10 days. For *H. influenzae* infections, erythromycin ethylsuccinate is administered with sulfisoxazole 150 mg/kg daily. *Maximum:* Adult dosage, or 6 g daily for erythromycin ethylsuccinate.

▶ *To treat lower respiratory tract infections caused by* S. pneumoniae *or* S. pyogenes *(group A beta-hemolytic streptococcus)*

I.V. INFUSION

Adults. 250 to 500 mg (base) q 6 hr for 10 days.

Children. 250 to 500 mg (base) q.i.d. or 20 to 50 mg (base)/kg daily in divided doses for 10 days. *Maximum:* Adult dosage.

▶ *To treat respiratory tract infections caused by* Mycoplasma pneumoniae

I.V. INFUSION

Adults. 500 mg (base) q 6 hr for 5 to 10 days or up to 3 wk for severe infections.

▶ *To treat mild to moderate skin and soft-tissue infections caused by* S. pyogenes *or* Staphylococcus aureus

I.V. INFUSION

Adults. 250 mg (base) q 6 hr or 500 mg (base) q 12 hr for 10 days. *Maximum:* 4 g (base) daily.

Children. 250 to 500 mg (base) q.i.d. or 20 to 50 mg (base)/kg daily in divided doses for 10 days. *Maximum:* Adult dosage.

▶ *To treat pertussis (whooping cough) caused by* Bordetella pertussis

I.V. INFUSION

Children. 500 mg (base) q.i.d. or 40 to 50 mg (base)/kg daily in divided doses for 5 to 14 days.

▶ *To treat diphtheria*

I.V. INFUSION

Adults and children. 500 mg (base) q 6 hr for 10 days.

▶ *To treat erythrasma*
I.V. INFUSION
Adults and children. 250 mg (base) t.i.d. for 21 days.
▶ *To treat intestinal amebiasis*
I.V. INFUSION
Adults. 250 mg (base) q 6 hr for 10 to 14 days.
Children. 30 to 50 mg (base)/kg daily in divided doses for 10 to 14 days
▶ *To treat pelvic inflammatory disease caused by* Neisseria gonorrhoeae
I.V. INFUSION
Adults. 500 mg (base) I.V. q 6 hr for 3 days and then 250 mg (base) P.O. or I.V. q 6 hr for 7 days.
▶ *To treat conjunctivitis in newborns*
I.V. INFUSION
Neonates. 50 mg (base)/kg daily in four divided doses for 14 days.
▶ *To treat pneumonia in neonates*
I.V. INFUSION
Neonates. 50 mg (base)/kg daily in divided doses for 21 days.
▶ *To treat Legionnaire's disease*
I.V. INFUSION
Adults. 1 to 4 g (base) daily in divided doses for 10 to 14 days.
▶ *To treat rheumatic fever*
I.V. INFUSION
Adults. 250 mg (base) q 12 hr.
▶ *To prevent bacterial endocarditis in patients with penicillin allergy who plan dental or upper respiratory tract surgery*
I.V. INFUSION
Adults. 1 g (base) given 1 to 2 hr before procedure and then 500 mg (base) 6 hr after initial dose.
Children. 20 mg (base)/kg given 2 hr before procedure and then 10 mg (base)/kg 6 hr after initial dose.
▶ *To treat listeriosis*
I.V. INFUSION
Adults. 250 mg (base) q 6 hr or 500 mg (base) q 12 hr. *Maximum:* 4 g (base) daily.

Contraindications
Astemizole, cisapride, pimozide, or terfenadine therapy; hypersensitivity to erythromycin, macrolide antibiotics, or their components

Mechanism of Action

Binds with the 50S ribosomal subunit of the 70S ribosome in many types of aerobic, anaerobic, gram-positive, and gram-negative bacteria. This action inhibits RNA-dependent protein synthesis in bacterial cells, causing them to die.

Interactions

DRUGS

alfentanil: Decreased alfentanil clearance, prolonged alfentanil action
astemizole, cisapride, terfenadine: Increased risk of cardiotoxicity, torsades de pointes, ventricular tachycardia, and death
atorvastatin, lovastatin, pravastatin, simvastatin: Increased risk of rhabdomyolysis
carbamazepine, valproic acid: Possibly inhibited metabolism of these drugs, increasing their blood levels and risk of toxicity
chloramphenicol, lincomycins: Antagonized effects of these drugs
cyclosporine: Increased risk of nephrotoxicity
digoxin: Increased serum digoxin level and risk of digitalis toxicity
diltiazem, verapamil: Increased risk of life-threatening cardiac events
ergotamine: Decreased ergotamine metabolism, increased risk of vasospasm from ergotamine use
hepatotoxic drugs: Increased risk of hepatotoxicity
midazolam, triazolam: Increased pharmacologic effects of these drugs
oral contraceptives: Failed contraception, hepatotoxicity
ototoxic drugs: Increased risk of ototoxicity if patient with impaired renal function receives high doses of erythromycin
penicillins: Interference with bactericidal effects of penicillins
sildenafil: Increased effects of sildenafil
warfarin: Prolonged PT and risk of hemorrhage, especially in elderly patients
xanthines (except dyphylline): Increased serum theophylline level and risk of theophylline toxicity

ACTIVITIES

alcohol use: Increased alcohol level (by 40%) with I.V. erythromycin

Adverse Reactions

CNS: Fatigue, fever, malaise, weakness

CV: Prolonged QT interval, torsades de pointes, ventricular arrhythmias
EENT: Hearing loss, oral candidiasis
GI: Abdominal cramps and pain, diarrhea, hepatotoxicity, nausea, vomiting
GU: Vaginal candidiasis
SKIN: Erythema, jaundice, pruritus, rash
Other: Fluid overload (from I.V. infusion), injection site inflammation and phlebitis

Nursing Considerations

- Use erythromycin cautiously in patients with impaired hepatic function because drug is metabolized by the liver.
- Before administering the first erythromycin dose, expect to obtain body fluid or tissue sample for culture and sensitivity testing.
- Reconstitute parenteral form before administration. Add at least 10 ml of preservative-free sterile water for injection to each 500-mg vial or at least 20 ml of diluent to each 1-g vial.
- For prolonged infusion, expect to infuse a buffered solution up to 24 hours after dilution.
- For intermittent infusion, dilute the dose if needed in 100 to 250 ml of normal saline solution or D_5W and administer slowly over 20 to 60 minutes.
- When giving I.V. erythromycin gluceptate, dilute the solution if needed to 1 g/L in normal saline solution or D_5W injection for slow, continuous infusion. Diluted solution remains potent for 7 days if refrigerated.
- When giving I.V. erythromycin lactobionate, dilute the solution if needed to 1 to 5 mg/ml in normal saline, lactated Ringer's, or other electrolyte solution for slow, continuous infusion. Diluted solution remains potent for 14 days if refrigerated and for 24 hours at room temperature.
- Be aware that infusions prepared in piggyback infusion bottles remain potent for 30 days if frozen, 24 hours if refrigerated, or 8 hours at room temperature. Don't store infusions prepared in the ADD-vantage system.
- Don't use diluent with benzyl alcohol if parenteral erythromycin is for a neonate. It may cause a fatal toxic syndrome of CNS depression, hypotension, metabolic acidosis, renal failure, respiratory problems, and, possibly, seizures and intracranial hemorrhage.

- Periodically monitor liver function test results to detect hepatotoxicity, which is most common with erythromycin estolate. Signs typically appear within 2 weeks after continuous therapy starts and resolve when it stops.
- Assess hearing regularly, especially in elderly patients and those who receive 4 g or more daily or have hepatic or renal disease. Hearing impairment begins 36 hours to 8 days after treatment starts and usually begins to improve 1 to 14 days after treatment stops.
- During I.V. therapy, watch for signs of fluid overload, such as acute dyspnea and crackles.
- Monitor infants for vomiting or irritability with feeding because infantile hypertrophic pyloric stenosis has been reported.
- Monitor myasthenia gravis patients for weakness because drug may aggravate it.
- Monitor patient closely for signs and symptoms of superinfection. If they occur, notify prescriber and expect to stop drug and provide appropriate therapy.
- If patient receives an order for urine catecholamine analysis, notify prescriber; erythromycin interferes with fluorometric measurement of urine catecholamines.

PATIENT TEACHING

- Instruct patient to promptly notify prescriber about allergic reactions, hearing changes, or signs of hepatic dysfunction.

esmolol hydrochloride

Brevibloc

Class and Category

Chemical: Beta blocker
Therapeutic: Antiarrhythmic, antihypertensive
Pregnancy category: C

Indications and Dosages

▶ *To treat supraventricular tachycardia*

I.V. INFUSION

Adults. *Loading:* 500 mcg/kg over 1 min. *Maintenance:* If response to loading dose is adequate after 5 min, 50 mcg/kg/min infused for 4 min. If response is inadequate after 5 min, another 500 mcg/kg may be given over 1 min, followed by 100 mcg/kg/min for 4 min. Sequence repeated, as needed, until adequate response occurs, increasing maintenance dosage by 50 mcg/kg/min at each step. *Maximum:* 200 mcg/kg/min for 48 hr.

Children. 50 mcg/kg/min, titrated q 10 min up to 300 mcg/kg/min.

▶ *To treat intraoperative and postoperative tachycardia and hypertension*

I.V. INFUSION

Adults. *Initial:* 250 to 500 mcg/kg over 1 min. *Maintenance:* 50 mcg/kg/min infused over 4 min. If response is inadequate after 5 min, another 250 to 500 mcg/kg may be given over 1 min, followed by 100 mcg/kg/min for 4 min. Sequence repeated, as needed, up to 4 times, increasing by 50 mcg/kg/min each time. *Maximum:* 200 mcg/kg/min for 48 hr.

DOSAGE ADJUSTMENT Subsequent loading doses omitted, increments decreased to 25 mcg/kg/min, and titration intervals increased to 10 min as heart rate approaches desired level or if blood pressure decreases too much.

Route	Onset	Peak	Duration
I.V.	Immediate	Unknown	10 to 20 min

Mechanism of Action

Inhibits stimulation of $beta_1$ receptors primarily in the heart, which decreases cardiac excitability, cardiac output, and myocardial oxygen demand. Esmolol also decreases renin release from the kidneys, which helps reduce blood pressure.

Incompatibilities

Don't mix esmolol with 5% sodium bicarbonate injection.

Contraindications

Cardiogenic shock, hypersensitivity to beta blockers, overt heart failure, second- or third-degree heart block, sinus bradycardia

Interactions

DRUGS

antihypertensives: Possibly hypotension

digoxin: Increased blood digoxin level

insulin, oral antidiabetic drugs: Possibly masking of signs and symptoms of hypoglycemia caused by these drugs

MAO inhibitors: Possibly severe hypertension if esmolol is administered within 14 days of discontinuing MAO inhibitor therapy

neuromuscular blockers: Possibly potentiated and prolonged action of these drugs

phenytoin: Possibly increased cardiac depression
reserpine and other catecholamine-depleting drugs: Possibly bradycardia and hypotension
sympathomimetics, xanthine derivatives: Possibly inhibited therapeutic effects of both drugs, decreased theophylline clearance

Adverse Reactions

CNS: Anxiety, confusion, depression, dizziness, drowsiness, fatigue, fever, headache, syncope
CV: Bradycardia, chest pain, decreased peripheral circulation, heart block, hypotension
GI: Nausea, vomiting
RESP: Dyspnea, wheezing
SKIN: Diaphoresis, flushing, pallor
Other: Infusion site pain, redness, and swelling

Nursing Considerations

- Be aware that esmolol is not administered for intraoperative or postoperative hypertension that results mainly from vasoconstriction caused by hypothermia.
- Expect to give lowest possible dose to patients with allergies, asthma, bronchitis, or emphysema. If bronchospasm occurs, expect to discontinue infusion immediately and give a $beta_2$-stimulating drug, as ordered.
- **WARNING** Examine esmolol label closely to make sure you're using correct concentration; concentrations of 10 mg/ml (100 mg/10-ml vial) and 250 mg/ml (2,500 mg/10-ml vial) are available. The 250-mg/ml concentration is not for direct I.V. injection.
- Before administering esmolol, inspect it for particles or discoloration.
- Don't give 250-mg/ml (2,500-mg/10 ml) concentration by direct I.V. push. Dilute it to a 10-mg/ml infusion by first removing 20 ml from 500 ml of a compatible I.V. solution, such as D_5W or dextrose 5% in normal saline solution, and then adding 5 g of esmolol to the solution.
- Use diluted solution within 24 hours if stored at room temperature.
- Use a 100-mg vial (prediluted to 10 mg/ml) to give loading dose. For a 70-kg (154-lb) patient, loading dose for 500 mcg/kg/minute would be 3.5 ml.
- Monitor blood pressure and heart rate frequently during therapy. Keep in mind that hypotension can occur at any dose but

usually is dose-related. Hypotension typically reverses within 30 minutes after dose is decreased or infusion is stopped.
- Monitor patient for signs of increased adverse reactions in patients with supraventricular arrhythmias, decreased cardiac output, hypotension, or other symptoms of hemodynamic compromise and in those who are taking drugs that decrease peripheral resistance or myocardial filling, contractility, or impulse generation.
- Also monitor for signs of increased adverse reactions in patients with impaired renal function, especially those with end-stage renal disease, because drug is excreted by the kidneys.
- Inspect infusion site regularly for evidence of thrombophlebitis (pain, redness, or swelling at site). Infusions of 20-mg/ml concentration are more likely to cause serious vein irritation than those of 10-mg/ml concentration. Extravasation of 20-mg/ml concentration may cause a serious local reaction and, possibly, skin necrosis. Don't infuse more than 10 mg/ml into a small vein or through a butterfly catheter.
- Before diluting drug, store it at 15° to 30° C (59° to 86° F). Avoid elevated temperatures.

PATIENT TEACHING
- Urge patient receiving esmolol to report adverse reactions immediately.
- Reassure patient that his blood pressure, heart rate, and response to therapy will be monitored throughout esmolol therapy.

esomeprazole magnesium
Nexium I.V.

Class and Category
Chemical: Substituted benzimidazole
Therapeutic: Antiulcer agent
Pregnancy category: B

Indications and Dosages
▶ *To treat gastroesophageal reflux disease in a patient with a history of erosive esophagitis who can't take the drug by mouth*

I.V. INFUSION, I.V. INJECTION

Adults. 20 or 40 mg daily infused for at least 3 min (I.V. injection) or 10 to 30 min (I.V. infusion).

DOSAGE ADJUSTMENT Maximum, 20 mg daily for patients with severe hepatic insufficiency.

Mechanism of Action

Interferes with gastric acid secretion by inhibiting the hydrogen-potassium-adenosine triphosphatase (H^+-K^+-ATPase) enzyme system, or proton pump, in gastric parietal cells. Normally, the proton pump uses energy from the hydrolysis of ATPase to drive H^+ and chloride (Cl^-) out of parietal cells and into the stomach lumen in exchange for potassium (K^+), which leaves the stomach lumen and enters parietal cells. After this exchange, H^+ and Cl^- combine in the stomach to form hydrochloric acid (HCl). Esomeprazole irreversibly inhibits the final step in gastric acid production by blocking the exchange of intracellular H^+ and extracellular K^+, thus preventing H^+ from entering the stomach and additional HCl from forming.

Incompatibilities

Don't give esomeprazole with any other drug through the same I.V. site or tubing.

Contraindications

Hypersensitivity to esomeprazole or its components

Interactions

DRUGS

antimicrobials: Increased blood esomeprazole levels
atazanavir: Possibly reduced blood atazanavir levels
diazepam: Possibly increased blood diazepam level
digoxin, iron salts, ketoconazole: Possibly decreased absorption of these drugs
warfarin: Possibly increased INR and PT, leading to abnormal bleeding

FOODS

all foods: Decreased bioavailability of esomeprazole

Adverse Reactions

CNS: Aggression, agitation, depression, dizziness, encephalopathy, hallucinations, headache
EENT: Blurred vision, dry mouth, sinusitis, taste disturbance
ENDO: Gynecomastia
GI: Abdominal pain, constipation, diarrhea, dyspepsia, flatulence, GI candidiasis, hepatic failure, hepatitis, jaundice, nausea, pancreatitis, stomatitis
GU: Interstitial nephritis
HEME: Agranulocytosis, pancytopenia
MS: Myalgia

RESP: Bronchospasm, respiratory tract infection
SKIN: Alopecia, erythema multiforme, excessive perspiration, Stevens-Johnson syndrome, toxic epidermal necrolysis
Other: Anaphylaxis, infusion site redness or pruritus

Nursing Considerations

- **WARNING** If patient takes drug with amoxicillin or clarithromycin for *Helicobacter pylori*–related ulcer, severe diarrhea may indicate pseudo-membranous colitis. Obtain stool cultures, as ordered.
- Always flush I.V. line with normal saline injection, lactated Ringer's injection, or 5% dextrose injection before and after giving esomeprazole intravenously.
- For I.V. injection, reconstitue powder with 5 ml of normal saline injection and give as a bolus dose over 3 or more minutes. Once reconstituted, drug may be stored at room temperature for up to 12 hours.
- For I.V. infusion, reconstitute powder with 5 ml of normal saline injection, lactated Ringer's injection, or dextrose 5% injection. Further dilute reconstituted solution to make a final volume of 50 ml, and infuse solution over 10 to 30 minutes. Reconstituted drug may be stored at room temperature up to 6 hours if mixed with 5% dextrose injection or up to 12 hours if mixed with normal saline injection or lactated Ringer's injection.
- Be aware that patient receiving I.V. esomeprazole should be switched to oral form as soon as possible.

PATIENT TEACHING

- Urge patient to tell prescriber if he experiences any adverse reactions.

estrogens (conjugated)

Premarin

Class and Category

Chemical: Estrogen derivative, steroid hormone
Therapeutic: Antiosteoporotic, ovarian hormone replacement
Pregnancy category: X

Indications and Dosages

▶ *To treat dysfunctional uterine bleeding*

I.V. INFUSION

Adults. 25 mg, repeated in 6 to 12 hr if needed.

Mechanism of Action

Increase the rate of DNA and RNA synthesis in the cells of female reproductive organs, hypothalamus, pituitary glands, and other target organs. In the hypothalamus, estrogens reduce the release of gonadotropin-releasing hormone, which decreases pituitary release of follicle-stimulating hormone and luteinizing hormone. In women, these hormones are required for normal genitourinary and other essential body functions. At the cellular level, estrogens increase cervical secretions, cause endometrial cell proliferation, and increase uterine tone. Estrogen replacement helps maintain genitourinary function and reduce vasomotor symptoms when estrogen production declines from menopause, surgical removal of ovaries, or other estrogen deficiency. It also may help prevent osteoporosis by keeping bone resorption from exceeding bone formation.

In men, estrogens inhibit pituitary secretion of luteinizing hormone and decrease testicular secretion of testosterone. These actions may decrease prostate tumor growth and lower the level of prostate-specific antigen.

Contraindications

Active deep vein thrombosis, pulmonary embolism, or history of these conditions; active or recent (within past year) arterial thromboembolic disease such as MI or stroke; hypersensitivity to estrogens or their components; known or suspected breast cancer or history of breast cancer; known or suspected estrogen-dependent cancer; liver dysfunction or disease; pregnancy; undiagnosed abnormal genital bleeding

Incompatibilities

Don't combine I.V. estrogens with acid solutions, ascorbic acid, and protein hydrolysate because they're incompatible.

Interactions

DRUGS

aminocaproic acid: Possibly increased level of hypercoagulability caused by amino-caproic acid

barbiturates, carbamazepine, hydantoins, rifabutin, rifampin: Possibly reduced activity of estrogen and medroxyprogesterone

bromocriptine: Possibly interference with bromocriptine's therapeutic effects

calcium: Possibly increased calcium absorption

corticosteroids: Increased therapeutic and toxic effects of corticosteroids

cyclosporine: Increased risk of hepatotoxicity and nephrotoxicity

didanosine, lamivudine, zalcitabine: Possibly pancreatitis
hepatotoxic drugs, such as isoniazid: Increased risk of hepatitis and hepatotoxicity
oral antidiabetic drugs: Decreased therapeutic effects of these drugs
somatrem, somatropin: Possibly accelerated epiphyseal maturation
tamoxifen: Possibly interference with tamoxifen's therapeutic effects
warfarin: Decreased anticoagulant effect
ACTIVITIES
smoking: Increased risk of CVA, pulmonary embolism, thrombophlebitis, and transient ischemic attack

Adverse Reactions

CNS: CVA, dementia, depression, dizziness, headache, migraine headache
CV: Hypertriglyceridemia, MI, peripheral edema, pulmonary embolism, thromboembolism, thrombophlebitis
EENT: Intolerance of contact lenses, retinal vascular thrombosis
ENDO: Breast enlargement, pain, tenderness, or tumors; gynecomastia; hyperglycemia
GI: Abdominal cramps or pain, anorexia, constipation, diarrhea, gallbladder obstruction, hepatitis, increased appetite, nausea, pancreatitis, vomiting
GU: Amenorrhea, breakthrough bleeding, cervical erosion, clear vaginal discharge, decreased libido (males), dysmenorrhea, endometrial cancer, impotence, increased libido (females), ovarian cancer, prolonged or heavy menstrual bleeding, testicular atrophy, vaginal candidiasis
SKIN: Acne, alopecia, hirsutism, jaundice, melasma, oily skin, purpura, rash, seborrhea, urticaria
Other: Angioedema, folic acid deficiency, hypercalcemia (in metastatic bone disease), weight gain

Nursing Considerations

- Use conjugated estrogens cautiously in patients with severe hypocalcemia because a sudden increase in serum calcium levels may cause adverse effects.
- Reconstitute conjugated estrogens with normal saline solution, dextrose, or invert sugar solution and use within a few hours. Discard solution that contains precipitate.
- Monitor serum calcium level to detect severe hypercalcemia in patients with bone metastasis from breast cancer.

- Watch for elevated liver function test values because estrogen and progestins may worsen such conditions as acute intermittent or variegate hepatic porphyria.
- Assess hypertensive patients for increases in blood pressure because estrogens may cause fluid retention.
- Monitor patients with asthma, diabetes mellitus, endometriosis, heart disease, renal disease, migraine headaches, seizure disorder, or lupus erythematosus for worsening of these conditions.
- If patient takes warfarin, assess PT test results as prescribed for loss of anticoagulant effects because estrogens increase production of clotting factors and promote platelet aggregation.
- Expect to stop estrogen combination therapy if woman develops evidence of dementia, cancer, or cardiovascular disease, such as CVA, MI, pulmonary embolism, or venous thrombosis.

PATIENT TEACHING

- Explain the risks of estrogen therapy, including increased risk of cardiovascular disease; dementia; breast, endometrial, or ovarian cancer; and gallbladder disease.
- Urge patient to immediately report breakthrough bleeding.
- Instruct patient to perform a monthly breast self-examination and to comply with all prescribed follow-up examinations.
- Warn female patient that long-term use may increase risk of dementia, heart disease, CVA, gallbladder disease, and breast or endometrial cancer.

ethacrynate sodium

Edecrin

Class and Category

Chemical: Ketone derivative of anyloxyacetic acid
Therapeutic: Diuretic
Pregnancy category: B

Indications and Dosages

▶ *To promote diuresis in heart failure; hepatic cirrhosis; renal disease; ascites of short duration caused by cancer, idiopathic edema, or lymphedema; and edema in children (excluding infants with congenital heart disease or nephrotic syndrome)*

I.V. INFUSION

Adults. *Initial:* 50 mg or 0.5 to 1 mg/kg. Dose repeated in 2 to 4 hr, if needed, then q 4 to 6 hr based on patient response. In an emergency, dose repeated q 1 hr, if needed. *Maximum:* 100 mg as a single dose.

Route	Onset	Peak	Duration
I.V.	5 min	15 to 30 min	2 hr

Mechanism of Action
May inhibit the sulfhydryl-catalyzed enzyme systems that cause sodium and chloride resorption in the proximal and distal tubules and the ascending limb of the loop of Henle. These inhibitory effects increase urinary excretion of sodium, chloride, and water, causing profound diuresis. The drug also increases the excretion of potassium, hydrogen, calcium, magnesium, bicarbonate, ammonium, and phosphate.

Incompatibilities
Don't mix or infuse ethacrynate sodium with whole blood or its derivatives.

Contraindications
Anuria; hypersensitivity to ethacrynate sodium, ethacrynic acid, sulfonylureas, or their components; infancy; severe diarrhea

Interactions
DRUGS
ACE inhibitors, antihypertensives: Possibly hypotension
aminoglycosides: Increased risk of ototoxicity
amiodarone: Increased risk of arrhythmias
amphotericin B: Increased risk of electrolyte imbalances, nephrotoxicity, and ototoxicity
anticoagulants, thrombolytics: Possibly potentiated anticoagulation and risk of hemorrhage
corticosteroids: Increased risk of gastric hemorrhage
digoxin: Increased risk of digitalis toxicity
insulin, oral antidiabetic drugs: Possibly increased blood glucose level and decreased therapeutic effects of these drugs
lithium: Increased risk of lithium toxicity
neuromuscular blockers: Possibly increased neuromuscular blockade effects
NSAIDs: Possibly decreased effects of ethacrynate sodium
sympathomimetics: Possibly interference with hypotensive effects of ethacrynate sodium
ACTIVITIES
alcohol use: Possibly potentiated hypotensive and diuretic effects of ethacrynate sodium

Adverse Reactions

CNS: Confusion, fatigue, headache, malaise, nervousness
CV: Orthostatic hypotension
EENT: Blurred vision, hearing loss, ototoxicity (ringing or buzzing in ears), sensation of fullness in ears, yellow vision
ENDO: Hyperglycemia, hypoglycemia
GI: Abdominal pain, anorexia, diarrhea, dysphagia, GI bleeding, nausea, vomiting
GU: Hematuria, interstitial nephritis, polyuria
HEME: Agranulocytosis, severe neutropenia, thrombocytopenia
SKIN: Rash
Other: Hyperuricemia, hypochloremic alkalosis, hypokalemia, hypomagnesemia, hyponatremia, hypovolemia, infusion site irritation and pain

Nursing Considerations

- Dilute ethacrynate sodium with D_5W or normal saline solution for I.V. infusion. Discard unused portion after 24 hours. Don't use diluted solution that is cloudy or opalescent. Infuse slowly over 30 minutes.
- Weigh patient daily and assess for signs of electrolyte imbalance and dehydration. Monitor blood pressure and fluid intake and output, and check laboratory test results. Be aware that elderly patients may be more sensitive to drug's effects. Notify prescriber about significant changes, which may require dosage reduction or temporary drug discontinuation.
- If patient develops hypokalemia, administer replacement potassium, as ordered.
- **WARNING** Monitor hepatic function test results in patients with advanced hepatic cirrhosis, especially those with a history of electrolyte imbalance or hepatic encephalopathy, because drug may lead to life-threatening hepatic coma.
- Monitor blood glucose level frequently, especially if patient has diabetes mellitus, because drug may cause hyperglycemia or hypoglycemia.
- Notify prescriber if patient experiences hearing loss, vertigo, or ringing, buzzing, or sense of fullness in his ears. Drug may need to be discontinued.
- Store drug between 15° and 30° C (59° and 86° F).

PATIENT TEACHING

- Instruct patient to immediately report diarrhea; buzzing, fullness, or ringing in ears; hearing loss; severe nausea; vertigo; or

vomiting because ethacrynate sodium therapy may need to be discontinued.
- Advise patient to change position slowly to minimize effects of orthostatic hypotension, especially if he takes an antihypertensive.
- Caution patient not to drink alcohol, stand for prolonged periods, or exercise during hot weather because these activities may exacerbate orthostatic hypotension.
- Unless contraindicated, urge patient to eat more high-potassium foods and to take a potassium supplement, if prescribed, to prevent hypokalemia.
- Inform diabetic patient that his blood glucose level will be checked frequently to detect alterations.

etidronate disodium

Didronel

Class and Category

Chemical: Bisphosphonate
Therapeutic: Antihypercalcemic, bone resorption inhibitor
Pregnancy category: C

Indications and Dosages

▶ *To treat moderate to severe hypercalcemia caused by cancer*

I.V. INFUSION

Adults. *Initial:* 7.5 mg/kg daily infused over at least 2 hr for 3 to 7 successive days. Oral etidronate therapy may begin at 20 mg/kg daily for 30 days on the day after last infusion.

DOSAGE ADJUSTMENT Dosage reduced if patient has renal impairment. Drug not given if serum creatinine level exceeds 5 mg/dl.

Mechanism of Action

Inhibits normal and abnormal bone resorption by reducing bone turnover and slowing the remodeling of pagetic or heterotopic bone. Etidronate also decreases the elevated cardiac output that's seen in Paget's disease of bone and reduces local increases in skin temperature. It also inhibits the abnormal bone resorption that may occur with cancer and reduces the amount of calcium that enters the blood from resorbed bone.

Contraindications

Hypersensitivity to etidronate, bisphosphonates, or their components; severe renal impairment

Interactions

DRUGS

aluminum-, calcium-, or magnesium-containing antacids; aluminum-, calcium-, iron-, or magnesium-containing vitamin and mineral supplements: Decreased etidronate absorption

FOODS

high-calcium food, such as milk and other dairy products: Decreased etidronate absorption

Adverse Reactions

EENT: Altered taste, metallic taste
GI: Diarrhea, elevated liver function test results, nausea
GU: Nephrotoxicity
MS: Bone fractures, bone pain, jaw osteonecrosis
Other: Hypocalcemia

Nursing Considerations

- Anticipate beginning etidronate therapy as soon as possible after spinal cord injury, preferably before evidence of heterotopic ossification exists.
- Dilute parenteral form in at least 250 ml of normal saline solution.
- Give parenteral form slowly over at least 2 hours.
- Store diluted parenteral solution at room temperature for up to 48 hours.
- **WARNING Monitor for hypocalcemia if patient receives parenteral form for more than 3 days.**
- When treating hypercalcemia, expect to continue drug for up to 90 days if serum calcium level remains within acceptable range.

PATIENT TEACHING

- Instruct patient to notify prescriber if adverse reactions occur.

etoposide

Toposar, VePesid

etoposide phosphate

Etopophos

Class and Category

Chemical: Podophyllotoxin derivative

Therapeutic: Antineoplastic
Pregnancy category: D

Indications and Dosages

▶ *To treat germ cell testicular cancer*

I.V. INFUSION

Adults. 50 to 100 mg (base)/m^2 daily for 5 days to 100 mg/m^2 on days 1, 3, and 5. Course repeated q 3 to 4 wk.

▶ *To treat small-cell lung cancer*

I.V. INFUSION

Adults. 35 mg (base)/m^2 daily for 4 days to 50 mg/m^2 daily for 5 days. Course repeated q 3 to 4 wk.

Mechanism of Action

May act at the premitotic stage of cell division to inhibit DNA synthesis by blocking topoisomerase II, an enzyme responsible for uncoiling and repairing damaged DNA. Etoposide is cell-cycle dependent and cell-cycle–phase specific, exerting maximum effect on the S and G_2 phases of cell division.

Contraindications

Hypersensitivity to etoposide, etoposide phosphate, or their components

Interactions

DRUGS

blood-dyscrasia–causing drugs (such as cephalosporins and sulfasalazine): Increased risk of leukopenia and thrombocytopenia

bone marrow depressants (such as carboplatin and lomustine): Possibly additive bone marrow depression

cyclosporine: Possibly increased blood etoposide level and increased risk of adverse reactions

phosphatase activity inhibitors (such as levamisole): Possibly inhibition of etoposide phosphate

vaccines, killed virus: Possibly decreased antibody response to vaccine

vaccines, live virus: Possibly decreased antibody response to vaccine, increased adverse effects of vaccine, and severe infection

Adverse Reactions

CNS: CNS toxicity, neurotoxicity

CV: Hypotension, thrombophlebitis

EENT: Stomatitis

GI: Anorexia, diarrhea, hepatotoxicity, nausea, vomiting

HEME: Anemia, leukopenia, myelosuppression (dose-related), thrombocytopenia
SKIN: Alopecia, phlebitis, pruritus, rash
Other: Anaphylaxis-like reaction, metabolic acidosis

Nursing Considerations

- Follow facility protocols for preparation and handling of antineoplastic drugs and for appropriate disposal of used equipment.
- Monitor CBC, including hematocrit, platelet count, and WBC with differential, before and intermittently during etoposide therapy.
- Be aware that adverse reactions can vary when etoposide is administered in combination therapy. Review information for all drugs administered as part of a specific regimen, including drug interactions and adverse effects.
- Anticipate dosage adjustment in patients with impaired renal or hepatic function because they may experience decreased hepatic clearance or elimination of etoposide.
- Dilute etoposide injection with D_5W or normal saline solution to a concentration of 0.2 to 0.4 mg/ml (200 to 400 mcg/ml). Be aware that a precipitate may form if concentration exceeds 0.4 mg/ml. Use 0.2-mg/ml concentration within 96 hours and 0.4-mg/ml concentration within 24 hours when stored at 25° C (77° F) under normal fluorescent light. Be aware that cracking and leaking of container has been observed when *undiluted* etoposide is placed in a plastic container made of ABS (acrylonitrile, butadiene, and styrene).
- Reconstitute etoposide phosphate for injection using 5 or 10 ml of sterile water for injection, 5% dextrose injection, normal saline injection, bacteriostatic water for injection with benzyl alcohol, or bacteriostatic sodium chloride for injection with benzyl alcohol to a concentration of 20 mg/ml or 10 mg/ml, respectively. Drug may be administered as reconstituted or further diluted with D_5W or normal saline solution to a final concentration as low as 0.1 mg/ml. Use reconstituted or diluted solution within 24 hours when stored at 20° to 25° C (68° to 77° F) or 2° to 8° C (36° to 46° F). Allow refrigerated solution to warm to room temperature before use.
- Administer an antiemetic, as prescribed, before administering etoposide to minimize nausea and vomiting.
- Inspect patient's mouth for signs of stomatitis before giving each etoposide dose.

- To prevent hypotension, give etoposide slowly over 30 to 60 minutes (infusion). Give etoposide phosphate injection over 5 to 10 minutes.
- **WARNING** Monitor patient for hypotension, which can result from too-rapid infusion. If hypotension occurs, stop infusion and notify prescriber immediately. Expect to administer fluids and other supportive treatment and then resume etoposide infusion at a slower rate.
- If etoposide solution comes in contact with your skin or mucosa, wash it off thoroughly with warm water.
- Monitor serum albumin level, as ordered. Low serum albumin level increases the risk of drug-related toxicity.
- **WARNING** Monitor patient for hypersensitivity reactions, such as rash, pruritus, wheezing, and dysphagia from laryngeal edema. If such reactions occur, stop infusion and notify prescriber immediately. If anaphylaxis occurs, administer epinephrine, antihistamines, and corticosteroids, as prescribed.
- Monitor patients who have or have recently been exposed to chicken pox or who have herpes zoster for signs and symptoms of severe, generalized disease.
- Be aware that patients who are receiving concurrent or consecutive radiation therapy are at risk for additive bone marrow depression.
- If patient develops thrombocytopenia, implement protective precautions according to facility policy.
- Assess for signs of infection, such as fever, if patient develops leukopenia. Expect to obtain appropriate specimens for culture and sensitivity testing.
- Before diluting etoposide injection, store it at a controlled room temperature. Store etoposide phosphate for injection at 2° to 8° C (36° to 46° F); don't freeze.

PATIENT TEACHING

- Advise patient to have dental work completed before beginning etoposide treatment, if possible, or to defer needed dental work until blood counts return to normal because etoposide can delay healing and cause gingival bleeding. Teach patient to perform proper oral hygiene, and advise him to use a soft-bristled toothbrush.
- Advise patient to immediately report GI upset.
- Instruct patient who develops bone marrow depression to avoid people with infections. Advise him to report fever, chills, cough, hoarseness, lower back or side pain, or painful or difficult uri-

nation because these signs and symptoms may signal an infection.

- Advise patient to immediately report unusual bleeding or bruising, black or tarry stools, blood in urine or stool, or red pinpoint spots on skin.
- Stress the importance of avoiding accidental cuts from sharp objects, such as razor blades or fingernail clippers, because excessive bleeding or infection may occur.
- Caution patient to avoid contact sports and other activities that put him at risk for bruising or injury.
- Instruct patient to avoid touching his eyes or inside of his nose unless he washes his hands immediately beforehand.
- Advise patient with stomatitis to eat bland, soft foods served cold or at room temperature to decrease irritation.
- Advise patient to use contraception to avoid pregnancy during etoposide therapy and to notify prescriber immediately if pregnancy occurs.
- Stress the importance of complying with the dosage regimen and keeping follow-up medical appointments and appointments for laboratory tests.
- Caution patient to avoid receiving immunizations unless approved by prescriber. Instruct him to avoid people who have recently received vaccines or to wear a protective mask over his nose and mouth when in their presence.

famotidine

Pepcid

Class and Category

Chemical: Thiazole derivative
Therapeutic: Antiulcer agent, gastric acid secretion inhibitor
Pregnancy category: B

Indications and Dosages

▶ *To provide short-term treatment of active duodenal ulcer*

I.V. INFUSION OR INJECTION

Adults and adolescents over age 16. 20 mg q 12 hr, infused over 15 to 30 min or injected over at least 2 min.

Children ages 1 to 16. *Initial:* 0.25 mg/kg q 12 hr, infused over 15 to 30 min or injected over at least 2 min. *Maximum:* 40 mg daily.

▶ *To provide short-term treatment for active, benign gastric ulcer*

I.V. INFUSION OR INJECTION
Adults and adolescents over age 16. 20 mg q 12 hr.
Children ages 1 to 16. *Initial:* 0.25 mg/kg q 12 hr. *Maximum:* 40 mg daily.

▶ *To treat gastroesophageal reflux disease*

I.V. INFUSION OR INJECTION
Children ages 1 to 16. *Initial:* 0.25 mg/kg q 12 hr. *Maximum:* 40 mg daily.

▶ *To treat gastric hypersecretory conditions, such as Zollinger-Ellison syndrome*

I.V. INFUSION OR INJECTION
Adults and adolescents. 20 mg q 12 hr.

DOSAGE ADJUSTMENT Parenteral dosage reduced or interval increased (to 36 to 48 hr), if needed, in patients with renal insufficiency and creatinine clearance of 49 ml/min/1.73 m^2 or less.

Route	Onset	Peak	Duration
I.V.	In 30 min	30 min to 3 hr	10 to 12 hr

Mechanism of Action

In normal digestion, parietal cells in the gastric epithelium secrete hydrogen (H^+) ions, which combine with chloride ions (Cl^-) to form hydrochloric acid (HCl), as shown below left. However, HCl can inflame, ulcerate, and perforate the gastric and intestinal mucosa that's normally protected by mucus. Famotidine, an H_2-receptor antagonist, reduces HCl formation by preventing histamine from binding with H_2 receptors on the surface of parietal cells, as shown below right. By doing so, the drug helps prevent peptic ulcers from forming and helps heal existing ones.

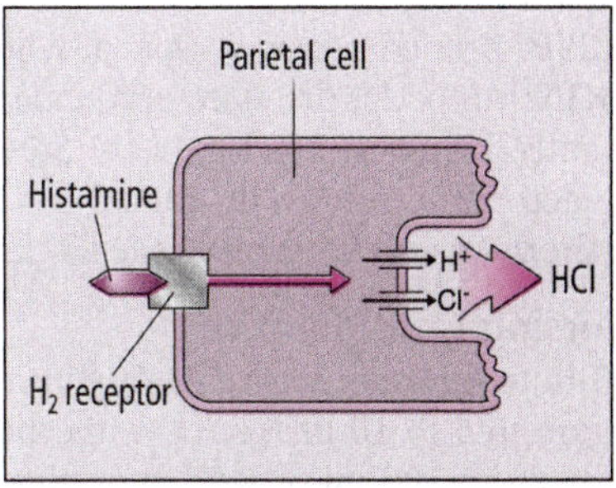

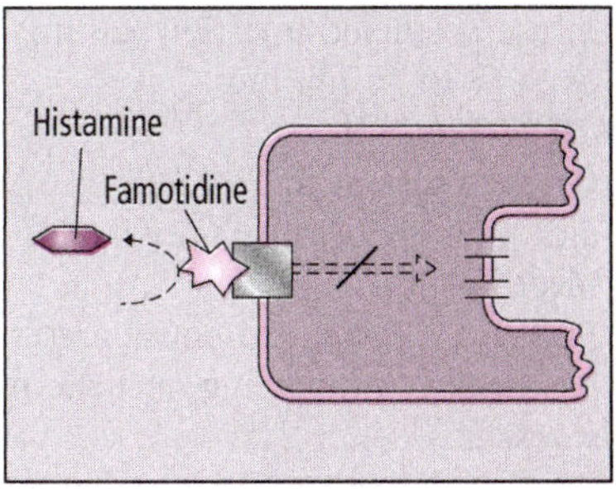

Contraindications

Hypersensitivity to famotidine, other H_2-receptor antagonists, or their components

Interactions

DRUGS

antacids, sucralfate: Possibly decreased absorption of famotidine
bone marrow depressants: Increased risk of blood dyscrasias
itraconazole, ketoconazole: Possibly decreased absorption of these drugs

ACTIVITIES

alcohol use: Possibly increased blood alcohol level

Adverse Reactions

CNS: Agitation (infants), dizziness, fever, headache, insomnia, mental or mood changes
CV: Arrhythmias, palpitations
EENT: Dry mouth, laryngeal edema, tinnitus
GI: Abdominal pain, anorexia, constipation, diarrhea, hepatitis, nausea, vomiting
HEME: Aplastic anemia, leukopenia, neutropenia, pancytopenia, thrombocytopenia
RESP: Bronchospasm, dyspnea, wheezing
SKIN: Alopecia, dry skin, erythema multiforme, exfoliative dermatitis, jaundice, pruritus, rash, Stevens-Johnson syndrome, toxic epidermal necrolysis, urticaria
Other: Anaphylaxis, angioedema, facial edema, hyperuricemia

Nursing Considerations

- Dilute injection form (2 ml) with normal saline or other solution to 5 to 10 ml; give I.V. injection over at least 2 minutes. Or dilute in 100 ml of D_5W and infuse over 15 to 30 minutes. Or infuse premixed injection (20 mg/50 ml normal saline solution) over 15 to 30 minutes.

PATIENT TEACHING

- Caution patient to avoid alcohol and smoking during famotidine therapy because they irritate the stomach and can delay ulcer healing.
- Encourage patient to notify prescriber if she develops pain or has trouble swallowing or if she has bloody vomit or black stools.
- Caution patient not to take famotidine with other acid-reducing products.

fenoldopam mesylate

Corlopam

Class and Category

Chemical: Dopamine agonist
Therapeutic: Antihypertensive
Pregnancy category: B

Indications and Dosages

▶ *To treat severe hypertension when rapid, but quickly reversible, emergency reduction of blood pressure is clinically indicated, including malignant hypertension with deteriorating end-organ function*

I.V. INFUSION

Adults. *Initial:* 0.025 to 0.3 mcg/kg/min, individualized according to patient weight and desired effect. *Usual:* 0.01 to 1.6 mcg/kg/min. *Maximum:* 1.6 mcg/kg/min for up to 48 hr.

Route	Onset	Peak	Duration
I.V.	Rapid	Unknown	Unknown

Mechanism of Action

Stimulates dopamine-1 postsynaptic receptors, which mediate renal and mesenteric vasodilation. Vasodilation lowers blood pressure and total peripheral resistance while increasing renal blood flow.

Contraindications

Hypersensitivity to fenoldopam or its components

Interactions

DRUGS

antihypertensives: Additive hypotensive effect
beta blockers: Increased risk of hypotension
dopamine antagonists, metoclopramide: Possibly decreased effects of fenoldopam

Adverse Reactions

CNS: Anxiety, headache, light-headedness
CV: Hypotension, ST- and T-wave changes, tachycardia
EENT: Increased intraocular pressure
GI: Abdominal pain, nausea
SKIN: Diaphoresis, flushing
Other: Hypokalemia, injection site pain

Nursing Considerations

- Reconstitute by adding 40 mg of fenoldopam (4 ml of concentrate) to 1,000 ml of normal saline solution or D_5W, or 20 mg of fenoldopam (2 ml of concentrate) to 500 ml of normal saline solution or D_5W, or 10 mg of fenoldopam (1 ml of concentrate) to 250 ml of normal saline solution or D_5W to produce a final fenoldopam concentration of 40 mcg/ml.
- Infuse through a mechanical infusion pump for proper control of infusion rate.
- Expect to titrate dosage in increments of 0.05 to 0.1 mcg/kg/min, as prescribed.
- Expect to monitor heart rate and blood pressure every 15 minutes during fenoldopam therapy because most of drug's effect on blood pressure occurs within 15 minutes of any dosage change.
- Be aware that patient may be started on oral antihypertensive therapy, as prescribed, any time after blood pressure is stable during fenoldopam infusion.
- Discard any reconstituted solution not used within 24 hours.
- **WARNING** Assess patient for signs of increased myocardial oxygen demand, especially if patient has heart failure or a history of angina, because fenoldopam may produce a rapid decline in blood pressure, resulting in symptomatic hypotension and a dose-dependent increase in heart rate.
- Monitor serum potassium level because fenoldopam decreases serum potassium concentrations, which may result in hypokalemia, exacerbate arrhythmias, or precipitate conduction abnormalities, especially in patients with cardiac disease.
- Monitor patients with glaucoma or increased intraocular pressure for changes in vision because fenoldopam may cause a dose-dependent increase in intraocular pressure.
- Be alert for possible allergic- or anaphylactic-type reaction to sodium metabisulfite, a component of fenoldopam injection, especially in patients with asthma.

PATIENT TEACHING

- Inform patient that she'll be switched to an oral antihypertensive once her blood pressure is controlled.
- Instruct patient to expect frequent monitoring of vital signs.

fentanyl citrate

Sublimaze

Class, Category, and Schedule

Chemical: Opioid, phenylpiperidine derivative
Therapeutic: Analgesic, anesthesia adjunct
Pregnancy category: C
Controlled substance: Schedule II

Indications and Dosages

▶ *As adjunct to regional anesthesia*

I.V. INJECTION

Adults. 0.05 to 0.1 mg I.M. or slow I.V. over 1 to 2 min.

Route	Onset	Peak	Duration
I.V.	1 to 2 min	3 to 5 min	30 to 60 min

Mechanism of Action

Binds to opioid receptor sites in the CNS, altering perception of and emotional response to pain by inhibiting ascending pain pathways. Fentanyl may alter neurotransmitter release from afferent nerves responsive to painful stimuli, and it causes respiratory depression by acting directly on respiratory centers in the brain stem.

Contraindications

Asthma, children younger than age 2, hypersensitivity to narcotics, myasthenia gravis, patients who aren't opioid-tolerant, significant respiratory depression, upper airway obstruction (I.V. or I.M. form); acute or chronic pain, body weight less than 10 kg (22 lb), doses above 5 mcg/kg in adults or 15 mcg/kg in children (transmucosal form); acute or postoperative pain, age less than 12 (or less than 18 if weight is less than 50 kg [110 lb]), dosage that exceeds 25 mcg/hr at the start of therapy, hypersensitivity to fentanyl (or alfentanil, sufentanil, or adhesives), treatment of mild to moderate pain responsive to nonopioid drugs (transdermal form)

Interactions

DRUGS

anticholinergics, antidiarrheals (such as loperamide and paregoric): Increased risk of severe constipation
antihypertensives, diuretics: Possibly potentiated hypotension
benzodiazepines: Possibly reduced fentanyl dose required for anesthesia induction
buprenorphine: Possibly decreased effects of buprenorphine

clarithromycin, erythromycin, itraconazole, ketoconazole, nefazodone, nelfinavir, ritonavir, troleandomycin: Possibly increased opioid effect of transdermal fentanyl leading to increased or prolonged adverse effects, including severe respiratory depression
CNS depressants: Possibly increased CNS and respiratory depression and hypotension
cytochrome P-450 inducers (such as rifampin, carbamazepine, and phenytoin): Possibly induced metabolism and increased clearance of fentanyl
hydroxyzine: Possibly increased analgesic effect of fentanyl and increased CNS depression and hypotension
MAO inhibitors: Possibly unpredictable, even fatal, effects if taken within 14 days of fentanyl
metoclopramide: Possibly antagonized effect of metoclopramide on gastric motility
nalbuphine, pentazocine: Possibly antagonized analgesic, respiratory depressant, and CNS depressant effects of fentanyl; possibly additive hypotensive and CNS and respiratory depressant effects of both drugs
naloxone: Antagonized analgesic, hypotensive, CNS, and respiratory depressant effects of fentanyl
naltrexone: Possibly blocked therapeutic effects of fentanyl
neuromuscular blockers: Possibly prevention or reversal of muscle rigidity by fentanyl
ACTIVITIES
alcohol use: Increased CNS and respiratory depression and hypotension

Adverse Reactions

CNS: Agitation, amnesia, anxiety, asthenia, ataxia, confusion, delusions, depression, dizziness, drowsiness, euphoria, fever, hallucinations, headache, lack of coordination, light-headedness, nervousness, paranoia, sedation, seizures, sleep disturbance, slurred speech, syncope, tremor, weakness, yawning
CV: Asystole, bradycardia, chest pain, edema, hypotension, orthostatic hypotension, tachycardia
EENT: Blurred vision, dental caries, dry mouth, gum line erosion, laryngospasm, rhinitis, sneezing, tooth loss
GI: Anorexia, constipation, ileus, indigestion, nausea, vomiting
GU: Anorgasmia, decreased libido, ejaculatory difficulty, urinary hesitancy, urine retention
RESP: Apnea, depressed cough reflex, dyspnea, hypoventilation, respiratory depression

SKIN: Diaphoresis, exfoliative dermatitis, localized skin redness and swelling (with transdermal form), pruritus, rash
Other: Drug tolerance, physical or psychological dependence with long-term use, weight loss

Nursing Considerations

- **WARNING** Monitor patient's respiratory status closely, especially during the first 24 to 72 hours after therapy starts or dosage increases, because severe hypoventilation may occur without warning at any time during therapy.
- To prevent withdrawal symptoms after long-term use, expect to taper drug dosage gradually, as prescribed.
- Assess patient for withdrawal symptoms after dosage reduction or conversion to another opioid analgesic.
- For patient with bradycardia, implement cardiac monitoring, as ordered, and assess heart rate and rhythm frequently during fentanyl therapy because drug may further slow heart rate.
- **WARNING** Expect respiratory depressant effects to last longer than analgesic effects. Also be prepared for residual drug to potentiate the effects of subsequent doses. Residual drug can be detected for at least 6 hours after I.V. dose. Monitor patient closely for at least 24 hours after therapy ends.

PATIENT TEACHING

- Reassure patient that he will be monitored closely throughout fentanyl therapy.

filgrastim
(granulocyte colony-stimulating factor, rG-CSF)

Neupogen

Class and Category

Chemical: Granulocyte colony-stimulating factor
Therapeutic: Antineutropenic, hematopoietic stimulator
Pregnancy category: C

Indications and Dosages

▶ *To prevent infection after myelosuppressive chemotherapy*

I.V. INFUSION

Adults. 5 mcg/kg daily over 15 to 30 min. Increased, if needed, by 5 mcg/kg with each chemotherapy cycle.

▶ *To reduce the duration of neutropenia after bone marrow transplantation*

I.V. INFUSION
Adults. 10 mcg/kg daily over 4 hr or as a continuous infusion over 24 hr.
DOSAGE ADJUSTMENT Dosage reduced for patients whose absolute neutrophil count remains above $10,000/mm^3$.

Route	Onset	Peak	Duration
I.V.	In 5 min	Unknown	Unknown

Mechanism of Action
Is pharmacologically identical to human granulocyte colony-stimulating factor, an endogenous hormone synthesized by monocytes, endothelial cells, and fibroblasts. Filgrastim induces the formation of neutrophil progenitor cells by binding directly to receptors on the surface of granulocytes, which then divide and differentiate. It also potentiates the effects of mature neutrophils, which reduces fever and the risk of infection raised by severe neutropenia.

Incompatibilities
Don't mix filgrastim in vial or syringe with normal saline solution because precipitate will form.

Contraindications
Hypersensitivity to filgrastim, its components, or proteins derived from *Escherichia coli*

Interactions
DRUGS
lithium: Increased neutrophil production

Adverse Reactions
CNS: Fever, headache
CV: Transient supraventricular tachycardia
GI: Splenic rupture, splenomegaly
HEME: Leukocytosis
MS: Arthralgia; myalgia; pain in arms, legs, lower back, or pelvis
SKIN: Pruritus, rash
Other: Anaphylaxis, injection site pain and redness

Nursing Considerations
- Warm filgrastim to room temperature before injection. Discard drug if stored longer than 6 hours at room temperature or 24 hours in refrigerator.

- Withdraw only one dose from a vial; don't repuncture the vial.
- Don't shake the solution.
- For continuous infusion, dilute in D_5W (not normal saline solution) to produce less than 15 mcg/ml.
- After chemotherapy, give filgrastim over 15 to 30 minutes. Don't give within 24 hours before or after cytotoxic chemotherapy.
- Monitor CBC, hematocrit, and platelet count two or three times weekly, as appropriate.
- Inform prescriber and expect to stop drug if leukocytosis develops or absolute neutrophil count consistently exceeds 10,000/mm^3.
- Anticipate decreased response to drug if patient has received extensive radiation therapy or long-term chemotherapy.

PATIENT TEACHING

- Provide patient with puncture-resistant container for needle and syringe disposal.
- Advise patient to promptly report left-upper-quadrant abdominal pain or shoulder-tip pain.
- Stress the importance of returning for follow-up laboratory tests.

fluconazole

Diflucan

Class and Category

Chemical: Triazole derivative
Therapeutic: Antifungal
Pregnancy category: C

Indications and Dosages

▶ *To treat oral and esophageal candidiasis*

I.V. INJECTION

Adults and adolescents. 200 mg on day 1 followed by 100 mg daily for at least 2 (oral) or 3 (esophageal) wk after symptoms resolve.

Children. 3 mg/kg daily for at least 2 (oral) or 3 (esophageal) wk and then for 2 wk after esophageal symptoms resolve.

▶ *To treat systemic candidiasis*

I.V. INJECTION

Adults and adolescents. 400 mg on day 1, followed by 200 mg daily for at least 4 wk and then for 2 wk after symptoms resolve.

▶ *To treat cryptococcal meningitis*

I.V. INJECTION

Adults and adolescents. 400 mg daily until patient responds to treatment; then 200 to 400 mg daily for 10 to 12 wk after CSF culture is negative. *Maintenance:* 200 mg daily to suppress relapse.
Children. 6 to 12 mg/kg daily for 10 to 12 wk after CSF culture is negative.

▶ *To prevent candidiasis after bone marrow transplantation*

I.V. INJECTION

Adults and adolescents. 400 mg daily starting several days before procedure if severe neutropenia is expected and continued for 7 days after absolute neutrophil count exceeds 1,000/mm^3.

DOSAGE ADJUSTMENT Dosage reduced for patients with hepatic or renal impairment. Dosage reduced by 50% for patients with creatinine clearance of 11 to 50 ml/min/1.73 m^2.

Mechanism of Action

Damages fungal cells by interfering with a cytochrome P-450 enzyme needed to convert lanosterol to ergosterol, an essential part of the fungal cell membrane.

Decreased ergosterol synthesis causes increased cell permeability, which allows cell contents to leak. Fluconazole also may inhibit endogenous respiration, interact with membrane phospholipids, inhibit transformation of yeasts to mycelial forms, inhibit purine uptake, and impair biosynthesis of triglycerides and phospholipids.

Incompatibilities

Don't add fluconazole to I.V. bag that contains any other drug.

Contraindications

Hypersensitivity to fluconazole or its components

Interactions

DRUGS

astemizole, terfenadine: Increased blood levels of these drugs
benzodiazepines (short-acting): Possibly increased blood benzodiazepine level and psychomotor effects
cimetidine: Decreased blood fluconazole level
cisapride: Possibly increased QT interval, leading to torsades de pointes
cyclosporine: Increased blood cyclosporine level
glipizide, glyburide, tolbutamide: Increased risk of hypoglycemia
hydrochlorothiazide: Increased blood fluconazole level from decreased excretion

isoniazid, rifampin: Decreased fluconazole effects
nonsedating antihistamines: Increased blood antihistamine level, increased risk of cardiotoxicity
oral anticoagulants: Increased anticoagulant effects
phenytoin: Increased blood phenytoin level
rifabutin: Increased blood rifabutin level
theophylline: Increased blood theophylline level
zidovudine: Increased blood zidovudine level

Adverse Reactions

CNS: Chills, dizziness, drowsiness, fever, headache, seizures
CV: Prolonged QT interval, torsades de pointes
GI: Abdominal pain, anorexia, constipation, diarrhea, hepatic failure, nausea, vomiting
HEME: Agranulocytosis, leukopenia, thrombocytopenia
SKIN: Exfoliative dermatitis, photosensitivity, pruritus, rash
Other: Anaphylaxis, angioedema

Nursing Considerations

- Use fluconazole cautiously in patients with potentially proarrhythmic conditions because drug may prolong the QT interval, which can lead to life-threatening torsades de pointes.
- Expect to obtain BUN and serum creatinine levels and culture and sensitivity and liver function test results before therapy starts.
- Discard I.V. solution that's cloudy or contains precipitate. Don't infuse more than 200 mg/hr or add supplemental drugs to infusion.
- Monitor hepatic and renal function periodically during therapy, and notify prescriber if you detect signs of dysfunction.
- Assess for rash every 8 hours during therapy, and notify prescriber if rash occurs.
- If patient receives an oral anticoagulant, monitor coagulation test results and assess patient for bleeding.
- Monitor patient for symptoms of overdose, such as hallucinations and paranoia. If they occur, provide supportive treatment, gastric lavage, and, possibly, hemodialysis, which can reduce blood fluconazole level by half after about 3 hours.

PATIENT TEACHING

- If patient takes an oral antidiabetic drug, caution her to monitor blood glucose level frequently because of increased risk of hypoglycemia.
- Alert patient that fluconazole may change the taste of food.

- Advise patient to notify prescriber immediately about diarrhea, headache, nausea, rash, right-upper-quadrant abdominal pain, yellow skin or whites of eyes, or vomiting.
- Suggest that breast-feeding patient consult prescriber because breast-feeding may need to be stopped during therapy.

flumazenil

Anexate (CAN), Romazicon

Class and Category

Chemical: Imidazobenzodiazepine derivative
Therapeutic: Benzodiazepine antidote
Pregnancy category: C

Indications and Dosages

▶ *To reverse sedation from benzodiazepine therapy*

I.V. INJECTION

Adults. 0.2 mg, repeated after 45 to 60 sec if response is inadequate and then repeated q 1 min, if needed. If sedation recurs, regimen is repeated q 20 min or more. *Maximum:* 1 mg over 5 min or 3 mg in 1-hr period.

▶ *To reverse benzodiazepine toxicity or suspected overdose*

I.V. INJECTION

Adults. 0.2 mg followed by 0.3 mg 30 to 60 sec later if response is inadequate and then 0.5 mg repeated q 1 min. If sedation recurs, regimen is repeated q 20 min. *Maximum:* 3 mg in 1-hr period.

Route	Onset	Peak	Duration
I.V.	1 to 2 min	6 to 10 min	Variable

Mechanism of Action

Antagonizes the CNS effects of benzodiazepines by competing for their binding sites.

Contraindications

Evidence of tricyclic antidepressant overdose; hypersensitivity to flumazenil, benzodiazepines, or their components; use of benzodiazepine to control intracranial pressure, status epilepticus, or a potentially life-threatening condition

Interactions

DRUGS

benzodiazepines: Benzodiazepine withdrawal symptoms, including seizures

nonbenzodiazepine agonists: Loss of effectiveness of these drugs

tetracyclic or tricyclic antidepressant overdose: High risk of seizures

FOODS

all foods: Increased flumazenil clearance (by half) with food ingestion during I.V. injection

Adverse Reactions

CNS: Agitation, anxiety, ataxia, confusion, dizziness, drowsiness, emotional lability, fatigue, headache, hypoesthesia, insomnia, paresthesia, resedation, seizures, tremor, vertigo

CV: Hot flashes, hypertension, palpitations

EENT: Blurred vision, diplopia, dry mouth

GI: Nausea, vomiting

RESP: Dyspnea, hyperventilation, hypoventilation

SKIN: Diaphoresis, flushing, rash

Other: Injection site pain and thrombophlebitis

Nursing Considerations

- Use flumazenil cautiously in patients with cardiac disease. Assess patient for increased stress or anxiety from benzodiazepine withdrawal because, in patient with cardiac disease, blood pressure may rise.
- Give flumazenil undiluted or diluted in a syringe with D_5W, normal saline solution, or lactated Ringer's solution. Administer over 15 to 30 seconds directly into tubing of a free-flowing compatible I.V. solution. Use a large vein, if possible, to minimize pain at site. Avoid extravasation because drug may irritate tissue.
- Be aware that drug may cause signs of benzodiazepine withdrawal in drug-dependent patient. Also, abrupt awakening from benzodiazepine overdose can cause agitation, dysphoria, and increased adverse reactions.
- Be aware that benzodiazepine reversal may cause an anxiety or a panic attack for patient with a history of these episodes. Expect to adjust dosage carefully.
- Monitor for signs of resedation and hypoventilation for at least 2 hours after giving flumazenil because drug has a short half-life. Be aware that patient shouldn't be discharged until the risk of resedation has resolved.

PATIENT TEACHING

- Caution patient to avoid alcohol and OTC drugs for 10 to 24 hours after taking flumazenil.
- Advise patient to avoid hazardous activities for 18 to 24 hours after discharge.
- Inform patient and family that agitation, emotional lability, fear, and panic attack (if patient has a history of them) may occur. Tell them to seek medical care if patient develops depression, trouble breathing, flushing, hyperventilation, insomnia, palpitations, or tremor.
- Because drug doesn't always reverse postprocedure amnesia, provide written instructions or instructions to caregiver even if patient is alert.

fluorouracil

(5-FU)

Adrucil

Class and Category

Chemical: Pyrimidine analogue antimetabolite
Therapeutic: Antineoplastic
Pregnancy category: D

Indications and Dosages

▶ *To treat colorectal, breast, gastric, or pancreatic cancer*

I.V. INFUSION

Adults and adolescents. *Initial:* 7 to 12 mg/kg daily for 4 days; then, after 3 days, if no toxicity has occurred, 7 to 10 mg/kg q 3 days for a total course of 2 wk. Or, 12 mg/kg daily for 4 days; then, after 1 day, if no toxicity has occurred, 6 mg/kg q other day for 4 or 5 doses (days 6, 8, 10, and 12) for a total of 12 days. *Maintenance:* 7 to 12 mg/kg q 7 to 10 days or 300 to 500 mg/m^2 daily for 4 to 5 days, repeated monthly. *Maximum adult dose:* 800 mg daily (400 mg daily for poor-risk patients).

Adults and adolescents who have not received a loading dose. 15 mg/kg or 500 to 600 mg/m^2 q wk.

DOSAGE ADJUSTMENT For poor-risk patients, dosage adjusted to 3 to 6 mg/kg daily for 3 days; then, after 1 day, if no toxicity occurs, 3 mg/kg q other day for 3 doses. Dosage also may be adjusted for patients who have received cytotoxic drug therapy with alkylating agents or high-dose pelvic radiation and for patients with impaired renal or hepatic function.

Mechanism of Action

Inhibits the formation of thymidylate from uracil, which interferes with DNA synthesis and, to a lesser extent, RNA formation. This may create a thymine deficiency, which provokes unbalanced cell growth and death, most markedly in cells that grow rapidly and take up fluorouracil at a rapid rate. Fluorouracil is cell-cycle–phase specific; it's active during the S phase of cell division.

Contraindications

Bone marrow depression, hypersensitivity to fluorouracil, major surgery within 1 month before fluorouracil administration, poor nutritional status, potentially serious infection

Interactions

DRUGS

blood-dyscrasia–causing drugs (such as cephalosporins and sulfasalazine): Increased risk of leukopenia and thrombocytopenia
bone marrow depressants (such as carboplatin and lomustine): Possibly additive bone marrow depression
cimetidine: Possibly increased peak concentrations of fluorouracil
leucovorin: Possibly increased therapeutic and toxic fluorouracil effects
vaccines, killed virus: Possibly decreased antibody response to vaccine
vaccines, live virus: Possibly decreased antibody response to vaccine, increased adverse effects of vaccine, and severe infection
warfarin and other coumarin-derived anticoagulants: Increased anticoagulant effect

Adverse Reactions

CNS: Acute cerebellar syndrome, confusion, disorientation, euphoria, headache, weakness
CV: Angina, myocardial ischemia, thrombophlebitis
EENT: Nystagmus, stomatitis
GI: Anorexia, diarrhea, esophogopharyngitis, GI ulceration, nausea, vomiting
HEME: Agranulocytosis, anemia, bone marrow depression, leukopenia, pancytopenia, thrombocytopenia
RESP: Pneumopathy
SKIN: Alopecia, dry skin and fissuring, maculopapular rash, palmar-plantar erythrodysesthesia syndrome, pruritus
Other: Anaphylaxis, infection

Nursing Considerations

- Follow facility protocols for preparation and handling of antineoplastic drugs and for appropriate disposal of used equipment.
- Be aware that fluorouracil should be administered only under the supervision of a qualifed physician. Expect patient to be hospitalized at least during the first course of therapy.
- Be aware that estimated lean body mass (dry weight) may be used to calculate dosage for obese patients and for those with weight gain secondary to abnormal fluid retention, ascites, or edema. Maximum fluorouracil daily dose for any patient should not exceed 800 mg.
- Monitor CBC, including hematocrit, platelet count, and WBC with differential, and liver function tests, including bilirubin and LDH values, before and intermittently during fluorouracil therapy, as ordered. Inspect patient's mouth for stomatitis before each dose.
- **WARNING** Be aware that adverse reactions can vary when fluorouracil is administered in combination therapy and that some reactions, such as severe diarrhea with dehydration and electrolyte imbalances, may be life-threatening. Review information for all drugs given as part of a specific regimen, including drug interactions and adverse effects. Expect increased patient evaluation and dosage adjustments based on combination used and incidence and severity of adverse reactions.
- Dilute fluorouracil with D_5W or normal saline solution. If using the 50-ml vial, don't use a syringe or needle to avoid leakage and contamination; instead, use a sterile dispensing device or a transfer set that accepts a syringe hub. Use proper aseptic technique under a laminar flow hood. Use diluted solution within 8 hours.
- Be aware that slight discoloration doesn't affect drug's potency or safety.
- **WARNING** Be aware that fluorouracil should not be administered intrathecally because of the increased risk of neurotoxicity.
- Infuse fluorouracil slowly, over 2 to 24 hours, to reduce the risk of toxicity. However, be aware that rapid injection (over 1 to 2 minutes) may be more effective.
- **WARNING** Because of fluorouracil's extremely toxic effects, expect to discontinue infusion if patient develops any of the following adverse reactions: diarrhea, esophagopharyngitis

(heartburn with potential for sloughing and ulceration), GI bleeding or ulceration, hemorrhage (from any site), intractable vomiting, marked leukopenia or rapidly falling leukocyte count, stomatitis, or thrombocytopenia. Expect to restart infusion at a lower dose when adverse reactions subside.

- Monitor patients who have, or have recently been exposed to, chicken pox or who have herpes zoster for signs and symptoms of severe, generalized disease.
- Assess for signs of infection, such as fever, if patient develops leukopenia. Expect to obtain appropriate specimens for culture and sensitivity testing.
- **WARNING** Be aware that myocardial ischemia can occur several hours after a dose (even later doses). Continue to assess patient for signs of ischemia throughout the course of treatment.
- Be aware that patients who are receiving concurrent or consecutive radiation therapy are at risk for additive bone marrow depression.
- Assess patient for signs of palmar-plantar erythrodysesthesia syndrome (also known as hand-foot syndrome), characterized by tingling of hands and feet, followed by pain, erythema, and swelling. Expect symptoms to subside 5 to 7 days after interruption of therapy.
- Store drug at 15° to 30° C (59° to 86° F); protect from freezing and light. Heat solution to 60° C (140° F) and shake vigorously to dissolve precipitates formed at low temperatures. Allow solution to cool to body temperature before use.

PATIENT TEACHING

- Advise patient to have dental work completed before beginning fluorouracil treatment, if possible, or to defer such work until blood counts return to normal because drug can delay healing and cause gingival bleeding. Teach patient proper oral hygiene, and advise her to use a soft-bristled toothbrush.
- Instruct patient who develops bone marrow depression to avoid persons with infections. Advise her to report fever, chills, cough, hoarseness, lower back or side pain, or painful or difficult urination because these signs and symptoms may signal an infection.
- Advise patient to immediately report unusual bleeding or bruising, black or tarry stools, blood in urine or stool, or red pinpoint spots on skin.

- Stress the importance of avoiding accidental cuts from sharp objects, such as razor blades or fingernail clippers, because excessive bleeding or infection may occur.
- Urge patient to avoid contact sports or other activities that put her at risk for bruising or injury.
- Instruct patient to avoid touching her eyes or inside of her nose unless she washes her hands immediately beforehand.
- Advise patient to use contraception to avoid pregnancy during therapy and to notify prescriber immediately if pregnancy occurs.
- Advise patient with stomatitis to eat bland, soft foods served cold or at room temperature to decrease irritation.
- Stress the importance of complying with the dosage regimen and of keeping follow-up medical appointments and appointments for laboratory tests.
- Caution patient to avoid receiving immunizations unless approved by prescriber. Instruct her to avoid people who have recently received vaccines or to wear a protective mask over her nose and mouth when in their presence.

folic acid
(vitamin B_9)
Folvite

Class and Category
Chemical: Water-soluble B-complex vitamin
Therapeutic: Nutritional supplement
Pregnancy category: A

Indications and Dosages
▶ *To prevent deficiency based on U.S. and Canadian recommended daily allowances*

I.V INFUSION

Adults and children age 11 and over. Dosage individualized based on patient need and given as part of total parenteral nutrition solution.

▶ *To treat deficiency*

I.V. INFUSION

Adults and children age 11 and over. 0.25 to 1 mg daily until hematologic response occurs.

Contraindications
Hypersensitivity to folic acid or its components

Mechanism of Action

Acts as a catalyst for normal production of RBCs, helping to prevent megaloblastic anemia, and helps maintain normal homocysteine levels. After being converted to tetrahydrofolic acid in the intestines, folic acid promotes synthesis of several enzymes, including purine and thymidylates; metabolism of amino acids, including glycine and methionine; and metabolism of histidine—all of which are essential for normal cell structure and growth.

Interactions

DRUGS

analgesics, carbamazepine, estrogens (including oral contraceptives), phenobarbital, primidone: Possibly increased folic acid requirements
hydantoin anticonvulsants: Possibly decreased effectiveness of these drugs, possibly increased folic acid requirements
methotrexate, pyrimethamine, triamterene, trimethoprim: Possibly decreased effectiveness of folic acid
sulfasalazine: Possibly decreased folic acid absorption

Adverse Reactions

Other: Allergic reaction (bronchospasm, erythema, fever, malaise, rash, pruritus)

Nursing Considerations

- **WARNING** Don't administer injection form of folic acid containing benzyl alcohol to neonates or premature infants because they may develop a fatal toxic syndrome characterized by CNS, respiratory, circulatory, and renal impairment and metabolic acidosis.
- Be aware that although folic acid will correct hematologic disorders associated with pernicious anemia, neurologic problems will progressively worsen.
- Store drug at 15° to 30° C (59° to 86° F); protect from freezing and light.

PATIENT TEACHING

- Inform patient that folic acid supplements are not a substitute for proper diet. Teach her that the best sources of dietary folic acid are green vegetables, potatoes, cereals, and organ meats. Recommend that she eat raw green vegetables because cooking destroys up to 90% of folic acid found in food.
- Explain to patients with pernicious anemia that folic acid won't affect the neurologic symptoms associated with the disease.

foscarnet sodium

Foscavir

Class and Category

Chemical: Organic pyrophosphate analogue
Therapeutic: Antiviral
Pregnancy category: C

Indications and Dosages

▶ *To treat cytomegalovirus retinitis*

I.V. INFUSION

Adults. *Induction:* 90 mg/kg over 1½ to 2 hr q 12 hr, or 60 mg/kg over 1 hr q 8 hr, for 14 to 21 days. *Maintenance:* 90 to 120 mg/kg over 2 hr daily.

DOSAGE ADJUSTMENT To achieve induction dose equivalent of 90 mg/kg q 12 hr in patients with impaired renal function, dosage reduced as follows: for creatinine clearance greater than 1 to 1.4 ml/min/kg, 70 mg/kg q 12 hr; for clearance greater than 0.8 to 1 ml/min/kg, 50 mg/kg q 12 hr; for clearance greater than 0.6 to 0.8 ml/min/kg, 80 mg/kg q 24 hr; for clearance greater than 0.5 to 0.6 ml/min/kg, 60 mg/kg q 24 hr; for clearance greater than or equal to 0.4 to 0.5 ml/min/kg, 50 mg/kg q 24 hr; and for clearance less than 0.4 ml/min/kg, use not recommended.

To achieve induction dose equivalent of 60 mg/kg q 8 hr in patients with impaired renal function, dosage reduced as follows: for creatinine clearance greater than 1 to 1.4 ml/min/kg, 45 mg/kg q 8 hr; for clearance greater than 0.8 to 1 m/min/kg, 50 mg/kg q 12 hr; for clearance greater than 0.6 to 0.8 ml/min/kg, 40 mg/kg q 12 hr; for clearance greater than 0.5 to 0.6 ml/min/kg, 60 mg/kg q 24 hr; for clearance greater than or equal to 0.4 to 0.5 ml/min/kg, 50 mg/kg q 24 hr; and for clearance less than 0.4 ml/min/kg, use not recommended.

DOSAGE ADJUSTMENT For patients with impaired renal function who are receiving 90-mg/kg daily maintenance dose, dosage reduced as follows: for creatinine clearance greater than 1 to 1.4 ml/min/kg, 70 mg/kg daily; for clearance greater than 0.8 to 1 ml/min/kg, 50 mg/kg daily; for clearance greater than 0.6 to 0.8 ml/min/kg, 80 mg/kg q 48 hr; for clearance greater than 0.5 to 0.6 ml/min/kg, 60 mg/kg q 48 hr; for clearance greater than or equal to 0.4 to 0.5 ml/min/kg, 50 mg/kg q 48 hr; and for clearance less than 0.4 ml/min/kg, use not recommended.

For patients with impaired renal function who are receiving 120-mg/kg daily maintenance dose, dosage reduced as follows: for creatinine clearance greater than 1 to 1.4 ml/min/kg, 90 mg/kg q day; for clearance greater than 0.8 to 1 ml/min/kg, 65 mg/kg q day; for clearance greater than 0.6 to 0.8 ml/min/kg, 105 mg/kg q 48 hr; for clearance greater than 0.5 to 0.6 ml/min/kg, 80 mg/kg q 48 hr; for clearance greater than or equal to 0.4 to 0.5 ml/min/kg, 65 mg/kg q 48 hr; and for clearance less than 0.4 ml/min/kg, use not recommended.

▶ *To treat acyclovir-resistant mucocutaneous herpes simplex*

I.V. INFUSION

Adults. 40 mg/kg over 1 hr q 8 or 12 hr for 14 to 21 days or until healed.

DOSAGE ADJUSTMENT For patients with impaired renal function who are receiving 40-mg/kg dose q 8 hr, dosage reduced as follows: for creatinine clearance greater than 1 to 1.4 ml/min/kg, 30 mg/kg q 8 hr; for clearance greater than 0.8 to 1 ml/min/kg, 35 mg/kg q 12 hr; for clearance greater than 0.6 to 0.8 ml/min/kg, 25 mg/kg q 12 hr; for clearance greater than 0.5 to 0.6 ml/min/kg, 40 mg/kg q 24 hr; for clearance greater than or equal to 0.4 to 0.5 ml/min/kg, 35 mg/kg q 24 hr; and for clearance less than 0.4 ml/min/kg, use not recommended.

For patients with impaired renal function who are receiving 40-mg/kg dose q 12 hr, dosage reduced as follows: for creatinine clearance greater than 1 to 1.4 ml/min/kg, 30 mg/kg q 12 hr; for clearance greater than 0.8 to 1 ml/min/kg, 20 mg/kg q 12 hr; for clearance greater than 0.6 to 0.8 ml/min/kg, 35 mg/kg q 24 hr; for clearance greater than 0.5 to 0.6 ml/min/kg, 25 mg/kg q 24 hr; for clearance greater than or equal to 0.4 to 0.5 ml/min/kg, 20 mg/kg q 24 hr; and for clearance less than 0.4 ml/min/kg, use not recommended.

Incompatibilities

Don't mix foscarnet through the same I.V. line or concurrently through the same catheter as any other solution or drug. Foscarnet is incompatible with solutions containing calcium, 30% dextrose solution, or LR. To avoid precipitation, don't mix foscarnet with acyclovir, amphotericin B, co-trimoxazole, dobutamine, droperidol, ganciclovir, haloperidol, pentamidine, trimetrexate, or vancomycin. To avoid gas production, don't mix foscarnet with diazepam, digoxin, lorazepam, midazolam, or promethazine hydrochloride. To avoid cloudiness or color change, don't mix foscarnet with diphenhydramine, leucovorin, or prochlorperazine.

Mechanism of Action

Inhibits replication of herpes simplex virus types 1 and 2, Epstein-Barr virus, cytomegalovirus, human herpes virus 6, and varicella-zoster virus by selectively inhibiting the pyrophosphate-binding site of viral DNA polymerase, an enzyme used in the viral DNA replication process. Viral replication resumes when drug therapy stops.

Contraindications

Clinically significant hypersensitivity to foscarnet sodium

Interactions

DRUGS

aminoglycosides, amphotericin B, cidofovir, and other nephrotoxic drugs: Increased risk of nephrotoxicity

pentamidine (I.V.): Hypocalcemia, hypomagnesemia, and nephrotoxicity

ritonavir, saquinavir: Abnormal renal function

zidovudine: Possibly increased risk of anemia

Adverse Reactions

CNS: Headache, neurotoxicity (including dizziness, paresthesia, seizures)

CV: Phlebitis

EENT: Mouth or throat ulcers

GI: Abdominal pain, anorexia, diarrhea, nausea, vomiting

GU: Elevated serum creatinine level, genital ulcers, nephrotoxicity

HEME: Anemia, granulocytopenia, leukopenia

Other: Hypocalcemia, hypophosphatemia, hyperphosphatemia, hypomagnesemia, hypokalemia

Nursing Considerations

- Expect to hydrate patient with ½ to 1 L of normal saline solution or D_5W, as ordered, before first dose of foscarnet and with each subsequent dose to avoid nephrotoxicity.
- Prepare peripheral infusion by diluting with an equal amount of D_5W or normal saline solution, which will result in a concentration of 12 mg/ml. Use diluted drug within 24 hours, and

discard any unused portion. Infuse undiluted foscarnet (24 mg/ml) by central line to prevent venous irritation.
- Administer 60-mg/kg doses over at least 1 hour and higher doses over at least 2 hours.
- **WARNING** Always administer foscarnet at a steady rate using an infusion pump; rapid infusion may result in increased blood level of foscarnet, which can lead to acute hypocalcemia or another toxicity.
- Monitor patient's serum electrolyte levels, especially calcium, magnesium, phosphate, and potassium, 2 to 3 times a week during induction and weekly during maintenance therapy, as ordered. Be aware that patient may have decreased ionized calcium level even if serum calcium level seems to be normal. Assess patient for signs of hypocalcemia, such as perioral tingling, numbness, and paresthesia. Be aware that electrolyte abnormalities can cause severe effects, such as arrhythmias, seizures, and tetany.
- Obtain patient's baseline BUN and serum creatinine levels; then monitor these levels 2 to 3 times a week during induction therapy and at least once a week during maintenance therapy, as ordered. Assess input and output of patients who are dehydrated, are using other nephrotoxic drugs, or have preexisting impaired renal function because foscarnet increases the risk of nephrotoxicity. Monitor elderly patients closely because they are more likely to have decreased renal function.
- Monitor CBC periodically during foscarnet therapy, especially in patients with preexisting anemia, because foscarnet may decrease hemoglobin concentration.
- Store drug at 15° to 30° C (59° to 86° F); don't freeze. Discard drug if it becomes frozen because a precipitate will form.

PATIENT TEACHING
- Advise patient receiving foscarnet to immediately report signs of hypocalcemia, such as tingling around mouth or numbness of arms or legs, as well as other adverse reactions, such as changes in urination pattern or increased eye pain.
- Stress the importance of keeping follow-up medical appointments and appointments for laboratory tests.
- Inform patient that retinitis may continue to progress and vision loss may occur during treatment. Encourage her to undergo follow-up ophthalmic examinations, even after she has completed treatment.

fosphenytoin sodium

Cerebyx

Class and Category

Chemical: Hydantoin derivative
Therapeutic: Anticonvulsant
Pregnancy category: D

Indications and Dosages

▶ *To treat status epilepticus*

I.V. INFUSION

Adults and adolescents. *Initial:* 15 to 20 mg of phenytoin equivalent (PE)/kg at 100 to 150 PE/min. *Maintenance:* 4 to 6 mg PE/kg daily in divided doses b.i.d. to q.i.d. *Maximum:* 30 mg PE/kg as total loading dose.

Children. *Initial:* 15 to 20 mg PE/kg given at up to 3 mg PE/kg/min. *Maintenance:* 4 to 6 mg PE/kg daily in divided doses b.i.d. to q.i.d.

▶ *To prevent or treat seizures during and after neurosurgery*

I.V. INFUSION

Adults and adolescents. *Initial:* 10 to 20 mg PE/kg, not to exceed 150 mg PE/min. *Maintenance:* 4 to 6 mg PE/kg daily in divided doses b.i.d. to q.i.d. *Maximum:* 30 mg PE/kg as total loading dose.

Mechanism of Action

Is converted from fosphenytoin (a prodrug) to phenytoin, which limits the spread of seizure activity and the start of new seizures. Phenytoin does so by regulating voltage-dependent sodium and calcium channels in neurons, inhibiting calcium movement across neuronal membranes, and enhancing the sodium-potassium–adenosine triphosphatase activity in neurons and glial cells. These actions may stem from phenytoin's ability to slow the recovery rate of inactivated sodium channels.

Contraindications

Hypersensitivity to fosphenytoin, phenytoin, other hydantoins, or their components

Interactions

DRUGS

acetaminophen (long-term use): Increased risk of hepatotoxicity
acyclovir: Decreased blood phenytoin level, loss of seizure control

alfentanil: Increased clearance and decreased effectiveness of alfentanil
amiodarone, fluoxetine: Possibly increased blood phenytoin level and risk of toxicity
antacids: Possibly decreased phenytoin effectiveness
antineoplastics: Increased phenytoin metabolism
beta blockers: Increased myocardial depression
bupropion, clozapine, loxapine, MAO inhibitors, maprotiline, phenothiazines, pimozide, thioxanthenes: Possibly lowered seizure threshold and decreased therapeutic effects of phenytoin, possibly intensified CNS depressant effects of these drugs
calcium: Possibly impaired phenytoin absorption
calcium channel blockers: Possibly increased blood phenytoin level
carbamazepine: Decreased blood carbamazepine level, possibly increased blood phenytoin level and risk of toxicity
chloramphenicol, cimetidine, disulfiram, isoniazid, methylphenidate, metronidazole, phenylbutazone, ranitidine, salicylates, sulfonamides, trimethoprim: Possibly impaired metabolism of these drugs, increased risk of phenytoin toxicity
CNS depressants: Possibly increased CNS depression
corticosteroids, cyclosporine, digoxin, disopyramide, doxycycline, furosemide, levodopa, mexiletine, quinidine: Decreased therapeutic effects of these drugs
diazoxide: Possibly decreased therapeutic effects of both drugs
dopamine: Possibly sudden hypotension or cardiac arrest after I.V. fosphenytoin administration
estrogen- and progestin-containing contraceptives: Possibly breakthrough bleeding and decreased contraceptive effectiveness
estrogens, progestins: Decreased therapeutic effects, increased blood phenytoin level
felbamate: Possibly impaired metabolism and increased blood level of phenytoin
fluconazole, itraconazole, ketoconazole, miconazole: Increased blood phenytoin level
folic acid: Increased phenytoin metabolism, decreased seizure control
haloperidol: Possibly lowered seizure threshold and decreased therapeutic effects of fosphenytoin; possibly decreased blood haloperidol level
insulin, oral antidiabetic drugs: Possibly increased blood glucose level and decreased therapeutic effects of these drugs
lamotrigine: Possibly decreased therapeutic effects of lamotrigine

lidocaine: Possibly decreased blood lidocaine level, increased myocardial depression
lithium: Increased risk of lithium toxicity
methadone: Possibly increased methadone metabolism, leading to withdrawal symptoms
molindone: Possibly lowered seizure threshold, impaired absorption, and decreased therapeutic effects of phenytoin
omeprazole: Possibly increased blood phenytoin level
oral anticoagulants: Possibly impaired metabolism of these drugs and increased risk of phenytoin toxicity; possibly increased anticoagulant effects initially and then decreased effects with prolonged therapy
rifampin: Possibly decreased therapeutic effects of phenytoin
streptozocin: Possibly decreased therapeutic effects of streptozocin
sucralfate: Possibly decreased phenytoin absorption
tricyclic antidepressants: Possibly lowered seizure threshold and decreased therapeutic effects of phenytoin; possibly decreased blood antidepressant level
valproic acid: Decreased blood phenytoin level, increased blood valproic acid level
vitamin D analogues: Decreased vitamin D analogue activity
xanthines: Possibly inhibited phenytoin absorption and increased clearance of xanthines
zaleplon: Increased clearance and decreased effectiveness of zaleplon
ACTIVITIES
alcohol use: Possibly decreased phenytoin effectiveness

Adverse Reactions

CNS: Agitation, amnesia, asthenia, ataxia, cerebral edema, chills, coma, confusion, CVA, delusions, depression, dizziness, emotional lability, encephalitis, encephalopathy, extrapyramidal reactions, fever, headache, hemiplegia, hostility, hypoesthesia, lack of coordination, malaise, meningitis, nervousness, neurosis, paralysis, personality disorder, positive Babinski's sign, seizures, somnolence, speech disorders, stupor, subdural hematoma, syncope, transient paresthesia, tremor, vertigo
CV: Atrial flutter, bradycardia, bundle-branch block, cardiac arrest, cardiomegaly, edema, heart failure, hypertension, hypotension, orthostatic hypotension, palpitations, PVCs, shock, tachycardia, thrombophlebitis
EENT: Amblyopia, conjunctivitis, diplopia, dry mouth, earache, epistaxis, eye pain, gingival hyperplasia, hearing loss, hyperacusis,

increased salivation, loss of taste, mydriasis, nystagmus, pharyngitis, photophobia, rhinitis, sinusitis, taste perversion, tinnitus, tongue swelling, visual field defects
ENDO: Diabetes insipidus, hyperglycemia, ketosis
GI: Anorexia, constipation, diarrhea, dysphagia, elevated liver function test results, flatulence, gastritis, GI bleeding, hepatic necrosis, hepatitis, ileus, indigestion, nausea, vomiting
GU: Albuminuria, dysuria, incontinence, oliguria, polyuria, renal failure, urine retention, vaginal candidiasis
HEME: Anemia, easy bruising, leukopenia, thrombocytopenia
MS: Arthralgia, back pain, leg cramps, muscle twitching, myalgia, myasthenia, myoclonus, myopathy
RESP: Apnea, asthma, atelectasis, bronchitis, dyspnea, hemoptysis, hyperventilation, hypoxia, increased cough, increased sputum production, pneumonia, pneumothorax
SKIN: Contact dermatitis, diaphoresis, maculopapular or pustular rash, nodules, photosensitivity, skin discoloration, Stevens-Johnson syndrome, transient pruritus, urticaria
Other: Cachexia, cryptococcosis, dehydration, facial edema, flu-like symptoms, hyperkalemia, hypokalemia, hypophosphatemia, infection, injection site reaction, lymphadenopathy, sepsis

Nursing Considerations

- **WARNING** Express the dosage, concentration, and infusion rate of fosphenytoin in PE units. Misreading an order or a label could result in a massive overdose.
- Dilute drug in D_5W or normal saline solution to 1.5 to 25 mg PE/ml. Use within 8 hours if stored at room temperature or within 24 hours if refrigerated.
- Inspect parenteral solution before administration. Discard solution that contains particles or is discolored.
- Be aware that drug is also administered by I.M. injection for maintenance doses. I.M. injection shouldn't be given for status epilepticus because I.V. route allows faster onset and peak.
- Keep in mind that I.V. fosphenytoin administration doesn't require use of a filter, as does phenytoin administration.
- Don't administer fosphenytoin solution at a rate exceeding 150 mg PE/minute because of the risk of hypotension. For a 50-kg (110-lb) patient, infusion typically takes 5 to 7 minutes. Be aware that I.V. fosphenytoin may be administered more rapidly than I.V. phenytoin.
- Follow loading dose with maintenance dosage of oral or parenteral phenytoin or parenteral fosphenytoin, as prescribed.

- As prescribed, give an I.V. benzodiazepine (such as lorazepam or diazepam) with fosphenytoin; otherwise, drug's full antiepileptic effect won't be immediate.
- Monitor ECG, blood pressure, and respiratory function during fosphenytoin infusion and for 10 to 20 minutes afterward.
- Expect to obtain blood fosphenytoin (phenytoin) level 2 hours after infusion. Therapeutic level generally ranges from 10 to 20 mcg/ml; steady state may be reached after several days to several weeks.
- Be aware that fosphenytoin may be substituted for oral phenytoin sodium at same total daily dose and frequency. If prescribed, give daily amount in two or more divided doses to maintain seizure control.
- When switching between phenytoin and fosphenytoin, remember that small differences in phenytoin bioavailability can lead to significant changes in blood phenytoin level and an increased risk of toxicity.
- If drug causes transient, infusion-related paresthesia and pruritus, decrease dosage or discontinue infusion, as ordered.
- Monitor CBC for thrombocytopenia or leukopenia—signs of hematologic toxicity. Also monitor serum albumin level and results of renal and liver function tests.
- Anticipate increased frequency and severity of adverse reactions after I.V. administration in patients with hepatic or renal impairment or hypoalbuminemia.
- Discontinue drug, as ordered, if patient develops signs of hypersensitivity—such as acute hepatotoxicity (hepatic necrosis and hepatitis), fever, lymphadenopathy, and skin reactions—during first 2 months of therapy.
- Monitor blood phenytoin level to detect early signs of toxicity, such as diplopia, nausea, confusion, slurred speech, and vomiting. Expect to reduce dosage or stop drug if such signs occur.
- **WARNING** Monitor for seizures because phenytoin is excitatory at toxic levels.
- **WARNING** If patient has bradycardia or heart block rhythm, notify prescriber and expect to withhold drug because severe CV reactions and death have occurred.
- Expect to provide vitamin D supplement if patient has inadequate dietary intake and is receiving long-term anticonvulsant treatment.
- Document type, onset, and characteristics of seizures as well as response to treatment.

- Before diluting fosphenytoin, store it at 2° to 8° C (36° to 46° F); don't freeze.

PATIENT TEACHING

- Inform patient that fosphenytoin typically is used for short-term treatment.
- Instruct patient to immediately report bothersome symptoms, especially rash and swollen glands.
- Because gingival hyperplasia may develop during long-term therapy, emphasize the importance of good oral hygiene and gum massage.
- Urge patient to consume an adequate amount of vitamin D–rich foods.

furosemide

Lasix, Lasix Special (CAN), Uritol (CAN)

Class and Category

Chemical: Sulfonamide
Therapeutic: Antihypertensive, diuretic
Pregnancy category: C

Indications and Dosages

▶ *To reduce edema caused by cirrhosis, heart failure, and renal disease, including nephrotic syndrome*

I.V. INFUSION OR INJECTION

Adults. 20 to 40 mg as a single dose, increased by 20 mg q 2 hr until desired response occurs.

Children. 1 mg/kg as a single dose, increased by 1 mg/kg q 2 hr until desired response occurs. *Maximum:* 6 mg/kg/dose.

DOSAGE ADJUSTMENT Initial single dose limited to 20 mg for elderly patients.

▶ *To manage mild to moderate hypertension, as adjunct to treat acute pulmonary edema and hypertensive crisis*

I.V. INFUSION OR INJECTION

Adults with normal renal function. 40 to 80 mg as a single dose over several min.

Adults with acute renal failure or pulmonary edema. 100 to 200 mg as a single dose over several min.

DOSAGE ADJUSTMENT For patients with acute pulmonary edema without hypertensive crisis, dosage reduced to 40 mg, followed by 80 mg 1 hr later if therapeutic response doesn't occur.

Route	Onset	Peak	Duration
I.V.	5 min	30 min	2 hr

Mechanism of Action

Inhibits sodium and water reabsorption in the loop of Henle and increases urine formation. As the body's plasma volume decreases, aldosterone production increases, which promotes sodium reabsorption and the loss of potassium and hydrogen ions. Furosemide also increases the excretion of calcium, magnesium, bicarbonate, ammonium, and phosphate. By reducing intracellular and extracellular fluid volume, the drug reduces blood pressure and decreases cardiac output. Over time, cardiac output returns to normal.

Incompatibilities

Don't mix furosemide (a milky, buffered alkaline solution) with highly acidic solutions.

Contraindications

Anuria unresponsive to furosemide; hypersensitivity to furosemide, sulfonamides, or their components

Interactions

DRUGS

ACE inhibitors: Possibly first-dose hypotension
aminoglycosides, cisplatin: Increased risk of ototoxicity
amiodarone: Increased risk of arrhythmias from hypokalemia
chloral hydrate: Possibly diaphoresis, hot flashes, and hypertension
digoxin: Increased risk of digitalis toxicity related to hypokalemia
insulin, oral antidiabetic drugs: Increased blood glucose level
lithium: Increased risk of lithium toxicity
NSAIDs: Possibly decreased diuresis
phenytoin, probenecid: Possibly decreased therapeutic effects of furosemide
propranolol: Possibly increased blood propranolol level
thiazide diuretics: Possibly profound diuresis and electrolyte imbalance

ACTIVITIES

alcohol use: Possibly increased hypotensive and diuretic effects of furosemide

Adverse Reactions

CNS: Dizziness, fever, headache, paresthesia, restlessness, vertigo, weakness

CV: Orthostatic hypotension, shock, thromboembolism, thrombophlebitis
EENT: Blurred vision, ototoxicity, stomatitis, tinnitus, transient hearing loss (rapid I.V. injection), yellow vision
ENDO: Hyperglycemia
GI: Abdominal cramps, anorexia, constipation, diarrhea, indigestion, nausea, pancreatitis, vomiting
GU: Bladder spasms, glycosuria
HEME: Agranulocytosis (rare), anemia, aplastic anemia (rare), azotemia, hemolytic anemia, leukopenia, thrombocytopenia
MS: Muscle spasms
SKIN: Erythema multiforme, exfoliative dermatitis, jaundice, photosensitivity, pruritus, purpura, rash, urticaria
Other: Allergic reaction (interstitial nephritis, necrotizing vasculitis, systemic vasculitis), dehydration, hyperuricemia, hypochloremia, hypokalemia, hyponatremia, hypovolemia

Nursing Considerations

- Obtain patient's weight before and periodically during furosemide therapy to monitor fluid loss.
- For once-a-day dosing, give drug in the morning so patient's sleep won't be interrupted by increased need to urinate.
- Prepare drug for infusion with normal saline solution, lactated Ringer's solution, or D_5W. Use within 24 hours.
- Administer drug slowly over 1 to 2 minutes to prevent ototoxicity. Expect to administer high doses by controlled I.V. infusion at a rate not exceeding 4 mg/minute.
- Expect patient to have periodic hearing tests during prolonged or high-dose I.V. therapy.
- Monitor blood pressure and hepatic and renal function as well as BUN, blood glucose, and serum creatinine, electrolyte, and uric acid levels, as appropriate.
- Be aware that elderly patients are more susceptible to drug's hypotensive and electrolyte-altering effects and thus are at greater risk for shock and thromboembolism.
- **WARNING** Be aware that furosemide use in patients with advanced hepatic cirrhosis, especially those who also have a history of electrolyte imbalance or hepatic encephalopathy, may lead to lethal hepatic coma. Assess patient with cirrhosis for signs of deteriorating hepatic function, such as confusion, decreasing mental alertness, lethargy, and asterixis.
- If patient is at high risk for hypokalemia, give potassium supplements along with furosemide, as prescribed.

- Expect to discontinue furosemide at maximum dosage if oliguria persists for longer than 24 hours.
- Be aware that furosemide may worsen left ventricular hypertrophy and adversely affect glucose tolerance and lipid metabolism.
- Notify prescriber if patient experiences hearing loss, vertigo, or ringing, buzzing, or sense of fullness in her ears. Drug may need to be discontinued.
- Store drug at 15° to 30° C (59° to 86° F); protect from freezing and light.

PATIENT TEACHING

- Advise patient receiving furosemide to change position slowly to minimize effects of orthostatic hypotension, and to take furosemide with food or milk to reduce GI distress.
- Caution patient against drinking alcoholic beverages, standing for prolonged periods, and exercising in hot weather because these actions increase the hypotensive effect of furosemide.
- Emphasize the importance of controlling weight and diet, especially of limiting sodium intake.
- Unless contraindicated, urge patient to eat more high-potassium foods and to take a potassium supplement, if prescribed, to prevent hypokalemia.
- Instruct patient to keep follow-up appointments with prescriber to monitor progress. Urge her to report persistent, severe nausea, vomiting, and diarrhea because these reactions may cause dehydration.
- Inform diabetic patient that her blood glucose level will be checked often.

G•H

ganciclovir sodium

Cytovene (CAN), Cytovene-IV

Class and Category

Chemical: Acyclic guanosine analogue
Therapeutic: Antiviral
Pregnancy category: C

Indications and Dosages

▶ *To treat cytomegalovirus (CMV) retinitis in immunocompromised patients, including patients with AIDS*

I.V. INFUSION

Adults and adolescents. *Induction:* 5 mg/kg over at least 1 hr q 12 hr for 14 to 21 days. *Maintenance:* 5 mg/kg over at least 1 hr daily for 7 days/wk, or 6 mg/kg over at least 1 hr daily for 5 days/wk.

▶ *To prevent CMV disease in transplant recipients at risk for it*

I.V. INFUSION

Adults and adolescents. *Induction:* 5 mg/kg over at least 1 hr q 12 hr for 7 to 14 days. *Maintenance:* 5 mg/kg over at least 1 hr daily for 7 days/wk or 6 mg/kg over at least 1 hr daily for 5 days/wk.

DOSAGE ADJUSTMENT For patients with impaired renal function, dosage reduced as follows: for creatinine clearance of 50 to 69 ml/min/1.73 m^2, induction and maintenance dosages reduced to 2.5 mg/kg q 12 hr; for clearance of 25 to 49 ml/min/1.73 m^2, induction dosage reduced to 2.5 mg/kg q 24 hr and maintenance dosage reduced to 1.25 mg/kg q 24 hr; for clearance of 10 to 24 ml/min/1.73 m^2, induction dosage reduced to 1.25 mg/kg q 24 hr and maintenance dosage reduced to 0.625 mg/kg q 24 hr; and for clearance of less than 10 ml/min/1.73 m^2, induction dosage reduced to 1.25 mg/kg three times/wk after dialysis and maintenance dosage reduced to 0.625 mg/kg three times/wk after dialysis.

Mechanism of Action

Inhibits replication of CMV. Infected cells take up ganciclovir, which is then converted by cellular enzymes to ganciclovir triphosphate. Ganciclovir triphosphate is incorporated into the DNA chain and inhibits viral DNA polymerase, an enzyme used in the viral DNA replication process. This inhibits DNA synthesis by suppressing the ability of the DNA chain to elongate, which is part of the cellular replication process. Uninfected cells also take up ganciclovir and produce low levels of ganciclovir triphosphate, but the drug inhibits viral DNA polymerase more effectively than it inhibits cellular polymerase.

Incompatibilities

Don't mix ganciclovir with bacteriostatic water for injection containing parabens because a precipitate may form.

Contraindications

Hypersensitivity to ganciclovir or acyclovir

Interactions

DRUGS

blood-dyscrasia–causing drugs (such as cephalosporins and sulfasalazine), bone marrow depressants (such as carboplatin and lomustine): Possibly additive bone marrow depression

didanosine: Increased blood didanosine level, possibly increased blood ganciclovir level

imipenem and cilastatin: Possible risk of generalized seizures

nephrotoxic drugs (such as amphotericin B, cyclosporine, and tacrolimus): Possibly increased serum creatinine level, increased risk of impaired renal function, decreased ganciclovir elimination, and increased risk of ganciclovir toxicity

probenecid: Possibly decreased ganciclovir elimination and increased risk of ganciclovir toxicity

zidovudine: Possibly hematologic toxicity

Adverse Reactions

CNS: Fever, mental and mood changes, nervousness, neuropathy, tremors

GI: Abdominal pain, anorexia, diarrhea, elevated liver function test results, nausea, vomiting

HEME: Anemia, granulocytopenia, leukopenia, neutropenia, thrombocytopenia

SKIN: Rash

Other: Infusion site pain

Nursing Considerations

- Monitor CBC and platelet count before initiating ganciclovir therapy, every 2 days during induction, and at least once a week thereafter. Expect to perform daily neutrophil and platelet counts in patients undergoing hemodialysis, patients with neutrophil counts less than $1,000/mm^3$ at beginning of treatment, and patients who have had leukopenia during previous treatment with ganciclovir or other nucleoside analogues.
- Be aware that ganciclovir shouldn't be given to patient with neutrophil count of less than $500/mm^3$ or platelet count of less than $25,000/mm^3$.
- Be aware that ganciclovir shares some mutagenic and carcinogenic properties of antineoplastics. Follow facility protocols for preparation and handling of such drugs and for appropriate disposal of used equipment.
- **WARNING** Avoid inhaling, ingesting, or coming in direct contact with ganciclovir. If ganciclovir solution comes in contact with your skin or mucosa, wash it off thoroughly with soap and water. If drug comes in contact with your eye, irrigate it thoroughly with plain water.
- To reconstitute ganciclovir, add 10 ml of sterile water for injection to 500-mg vial to yield a concentration of 50 mg/ml. Don't use bacteriostatic water for injection containing parabens to reconstitute ganciclovir because a precipitate may form. Shake vial until solution is clear. Store at room temperature and use within 12 hours.
- Further dilute reconstituted ganciclovir, typically with 100 ml of normal saline solution, D_5W, lactated Ringer's solution, or Ringer's solution, to a final concentration of 10 mg/ml or less. Refrigerate if not given immediately. Use within 24 hours.
- Infuse ganciclovir at a constant rate, over at least 1 hour, through a central or peripheral line. Ensure that patient is adequately hydrated, as ordered.
- Expect to administer no more than 1.25 mg/kg/24 hours if patient receives hemodialysis. Administer ganciclovir dose after hemodialysis to prevent decreased plasma ganciclovir level.
- Be aware that reinduction treatment may be ordered if CMV retinitis progresses while patient is on maintenance therapy.
- Monitor renal and liver function tests, as ordered. Anticipate a dosage adjustment or increased dosing intervals if renal function test results are elevated.

- Observe patient for fever, chills, pharyngitis, tiredness or weakness, or unusual bleeding or ecchymosis. Be aware that granulocytopenia typically occurs during the first week of treatment but may occur at any time.
- Be aware that patients receiving concurrent radiation therapy are at risk for additive bone marrow depression.
- Store unopened vials below 40° C (104° F).

PATIENT TEACHING

- Inform patient that ganciclovir is not a cure for CMV retinitis and that the disease may progress during or after treatment. Explain that maintenance therapy is used to help prevent relapse.
- Advise patient to contact prescriber immediately if he notices unusual bleeding or bruising, black or tarry stools, blood in urine or stool, or red pinpoint spots on skin.
- Teach patient proper oral hygiene and encourage him to use a soft-bristled toothbrush because ganciclovir can delay healing, increase the risk of infection, and cause gingival bleeding. Advise patient to check with prescriber before undergoing any dental work.
- Stress the importance of avoiding accidental cuts from sharp objects, such as razors or fingernail clippers, because excessive bleeding or infection may occur.
- Teach patient about the need for contraception during ganciclovir treatment because drug has caused birth defects in animals. Advise female patients to use effective contraceptive method during treatment and male patients to use barrier protection during treatment and for 90 days afterward. Inform patient that ganciclovir may cause infertility.
- Stress the importance of keeping follow-up appointments, including those for ophthalmic examinations, which may be scheduled weekly during induction and every 4 weeks during maintenance therapy.

gentamicin sulfate

Cidomycin (CAN), Garamycin, G-Mycin, Jenamicin

Class and Category

Chemical: Aminoglycoside derived from *Micromonospora purpurea*
Therapeutic: Antibiotic
Pregnancy category: D

Indications and Dosages

▶ *To treat serious bacterial infections caused by aerobic gram-negative organisms and some gram-positive organisms, including* Citrobacter *sp.,* Enterobacter *sp.,* Escherichia coli, Klebsiella *sp.,* Proteus *sp.,* Pseudomonas aeruginosa, Serratia *sp.,* Staphylococcus aureus, *and many strains of* Streptococcus *sp.*

I.V. INFUSION

Adults and adolescents. 1 to 1.7 mg/kg q 8 hr for 7 to 10 days.
Children. 2 to 2.5 mg/kg q 8 hr for 7 to 10 days.
Infants. 2.5 mg/kg q 8 to 16 hr for 7 to 10 days.
Premature or full-term neonates up to age 1 week. 2.5 mg/kg q 12 to 24 hr for 7 to 10 days.

▶ *To treat uncomplicated UTI*

I.V. INFUSION

Adults and adolescents weighing 60 kg (132 lb) or more. 160 mg daily or 80 mg q 12 hr.
Adults and adolescents weighing less than 60 kg. 3 mg/kg daily or 1.5 mg/kg q 12 hr.

DOSAGE ADJUSTMENT Supplemental dose of 1 to 1.7 mg/kg (2 to 2.5 mg/kg for children) given after hemodialysis, based on severity of infection.

Mechanism of Action

Binds to negatively charged sites on the outer cell membrane of bacteria, thereby disrupting the membrane's integrity. Gentamicin also binds to bacterial ribosomal subunits and inhibits protein synthesis. Both actions lead to cell death.

Incompatibilities

Don't administer gentamicin through same I.V. line as other drugs, especially beta-lactam antibiotics (penicillins and cephalosporins), because substantial mutual inactivation may occur. Give drugs through separate sites.

Contraindications

Hypersensitivity to gentamicin or its components, hypersensitivity or serious toxic reaction to other aminoglycosides

Interactions

DRUGS

aminoglycosides (concurrent use of two or more): Decreased bacterial

uptake of each drug, increased risk of ototoxicity and nephrotoxicity
cephalosporins, enflurane, methoxyflurane, vancomycin: Increased risk of nephrotoxicity
loop diuretics: Increased risk of ototoxicity and nephrotoxicity
neuromuscular blockers: Prolonged respiratory depression, increased neuromuscular blockade
penicillins: Inactivation of gentamicin by certain penicillins, increased risk of nephrotoxicity

Adverse Reactions

CNS: Acute organic mental syndrome, confusion, depression, fever, headache, increased protein in cerebrospinal fluid, lethargy, myasthenia gravis–like syndrome, neurotoxicity (dizziness, hearing loss, tinnitus, vertigo), peripheral neuropathy or encephalopathy (muscle twitching, numbness, seizures, skin tingling), pseudotumor cerebri
CV: Hypertension, hypotension, palpitations
EENT: Blurred vision, increased salivation, laryngeal edema, ototoxicity, stomatitis, vision changes
GI: Anorexia, nausea, splenomegaly, transient hepatomegaly, vomiting
GU: Nephrotoxicity
HEME: Anemia, eosinophilia, granulocytopenia, increased or decreased reticulocyte count, leukopenia, thrombocytopenia
MS: Arthralgia, leg cramps
RESP: Pulmonary fibrosis, respiratory depression
SKIN: Alopecia, generalized burning sensation, pruritus, purpura, rash, urticaria
Other: Anaphylaxis, injection site pain, superinfection, weight loss

Nursing Considerations

- Before gentamicin therapy begins, expect to obtain a body fluid or tissue specimen for culture and sensitivity testing, as ordered.
- Dilute each dose with 50 to 200 ml of normal saline solution or D_5W to yield no more than 1 mg/ml. Be aware that no further dilution is needed if premixed flexible bags are used. Don't use an I.V. line with series connections when administering drug from a premixed flexible container to decrease the risk of air embolism. Don't administer if solution is discolored or contains precipitate. Administer slowly over 30 to 60 minutes.
- Expect to adjust dosage based on peak and trough blood drug levels drawn after third maintenance dose, as prescribed.

- Don't give gentamicin to pregnant women because drug can cause hearing loss in fetus.
- **WARNING** Be alert for allergic reactions—including anaphylaxis and, possibly, life-threatening asthmatic episodes—because some forms of drug contain sodium bisulfite.
- Assess for signs of other infections because gentamicin may cause overgrowth of nonsusceptible organisms.
- Be aware that premature infants, neonates, elderly patients, patients with impaired renal function, and dehydrated patients are at increased risk for nephrotoxicity.
- Be aware that premixed form contains 19.6 mEq of sodium per 50 ml. Take this into consideration if patient is on a sodium-restricted diet.
- Be aware that infants with botulism and patients with myasthenia gravis or Parkinson's disease may experience increased muscle weakness.
- Be aware that patients with impairment of cranial nerve VIII are at increased risk for ototoxicity or vestibular toxicity.
- Store vial at 15° to 30° C (59° to 86° F); store flexible bag at 2° to 30° C (36° to 86° F). Don't freeze gentamicin.

PATIENT TEACHING

- Stress the importance of completing the full course of gentamicin therapy.
- Instruct patient to immediately report adverse reactions, such as hearing loss, to avoid permanent effects.
- Emphasize the importance of keeping follow-up appointments and having diagnostic tests, such as audiometric tests and renal function tests, if ordered.

glucagon

Glucagon Diagnostic Kit, Glucagon Emergency Kit

Class and Category

Chemical: Synthetic hormone
Therapeutic: Antihypoglycemic, diagnostic aid adjunct
Pregnancy category: B

Indications and Dosages

▶ *To provide emergency treatment of severe hypoglycemia*

I.V. INJECTION

Adults and children weighing more than 20 kg (44 lb). 1 mg, repeated in 15 min if needed.

Children weighing 20 kg or less. 0.5 mg, or 0.02 to 0.03 mg/kg, repeated in 15 min, if needed.

▶ *To provide diagnostic assistance by inhibiting bowel peristalsis in radiologic examination of GI tract*

I.V. INJECTION

Adults. 0.25 to 2 mg before procedure. Dose, route, and timing vary with segment of GI tract examined and length of procedure.

Route	Onset	Peak	Duration
I.V.	5 to 20 min*†	Unknown	90 min*‡

Mechanism of Action

Increases production of adenylate cyclase, which catalyzes the conversion of adenosine triphosphate to cAMP, a process that in turn activates phosphorylase. Phosphorylase promotes the breakdown of glycogen to glucose (glycogenolysis) in the liver. As a result, the blood glucose level increases and GI smooth muscles relax.

Incompatibilities

Don't mix glucagon with sodium chloride or solutions that have a pH of 3.0 to 9.5; use with dextrose solutions instead.

Contraindications

Hypersensitivity to glucagon or its components, pheochromocytoma

Interactions

DRUGS

oral anticoagulants: Possibly increased anticoagulant effects

Adverse Reactions

CV: Hypertension, hypotension (with hypersensitivity reaction), tachycardia

GI: Nausea, vomiting

RESP: Bronchospasm, respiratory distress

SKIN: Urticaria

Nursing Considerations

- Rouse patient as quickly as possible because prolonged hypoglycemia can cause cerebral damage.

* For antihypoglycemic action.

† 45 sec to 1 min for smooth-muscle relaxation.

‡ 9 to 25 min for smooth-muscle relaxation.

- For I.V. use, reconstitute a 1-mg vial of glucagon with 1 ml of diluent or a 10-mg vial with 10 ml of diluent. Don't give more than 1 mg/ml. For large doses, dilute with sterile water for injection.
- Before injecting glucagon, place unconscious patient on his side to prevent aspiration of vomitus when he regains consciousness.
- Administer by slow I.V. injection to decrease the risk of adverse reactions, such as tachycardia and vomiting.
- If patient doesn't respond to glucagon, expect to administer I.V. dextrose.
- When patient has regained consciousness or as soon as diagnostic procedure is completed, give him oral carbohydrates to restore hepatic glycogen stores and prevent secondary hypoglycemia.
- Keep in mind that glucagon isn't effective in patients with depleted hepatic glycogen stores caused by such conditions as adrenal insufficiency, chronic hypoglycemia, and starvation.

PATIENT TEACHING

- Instruct patient to monitor his blood glucose level, especially when signs of hypoglycemia occur.
- Teach patient and family members how to recognize signs of hypoglycemia and when to notify prescriber.
- Advise patient to carry candy or other simple sugars with him to treat early hypoglycemia.
- Emphasize the importance of a consistent diet, regular exercise, and proper use of insulin or an oral antidiabetic drug.
- Make sure unstable diabetic patients and family members know how to give glucagon subcutaneously in case of hypoglycemia. Instruct family members to keep patient on his side and give him a carbohydrate when he awakens. Advise against giving fluids by mouth until patient is fully conscious.
- Instruct patient and family members to call for emergency medical assistance after glucagon treatment, especially if patient can't ingest oral glucose or if he's taking the sulfonylurea chlorpropamide, in case secondary hypoglycemia occurs.

glycopyrrolate

Robinul

Class and Category

Chemical: Quaternary ammonium compound

Therapeutic: Antiarrhythmic, anticholinergic, cholinergic adjunct
Pregnancy category: B

Indications and Dosages

▶ *To treat peptic ulcer disease*

I.V, INJECTION

Adults and adolescents. 0.1 to 0.2 mg q 4 hr, p.r.n. *Maximum:* 4 doses daily.

▶ *To counteract intraoperative and anesthesia-induced arrhythmias*

I.V. INJECTION

Adults and adolescents. 0.1 mg, repeated q 2 to 3 min, if needed.

Children over age 2. 0.0044 mg/kg, repeated q 2 to 3 min, if needed. *Maximum:* 0.1 mg as a single dose.

▶ *As cholinergic adjunct in curariform block*

I.V. INJECTION

Adults and children over age 2. 0.2 mg glycopyrrolate for each 1 mg neostigmine or 5 mg pyridostigmine when given together.

Route	Onset	Peak	Duration
I.V.	1 min	Unknown	2 to 3 hr*

Mechanism of Action

Inhibits acetylcholine's action on postganglionic muscarinic receptors throughout the body. Depending on the receptors' location, glycopyrrolate produces various effects, such as:

- reducing the volume and acidity of gastric secretions
- controlling excessive bronchial, pharyngeal, and tracheal secretions and dilating the bronchi
- inhibiting vagal stimulation of the heart
- relaxing smooth muscle in the GI and GU tracts.

Incompatibilities

Don't mix glycopyrrolate with alkaline drugs or solutions with a pH over 6.0 because drug stability may be affected. A pH over 6.0 may occur if glycopyrrolate is mixed with dexamethasone sodium phosphate or LR solution. Gas or precipitate may form if glycopyrrolate is mixed in same syringe as chloramphenicol, diazepam,

* For vagal blocking effect.

dimenhydrinate, methohexital sodium, pentobarbital sodium, secobarbital sodium, sodium bicarbonate, or thiopental sodium.

Contraindications

Angle-closure glaucoma, asthma, hemorrhage with unstable cardiovascular status, hepatic disease, hypersensitivity to anticholinergics, ileus, intestinal atony, myasthenia gravis, obstructive GI or urinary disorders, severe ulcerative colitis, toxic megacolon

Interactions

DRUGS

anticholinergics, antiparkinsonian drugs, phenothiazines, tricyclic antidepressants: Possibly increased anticholinergic effects
antidiarrheals (adsorbent): Decreased glycopyrrolate absorption, leading to decreased therapeutic effectiveness
antimyasthenics: Possibly reduced intestinal motility
atenolol: Possibly potentiated atenolol effects
calcium- or magnesium-containing antacids, carbonic anhydrase inhibitors, citrates, sodium bicarbonate: Possibly reduced excretion of glycopyrrolate and increased therapeutic and adverse effects
cyclopropane: Possibly ventricular arrhythmias
digoxin: Possibly potentiated digoxin effects
haloperidol, phenothiazines: Possibly decreased effectiveness of these drugs
ketoconazole: Possibly decreased ketoconazole absorption
metoclopramide: Possibly antagonized effects of metoclopramide
opioids: Possibly severe constipation and urine retention, risk of ileus
potassium chloride: Possibly increased severity of potassium chloride–induced gastric lesions

Adverse Reactions

CNS: Confusion, dizziness, drowsiness, headache, insomnia, nervousness, weakness
CV: Bradycardia (low doses), heart block, palpitations, prolonged QT interval, tachycardia (high doses)
EENT: Blurred vision, cycloplegia, dilated pupils, dry mouth, increased intraocular pressure, loss of taste, mydriasis, nasal congestion, photophobia, taste perversion
GI: Abdominal distention, constipation, dysphagia, nausea, vomiting
GU: Impotence, urinary hesitancy, urine retention
RESP: Dyspnea

SKIN: Decreased sweating (heat exhaustion), dry skin, flushing, pruritus, urticaria
Other: Anaphylaxis

Nursing Considerations

- Use glycopyrrolate cautiously in patients with autonomic neuropathy, hepatic disease, mild to moderate ulcerative colitis, prostatic hypertrophy, or hiatal hernia because drug's anticholinergic effect can worsen these conditions; gastric ulcer because drug may delay gastric emptying; and renal disease because drug excretion may be altered.
- For I.V. use, administer by direct injection without diluting. Or inject into tubing of a flowing I.V. solution unless it contains an alkaline drug or sodium bicarbonate.
- Closure system contains dry natural rubber that may cause hypersensitivity reaction if handled by or used to inject someone with latex sensitivity.
- Use continuous cardiac monitoring, as ordered, to assess patient for arrhythmias during drug administration.
- **WARNING** Check all doses carefully because even a slight overdose can lead to toxicity.
- To prevent overheating caused by decreased sweating, adjust the room temperature and make sure patient is well hydrated.

PATIENT TEACHING

- Caution patient about possible drowsiness and dizziness and need to avoid hazardous activities until drug effects are known.
- Suggest that he use sugarless hard candy, ice, or saliva substitute to relieve dry mouth.
- Tell patient to notify prescriber about abdominal distention, trouble breathing or urinating, eye pain, irregular heartbeat, sensitivity to light, or severe constipation.
- Inform male patient that reversible impotence may occur during therapy.
- If urinary hesitancy occurs, advise patient to void before taking each dose.

granisetron hydrochloride

Kytril

Class and Category

Chemical: Carbazole
Therapeutic: Antiemetic
Pregnancy category: B

Indications and Dosages

▶ *To prevent nausea and vomiting caused by chemotherapy*

I.V. INFUSION

Adults and adolescents. 10 mcg/kg diluted and infused over 5 min, starting 30 min before chemotherapy; or 10 mcg/kg undiluted and infused over 30 sec, starting 30 min before chemotherapy.

▶ *To prevent or treat postoperative nausea and vomiting*

I.V. INJECTION

Adults and adolescents. For prevention, 1 mg given over 30 sec before anesthesia induction or immediately before anesthesia reversal. For treatment, 1 mg given over 30 sec after surgery.

Mechanism of Action

Has a high affinity for serotonin receptors along vagal nerve endings in the intestines. Because of this affinity, granisetron prevents the nausea and vomiting that usually result when serotonin is released by damaged enterochromaffin cells.

Incompatibilities

Don't mix granisetron in same solution as other drugs.

Contraindications

Hypersensitivity to granisetron or its components

Interactions

DRUGS

ketoconazole: May inhibit effectiveness of granisetron

phenobarbital: Increased total plasma clearance of I.V. granisetron

Adverse Reactions

CNS: Asthenia, chills, CNS stimulation, drowsiness, fever, headache, insomnia, somnolence

CV: Hypertension

EENT: Taste perversion

GI: Abdominal pain, anorexia, constipation, diarrhea, elevated liver function test results, nausea, vomiting

HEME: Anemia, leukopenia, thrombocytopenia

SKIN: Alopecia

Nursing Considerations

- For use with chemotherapy, dilute I.V. preparation of granisetron with normal saline solution or D_5W to a total volume of 20 to 50 ml. Mixture may be stored for up to 24 hours. Use only on days when chemotherapy is given.

PATIENT TEACHING

- Inform patient that granisetron is given I.V. before chemotherapy to help prevent nausea.
- Advise patient to report constipation, fever, severe diarrhea, or severe headache to prescriber. Also caution him about possible drowsiness.

heparin calcium

Calcilean (CAN), Calciparine

heparin sodium

Hepalean (CAN), Heparin Leo (CAN), Heparin Lock Flush, Liquaemin

Class and Category

Chemical: Glycosaminoglycan
Therapeutic: Anticoagulant
Pregnancy category: C

Indications and Dosages

▶ *To prevent and treat deep vein thrombosis and pulmonary embolism, to treat peripheral arterial embolism, and to prevent thromboembolism before and after cardioversion of chronic atrial fibrillation*

I.V. INFUSION, I.V. INJECTION

Adults. *Loading:* 35 to 70 units/kg or 5,000 units by injection. Then 20,000 to 40,000 units infused over 24 hr.

Children. *Loading:* 50 units/kg by injection. Then 100 units/kg infused q 4 hr or 20,000 units/m^2 infused over 24 hr.

I.V. INJECTION

Adults. *Initial:* 10,000 units. *Maintenance:* 5,000 to 10,000 units q 4 to 6 hr.

Children. *Initial:* 50 units/kg. *Maintenance:* 100 units/kg/dose q 4 hr.

I.V. INJECTION

Adults. *Loading:* 5,000 units I.V.; then 10,000 to 20,000 units S.C. *Maintenance:* 8,000 to 10,000 units S.C. q 8 hr or 15,000 to 20,000 units S.C. q 12 hr.

▶ *To diagnose and treat disseminated intravascular coagulation (DIC)*

I.V. INFUSION, I.V. INJECTION

Adults. 50 to 100 units/kg q 4 hr. Drug may be discontinued if no improvement occurs in 4 to 8 hr.

Children. 25 to 50 units/kg q 4 hr. Drug may be discontinued if no improvement occurs in 4 to 8 hr.

▶ *To prevent clots in patients undergoing open-heart and vascular surgery*

I.V. INFUSION, I.V. INJECTION

Adults. 300 units/kg for procedures that last less than 60 min; 400 units/kg for procedures that last longer than 60 min. *Minimum:* 150 units/kg.

Children. 300 units/kg for procedures that last less than 60 min. Then dosage is based on coagulation test results. *Minimum:* 150 units/kg.

▶ *To maintain heparin lock patency*

I.V. INJECTION

Adults. 10 to 100 units/ml heparin flush solution (enough to fill device) after each use of device.

Route	Onset	Peak	Duration
I.V.	Immediate	Minutes	Unknown

Mechanism of Action

Binds with antithrombin III, enhancing antithrombin III's inactivation of the coagulation enzymes thrombin (factor IIa) and factors Xa and XIa. At low doses, heparin inhibits factor Xa and prevents the conversion of prothrombin to thrombin. Thrombin is necessary for the conversion of fibrinogen to fibrin; without fibrin, clots can't form. At high doses, heparin inactivates thrombin, preventing fibrin formation and existing clot extension.

Incompatibilities

Don't mix heparin with any other drug unless you have an order to do so and have checked with pharmacist. Heparin is incompatible with many drugs and solutions, especially ones that contain a phosphate buffer, sodium bicarbonate, or sodium oxalate.

Contraindications

Hypersensitivity to heparin or its components; severe thrombocytopenia; uncontrolled bleeding, except in DIC

Interactions

DRUGS

antihistamines, digoxin, nicotine, tetracyclines: Decreased anticoagulant effect of heparin

aspirin, NSAIDs, platelet aggregation inhibitors, sulfinpyrazone: Increased platelet inhibition and risk of bleeding
cefamandole, cefoperazone, cefotetan, methimazole, plicamycin, propylthiouracil, valproic acid: Possibly hypoprothrombinemia and increased risk of bleeding
chloroquine, hydroxychloroquine: Possibly thrombocytopenia and increased risk of hemorrhage
ethacrynic acid, glucocorticoids, salicylates: Increased risk of bleeding and GI ulceration and hemorrhage
nitroglycerin (I.V.): Possibly decreased anticoagulant effect of heparin
probenecid: Possibly increased anticoagulant effect of heparin
thrombolytics: Increased risk of hemorrhage
ACTIVITIES
smoking: Decreased anticoagulant effect of heparin

Adverse Reactions

CNS: Chills, dizziness, fever, headache, peripheral neuropathy
CV: Chest pain
EENT: Epistaxis, gingival bleeding, rhinitis
GI: Abdominal distention and pain, hematemesis, melena, nausea, vomiting
GU: Hematuria, hypermenorrhea
HEME: Easy bruising, excessive bleeding from wounds, thrombocytopenia
MS: Back pain, myalgia, osteoporosis
RESP: Dyspnea, wheezing
SKIN: Alopecia, cyanosis, petechiae, pruritus, urticaria
Other: Anaphylaxis; injection site hematoma, irritation, pain, redness, and ulceration

Nursing Considerations

- Use heparin cautiously in alcoholics; menstruating women; patients over age 60, especially women; and patients with mild hepatic or renal disease or a history of allergies, asthma, or GI ulcer.
- **WARNING** Give heparin only S.C. or I.V.; I.M. use causes hematoma, irritation, and pain.
- Avoid injecting any drugs by I.M. route during heparin therapy to decrease the risk of bleeding and hematoma.
- To prepare heparin for continuous infusion, invert container at least six times to prevent drug from pooling. Anticipate slight discoloration of prepared solution; this doesn't indicate a change in potency.

- During continuous I.V. therapy, expect to obtain APTT after 8 hours of therapy. Use the arm opposite the infusion site.
- For intermittent I.V. therapy, expect to adjust dose based on coagulation test results performed 30 minutes earlier. Therapeutic range is typically 1.5 to 2.5 times the control.
- Take safety precautions to prevent bleeding, such as having patient use a soft-bristled toothbrush and an electric razor.
- Monitor blood test results and observe for signs of bleeding, such as ecchymosis, epistaxis, hematemesis, hematuria, melena, and petechiae.
- Make sure all health care providers know that patient is receiving heparin.
- Keep protamine sulfate on hand to use as an antidote for heparin. Be aware that each milligram of protamine sulfate neutralizes 100 units of heparin.
- Be aware that prescriber may order oral anticoagulants before discontinuing heparin to avoid increased coagulation caused by heparin withdrawal. Heparin may be discontinued when full therapeutic effect of oral anticoagulant is achieved.
- Know that women over age 60 have the highest risk of hemorrhage during therapy.

PATIENT TEACHING

- Explain that heparin can't be taken orally.
- Inform patient about the increased risk of bleeding; urge her to avoid injuries and to use a soft-bristled toothbrush and an electric razor.
- Advise patient to avoid drugs that interact with heparin, such as aspirin and ibuprofen.
- Instruct patient and family to watch for and report abdominal or lower back pain, black stools, bleeding gums, bloody urine, excessive menstrual bleeding, nosebleeds, and severe headaches.
- Inform patient that temporary hair loss may occur.
- Advise patient to wear or carry appropriate medical identification.

hydralazine hydrochloride

Apresoline (CAN)

Class and Category

Chemical: Phthalazine derivative
Therapeutic: Antihypertensive, vasodilator

Pregnancy category: C

Indications and Dosages

▶ *To manage severe essential hypertension when drug can't be taken orally or when need to reduce blood pressure is urgent*

I.V. INJECTION

Adults. 5 to 40 mg, repeated as needed.

Children. 1.7 to 3.5 mg/kg daily in divided doses q 4 to 6 hr, as needed.

Route	Onset	Peak	Duration
I.V.	5 to 20 min	10 to 80 min	2 to 6 hr

Mechanism of Action

May act in a manner that resembles organic nitrates and sodium nitroprusside, except that hydralazine is selective for arteries. This drug:

- exerts a direct vasodilating effect on vascular smooth muscle
- interferes with calcium movement in vascular smooth muscle by altering cellular calcium metabolism
- dilates arteries rather than veins, which minimizes orthostatic hypotension and increases cardiac output and cerebral blood flow
- causes a reflex autonomic response that increases heart rate, cardiac output, and left ventricular ejection fraction
- has a positive inotropic effect on the heart.

Incompatibilities

Don't mix hydralazine in I.V. infusion solutions.

Contraindications

Coronary artery disease, hypersensitivity to hydralazine or its components, mitral valve disease

Interactions

DRUGS

beta blockers: Increased effects of both drugs

diazoxide, MAO inhibitors, other antihypertensives: Risk of severe hypotension

epinephrine: Possibly decreased vasopressor effect of epinephrine

NSAIDs: Decreased hydralazine effects

sympathomimetics: Possibly decreased antihypertensive effect of hydralazine

Adverse Reactions

CNS: Chills, fever, headache, peripheral neuritis
CV: Angina, edema, orthostatic hypotension, palpitations, tachycardia
EENT: Lacrimation, nasal congestion
GI: Anorexia, constipation, diarrhea, nausea, vomiting
RESP: Dyspnea
SKIN: Blisters, flushing, pruritus, rash, urticaria
Other: Lupuslike symptoms (especially with high doses), lymphadenopathy

Nursing Considerations

- Monitor CBC, lupus erythematosus cell preparation, and ANA titer before hydralazine therapy and periodically, as appropriate, during long-term treatment.
- Use drug immediately after opening ampule.
- Anticipate that drug may change color in solution. Consult pharmacist if color change occurs.
- Be aware that hydralazine also may undergo color changes when exposed to a metal filter.
- Monitor blood pressure and pulse rate regularly and weigh patient daily during therapy.
- Check blood pressure with patient in lying, sitting, and standing positions, and watch for signs of orthostatic hypotension. Expect orthostatic hypotension to be most common in the morning, during hot weather, and with exercise.
- **WARNING** Expect to discontinue drug immediately if patient experiences lupuslike symptoms, such as arthralgia, fever, myalgia, pharyngitis, and splenomegaly.
- Expect prescriber to withdraw drug gradually to avoid a rapid increase in blood pressure.
- Before opening ampule, store it at 15° to 30° C (59° to 86° F); don't freeze.
- Expect to treat peripheral neuritis with pyridoxine.

PATIENT TEACHING

- Advise patient to change position slowly, especially in the morning, while receiving hydralazine. Caution her that hot showers may increase hypotension.
- Instruct patient to immediately report fever, aching muscles and joints, and sore throat.
- Urge patient to report numbness and tingling in the limbs, which may require treatment with another drug.

hydrocortisone sodium phosphate

Hydrocortone Phosphate

hydrocortisone sodium succinate

A-hydroCort, Solu-Cortef

Class and Category

Chemical: Glucocorticoid
Therapeutic: Adrenocorticoid replacement, anti-inflammatory
Pregnancy category: Not rated

Indications and Dosages

▶ *To treat severe inflammation or acute adrenal insufficiency*

I.V. INFUSION OR INJECTION (HYDROCORTISONE SODIUM PHOSPHATE)

Adults. 15 to 240 mg daily as a single dose or in divided doses. *Usual:* One-half to one-third the oral dose.

DOSAGE ADJUSTMENT Dosage increased to more than 240 mg daily if needed to treat acute disease.

I.V. INFUSION OR INJECTION (HYDROCORTISONE SODIUM SUCCINATE)

Adults. 100 to 500 mg q 2, 4, or 6 hr.

Route	Onset	Peak	Duration
I.V. (phosphate, succinate)	Rapid	Unknown	Unknown

Mechanism of Action

Binds to intracellular glucocorticoid receptors and suppresses the inflammatory and immune responses by:

- inhibiting neutrophil and monocyte accumulation at the inflammation site and suppressing their phagocytic and bactericidal activity
- stabilizing lysosomal membranes
- suppressing the antigen response of macrophages and helper T cells
- inhibiting the synthesis of cellular mediators of the inflammatory response, such as cytokines, interleukins, and prostaglandins.

Contraindications

Hypersensitivity to hydrocortisone or its components, recent vaccination with live-virus vaccine, systemic fungal infection

Interactions

DRUGS

acetaminophen: Increased risk of hepatotoxicity
amphotericin B, carbonic anhydrase inhibitors: Possibly severe hypokalemia

anabolic steroids, androgens: Increased risk of edema and severe acne
anticholinergics: Possibly increased intraocular pressure
anticoagulants, thrombolytics: Increased risk of GI ulceration and hemorrhage, possibly decreased therapeutic effects of these drugs
asparaginase: Increased risk of hyperglycemia and toxicity
aspirin, NSAIDs: Increased risk of GI distress and bleeding
digoxin: Possibly hypokalemia-induced arrhythmias and digitalis toxicity
ephedrine, phenobarbital, phenytoin, rifampin: Decreased blood hydrocortisone level
estrogens, oral contraceptives: Possibly increased therapeutic and toxic effects of hydrocortisone
isoniazid: Possibly decreased therapeutic effects of isoniazid
mexiletine: Possibly decreased blood mexiletine level
neuromuscular blockers: Possibly increased neuromuscular blockade, causing respiratory depression or apnea
potassium-depleting drugs (such as thiazide diuretics): Possibly severe hypokalemia
potassium supplements: Possibly decreased effects of these supplements
salicylates: Possibly decreased effectiveness and blood level of salicylates
somatrem, somatropin: Possibly decreased therapeutic effects of these drugs
streptozocin: Increased risk of hyperglycemia
vaccines: Decreased antibody response and increased risk of neurologic complications
ACTIVITIES
alcohol use: Increased risk of GI distress and bleeding

Adverse Reactions

CNS: Ataxia, behavioral changes, depression, dizziness, euphoria, fatigue, headache, increased ICP with papilledema, insomnia, malaise, mood changes, paresthesia, seizures, steroid psychosis, syncope, vertigo
CV: Arrhythmias (from hypokalemia), fat embolism, heart failure, hypertension, hypotension, thromboembolism, thrombophlebitis
EENT: Exophthalmos, glaucoma, increased intraocular pressure, nystagmus, posterior subcapsular cataracts
ENDO: Adrenal insufficiency during stress, cushingoid symptoms (buffalo hump, central obesity, moon face, supraclavicular fat pad enlargement), diabetes mellitus, growth suppression in children, hyperglycemia, negative nitrogen balance from protein catabolism

GI: Abdominal distention, hiccups, increased appetite, nausea, pancreatitis, peptic ulcer, ulcerative esophagitis, vomiting
GU: Amenorrhea, glycosuria, menstrual irregularities, perineal burning or tingling
HEME: Easy bruising, leukocytosis
MS: Arthralgia; aseptic necrosis of femoral and humeral heads; compression fractures; muscle atrophy, twitching, or weakness; myalgia; osteoporosis; spontaneous fractures; steroid myopathy; tendon rupture
SKIN: Acne; altered skin pigmentation; diaphoresis; erythema; hirsutism; necrotizing vasculitis; petechiae; purpura; rash; scarring; sterile abscess; striae; subcutaneous fat atrophy; thin, fragile skin; urticaria
Other: Anaphylaxis, hypocalcemia, hypokalemia, hypokalemic alkalosis, impaired wound healing, masking of signs of infection, metabolic alkalosis, suppressed skin test reaction, weight gain

Nursing Considerations

- Be aware that systemic hydrocortisone shouldn't be given to immunocompromised patients, such as those with fungal and other infections, including amebiasis, hepatitis B, tuberculosis, vaccinia, and varicella.
- **WARNING** Don't give hydrocortisone containing benzyl alcohol to neonates or premature infants because they may develop a fatal toxic syndrome characterized by CNS, respiratory, circulatory, and renal impairment and metabolic acidosis.
- Give daily dose of hydrocortisone in the morning to mimic the normal peak in adrenocortical secretion of corticosteroids.
- Don't give acetate injectable suspension by I.V. route. This form is used for intra-articular, intralesional, and soft-tissue injection.
- Give hydrocortisone sodium succinate as direct I.V. injection over 30 seconds to several minutes, or as intermittent or continuous infusion. For infusion, dilute to 1 mg/ml or less with D_5W, normal saline solution, or dextrose 5% in normal saline solution. Use reconstituted hydrocortisone sodium succinate within 3 days. Protect reconstituted solution from light; discard if not clear.
- **WARNING** Avoid rapid admnistration of high hydrocortisone doses, which may cause anaphylaxis, angioedema, seizures, and possibly sudden death. Maintain ECG monitoring, as prescribed, and have emergency equipment and drugs readily available.

- Dilute hydrocortisone sodium phosphate with D_5W or normal saline solution, and use diluted solution within 24 hours.
- Be aware that high-dose therapy shouldn't be given for longer than 48 hours. Be alert for depression or psychotic episodes during high-dose therapy.
- Regularly monitor weight, blood pressure, and serum electrolyte levels during therapy.
- Expect hydrocortisone to exacerbate infections or mask their signs and symptoms.
- Monitor blood glucose level in diabetic patients, and increase insulin or oral antidiabetic drug dosage, as prescribed.
- Know that elderly patients are at high risk for osteoporosis during long-term therapy.
- Anticipate the possibility of acute adrenal insufficiency with stress, such as emotional upset, fever, surgery, and trauma. Increase hydrocortisone dosage, as prescribed.
- **WARNING** Avoid withdrawing drug suddenly after long-term use because adrenal crisis can result. Expect to reduce dosage gradually and to monitor patient's response.
- Store hydrocortisone at 15° to 30° C (59° to 86° F); don't freeze.

PATIENT TEACHING

- Instruct patient receiving hydrocortisone to report early signs of adrenal insufficiency: anorexia, difficulty breathing, dizziness, fainting, fatigue, joint pain, muscle weakness, and nausea.
- Inform patient that she may bruise easily.
- Advise patient on long-term therapy to have periodic ophthalmic examinations and to carry or wear medical identification.

hydromorphone hydrochloride (dihydromorphinone)

Dilaudid, Dilaudid-HP

Class, Category, and Schedule

Chemical: Phenanthrene derivative, semisynthetic opioid derivative
Therapeutic: Opioid analgesic
Pregnancy category: C
Controlled substance: Schedule II

Indications and Dosages

▶ *To relieve moderate to severe pain*

I.V. INJECTION

Adults. 1 mg q 3 hr, p.r.n.

Route	Onset	Peak	Duration
I.V.	10 to 15 min	15 to 30 min	2 to 3 hr

Mechanism of Action

May bind with opioid receptors in the spinal cord and higher levels in the CNS. In this way, hydromorphone is believed to stimulate mu and kappa receptors, thus altering the perception of, and emotional response to, pain.

Contraindications

Acute asthma; hypersensitivity to hydromorphone, other opioid analgesics, or their components; increased ICP; severe respiratory depression; upper respiratory tract obstruction

Interactions

DRUGS

anticholinergics: Increased risk of ileus, severe constipation, or urine retention
antihypertensives, diuretics, guanadrel, guanethidine, mecamylamine: Increased risk of orthostatic hypotension
barbiturate anesthetics: Increased sedative effect of hydromorphone
belladonna alkaloids, difenoxin and atropine, diphenoxylate and atropine, kaolin pectin, loperamide, paregoric: Increased risk of CNS depression and severe constipation
buprenorphine, butorphanol, dezocine, nalbuphine, pentazocine: Possibly potentiated or suppressed symptoms of spontaneous opioid withdrawal
CNS depressants, other opioid analgesics: Additive CNS depression and hypotension
hydroxyzine: Increased analgesia, CNS depression, and hypotension
metoclopramide: Decreased effect of metoclopramide on GI motility
naloxone: Possibly withdrawal symptoms in physically dependent patients
naltrexone: Possibly prolonged respiratory depression, cardiac arrest
neuromuscular blockers: Additive CNS depression

ACTIVITIES

alcohol use: Increased CNS depression

Adverse Reactions

CNS: Anxiety, confusion, dizziness, drowsiness, euphoria, hallucinations, headache, nervousness, restlessness, sedation, somnolence, tremor, weakness

CV: Hypertension, orthostatic hypotension, palpitations, tachycardia
EENT: Blurred vision, diplopia, dry mouth, laryngeal edema, laryngospasm, nystagmus, tinnitus
GI: Abdominal cramps, anorexia, biliary tract spasm, constipation, hepatotoxicity, nausea, vomiting
GU: Dysuria, urine retention
RESP: Dyspnea, respiratory depression, wheezing
SKIN: Diaphoresis, flushing
Other: Injection site pain, redness, and swelling; physical and psychological dependence

Nursing Considerations

- To improve analgesic action, give hydromorphone before pain becomes intense.
- Instruct patient to lie down during hydromorphone administration and for a period afterward to lessen dizziness, lightheadedness, nausea, and vomiting.
- **WARNING** Administer hydromorphone slowly over several minutes. Rapid administration may cause serious adverse reactions, including anaphylaxis, severe respiratory depression, hypotension, peripheral circulatory collapse, and cardiac arrest. Make sure emergency equipment and drugs are available.
- Administer hydromorphone by direct injection over at least 2 minutes. For infusion, mix drug with D_5W, normal saline solution, or Ringer's solution.
- Watch for respiratory depression, especially in patients who are having an acute asthma attack and those with chronic respiratory disease. Children, elderly patients, and debilitated or seriously ill patients are at increased risk for respiratory depression. Keep resuscitation equipment and naloxone nearby.
- Monitor patient for evidence of drug-induced CNS depression or increased CSF pressure, such as altered LOC, restlessness, and irritability, in patients with a head injury, intracranial lesions, or other conditions that could cause these effects. Patients who are taking, or have recently taken, drugs that cause CNS depression are also more susceptible to these effects. Take appropriate safety precautions.
- Be aware that hydromorphone may induce or worsen arrhythmias or seizures in patients with a history of these conditions and may mask symptoms of acute abdominal conditions.
- Be aware that patients with a history of drug abuse (including acute alcoholism), emotional instability, or suicidal ideation or attempts are at increased risk for opioid abuse.

- Assess patient for constipation.
- Watch for signs of physical dependence or abuse.
- Anticipate that drug may mask or worsen gallbladder pain.
- Store drug at 15° to 30° C (59° to 86° F); protect from freezing and light.

PATIENT TEACHING

- Instruct patient receiving hydromorphone to report constipation, difficulty breathing, severe nausea, or vomiting.
- Inform patient that drug may cause drowsiness and sedation. Advise her to avoid potentially hazardous activities until drug's CNS effects are known.
- Advise patient to change position slowly to minimize effects of orthostatic hypotension.
- To prevent constipation, encourage patient to consume plenty of fluids and high-fiber foods, if not contraindicated by another condition.
- Instruct patient to report pain before it becomes severe.
- Caution patient to avoid alcohol and OTC drugs during therapy, unless prescriber approves.

hyoscyamine sulfate

Levsin

Class and Category

Chemical: Belladonna alkaloid, tertiary amine
Therapeutic: Antimuscarinic, antispasmodic
Pregnancy category: C

Indications and Dosages

▶ *To treat peptic ulcers and GI tract disorders caused by spasm*

I.V. INJECTION

Adults and adolescents. 0.25 to 0.5 mg q 4 to 6 hr.
Children. Dosage individualized by weight.

▶ *To control salivation and excessive secretions during surgical procedures*

I. V. INJECTION

Adults and adolescents. 0.5 mg 30 to 60 min before procedure.

Route	Onset	Peak	Duration
I.V.	2 to 3 min	15 to 30 min	4 hr

Contraindications

Acute hemorrhage and hemodynamic instability; angle-closure

glaucoma; hepatic disease; hypersensitivity to hyoscyamine, other anticholinergics, or their components; ileus; intestinal atony; myasthenia gravis; myocardial ischemia; obstructive GI disease; obstructive uropathy; renal disease; severe ulcerative colitis; tachycardia; toxic megacolon

Mechanism of Action

Competitively inhibits acetylcholine at autonomic postganglionic cholinergic receptors. Because the most sensitive receptors are in the salivary, bronchial, and sweat glands, hyoscyamine acts mainly to reduce salivary, bronchial, and sweat gland secretions. It also causes GI smooth muscle to contract and decreases gastric secretion and GI motility. In addition, hyoscyamine causes the bladder detrusor muscle to contract; reduces nasal and oropharyngeal secretions; and decreases airway resistance from relaxation of smooth muscle in the bronchi and bronchioles.

Interactions

DRUGS

anticholinergics: Possibly increased anticholingeric effects
calcium- and magnesium-containing antacids, carbonic anhydrase inhibitors, citrates, sodium bicarbonate, urinary alkalinizers: Possibly potentiated therapeutic and adverse effects of hyoscyamine
haloperidol: Possibly decreased therapeutic effects of haloperidol
ketoconazole: Possibly reduced ketoconazole absorption
metoclopramide: Possibly antagonized therapeutic effects of metoclopramide
opioid analgesics: Increased risk of severe constipation and ileus

Adverse Reactions

CNS: Drowsiness, insomnia
EENT: Blurred vision; dry mouth, nose, and throat; photophobia
ENDO: Decreased lactation
GI: Constipation
GU: Impotence, urine retention
SKIN: Decreased sweating
Other: Heatstroke, injection site redness and urticaria

Nursing Considerations

- Give hyoscyamine 30 to 60 minutes before meals and at bedtime. Give bedtime dose at least 2 hours after last meal.
- **WARNING** Expect an increased risk of drug-induced heatstroke in hot or humid weather because hyoscyamine de-

creases sweating.
- **WARNING** Be aware that lower doses may paradoxically decrease the heart rate and that higher doses affect nicotinic receptors in autonomic ganglia, causing delirium, disorientation, hallucinations, and restlessness.
- Monitor patients with the following conditions for exacerbations caused by drug's anticholinergic effects: arrhythmias, coronary artery disease, heart failure, hiatal hernia with reflux esophagitis, hypertension, hyperthyroidism, or tachycardia. Also monitor blood pressure in patients with toxemia from pregnancy because they're at risk for aggravated hypertension.
- Monitor urine output, and be alert for urine retention, especially in patients with autonomic neuropathy.
- Be aware that infants, patients with Down syndrome, and children with brain damage or spastic paralysis may be more sensitive to drug's effects.
- Be aware that elderly patients and patients with impaired renal function are at increased risk for adverse reactions.
- Store drug at 15° to 30° C (59° to 86° F); don't freeze.

PATIENT TEACHING
- Instruct patient to void before receiving each dose of hyoscyamine and to report trouble urinating during hyoscyamine therapy.
- Inform patient that drug may cause drowsiness. Advise her to avoid potentially hazardous activities until drug's CNS effects are known.
- If patient reports dry mouth, suggest using sugarless hard candy or gum.
- Inform male patient that drug may cause impotence. If it occurs, suggest that he discuss it with prescriber.
- Advise patient to avoid exposure to high temperatures and to increase fluid intake, unless contraindicated.

I•J

ibandronate sodium

Boniva

Class and Category

Chemical: Nitrogen-containing bisphosphonate
Therapeutic: Bone resorption inhibitor
Pregnancy category: C

Indications and Dosages

▶ *To prevent or treat osteoporosis in postmenopausal women*

I.V. INJECTION

Adults. 3 mg over 15 to 30 sec q 3 mo.

Route	Onset	Peak	Duration
I.V.	Unknown	30 min to 2 hr	Unknown

Mechanism of Action

Binds to calcified bone matrix because of its affinity for hydroxyapatite in the mineral matrix, thus reducing bone solubility, inhibiting osteoclast activity, and reducing bone resorption and turnover. In postmenopausal women, ibandronate also reduces the elevated rate of bone turnover, leading to, on average, a net gain in bone mass. These activities help prevent or alleviate the loss of bone mass in osteoporosis.

Incompatibilities

Do not give with calcium-containing solutions or other intravenous drugs.

Contraindications

Esophageal stricture or achlasia, hypersensitivity to ibandronate or its components, hypocalcemia, inability to stand or sit upright for at least 60 minutes (oral form only), severe renal impairment (parenteral form only), untreated vitamin D deficiency

Interactions

DRUGS

aspirin, NSAIDs: Increased risk of GI irritation
calcium-containing preparations, including antacids containing calcium, aluminum, magnesium, or iron: Impaired absorption of ibandronate

FOODS

all foods: Decreased ibandronate bioavailability

Adverse Reactions

CNS: Asthenia, dizziness, headache, insomnia, vertigo
CV: Hypercholesterolemia, hypertension
EENT: Conjunctivitis, nasopharyngitis, ocular pain, scleritis, uveitis, visual impairment
GI: Abdominal pain, constipation, diarrhea, dyspepsia, gastritis, nausea, vomiting
GU: UTI
MS: Arthritis; back, bone, extremity, joint, or muscle pain; joint dysfunction; localized osteoarthritis; muscle cramps; myalgia
RESP: Bronchitis, pneumonia, bronchitis, upper respiratory infection
SKIN: Rash
Other: Allergic reaction, angioedema, flulike symptoms, infection

Nursing Considerations

- Use needle provided with the prefilled syringe when giving ibandronate intravenously. Know that parenteral form of drug should be given only as an I.V. bolus over 15 to 30 seconds.
- Give supplemental calcium and vitamin D, as prescribed, during ibandronate therapy if patient's dietary intake of these nutrients is inadequate.
- Give calcium supplements and antacids at different time of day than ibandronate to avoid impaired drug absorption and altered effectiveness.
- Monitor patient for hypersensitivity skin reactions such as generalized rash or angioedema because such reactions, although rare, can be severe.
- Be aware that although ibandronate has not been linked to osteonecrosis, biphosphates as a group have been, especially osteonecrosis affecting the jaw. Monitor patient for complaints of jaw or bone pain, and report to prescriber.
- Know that biphosphates but not specifically ibandronate have caused severe, sometimes incapacitating bone, joint, and muscle pain. If these symptoms occur, notify prescriber and expect drug to be discontinued.

PATIENT TEACHING

- Instruct patient to take ibandronate with 6 to 8 oz of water, in an upright position, at least 1 hour before first food or drink of the day. Tell patient to avoid mineral waters that contain a higher concentration of calcium. Caution against lying down for at least 60 minutes after taking drug to prevent it from lodging in esophagus and causing irritation.
- Advise patient to report symptoms of esophageal irritation, such as new or worsening dysphagia, pain on swallowing, retrosternal pain, or heartburn.
- Tell patient not to chew or suck on tablet because of risk of oropharyngeal ulcer.
- Instruct patient taking the 150-mg tablet to do so on the same date each month. If patient misses the monthly dose and the next scheduled dose is more than 7 days away, tell patient to take one 150-mg tablet the morning after she remembers the missed dose. She should then resume the normal schedule. Caution her never to take two 150-mg tablets in the same week.
- Advise patient to take calcium supplements or antacids at different time of day than ibandronate.
- Tell patient to stop taking ibandronate and notify prescriber immediately if she has skin reactions, such as a rash, or swelling, especially of the face or throat.
- Advise patient to report jaw discomfort to prescriber.
- Urge woman of childbearing age to tell prescriber if she is, could be, or is considering pregnancy while taking ibandronate because of risk to the fetus, especially the skeleton.

ibutilide fumarate

Corvert

Class and Category

Chemical: Methanesulfonanilide derivative
Therapeutic: Class III antiarrhythmic
Pregnancy category: C

Indications and Dosages

▶ *To rapidly convert recent-onset atrial flutter or fibrillation to sinus rhythm*

I.V. INFUSION

Adults weighing 60 kg (132 lb) or more. 1 mg over 10 min. Repeated 10 min after first dose is finished if arrhythmia persists.

Adults weighing less than 60 kg. 0.01 mg/kg over 10 min. Repeated 10 min after first dose is finished if arrhythmia persists. **DOSAGE ADJUSTMENT** Infusion discontinued if arrhythmia is terminated or if sustained or nonsustained ventricular tachycardia or prolonged QT or QTc interval develops.

Mechanism of Action

May promote sodium movement through slow inward sodium channels in myocardial cell membranes. Ibutilide also may inhibit a component of potassium channels in myocardial cell membranes involved in cardiac repolarization. These actions prolong the cardiac action potential by delaying repolarization and increasing atrial and ventricular refractoriness. As a result, the sinus rate slows and AV conduction is delayed.

Contraindications

Hypersensitivity to ibutilide or its components

Interactions

DRUGS

amiodarone, astemizole, disopyramide, maprotiline, phenothiazines, procainamide, quinidine, sotalol, tricyclic antidepressants: Possibly prolonged QT interval, leading to increased risk of proarrhythmias

Adverse Reactions

CNS: Headache, syncope

CV: AV block, bradycardia, bundle-branch block, heart failure, hypertension, hypotension, idioventricular rhythm, orthostatic hypotension, palpitations, prolonged QT interval, sinus and supraventricular tachycardia, supraventricular arrhythmias, ventricular arrhythmias, ventricular tachycardia (sustained and nonsustained)

GI: Nausea

GU: Renal failure

Nursing Considerations

- Before giving ibutilide, check serum electrolyte levels and expect to correct abnormalities. Be especially alert for hypokalemia and hypomagnesemia, which can lead to arrhythmias.
- Give drug undiluted, or dilute it in 50 ml of normal saline solution or D_5W. Add contents of 10-ml vial (0.1 mg/ml) to 50 ml of solution to obtain 0.017 mg/ml. Use polyvinyl chloride plastic bags or polyolefin bags for ibutilide admixtures. Administer within 24 hours (48 hours if refrigerated).

- Infuse drug slowly over 10 minutes.
- As ordered, monitor cardiac rhythm continuously during drug infusion and for at least 4 hours afterward—longer if arrhythmias appear or if patient has abnormal hepatic function. Observe for ventricular ectopy.
- **WARNING** Be aware that ibutilide use is not recommended for patients with a history of prolonged QT interval or torsades de pointes. Also be aware that patients with bradycardia, heart failure, or a history of low left ventricular ejection fraction are at increased risk for torsades de pointes and those with a history of chronic atrial fibrillation are at increased risk for recurrence after conversion to sinus rhythm.
- Before preparing ibutilide, store it at 20° to 25° C (68° to 77° F).
- Make sure that a defibrillator and drugs to treat sustained ventricular tachycardia are available during therapy and when monitoring patient after therapy.

PATIENT TEACHING

- Inform patient that ibutilide will be given by I.V. infusion and that his heart rhythm will be monitored continuously.
- Ask patient to report chest pain, faintness, numbness, tingling, palpitations, and shortness of breath.
- Advise patient to keep appointments to monitor heart rhythm.

imipenem and cilastatin sodium

Primaxin (CAN), Primaxin ADD-Vantage, Primaxin IM, Primaxin IV

Class and Category

Chemical: Thienamycin derivative (imipenem), heptenoic acid derivative (cilastatin sodium)
Therapeutic: Antibiotic
Pregnancy category: C

Indications and Dosages

▶ *To treat severe or life-threatening bacterial infections (including endocarditis, pneumonia, and septicemia as well as bone, joint, intra-abdominal, skin, and soft-tissue infections) caused by gram-positive anaerobic organisms, such as most staphylococci and streptococci and some enterococci (including* Enterococcus faecalis*); most strains of Enterobacteriaceae (including* Citrobacter *sp.,* Enterobacter *sp.,* Escherichia coli, Klebsiella *sp.,* Morganella morganii, Proteus mirabilis, Providencia stuartii, *and* Serratia marcescens*); and many gram-negative aerobic and anaerobic species (including* Bacteroides *sp.,* Campylobacter *sp.,* Clostridium *sp.,* Haemophilus influenzae,

Legionella *sp.,* Neisseria gonorrhoeae, *and* Pseudomonas aeruginosa*)*
I.V. INFUSION (DOSAGES BASED ON IMIPENEM CONTENT)
Adults and adolescents. 500 mg q 6 hr to 1,000 mg q 6 to 8 hr. *Maximum:* 50 mg/kg or 4 g daily, whichever is lower.
Children age 3 months and over. 15 to 25 mg/kg q 6 hr. *Maximum:* 2,000 to 4,000 mg daily.
Infants ages 4 weeks to 3 months weighing 1,500 g (3 lb, 3 oz) or more. 25 mg/kg q 6 hr. *Maximum:* 2,000 to 4,000 mg daily.
Neonates ages 1 to 4 weeks weighing 1,500 g or more. 25 mg/kg q 8 hr. *Maximum:* 2,000 to 4,000 mg daily.
Neonates under age 1 week weighing 1,500 g or more. 25 mg/kg q 12 hr. *Maximum:* 2,000 to 4,000 mg daily.

▶ *To treat moderate infections caused by the organisms listed above*
I.V. INFUSION (DOSAGES BASED ON IMIPENEM CONTENT)
Adults and adolescents. 500 mg q 6 to 8 hr up to 1,000 mg q 8 hr. *Maximum:* 50 mg/kg or 4 g daily, whichever is lower.
Children age 3 months and older. 15 to 25 mg/kg q 6 hr. *Maximum:* 2,000 to 4,000 mg daily.
Infants ages 4 weeks to 3 months weighing 1,500 g or more. 25 mg/kg q 6 hr. *Maximum:* 2,000 to 4,000 mg daily.
Neonates ages 1 to 4 weeks weighing 1,500 g or more. 25 mg/kg q 8 hr. *Maximum:* 2,000 to 4,000 mg daily.
Neonates under age 1 week weighing 1,500 g or more. 25 mg/kg q 12 hr. *Maximum:* 2,000 to 4,000 mg daily.

▶ *To treat mild infections caused by the organisms listed above*
I.V. INFUSION (DOSAGES BASED ON IMIPENEM CONTENT)
Adults and adolescents. 250 to 500 mg q 6 hr. *Maximum:* 50 mg/kg or 4 g daily, whichever is lower.
Children age 3 months and over. 15 to 25 mg/kg q 6 hr. *Maximum:* 2,000 mg (for fully susceptible organisms) to 4,000 mg (for moderately susceptible organisms) daily.
Infants ages 4 weeks to 3 months weighing 1,500 g or more. 25 mg/kg q 6 hr. *Maximum:* 2,000 to 4,000 mg daily.
Neonates ages 1 to 4 weeks weighing 1,500 g or more. 25 mg/kg q 8 hr. *Maximum:* 2,000 to 4,000 mg daily.
Neonates under age 1 week weighing 1,500 g or more. 25 mg/kg q 12 hr. *Maximum:* 2,000 to 4,000 mg daily.

▶ *To treat uncomplicated UTI caused by the organisms listed above*
I.V. INFUSION (DOSAGES BASED ON IMIPENEM CONTENT)
Adults and adolescents. 250 mg q 6 hr. *Maximum:* 50 mg/kg or 4 g daily, whichever is lower.

▶ *To treat complicated UTI caused by the organisms listed above*
I.V. INFUSION (DOSAGES BASED ON IMIPENEM CONTENT)
Adults and adolescents. 500 mg q 6 hr. *Maximum:* 50 mg/kg or 4 g daily, whichever is lower.
DOSAGE ADJUSTMENT Dosage reduced based on creatinine clearance for patients with impaired renal function.

Mechanism of Action
Produces two related actions. During bacterial cell wall synthesis, imipenem selectively binds to penicillin-binding proteins that are responsible for cell wall formation. This action causes bacterial cells to rapidly lyse and die. Cilastatin sodium inhibits imipenem's breakdown in the kidneys, thus maintaining a high imipenem level in the urinary tract.

Incompatibilities
Don't administer imipenem and cilastatin through same I.V. line as beta-lactam antibiotics or aminoglycosides.

Contraindications
Hypersensitivity to imipenem, its components, other beta–lactam antibiotics, or amide-type local anesthetics (I.M.); meningitis (I.V.); severe heart block or shock (I.M.)

Interactions
DRUGS
cyclosporine: Increased adverse CNS effects of both drugs
ganciclovir: Increased risk of seizures
probenecid: Slightly increased blood level and half-life of imipenem

Adverse Reactions
CNS: Confusion, dizziness, fever, seizures, somnolence, tremor, weakness
CV: Hypotension
EENT: Oral candidiasis
GI: Diarrhea, hepatic failure, hepatitis, nausea, pseudomembranous colitis, vomiting
RESP: Wheezing
SKIN: Diaphoresis, pruritus, rash, urticaria
Other: Anaphylaxis, injection site thrombophlebitis

Nursing Considerations
- Obtain specimens for culture and sensitivity testing, as ordered, before giving imipenem and cilastatin.

- For I.V. administration, add about 10 ml of diluent to each 250- or 500-mg vial and shake well. Transfer this reconstituted drug to at least 100 ml of prescribed I.V. solution. After the transfer, add another 10 ml of diluent to each vial, shake, and then transfer to infusion container. Shake infusion container until clear. To reconstitute piggyback bottles, add 100 ml of diluent to each 250- or 500-mg infusion bottle, and shake well.
- Give reconstituted drug within 4 to 10 hours, depending on diluent used (24 to 48 hours if refrigerated). Color may range from clear to yellow; don't administer solution that contains particles.
- Infuse 500-mg or smaller dose over 20 to 30 minutes and 750- to 1,000-mg dose over 40 to 60 minutes.
- Expect increased risk of imipenem-induced seizures in patients with brain lesions, head trauma, or history of CNS disorders and in those receiving more than 2 g of drug daily.
- Assess patient for signs and symptoms of allergic reaction and bacterial or fungal superinfection.

PATIENT TEACHING

- Inform patient that drug must be given by infusion or injection.
- Instruct patient to report discomfort at I.V. insertion site.
- Advise patient to report itching, signs of superinfection (such as diarrhea and sore mouth), and hives.

immune globulin intravenous (human) (IGIV, immune serum globulin, ISG, IVIG)

Gamimune N 5% S/D, Gamimune N 10% S/D, Gammagard Liquid, Gammagard S/D, Gammagard S/D 0.5 g, Gammar-P IV, Gamunex 10%, Iveegam EN, Octagam 5%, Polygam S/D, Sandoglobulin, Venoglobulin-I, Venoglobulin-S 5%, Venoglobulin-S 10%, WinRho SDF

Class and Category

Chemical: Polyvalent antibody
Therapeutic: Antibacterial, anti–Kawasaki disease agent, antipolyneuropathy agent, antiviral, immunizing agent, platelet count stimulator
Pregnancy category: C

Indications and Dosages

▶ *To treat primary immunodeficiency*

I.V. INFUSION (GAMMAR-P IV)

Adults. 200 to 400 mg/kg q 3 to 4 wk.

Adolescents and children. 200 mg/kg q 3 to 4 wk.

I.V. INFUSION (IVEEGAM EN)

Adults. 200 mg/kg q mo.

I.V. INFUSION (SANDOGLOBULIN)

Adults and children. 200 mg/kg q mo. If response is inadequate, dose may be increased to 300 mg/kg or dosing frequency may be increased.

I.V. INFUSION (GAMIMUNE N 5% S/D OR 10% S/D)

Adults. 100 to 200 mg/kg q mo. If response is inadequate, dose may be increased to as high as 400 mg/kg or dosing frequency may be increased.

I.V. INFUSION (GAMMAGARD S/D, POLYGAM S/D)

Adults. 200 to 400 mg/kg initially, then at least 100 mg/kg q mo thereafter. If response is inadequate, dose or frequency may be adjusted.

I.V. INFUSION (OCTAGAM 5%)

Adults. *Initial:* 30 mg/kg/hr for first 30 minutes; increased, if tolerated, to 60 mg/kg/hr for second 30 minutes and, if tolerated, to 120 mg/kg/hr for another 30 minutes; followed by maintenance infusion of up to 200 mg/kg/hr.

I.V. INFUSION (GAMUNEX 10%)

Adults. 300 to 600 mg/kg q 3 or 4 wk.

I.V. INFUSION (VENOGLOBULIN-I)

Adults and children. 200 mg/kg q mo. If response is inadequate, dose may be increased to 300 to 400 mg/kg q mo or dosing frequency may be increased.

I.V. INFUSION (VENOGLOBULIN-S 5% OR 10%)

Adults and children. 200 mg/kg q mo. If response is inadequate, dose may be increased to as high as 400 mg/kg or dosing frequency may be increased.

▶ *To treat primary immunodeficiency disorders associated with defects in humoral immunity*

I.V. INFUSION (GAMMAGARD LIQUID)

Adults and children. 300 to 600 mg/kg daily q 3 to 4 wk.

▶ *To treat idiopathic thrombocytopenic purpura (ITP)*

I.V. INFUSION (GAMIMUNE N 5% S/D)

Adults and children. 400 mg/kg daily for 5 days. Or, 1,000 mg/kg for 1 or 2 days for patients not at risk for increased fluid volume.

I.V. INFUSION (GAMIMUNE N 10% S/D)

Adults and children. 1,000 mg/kg for 1 or 2 days for patients not at risk for increased fluid volume.

I.V. INFUSION (GAMUNEX 10%)

Adults. 1 g/kg daily for 2 consecutive days (second dose may be withheld if platelet count increases adequately 24 hours after first dose). Alternatively, 0.4 g/kg daily for 5 consecutive days.

DOSAGE ADJUSTMENT In acute ITP of childhood, I.V. Sandoglobulin therapy may be stopped after second day of 5-day course if initial platelet count response is adequate (30,000 to 50,000/mm^3). In chronic ITP, an additional I.V. infusion of 400 mg/kg (of either Sandoglobulin or Gamimune) may be prescribed if platelet count falls below 30,000/mm^3 or if patient develops significant bleeding. If response remains inadequate, an additional I.V. infusion of 800 to 1,000 mg/kg may be given.

I.V. INFUSION (GAMMAGARD S/D)

Adults. 1 g/kg. If response is inadequate, up to three separate doses may be administered on alternate days.

I.V. INFUSION (SANDOGLOBULIN)

Adults and adolescents. 400 mg/kg daily for 2 to 5 consecutive days.

I.V. INFUSION (VENOGLOBULIN-I)

Adults and children. *Induction:* Cumulative dose up to 2 g/kg over 2 to 7 consecutive days. *Maintenance (adults):* 2 g/kg as a single dose q 2 wk as needed to maintain platelet count above 30,000/mm^3 or prevent bleeding episodes. *Maintenance (children):* 1 g/kg as a single dose q 2 wk as needed to maintain platelet count above 30,000/mm^3 or prevent bleeding episodes.

I.V. INFUSION (VENOGLOBULIN-S 5% OR 10%)

Adults and children. Cumulative dose up to 2,000 mg/kg over 5 consecutive days.

DOSAGE ADJUSTMENT An additional I.V. infusion of 1,000 mg/kg may be given to maintain a platelet count of 30,000/mm^3 in children or 20,000/mm^3 in adults or to prevent bleeding episodes.

▶ *To treat acute or chronic pediatric immune thrombocytopenia purpura; to treat chronic adult-onset immune thrombocytopenia purpura; to treat prediatric- and adult-onset immune thrombocytopenia purpura secondary to HIV infection*

I.V. INJECTION (WINRHO SDF)

Adults and children. *Initial:* 250 international units/kg given as a single injection over 3 to 5 min. Or 125 international units/kg given as a single injection over 3 to 5 min and repeated once on a separate day. *Maintenance:* Frequency and dosage highly individualized based on patient's hemoglobin and platelet levels.

DOSAGE ADJUSTMENT For patients with a hemoglobin level less than 10 g/dl, dose reduced to 125 to 200 international units/kg.

▶ *As adjunct to treat Kawasaki disease*

I.V. INFUSION (GAMMAGARD S/D)

Adults and adolescents. 1 g/kg as a single dose; or, 400 mg/kg daily for 4 consecutive days.

I.V. INFUSION (IVEEGAM EN, VENOGLOBULIN-S 5% OR 10%)

Adults and adolescents. 2 g/kg as a single dose; alternatively, Iveegam EN may be given at 400 mg/kg daily for 4 days.

▶ *To decrease the risk of graft-versus-host disease, interstitial pneumonia, septicemia, and other infections during first 100 days after bone marrow transplantation*

I.V. INFUSION (GAMIMUNE N 5% S/D OR 10% S/D)

Adults over age 20. 500 mg/kg on 7th and 2nd days before transplant (or at time conditioning therapy for transplantation begins), and then weekly through 90th day after transplant.

▶ *As adjunct to treat bacterial infections secondary to B-cell chronic lymphocytic leukemia*

I.V. INFUSION (GAMMAGARD S/D, POLYGAM S/D)

Adults and adolescents. 400 mg/kg q 3 to 4 wk.

▶ *To prevent bacterial infection in children with HIV who are immunosuppressed*

I.V. INFUSION (GAMIMUNE N 5% S/D OR 10% S/D)

Children. 400 mg/kg daily every 28 days.

▶ *To suppress Rh isoimmunization*

I.V. INJECTION (WINRHO SDF)

Adult pregnant females. 1,500 international units as a single dose infused over 3 to 5 min at 28 wk gestation followed by 600 international units infused over 3 to 5 min within 72 hr after delivery of an Rh-positive newborn.

DOSAGE ADJUSTMENT For patients who are at more than 34 wk gestation and are having an abortion, amniocentesis, or other manipulative procedure, 600 international units given within 72 hr but preferably immediately after procedure. For patients who are 34 wk gestation or less and are having amniocentesis or chorionic villus sampling, 1,500 international units given immediately after procedure and repeated q 12 wk for duration of pregnancy. For patients with a threatened abortion at any stage of pregnancy, 1,500 international units given immediately.

▶ *To treat incompatible blood transfusions or massive fetal hemorrhage*

I.V. INJECTION (WINRHO SDF)
Adults exposed to Rh-positive whole blood. 3,000 international units infused over 3 to 5 min q 8 hr until total dose (45 international units/ml of blood) is given.
Adults exposed to Rh-positive RBCs. 3,000 international units infused over 3 to 5 min q 8 hr until total dose (90 international units/ml of cells) is given.

Route	Onset	Peak	Duration
I.V.	Unknown	Unknown	21 to 28 days

Mechanism of Action
Releases antibody-specific globulins to produce an antibody-antigen reaction that results in bacterial lysis and facilitates bacterial phagocytosis. In treatment of ITP, immune globulin blocks iron receptors on macrophages to increase immunoglobulin action. Immune globulin also increases cytokine production and improves B-cell immune function by regulating T-cell and macrophage activity. Newly formed antigen-antibody complexes produce split complement components that cause bacterial lysis.

In Kawasaki disease and bacterial infections secondary to B-cell chronic lymphocytic leukemia, immune globulin neutralizes bacterial and viral toxins that harm the immune and inflammatory responses.

Incompatibilities
Don't mix immune globulin with any other drugs, including other immune globulins, or with any I.V. solutions other than D_5W or manufacturer's supplied diluent because effects of doing so are unknown.

Contraindications
Hypersensitivity to immune globulin (human) or its components, IgA deficiency in patients with known antibody to IgA

Interactions
DRUGS
vaccines, live-virus: Possibly decreased response to vaccine

Adverse Reactions
CNS: Headache, malaise
CV: Tachycardia
GI: Nausea, vomiting
HEME: Disseminated intravascular coagulation, hemolysis

MS: Arthralgia, back pain, myalgia
RESP: Dyspnea

Nursing Considerations

- Before giving immune globulin, monitor patient's fluid volume and BUN and serum creatinine levels, as ordered, to determine if he's at risk for acute renal failure. Those at increased risk include patients with existing renal insufficiency, diabetes mellitus, volume depletion, sepsis, or paraproteinemia; those taking concomitant nephrotoxic drugs; and those over age 65. Expect drug to be discontinued if renal function deteriorates.
- When preparing drug for administration, verify that immune globulin intravenous for I.V. infusion is being used because the drug is also available as immune globulin intramuscular.
- To reconstitute drug (except Gammagard Liquid, which doesn't need reconstitution), follow manufacturer's guidelines and use only diluent recommended by manufacturer. Don't shake solution; excessive shaking causes foaming. If drug or diluent is cold, drug may take up to 20 minutes to dissolve.
- If drug is reconstituted outside of sterile laminar airflow conditions, administer it immediately and discard unused portions.
- Consult manufacturer's guidelines to determine appropriate flow rate for starting infusion. Expect to increase flow rate after 15 to 30 minutes, according to guidelines.
- **WARNING** Watch for an acute inflammatory reaction in patients who have never received immune globulin therapy before, in those whose last treatment was more than 8 weeks before, and in those whose initial infusion rate exceeded 1 ml/minute. Within 30 minutes to 1 hour after beginning of infusion, assess for chills, fever, facial flushing, feeling of tightness in chest, dizziness, nausea and vomiting, diaphoresis, and hypotension. Notify prescriber immediately if such symptoms occur, and be prepared to stop infusion until symptoms have subsided.
- **WARNING** After immune globulin administration, monitor patient closely for aseptic meningitis. Notify prescriber if patient develops drowsiness, fever, nausea and vomiting, nuchal rigidity, photophobia, painful eye movements, or severe headache.
- Be aware that immune globulin intravenous is made from human plasma and therefore may contain infectious agents, such as viruses. However, the risk of transmitting a virus by infusion

has been reduced by screening blood donors, testing donated blood, and inactivating or removing certain viruses from the product.

- For patient receiving WinRho SDF to treat immune thrombocytopenia purpura, assess clinical response by monitoring patient's platelet count, RBC count, hemoglobin level, and reticulocyte level.
- For patient receiving WinRho SDF for exposure to incompatible blood transfusions or massive fetal hemorrhage, give drug within 72 hours of incident.

PATIENT TEACHING

- Instruct patient to immediately report any symptoms he experiences after receiving immune globulin.
- Inform patient that he'll need to postpone live-virus vaccinations for up to 11 months after receiving immune globulin because drug may delay or inhibit his response to vaccine.

inamrinone lactate
(amrinone lactate)

Inocor

Class and Category

Chemical: Bipyridine derivative
Therapeutic: Cardiac inotrope
Pregnancy category: C

Indications and Dosages

▶ *To treat heart failure in patients who haven't responded sufficiently to digoxin, diuretics, or vasodilators*

I.V. INFUSION

Adults. *Initial:* 0.75 mg/kg by bolus administered over 2 to 3 min and repeated after 30 min, if needed. *Maintenance:* 5 to 10 mcg/kg/min by infusion. *Maximum:* 10 mg/kg daily.

Route	Onset	Peak	Duration
I.V.	2 to 5 min	In 10 min	30 min to 2 hr

Incompatibilities

Don't administer inamrinone through same I.V. line as furosemide to prevent precipitate formation. Don't dilute inamrinone in solution that contains dextrose because a chemical interaction occurs over 24 hours.

Mechanism of Action

Inhibits phosphodiesterase enzymes that normally degrade myocardial cAMP. This action increases intracellular levels of cAMP, which regulates intracellular and extracellular calcium balance. An increased intracellular cAMP level enhances the influx of calcium into the cell, thereby increasing the force of myocardial contractions. Inamrinone also acts directly on peripheral vascular smooth-muscle cells, causing relaxation and dilation. This action reduces preload and afterload.

Contraindications

Hypersensitivity to inamrinone, bisulfites, or their components; severe aortic or pulmonary valvular disease

Interactions

DRUGS

disopyramide: Possibly severe hypotension

Adverse Reactions

CNS: Fever

CV: Chest pain, hypotension, pericarditis, supraventricular tachycardia, ventricular arrhythmias

GI: Abdominal pain, anorexia, elevated liver function test results, hepatotoxicity, nausea, vomiting

HEME: Elevated erythrocyte sedimentation rate, thrombocytopenia (especially with high-dose or long-term treatment)

MS: Myositis

RESP: Hypoxemia, pleuritis

SKIN: Jaundice

Other: Infusion site burning

Nursing Considerations

- **WARNING** Be aware that inamrinone may increase the risk of ventricular arrhythmias in patients with atrial flutter or fibrillation. To minimize this risk, expect to pretreat such patients with digoxin.
- Administer inamrinone undiluted or diluted in normal saline solution or 0.45 normal saline solution to a concentration of 1 to 3 mg/ml, as prescribed. Use diluted solution within 24 hours. Don't use if solution is discolored or contains particles.
- **WARNING** Monitor vital signs regularly. If blood pressure falls significantly, slow or stop inamrinone infusion and notify prescriber.

- Monitor weight, cardiac index, central venous pressure, pulmonary artery wedge pressure, and fluid intake and output as appropriate to assess effectiveness of therapy.
- **WARNING** Assess frequently for signs of thrombocytopenia, such as bruising or bleeding and altered platelet count. If signs appear, expect to decrease inamrinone dose or discontinue drug.
- Store drug at 15° to 30° C (59° to 86° F), and protect it from light.

PATIENT TEACHING

- Instruct patient to report dizziness, which may indicate hypotension, or signs of an allergic reaction, such as a rash, facial swelling, or difficulty breathing or swallowing.

indomethacin sodium trihydrate

Indocid PDA (CAN), Indocin I.V.

Class and Category

Chemical: Indoleacetic acid derivative
Therapeutic: Antigout, anti-inflammatory, antirheumatic
Pregnancy category: Not rated

Indications and Dosages

► *To treat hemodynamically significant patent ductus arteriosus in premature infants weighing 500 to 1,750 g (1 to 3.9 lb)*

I.V. INJECTION

Infants over age 7 days. *Initial:* 200 mcg/kg (0.2 mg/kg) over 5 to 10 sec; 1 or 2 additional doses of 250 mcg/kg (0.25 mg/kg) given at 12- to 24-hr intervals, if needed.
Neonates ages 2 to 7 days. *Initial:* 200 mcg/kg (0.2 mg/kg) over 5 to 10 sec; 1 or 2 additional doses of 200 mcg/kg (0.2 mg/kg) given at 12- to 24-hr intervals, if needed.
Neonates under age 48 hours. *Initial:* 200 mcg/kg (0.2 mg/kg) over 5 to 10 sec; 1 or 2 additional doses of 100 mcg/kg (0.1 mg/kg) given at 12- to 24-hr intervals, if needed.

Mechanism of Action

Blocks the activity of cyclooxygenase, the enzyme needed to synthesize prostaglandins, which mediate the inflammatory response and cause local vasodilation, swelling, and pain. By blocking cyclooxygenase and inhibiting prostaglandins, this NSAID reduces inflammatory symptoms and helps relieve pain.

Incompatibilities

Don't give indomethacin suspension with alkaline antacids or liquids. Don't mix reconstituted indomethacin sodium with I.V. infusion solutions.

Contraindications

Allergy or hypersensitivity to aspirin, indomethacin, iodides, other NSAIDs, or their components; history of proctitis or recent rectal bleeding (suppositories)

Interactions

DRUGS

Note: All effects listed are for oral forms and suppositories unless indicated.

acetaminophen: Increased risk of adverse renal effects (with long-term use of both drugs)

aluminum- and magnesium-containing antacids: Possibly decreased blood indomethacin level

aminoglycosides: Increased risk of aminoglycoside toxicity

antihypertensives: Decreased effectiveness of these drugs

aspirin, other NSAIDs: Increased risk of adverse GI effects and non-GI bleeding

bone marrow depressants: Possibly increased leukopenic or thrombocytopenic effects of these drugs

cefamandole, cefoperazone, cefotetan: Increased risk of hypoprothrombinemia and bleeding

colchicine, platelet aggregation inhibitors: Increased risk of GI bleeding, hemorrhage, and ulcers

corticosteroids, potassium supplements: Increased risk of adverse GI effects

cyclosporine: Increased risk of nephrotoxicity from both drugs, increased blood cyclosporine level

diflunisal: Increased blood indomethacin level and risk of GI bleeding

digoxin: Increased blood digoxin level and risk of digitalis toxicity (all forms)

diuretics (thiazide, loop, and potassium-sparing): Decreased diuretic and antihypertensive effects

gold compounds, nephrotoxic drugs: Increased risk of adverse renal effects

heparin, oral anticoagulants, thrombolytics: Possibly increased anticoagulant effects and risk of hemorrhage

lithium: Increased blood lithium level and risk of toxicity

methotrexate: Increased risk of methotrexate toxicity
plicamycin, valproic acid: Increased risk of hypoprothrombinemia and GI bleeding, hemorrhage, and ulcers
probenecid: Increased blood level and effectiveness of indomethacin, increased risk of indomethacin toxicity
zidovudine: Increased blood zidovudine level and risk of toxicity, increased risk of indomethacin toxicity
ACTIVITIES
alcohol use: Increased risk of adverse GI effects

Adverse Reactions

CNS: Confusion, depression, dizziness, drowsiness, fatigue, hallucinations, headache, intraventricular hemorrhage, peripheral neuropathy, seizures, stroke, syncope, vertigo
CV: Arrhythmias, chest pain, edema, fluid retention (all forms), heart failure, hypertension, MI, pulmonary hypertension, tachycardia
EENT: Blurred vision, corneal and retinal damage, epistaxis, hearing loss, tinnitus
ENDO: Hypoglycemia
GI: Abdominal cramps or pain, abdominal distention, anorexia, constipation, diarrhea, diverticulitis, dyspepsia, dysphagia, epigastric discomfort, esophagitis, gastric perforation, gastritis, gastroenteritis, gastroesophageal reflux disease, GI bleeding and ulceration (all forms), hemorrhoids, hepatic dysfunction, hepatic failure, hiatal hernia, ileus, indigestion, melena, nausea, necrotizing enterocolitis, pancreatitis, peptic ulcer, perforation of stomach or intestine, stomatitis, vomiting (all forms)
GU: Acute renal failure, hematuria, interstitial nephritis, nephrotic syndrome, oliguria, proteinuria, renal dysfunction, vaginal bleeding
HEME: Agranulocytosis, anemia, aplastic anemia, bone marrow depression, disseminated intravascular coagulation, hemolytic anemia, iron deficiency anemia, leukopenia, neutropenia, pancytopenia, thrombocytopenia, unusual bleeding or bruising (all forms)
RESP: Asthma, respiratory depression
SKIN: Ecchymosis, erythema multiforme, erythema nodosum, photosensitivity, pruritus, rash, Stevens-Johnson syndrome, toxic epidermal necrolysis, urticaria
Other: Anaphylaxis, angioedema, hyperkalemia, hyponatremia, injection site irritation

Nursing Considerations

- Use indomethacin cautiously in patients with hypertension, and monitor blood pressure closely throughout therapy. Drug may cause hypertension or worsen it.
- To reconstitute I.V. form, add 1 to 2 ml of preservative-free sodium chloride for injection or preservative-free sterile water to vial. Solution made with 1 ml of diluent contains 100 mcg (0.1 mg) of indomethacin/0.1 ml. Solution made with 2 ml of diluent contains 50 mcg (0.05 mg) of indomethacin/0.1 ml. Use solution immediately because it contains no preservatives. Discard unused portion.
- Be aware that scheduled I.V. doses may be withheld if infant or neonate has anuria or a significant decrease in urine output (less than 0.6 ml/kg/hr).
- When using I.V. form, avoid extravasation to protect surrounding tissue.
- Anticipate a second course (another 3 doses) of I.V. indomethacin if patent ductus arteriosus fails to close or reopens. After two courses, surgery may be performed.
- **WARNING** Monitor patient closely for thrombotic events, including MI and stroke, because NSAIDs increase the risk.
- Monitor infant for necrotizing entercolitis such as abdomen distention, severe abdominal pain, and fever.
- Monitor CBC for decreased hemoglobin and hematocrit because drug may worsen anemia.
- **WARNING** If patient has bone marrow suppression or is receiving an antineoplastic drug, monitor laboratory results (including WBC count), and watch for evidence of infection because anti-inflammatory and antipyretic actions of indomethacin may mask signs and symptoms, such as fever and pain.
- Assess patient's skin regularly for signs of rash or other hypersensitivity reaction because indomethacin is an NSAID and may cause serious skin reactions without warning, even in patients with no history of NSAID sensivitity. At first sign of reaction, stop drug and notify prescriber.
- Because indomethacin causes sodium retention, monitor weight and blood pressure, especially if patient has hypertension.

PATIENT TEACHING

- Reassure parents that infant will be monitored closely throughout course of therapy.

infliximab

Remicade

Class and Category

Chemical: Monoclonal antibody
Therapeutic: Anti-inflammatory
Pregnancy category: C

Indications and Dosages

▶ *To control moderate to severe Crohn's disease long term*

I.V. INFUSION

Adults and children. *Induction:* 5 mg/kg over 2 hr, repeated 2 and 6 wk after first infusion. *Maintenance:* 5 mg/kg over 2 hr q 8 wk.

DOSAGE ADJUSTMENT For adult patients who respond and then lose response, dosage may be increased up to 10 mg/kg.

▶ *To reduce number of draining enterocutaneous and rectovaginal fistulas and to maintain fistula closure in fistulizing Crohn's disease*

I.V. INFUSION

Adults. *Induction:* 5 mg/kg over 2 hr, repeated 2 and 6 wk after first infusion. *Maintenance:* 5 mg/kg over 2 hr q 8 wk.

DOSAGE ADJUSTMENT For patients who respond and then lose response, dosage may be increased up to 10 mg/kg.

▶ *To reduce signs and symptoms, to induce and maintain remission and mucosal healing, and eliminate corticosteroid use in patients with moderate to severe active ulcerative colitis who have had an inadequate response to conventional therapy*

I.V. INFUSION

Adults. 5 mg/kg over 2 hr, repeated 2 and 6 wk after infusion. *Maintenance:* 5 mg/kg over 2 hr q 8 wk.

▶ *As adjunct to reduce signs and symptoms, inhibit progression of structural damage, and improve physical function in patients with moderate to severe active rheumatoid arthritis*

I.V. INFUSION

Adults. 3 mg/kg, with methotrexate, repeated 2 and 6 wk after first infusion and then q 8 wk thereafter.

DOSAGE ADJUSTMENT For patients with inadequate response to combination treatment, infliximab increased to 10 mg/kg or frequency increased to q 4 wk.

▶ *To treat active ankylosing spondylitis*

I.V. INFUSION

Adults. 5 mg/kg, repeated 2 and 6 wk after first infusion and then q 6 wk thereafter.

▶ *To reduce signs and symptoms, inhibit progression of structural damage, and improve physical function in patients with psoriatic arthritis*
I.V. INFUSION
Adults. 5 mg/kg, with or without methotrexate, repeated 2 and 6 wk after first infusion and then q 8 wk thereafter.
▶ *To treat chronic severe plaque psoriasis in patients who are candidates for systemic therapy when those therapies are medically less appropriate*
I.V. INFUSION
Adults. 5 mg/kg, repeated 2 and 6 wk after first infusion and then q 8 wk thereafter.

Mechanism of Action

Binds with cytokine tumor necrosis factor-alpha (TNF-alpha), preventing it from binding with its receptors. As a result, TNF-alpha can't produce proinflammatory cytokines and endothelial permeability. Infiltration of inflammatory cells into inflamed intestine and joints declines.

Incompatibilities

Don't infuse infliximab in same I.V. line with other drugs or through plasticized polyvinyl chloride infusion equipment or devices.

Contraindications

Breast-feeding, hypersensitivity to infliximab, murine proteins, or their components; moderate or severe (NYHA Class III or IV) heart failure

Drug Interactions

anakinra, etanercept: Increased risk of neutropenia and serious infections

Adverse Reactions

CNS: Chills, CVA, dizziness, fatigue, fever, Guillain-Barre syndrome, headache, meningitis, neuritis, numbness, paresthesia, pericardial effusion, syncope, tingling
CV: Arrhythmias, chest pain, hypertension, hypotension, MI, myelitis, neuropathies, systemic and cutaneous vasculitis, thrombophlebitis
EENT: Oral candidiasis, pharyngitis, rhinitis, sinusitis, visual changes
GI: Abdominal hernia; abdominal pain; acute hepatic failure; cholecystitis; cholestasis; diarrhea; dyspepsia; elevated amino-

transferases; gastrointestinal hemorrhage; hepatitis; hepatotoxicity; ileus; intestinal obstruction, perforation, or stenosis; melena; nausea; pancreatitis; splenic infarction; splenomegaly; vomiting
GU: Kidney infection, renal failure, ureteral obstruction, UTI, vaginal candidiasis, vaginitis
HEME: Anemia, leukopenia, neutropenia, pancytopenia, thrombocytopenia
MS: Arthralgia, back pain, extremity weakness, myalgia
RESP: Adult respiratory distress syndrome, bronchitis, cough, dyspnea, interstitial pneumonitis or fibrosis, pneumonia, pulmonary edema or embolism, tuberculosis, respiratory tract infection, wheezing
SKIN: Facial flushing, jaundice, pruritus, rash, urticaria
Other: Antibody formation to infliximab; bacterial, fungal or viral infections; infusion reactions; lupuslike symptoms; lymphadenopathy; lymphoma; sepsis

Nursing Considerations

- **WARNING** Avoid giving infliximab to patients with NYHA Class III or IV congestive heart failure (CHF) because it may worsen the condition or cause death. If patient does receive infliximab, expect to stop it if CHF worsens.
- Use cautiously in elderly patients because they are at higher risk for developing infections.
- **WARNING** Because infliximab increases the risk of developing tuberculosis or reactivating latent tuberculosis, expect prescriber to evaluate patient's risk and start tuberculosis treatment, as needed, before starting infliximab.
- **WARNING** Be aware that infliximab increases the risk of serious or fatal opportunistic infections, including histoplasmosis, listeriosis, and pneumocystosis. Expect prescriber to evaluate patient's risk before starting drug.
- To reconstitute infliximab, use a 21G (or smaller) needle to add 10 ml of sterile water for injection to each vial of drug. Swirl to mix; don't shake. Be aware that solution may foam and be clear or light yellow.
- Withdraw a volume equal to amount of reconstituted drug from a 250-ml glass bottle or polypropylene or polyolefin infusion bag of normal saline solution. Then add reconstituted infliximab to bottle to dilute to 250 ml. Use within 3 hours.
- Infuse over at least 2 hours using polyethylene-lined infusion set and in-line, sterile, nonpyrogenic, low–protein-binding filter with pores of 1.2 microns or less. Don't reuse.

- Be prepared to stop infusion if a hypersensitivity or CNS reaction occurs. Keep acetaminophen, antihistamines, corticosteroids, and epinephrine on hand. A reaction may occur 2 hours to 12 days after infusion.
- **WARNING** Watch for infection, especially if patient receives immunosuppressant therapy or has a chronic infection. Upper respiratory tract infections and UTIs are most common, but sepsis and fatal infections have occurred.
- Because severe hepatic reactions may occur, monitor liver function. Expect to stop infliximab if jaundice develops or liver enzymes are 5 times or more the upper limit of normal.

PATIENT TEACHING

- Explain that infliximab should take effect within 1 to 2 weeks.
- Urge patient to report signs of infection, such as painful urination, cough, and sore throat. Infusion reaction (chest pain, chills, dyspnea, facial flushing, fever, itching, headache, rash) may occur for up to 12 days.
- Explain that infliximab increases the risk of lymphoma; urge prompt medical attention for suspicious signs or symptoms.

insulin injection, regular

Regular Iletin II, Regular Insulin

insulin human injection, regular

Humulin R, Novolin ge Toronto (CAN), Novolin R

insulin human injection, buffered regular

Velosulin BR

Class and Category

Chemical: Polypeptide hormone
Therapeutic: Antidiabetic
Pregnancy category: B

Indications and Dosages

▶ *To treat diabetic ketoacidosis*

I.V. INJECTION OR INFUSION

Adults and adolescents. Loading dose of 0.15 USP Insulin Unit/kg, followed by 0.1 USP Insulin Unit/kg/hr by continuous infusion.

Route	Onset	Peak	Duration
I.V.*	10 to 30 min	15 to 30 min	30 to 60 min

*Individual responses vary.

Mechanism of Action

Controls the storage and metabolism of carbohydrates, proteins, and fats that bind to receptor sites on cellular plasma membranes, especially in the liver, muscle, and adipose tissues. In hyperglycemia, the body lacks sufficient insulin or is unable to use insulin to transport glucose through the cellular membranes. When this occurs, the body uses proteins and fats for energy. The liver produces excess ketone bodies, which accumulate in the blood; metabolic acidosis develops, resulting in diabetic ketoacidosis.

Insulin stimulates carbohydrate metabolism in skeletal and cardiac muscle and adipose tissue by facilitating transport of glucose into these cells. It also increases conversion of glucose to glycogen in the liver and suppresses hepatic glucose output.

Contraindications

Hypersensitivity to specific insulin preparation (animal or human)

Interactions

DRUGS

ACE inhibitors, anabolic steroids (such as stanozolol and oxandrolone), androgens, antidiabetic drugs, bromocriptine, clofibrate, ketoconazole, lithium, mebendazole, pyridoxine, sulfonamides, theophylline: Increased risk of hypoglycemia

beta blockers (systemic and oral), guanethidine, MAO inhibitors (such as furazolidone), procarbazine: Possibly hyperglycemia or hypoglycemia and masking of hypoglycemic adverse effects

calcium channel blockers, clonidine, corticosteroids, danazole, dextrothyroxine, diazoxide (parenteral), epinephrine, estrogen, glucagon, growth hormone, heparin, loop and thiazide diuretics, morphine, oral contraceptives (containing estrogen and progestin), phenytoin, sulfinpyrazone, thyroid hormones: Possibly hyperglycemia

carbonic anhydrase inhibitors (such as acetazolamide), sulfonylureas: Possibly increased hypoglycemic response

chloroquine, quinidine, quinine: Increased risk of hypoglycemia, increased blood insulin level

NSAIDs, salicylates (large doses): Increased hypoglycemic effect

octreotide: Possibly hyperglycemia or hypoglycemia

pentamidine: Possibly hyperglycemia, hypoglycemia, or hypoinsulinemia

tetracycline: Increased tissue sensitivity to insulin

ACTIVITIES
alcohol use: Increased hypoglycemic effect of insulin, increased risk of prolonged hypoglycemia
marijuana use, smoking: Possibly hyperglycemia

Adverse Reactions

CV: Edema
ENDO: Hypoglycemia
Other: Allergic reaction, weight gain

Nursing Considerations

- **WARNING** Be aware that the 100-USP unit concentration of regular insulin is the only type of insulin that should be used for I.V. infusion.
- Monitor patient's blood glucose level frequently, as ordered, before starting insulin infusion and at least hourly, as ordered, during the infusion.
- Don't use cloudy or viscous regular insulin. Use only clear, colorless solutions. In addition, use only syringes specifically calibrated to measure 100–USP unit concentrations when preparing for infusion.
- Be aware that insulin can be adsorbed to glass and plastic I.V. infusion containers and I.V. tubing. To minimize adsorption, allow 50 ml of diluted solution to run through the infusion apparatus before use and wait 30 minutes to administer a prepared solution. Follow facility protocols for preparing and administering insulin I.V. infusions.
- Monitor urine ketone and glucose levels, as ordered. Expect urine glucose level to return to normal more slowly than blood glucose level.
- Be aware that patients with impaired renal or hepatic function may require an increase or decrease in insulin dosage.
- Monitor blood pH and serum electrolyte levels, particularly potassium, sodium chloride, and phosphate, as ordered. After initially experiencing hyperkalemia due to decreased pH, patient may develop hypokalemia as potassium reenters cells with insulin administration.
- Expect to decrease infusion rate when blood glucose level is 300 mg/dl or less. Expect a separate infusion of D_5W to be ordered when blood glucose level is 250 mg/dl.
- Assess patient for signs and symptoms of hypoglycemia, including anxiety, behavioral changes, blurred vision, cold sweats, confusion, cool skin, decreased concentration, headache, hunger, nausea, nervousness, nightmares, restless sleep, pallor,

shakiness, slurred speech, tachycardia, tiredness, and weakness. Severe hypoglycemia may also cause coma or seizures.
- Anticipate an appropriate S.C. or I.M. dose of insulin to be ordered 30 minutes before discontinuation of insulin infusion.
- Store regular insulin at 2° to 8° C (36° to 46° F); protect from freezing and sunlight.

PATIENT TEACHING
- Advise patient receiving insulin infusion to immediately report signs of abnormal blood glucose level, including anxiety, tachycardia, blurred vision, and tremors.
- Review with patient events that may trigger a change in insulin requirements, including fever, infection, injury, psychological or physical stress, surgery, and medical conditions affecting food intake or absorption, such as vomiting and diarrhea.
- Stress the need to keep follow-up appointments, to use insulin as prescribed, and to monitor blood glucose level.
- Refer patient to an outpatient diabetes education program, if needed, for additional information and support.

interferon alfa-2b, recombinant

Intron A

Class and Category

Chemical: Cytokine
Therapeutic: Antineoplastic, immunomodulator
Pregnancy category: C

Indications and Dosages

▶ *To treat malignant melanoma*

I.V. INFUSION, S.C. INJECTION

Adults. *Initial:* 20 million international units/m^2 I.V. for 5 consecutive days/wk for 4 wk. *Maintenance:* 10 million international units/m^2 S.C. 3 times/wk for 48 wk.

Mechanism of Action

May exert a cytostatic effect, reducing the rate of cell proliferation by delaying RNA and protein production. This delay induces cells to enter a resting stage. Interferon alfa-2b also increases the action of human natural killer cells, which lyse certain tumor cells and normal targets. In addition, the drug selectively increases the number of cytotoxic T-cells, thereby affecting tumor growth, and increases phagocytic activity of macrophages.

Contraindications

Hypersensitivity to interferon alfa or its components

Interactions

DRUGS

barbiturates and other CNS depressants: Possibly increased CNS depression

blood-dyscrasia–causing drugs (such as cephalosporins and sulfasalazine): Increased risk of leukopenia and thrombocytopenia

bone marrow depressants (such as carboplatin and lomustine): Possibly increased bone marrow depression

theophylline: Risk of decreased theophylline clearance and increased blood theophylline level

vaccines, killed virus: Possibly decreased antibody response to vaccine

vaccines, live virus: Possibly decreased antibody response to vaccine, increased adverse effects of vaccine, and severe infection

ACTIVITIES

alcohol use: Increased risk of CNS depression

Adverse Reactions

CNS: Dizziness, fatigue, neurotoxicity, peripheral neuropathy
CV: Cardiotoxicity, hypotension
EENT: Altered taste, blurred vision, dry mouth, stomatitis
GI: Anorexia, diarrhea, hepatotoxicity, nausea, vomiting
HEME: Anemia, leukopenia, neutropenia, thrombocytopenia
MS: Leg cramps
SKIN: Alopecia, diaphoresis, dry skin, pruritus, rash
Other: Flulike symptoms, weight loss

Nursing Considerations

- **WARNING** Be aware that recombinant interferon alfa-2b is *not* interchangeable with other interferon preparations, including interferon alfa-2a, -n1, and -n3. Don't use interferon alfa-2b solution for injection for I.V. treatment of malignant melanoma; use the recombinant powder for injection.
- Monitor liver function tests, hematocrit, hemoglobin, platelet count, and total and differential leukocyte count before and periodically during therapy.
- Obtain an ECG before and during therapy, as ordered, in patients with a history of cardiac disease or advanced malignant melanoma.
- Anticipate the need to hydrate patient before therapy. Monitor blood pressure during therapy to detect hypotensive changes.

- Reconstitute interferon with appropriate amount of bacteriostatic water for injection provided by manufacturer. Agitate gently to dissolve. Expect liquid to be clear and colorless to light yellow. Use within 1 month if stored between 2° and 8° C (36° and 46° F).
- Be aware that patients receiving concurrent or consecutive radiation therapy and those who have received previous cytotoxic drug therapy are at risk for additive bone marrow depression. Expect prescriber to decrease dosage.
- If patient develops thrombocytopenia, implement protective precautions according to facility policy.
- Monitor patients with severe renal disease for exacerbation caused by fever and dehydrating effects of interferon alfa-2b. Monitor patients with cardiac disease (including recent MI), diabetes mellitus prone to ketoacidosis, or pulmonary disease for exacerbations of these conditions caused by interferon-induced fever and chills.
- Monitor patients with herpes zoster or recent or current chicken pox (including recent exposure) for signs and symptoms of severe generalized disease.
- Assess patients with a history of autoimmune disease for exacerbation of condition.
- Be aware that elderly patients may be more prone to drug's adverse effects because of underlying CNS, cardiac, or renal disease.
- Be aware that patients with a history of compromised CNS function, severe psychiatric conditions, or seizure disorders are at risk for severe CNS adverse reactions. Neuropsychiatric follow-up may be ordered, especially for patients receiving high doses of drug.
- Administer acetaminophen, as ordered, to prevent or treat flu-like symptoms, such as fever or headache.
- Be aware that interferon alfa-2b is also given S.C. in combination with ribavirin for treatment of chronic hepatitis. Consult manufacturer's insert for specific information, including contraindications, adverse reactions, and nursing considerations, relating to combination therapy.
- Store drug at 2° to 8° C (36° to 46° F).

PATIENT TEACHING

- Advise patient to avoid potentially hazardous activities until interferon alfa-2b's CNS effects are known.

- Instruct patient to avoid alcohol and CNS depressants during therapy.
- Advise patient to contact prescriber immediately if he notices unusual bleeding or bruising, black or tarry stools, blood in urine or stools, or red pinpoint spots on skin.
- Instruct patient to avoid touching his eyes or inside of nose unless he washes hands immediately beforehand.
- Urge patient to avoid people with infection if he develops bone marrow depression. Advise him to contact prescriber if he experiences fever, chills, cough, hoarseness, lower back or side pain, or painful or difficult urination because these signs and symptoms may signal an infection.
- Teach patient proper oral hygiene, and advise him to use a soft-bristled toothbrush because drug can delay healing, increase the risk of infection, and cause gingival bleeding. Advise patient to check with prescriber before undergoing any dental work.
- Stress the importance of avoiding accidental cuts from sharp objects, such as razors and fingernail clippers, because excessive bleeding or infection may occur. Also, caution patient to avoid contact sports and other activities that increase the risk of injury.
- If patient will self-administer interferon alpha-2b, teach him and his caregiver the proper administration technique, including bedtime administration to decrease effect of fatigue on daily activities.
- Caution patient and caregiver not to reuse needles or syringes, and teach them how to properly dispose of needles and syringes in puncture-resistant containers.
- Stress the importance of complying with the dosage regimen and of keeping follow-up medical appointments and appointments for laboratory tests.

irinotecan hydrochloride
Camptosar

Class and Category
Chemical: Synthetic camptothecin derivative
Therapeutic: Antineoplastic
Pregnancy category: D

Indications and Dosages
▶ *To treat colorectal cancer*

I.V. INFUSION

Adults receiving drug as a single agent. 125 mg/m^2 over 90 min q wk for 4 wk, followed by 2-wk rest period, then subsequent courses. Alternatively, 240 to 350 mg/m^2 over 90 min q 3 wk. *Maximum:* 150 mg/m^2/wk.

DOSAGE ADJUSTMENT Dosage is highly individualized, ranging from 50 to 150 mg/m^2, and may be adjusted in increments—typically of 25 to 50 mg/m^2. Doses may even be omitted, based on severity of adverse reactions, according to the National Cancer Institute's (NCI) Common Toxicity Criteria. (See *Selected Common Toxicity Criteria* in the appendices.) Expect initial dose to be decreased to 100 mg/m^2 or less for patients over age 65 with impaired hepatic function *and* a history of pelvic or abdominal irradiation.

Adults receiving drug in combination with fluorouracil and leucovorin. If administering fluorouracil-leucovorin boluses, 125 mg/m^2 over 90 minutes on days 1, 8, 15, and 22, with next course beginning on day 43. Alternatively, if administering fluorouracil-leucovorin infusions, 180 mg/m^2 over 90 minutes on days 1, 15, and 29, with next course beginning on day 43. *Maximum:* 125 mg/m^2/wk.

DOSAGE ADJUSTMENT Dosage reduced or doses omitted based on severity of adverse reactions, according to NCI's Common Toxicity Criteria.

Mechanism of Action

Inhibits the activity of topoisomerase I, an enzyme that allows single-strand breaks in the double-stranded DNA chain. Single-strand breaks during DNA replication, recombination, and repair decrease the torsional strain of the DNA configuration. Irinotrecan and its metabolite, SN-38, bind to the topoisomerase I complex and prevent religation of the single-strand breaks, which normally takes place after the DNA has relaxed. This action halts DNA replication, resulting in DNA damage and, eventually, in cell death.

Incompatibilities

Don't refrigerate irinotecan diluted with normal saline solution because a precipitate may form. Don't mix irinotecan with any other drugs.

Contraindications

Hypersensitivity to irinotecan

Interactions

DRUGS

blood-dyscrasia–causing drugs (such as cephalosporins and sulfasalazine): Increased risk of leukopenia and thrombocytopenia

bone marrow depressants (such as carboplatin and lomustine): Possibly additive bone marrow depression

corticosteroids, cyclosporine, and other immunosuppressive drugs: Increased risk of infection

dexamethasone: Possibly hyperglycemia, increased risk of lymphocytopenia

laxatives: Increased risk of severe diarrhea

vaccine, killed virus: Possibly decreased antibody response to vaccine

vaccine, live virus: Possibly decreased antibody response to vaccine, increased adverse effects of vaccine, and severe infection

Adverse Reactions

CNS: Asthenia, chills, fever, headache

CV: Bradycardia, edema, vasodilation (flushing)

EENT: Rhinitis, stomatitis

GI: Abdominal cramps or pain, abdominal distention, anorexia, bloating, constipation, diarrhea, indigestion, nausea, vomiting

HEME: Anemia, leukopenia, neutropenia, thrombocytopenia

RESP: Cough, dyspnea, upper respiratory tract infection

SKIN: Alopecia, diaphoresis, rash

Other: Allergic reaction, anaphylaxis, dehydration, infection (minor), weight loss

Nursing Considerations

- Be aware that irinotecan should be administered only under the supervision of a qualified physician and in a setting where appropriate diagnostic and treatment facilities are available.
- Expect to obtain hemoglobin level and leukocyte and platelet counts before beginning each course of therapy and periodically thereafter. Expect dosage to be adjusted if test results reveal hematologic toxicity—for example, a granulocyte count less than $1,500/mm^3$ or a platelet count less than $100,000/mm^3$.
- Follow facility policy for handling antineoplastic drugs and for appropriate disposal of used equipment. If irinotecan solution comes in contact with your skin, wash if off thoroughly with soap and water. If drug comes in contact with mucous membranes, irrigate the area thoroughly with water.
- Dilute irinotecan with D_5W (preferred) or normal saline solution to a concentration of 0.12 to 2.8 mg/ml. Discard unused portion in single-use vials (2 ml and 5 ml).

- Because drug contains no preservatives, use solutions prepared with D_5W within 6 hours if stored at room temperature or within 24 hours if refrigerated at 2° to 8° C (36° to 46° F).
- Use solutions made with normal saline solution within 6 hours if stored at room temperature. Don't refrigerate solutions diluted with normal saline solution because precipitate will form.
- Be aware that adverse reactions can vary when irinotecan is administered in combination therapy. Review information for all drugs administered as part of a specific regimen, including drug interactions and adverse effects. Expect dosage to be adjusted based on type of combination therapy used and on incidence and severity of adverse reactions.
- Assess patient often for diarrhea, which may occur immediately after or more than 24 hours after irinotecan dose. Expect to give loperamide at first sign of increased bowel movements.
- Monitor liver function test results periodically, as prescribed, to identify signs of hepatic function impairment.
- Monitor patients with herpes zoster or recent or current chicken pox (including recent exposure) for signs and symptoms of severe generalized disease.
- Assess for signs of infection, such as fever, if patient develops leukopenia. Expect to obtain appropriate specimens for culture and sensitivity testing. Be aware that patients with a preexisting infection may experience impaired recovery.
- Be aware that patients receiving concurrent or consecutive radiation therapy and those with preexisting bone marrow depression are at risk for increased bone marrow depression.
- If extravasation occurs, stop the infusion, flush the area with sterile water, and apply ice. Restart infusion in another vein.
- Monitor patients with drug-induced vomiting and diarrhea for signs of dehydration, such as decreased urine output, poor skin turgor, dry and furrowed tongue, and dry mucous membranes. Patients taking diuretics are at increased risk and may have diuretic withheld if vomiting or diarrhea occurs.
- Store drug at 15° to 30° C (59° to 86° F); protect from freezing and light.

PATIENT TEACHING

- Advise patient to have dental work completed before irinotecan treatment begins, if possible, or to defer such work until blood counts return to normal because drug can delay healing and cause gingival bleeding. Teach patient proper oral hygiene, and suggest that he use a toothbrush with soft bristles.

- Instruct patient to immediately report nausea, vomiting, or diarrhea during irinotecan therapy. Advise him to avoid foods that may irritate the GI system, including high-fiber foods (bran, whole grain breads, and raw fruits and vegetables) and fatty, spicy, or fried foods.
- Advise patient to report burning or other signs of extravasation, such as redness, at I.V. insertion site.
- Encourage patient to drink fluids as prescribed. Urge him to avoid alcohol and caffeinated beverages, such as coffee and cola, which can exacerbate dehydration.
- If patient develops thrombocytopenia, implement protective precautions according to facility policy.
- Urge patient to avoid people with infection if he develops bone marrow depression. Advise him to contact prescriber if he experiences fever, chills, cough, hoarseness, lower back or side pain, or painful or difficult urination because these signs and symptoms may signal an infection.
- Advise patient to contact prescriber immediately if he notices unusual bleeding or bruising, black or tarry stools, blood in urine or stools, or red pinpoint spots on skin.
- Instruct patient to avoid touching his eyes or inside of nose unless he washes hands immediately beforehand.
- Stress the importance of avoiding accidental cuts from sharp objects, such as razors or nail clippers, because excessive bleeding or infection may occur. Also, caution patient to avoid contact sports and other activities that increase the risk of injury.
- Caution patient to avoid receiving immunizations unless approved by prescriber. Instruct him to avoid people who have recently received vaccines or to wear a protective mask that covers his nose and mouth when he's around them.
- Advise patient with stomatitis to eat bland, soft foods served cold or at room temperature to decrease irritation.
- Stress the importance of complying with the dosage regimen and of keeping follow-up medical and laboraotry appointments.

iron dextran

(contains 50 mg of elemental iron per milliliter)
DexFerrum, DexIron (CAN), InFeD

Class and Category

Chemical: Iron salt, mineral
Therapeutic: Antianemic

Pregnancy category: C

Indications and Dosages

▶ *To treat iron deficiency anemia*

I.V. INFUSION

Adults and children weighing over 15 kg (33 lb). Dose (ml) = 0.0442 (desired hemoglobin − observed hemoglobin) × lean body weight (in kg) + (0.26 × lean body weight). Or, consult dosage table in package insert. *Maximum:* 2 ml (100 mg) daily.

Children over age 4 months weighing 5 to 15 kg (11 to 33 lb). Dose (ml) = 0.0442 (desired hemoglobin − observed hemoglobin) × weight (kg) + (0.26 × weight). Or, consult dosage table in package insert. *Maximum*: 1 ml (50 mg) daily.

▶ *To replace iron lost in blood loss*

I.V. INFUSION

Adults. Replacement iron (mg) = ml of blood loss × hematocrit.

Mechanism of Action

Restores hemoglobin and replenishes iron stores. Iron, an essential component of hemoglobin, myoglobin, and several enzymes (including cytochromes, catalase, and peroxidase), is needed for catecholamine metabolism and normal neutrophil function. In iron dextran therapy, iron binds to available protein parts after the drug has been split into iron and dextran by cells of the reticuloendothelial system. The bound iron forms hemosiderin or ferritin, physiologic forms of iron, and transferrin, which replenish hemoglobin and depleted iron stores. Dextran is metabolized or excreted.

Incompatibilities

Don't mix iron dextran with blood for transfusion, other drugs, or parenteral nutrition solutions for I.V. infusion.

Contraindications

Anemia other than iron deficiency, hypersensitivity to iron dextran or its components

Interactions

None known.

Adverse Reactions

CNS: Chills, disorientation, dizziness, fever, headache, malaise, paresthesia, seizures, syncope, unconsciousness, weakness

CV: Arrhythmias, bradycardia, chest pain, shock, hypotension, hypertension, tachycardia

EENT: Altered taste
GI: Abdominal pain, diarrhea, nausea, vomiting
GU: Hematuria
HEME: Leukocytosis
MS: Arthralgia, arthritis, backache, myalgia, rhabdomyolysis
RESP: Bronchospasm, dyspnea, respiratory arrest, wheezing
SKIN: Cyanosis, diaphoresis, rash, pruritus, purpura, urticaria
Other: Anaphylaxis, infusion site phlebitis

Nursing Considerations

- Expect oral iron therapy to be stopped before iron dextran therapy starts. Iron dextran is given only when oral therapy is not feasible; it also may be given by I.M. injection.
- Expect to monitor hemoglobin, hematocrit, serum ferritin, and transferrin saturation, as ordered, before, during, and after iron dextran therapy.
- **WARNING** Before starting therapy, administer a test dose of 0.5 ml of iron dextran gradually over 30 seconds, as prescribed, and watch closely for an anaphylactic reaction.
- Wait 1 to 2 hours before administering the remainder of the dose. Infuse undiluted iron dextran slowly, at a rate not to exceed 1 ml/minute (50 mg/minute).
- **WARNING** Monitor patient closely for signs and symptoms of anaphylaxis, such as severe hypotension, loss of consciousness, collapse, dyspnea, and seizures, during and after infusion. Patients with a history of asthma or known allergies are at increased risk for anaphylaxis and, possibly, death. Institute emergency resuscitation measures as needed, including epinephrine administration, as prescribed.
- **WARNING** Assess blood pressure frequently after drug administration because hypotension is a common adverse effect that may be related to infusion rate; avoid rapid infusion.
- Be aware that patient may exhibit adverse reactions, including arthralgia, backache, chills, and vomiting, 1 to 2 days after drug therapy. Symptoms should resolve within 3 to 4 days.
- Assess patients with a history of rheumatoid arthritis for exacerbation of joint pain and swelling.
- Monitor patients with cardiovascular disease for an exacerbation caused by drug's adverse effects.
- Assess patient for iron overload, characterized by sedation, decreased activity, pale eyes, and bleeding in GI tract and lungs.
- Store iron dextran at 15° to 30° C (59° to 86° F).

PATIENT TEACHING

- Instruct patient to immediately report adverse reactions, such as shortness of breath, wheezing, or rash, during iron dextran therapy.
- Advise patient not to take any oral iron preparations without first consulting prescriber.
- Inform patient that symptoms of iron deficiency may include decreased stamina, learning problems, shortness of breath, and fatigue. During periods of anemia, encourage patient to plan periods of activity and rest in order to avoid excessive fatigue.
- Stress the need to follow dosage regimen and keep follow-up medical and laboratory appointments.

iron sucrose
(contains 100 mg of elemental iron per 5 ml)

Venofer

Class and Category

Chemical: Iron salt, mineral
Therapeutic: Antianemic
Pregnancy category: B

Indications and Dosages

▶ ***To treat iron deficiency anemia in hemodialysis patients receiving erythropoietin***

I.V. INJECTION

Adults. *Initial:* 100 mg of elemental iron injected undiluted over 2 to 5 min during dialysis. *Usual:* 100 mg of elemental iron q wk to three times/wk to a total dose of 1,000 mg. Dosage repeated as needed to maintain target levels of hemoglobin and hematocrit and acceptable blood iron level. *Maximum:* 100 mg/dose.

I.V. INFUSION

Adults. *Initial:* 100 mg of elemental iron infused diluted over 15 min during dialysis. *Usual:* 100 mg of elemental iron q wk to three times/wk to a total dose of 1,000 mg. Dosage repeated as needed to maintain target levels of hemoglobin and hematocrit and acceptable blood iron level. *Maximum:* 100 mg/dose.

▶ ***To treat iron deficiency anemia in peritoneal dialysis patients receiving erythropoietin***

I.V. INFUSION

Adults. *Initial:* 300 mg of elemental iron infused diluted over 1.5 hr on days 1 and 14, followed by 400 mg of elemental iron infused over 2.5 hr on day 28. Dosage repeated as needed to maintain target levels of hemoglobin and hematocrit and acceptable blood iron level. *Maximum:* 1,000 mg/28 days.

▶ ***To treat iron deficiency anemia in nondialysis patients with chronic renal disease regardless of whether they're receiving erythropoietin***

I.V. INJECTION

Adults. *Initial:* 200 mg of elemental iron injected undiluted over 2 to 5 min and repeated four more times over a 14-day period for a total dose of 1,000 mg. Dosage repeated as needed to maintain target levels of hemoglobin and hematocrit and acceptable blood iron level. *Maximum:* 1,000 mg/14 days.

I.V. INFUSION

Adults. 500 mg of elemental iron infused diluted over 3.5 to 5 hr on days 1 and 14. Dosage repeated as needed to maintain target levels of hemoglobin and hematocrit and acceptable blood iron level. *Maximum:* 1,000 mg/14 days.

Mechanism of Action

Acts to replenish iron stores lost during dialysis because of increased erythropoiesis and insufficient absorption of iron from the GI tract. Iron is an essential component of hemoglobin, myoglobin, and several enzymes, including cytochromes, catalase, and peroxidase, and is needed for catecholamine metabolism and normal neutrophil function. Iron sucrose injection also normalizes RBC production by binding with hemoglobin or being stored as ferritin in reticuloendothelial cells of the liver, spleen, and bone marrow.

Incompatibilities

Don't mix with other drugs or parenteral nutrition solutions for I.V. infusion.

Contraindications

Anemia other than iron deficiency, hypersensitivity to iron salts or their components, iron overload

Interactions

DRUGS

chloramphenicol: Possibly decreased effectiveness of iron sucrose
oral iron preparations: Possibly reduced absorption of oral iron supplements

Adverse Reactions

CNS: Asthenia, dizziness, fatigue, fever, headache, hypoesthesia, malaise

CV: Chest pain, heart failure, hypertension, hypotension, peripheral edema
EENT: Conjunctivitis, ear pain, nasal congestion, nasopharyngitis, rhinitis, sinusitis, taste perversion
ENDO: Hyperglycemia, hypoglycemia
GI: Abdominal pain, constipation, diarrhea, dysgeusia, elevated liver function test results, nausea, occult-positive feces, peritoneal infection, vomiting
GU: UTI
MS: Arthralgia, arthritis, back pain, leg cramps, muscle pain or weakness, myalgia
RESP: Cough, dyspnea, pneumonia, upper respiratory tract infection, wheezing
SKIN: Pruritus, rash
Other: Anaphylaxis; fluid overload; gout; hypervolemia; infusion or injection site burning, pain, or redness; sepsis

Nursing Considerations

- To reconstitute iron sucrose injection for infusion, dilute 100 mg of elemental iron in no more than 100 ml (hemodialysis) or 250 ml (peritoneal or no dialysis) of normal saline solution immediately before infusion. Discard any unused diluted solution.
- Give drug directly into dialysis line by slow I.V. injection or by infusion.
- **WARNING** Monitor patient closely for evidence of anaphylaxis, such as severe hypotension, loss of consciousness, collapse, dyspnea, or seizures, during and after therapy. Institute emergency resuscitation measures as needed.
- **WARNING** Assess blood pressure often after giving drug. Hypotension is common and may be related to infusion rate (avoid rapid infusion) or total cumulative dose.
- Monitor hemoglobin, hematocrit, serum ferritin, and transferrin saturation, as ordered, before, during, and after iron sucrose therapy. Serum iron levels must be tested 48 hours after last dose. Notify prescriber and expect to stop therapy if blood iron levels are normal or elevated, to prevent iron toxicity.
- Watch for possible iron overload, characterized by sedation, decreased activity, pale eyes, and bleeding in GI tract and lungs.

PATIENT TEACHING

- Advise patient not to take any oral iron preparations during iron sucrose therapy without first consulting prescriber.
- Inform patient that iron deficiency may cause decreased stamina, learning problems, shortness of breath, and fatigue.

isoproterenol hydrochloride

Isuprel

Class and Category

Chemical: Catecholamine
Therapeutic: Antiarrhythmic, bronchodilator
Pregnancy category: C

Indications and Dosages

▶ *To manage bronchospasm during anesthesia*

I.V. INJECTION

Adults. 0.01 to 0.02 mg, repeated p.r.n.

▶ *To treat bradycardia with significant hemodynamic change, such as third-degree heart block or prolonged QT interval*

I.V. INFUSION

Adults. *Initial:* 2 mcg/min, titrated according to heart rate, as ordered. *Maximum:* 10 mcg/min.

Route	Onset	Peak	Duration
I.V.	In 5 min*	Unknown	10 min†

Mechanism of Action

Stimulates $beta_1$ receptors in the myocardium and cardiac conduction system, resulting in positive inotropic and chronotropic effects. Isoproterenol also shortens the AV conduction time and refractory period in patients with AV block. This action increases the ventricular rate and halts bradycardia and associated syncope.

In addition, isoproterenol attaches to $beta_2$ receptors on bronchial cell membranes. This action stimulates the intracellular enzyme adenylate cyclase to convert adenosine triphosphate to cAMP. An increased intracellular level of cAMP relaxes bronchial smooth-muscle cells, stabilizes mast cells, and inhibits histamine release.

Contraindications

Angina pectoris, heart block or tachycardia from digitalis toxicity, hypersensitivity to isoproterenol or its components (such as sulfite in some preparations), tachyarrhythmias, ventricular arrhythmias that require inotropic therapy

* For treatment of bradycardia; unknown for treatment of bronchospasm.
† For treatment of bradycardia; 1 to 2 hr for treatment of bronchospasm.

Interactions

DRUGS

alpha blockers, other drugs with alpha-blocking effects: Possibly decreased peripheral vasoconstricting and hypertensive effects of isoproterenol
astemizole, cisapride, drugs that prolong QTc interval, terfenadine: Possibly prolonged QTc interval
beta blockers (ophthalmic): Decreased effects of isoproterenol, increased risk of bronchospasm, wheezing, decreased pulmonary function, and respiratory failure
beta blockers (systemic): Increased risk of bronchospasm, decreased effects of both drugs
digoxin: Increased risk of arrhythmias, hypokalemia, and digitalis toxicity
diuretics, other antihypertensives: Possibly decreased antihypertensive effects
ergot alkaloids: Increased vasoconstriction and vasopressor effects
hydrocarbon inhalation anesthetics: Increased risk of atrial and ventricular arrhythmias
MAO inhibitors: Intensified and extended cardiac stimulation and vasopressor effects
quinidine, other drugs that affect myocardial reaction to sympathomimetics: Increased risk of arrhythmias
theophylline: Increased risk of cardiotoxicity, decreased blood theophylline level
thyroid hormones: Increased effects of both drugs, increased risk of coronary insufficiency in patients with coronary artery disease
tricyclic antidepressants: Increased vasopressor response, increased risk of prolonged QTc interval and arrhythmias

Adverse Reactions

CNS: Dizziness, headache, insomnia, nervousness, syncope, tremor, weakness
CV: Adams-Stokes syndrome, angina, arrhythmias, bradycardia, hypertension, hypotension, palpitations, tachycardia, ventricular arrhythmias
EENT: Blurred vision, oropharyngeal edema
ENDO: Hyperglycemia
GI: Nausea, vomiting
MS: Muscle spasms and twitching
RESP: Bronchospasm, dyspnea, wheezing
SKIN: Diaphoresis, erythema multiforme, pallor, pruritus, rash, Stevens-Johnson syndrome, urticaria

Other: Angioedema, hypokalemia

Nursing Considerations

- Expect to give lowest possible dose of isoproterenol for shortest possible time to minimize tolerance.
- Don't give drug if it is pink or brown or contains precipitate.
- Inspect label carefully to verify correct concentration, which ranges from 0.02 mg/ml (1:50,000) to 0.2 mg/ml (1:5,000).
- Administer infusion through large vein, and watch for signs of extravasation.
- Monitor blood pressure, cardiac rhythm, central venous pressure, and urine output during administration. Adjust infusion rate to response, as ordered.
- Notify prescriber immediately if heart rate increases significantly or exceeds 110 beats/minute during infusion.
- Know that drug may increase pulse pressure and cause hypotension. Expect to reduce infusion slowly to decrease the risk of hypotension.
- **WARNING** Be aware that isoproterenol markedly increases the risk of arrhythmias. If an arrhythmia occurs, expect to give a cardioselective beta blocker, such as atenolol, as prescribed.
- Be aware that isoproterenol isn't used regularly to treat asthma, decreased cardiac output, hypotension, or shock because it increases the risk of arrhythmias, hypotension, and ischemia.
- **WARNING** If isoproterenol aggravates a ventilation-perfusion problem, expect patient's blood oxygen level to fall even as his breathing seems to improve.
- Consult manufacturer's guidelines for storage information. Recommended temperature varies with form used.

PATIENT TEACHING

- Instruct patient receiving isoproterenol to report chest pain, difficulty breathing, dizziness, hyperglycemic symptoms (such as abdominal cramps, lethargy, nausea, and vomiting), insomnia, irregular heartbeat, palpitations, tremor, and weakness.

itraconazole

Sporanox

Class and Category

Chemical: Triazole derivative
Therapeutic: Antifungal
Pregnancy category: C

Indications and Dosages

▶ *To treat pulmonary and extrapulmonary blastomycosis, histoplasmosis, and refractory aspergillosis*

I.V. INFUSION

Adults and adolescents. 200 mg infused over 1 hr q 12 hr for 4 doses; then 200 mg daily Drug changed to P.O. form within 14 days and therapy continued for at least 3 mo.

DOSAGE ADJUSTMENT In life-threatening situations, loading dose adjusted to 200 mg P.O. or I.V. t.i.d. for 3 days. Be aware that I.V. itraconazole shouldn't be used in patients with creatinine clearance less than 30 ml/min/1.73 m^2.

Mechanism of Action

Inhibits the synthesis of ergosterol, an essential component of fungal cell membranes, by binding with a cytochrome P-450 enzyme needed to convert lanosterol to ergosterol. The lack of ergosterol results in increased cellular permeability and leakage of cell contents. Itraconazole also may lead to fungal cell death by inhibiting fungal respiration under aerobic conditions.

Incompatibilities

Don't give itraconazole through same I.V. line with other drugs. Don't mix I.V. itraconazole with D_5W or solutions that contain lactated Ringer's solution.

Contraindications

Concurrent therapy with cisapride, dofetilide, ergot alkaloids, HMG-CoA inhibitors (lovastatin and simvastatin), levomethadyl, oral midazolam, pimozide, quinidine, or triazolam; evidence of ventricular dysfunction, as in congestive heart failure (CHF) or a history of it (onychomycosis treatment); hypersensitivity to itraconazole or its components; planning for pregnancy during onychomycosis treatment

Interactions

DRUGS

alfentanil, buspirone, busulfan, carbamazepine, cyclosporine, digoxin, docetaxel, dofetilide, indinavir, methylprednisolone, phenytoin, pimozide, quinidine, rifabutin, ritonavir, saquinavir, sirolimus, tacrolimus, trimetrexate, vinca alkaloids: Possibly increased blood levels of these drugs

alprazolam, diazepam, oral midazolam, triazolam: Elevated blood levels and possibly prolonged sedative effects of these drugs

antacids, anticholinergics, H_2-receptor antagonists, omeprazole, sucralfate: Possibly decreased itraconazole absorption
atorvastatin, lovastatin, simvastatin: Increased blood levels of these drugs; possibly rhabdomyolysis
calcium channel blockers: Possibly edema and increased blood levels of these drugs
carbamazepine, isoniazid, nevirapine, phenobarbital, phenytoin, rifabutin, rifampin: Possibly decreased blood itraconazole level
cisapride, pimozide, levomethadyl, quinidine: Possibly life-threatening cardiovascular complications as well as sudden death
clarithromycin, erythromycin, indinavir, ritonavir: Possibly increased blood itraconazole level
didanosine: Possibly decreased therapeutic effects of itraconazole
oral antidiabetic drugs: Possibly increased blood levels of these drugs and risk of hypoglycemia
warfarin: Increased anticoagulant effect of warfarin

Adverse Reactions

CNS: Dizziness, drowsiness, fatigue, fever, headache, peripheral neuropathy, vertigo
CV: CHF, hypertriglyceridemia, hypertension, peripheral edema
GI: Abdominal pain, anorexia, constipation, diarrhea, elevated liver function test results, flatulence, hepatic failure, hepatitis, hepatotoxicity, hyperbilirubinemia, indigestion, nausea, vomiting
GU: Menstrual irregularities
HEME: Neutropenia
RESP: Cough, dyspnea, pulmonary edema
SKIN: Alopecia, diaphoresis, photosensitivity, pruritus, rash, Stevens-Johnson syndrome, urticaria
Other: Angioedema, anaphylaxis, hypokalemia

Nursing Considerations

- Because itraconazole has been linked to serious adverse cardiac and hepatic effects, expect to send appropriate nail specimens for laboratory testing to confirm onychomycosis before beginning therapy.
- Be aware that I.V. itraconazole is for infusion only. Don't administer by bolus.
- **WARNING** Keep in mind that itraconazole is a potent inhibitor of the cytochrome P-450 3A4 (CYP3A4) isoenzyme system, which may increase blood levels of drugs metabolized by this system. Patients using such drugs as cisapride with itraconazole or other CYP3A4 inhibitors have experienced life-threatening cardiovascular complications, such as pro-

longed QT interval, torsades de pointes, and ventricular tachycardia, as well as sudden death.

- Infuse each I.V. dose over 1 hour.
- Keep in mind that a patient with AIDS may have hypochlorhydria, which reduces drug absorption. For such a patient, expect to administer higher doses of itraconazole.
- Monitor liver function test results in patients with impaired hepatic function and those who have experienced hepatotoxicity with other drugs.
- If patient develops signs and symptoms of peripheral neuropathy or CHF, such as fatigue, dyspnea, and peripheral edema, expect to discontinue drug.
- Assess patient for rash every 8 hours during therapy; notify prescriber if rash occurs.
- If patient also receives warfarin, monitor PT and assess patient for signs and symptoms of bleeding.
- If patient also receives digoxin, monitor blood digoxin level as appropriate to detect toxic level, and assess patient for signs and symptoms of digitalis toxicity, such as nausea and yellow vision.

PATIENT TEACHING

- If patient also takes an oral antidiabetic drug, instruct him to monitor his blood glucose level frequently because of the increased risk of hypoglycemia.
- Advise patient to notify prescriber immediately of changes in other drugs, such as new drugs and dosage changes.
- Advise patient to notify prescriber immediately about abdominal pain, diarrhea, headache, nausea, peripheral neuropathy, rash, or vomiting.
- Instruct patient to notify prescriber if he experiences signs of liver problems, such as abdominal pain, dark urine, fatigue, loss of appetite, pale stools, weakness, or yellow eyes or skin.
- Caution breast-feeding patient to consult prescriber about continuation of breast-feeding during itraconazole therapy.

K•L

kanamycin sulfate

Kantrex

Class and Category

Chemical: Aminoglycoside
Therapeutic: Antibiotic
Pregnancy category: D

Indications and Dosages

▶ *To treat infections caused by gram-negative organisms (including* Acinetobacter *sp.,* Enterobacter aerogenes, Escherichia coli, Haemophilus influenzae, Klebsiella pneumoniae, Neisseria *sp.,* Proteus *sp.,* Providencia *sp.,* Salmonella *sp.,* Serratia marcescens, Shigella *sp., and* Yersinia *sp.) and gram-positive organisms (including* Staphylococcus aureus *and* Staphylococcus epidermidis*)*

I.V. INFUSION

Adults and children. 5 mg/kg q 8 hr or 7.5 mg/kg q 12 hr for 7 to 10 days. *Maximum:* 1.5 g daily.

DOSAGE ADJUSTMENT For elderly patients and those with renal failure, dosage reduced and blood kanamycin level and renal function test results monitored.

Route	Onset	Peak	Duration
I.V.	Rapid	Unknown	Unknown

Mechanism of Action

Binds to negatively charged sites on bacterial outer cell membranes, which disrupts cell membrane integrity. Kanamycin also binds to bacterial ribosomal subunits and inhibits protein synthesis; these actions lead to cell death.

Contraindications

Hypersensitivity to kanamycin, other aminoglycosides, or their components

Incompatibilities

Don't mix kanamycin in same syringe or administer through same I.V. line as other antibiotics.

Interactions

DRUGS

cephalosporins, vancomycin: Increased risk of nephrotoxicity
digoxin, loop diuretics: Increased ototoxic and nephrotoxic effects of kanamycin
general anesthetics, neuromuscular blockers: Increased risk of neuromuscular blockade
penicillins: Inactivation of kanamycin or synergistic effects

Adverse Reactions

CNS: Ataxia, dizziness, headache
EENT: Hearing loss
GI: Diarrhea
GU: Elevated BUN and serum creatinine levels, oliguria, proteinuria
MS: Muscle paralysis
RESP: Apnea
SKIN: Injection site irritation or pain, rash, pruritus, urticaria

Nursing Considerations

- Obtain body fluid or tissue specimen for culture and sensitivity testing before kanamycin therapy begins, as indicated. Therapy may begin before test results are available.
- Dilute 500-mg vial with 100 to 200 ml of normal saline solution or D_5W, or 1-g vial with 200 to 400 ml of normnal saline solution or D_5W, and infuse over 30 to 60 minutes. Adjust amount of diluent proportionately for pediatric doses. Be aware that vial contents may darken during storage but that this won't affect potency.
- Keep patient well hydrated before and during therapy.
- Monitor blood kanamycin level periodically during therapy, as appropriate.
- Be aware that prolonged treatment increases the risk of ototoxicity and nephrotoxicity. Monitor hearing and renal function if therapy lasts longer than 10 days.
- Store drug at 15° to 30° C (59° to 86° F); don't freeze.

PATIENT TEACHING

- Advise patient to report dizziness, hearing loss, and severe diarrhea or headache during kanamycin therapy.

- Explain the need to receive kanamycin at prescribed intervals around the clock until patient completes full course of therapy.

ketorolac tromethamine

Toradol

Class and Category

Chemical: Acetic acid derivative
Therapeutic: Analgesic, anti-inflammatory
Pregnancy category: C

Indications and Dosages

▶ *To treat moderate to severe pain*

I.V. INJECTION

Adults ages 16 to 64. *Initial:* 30 mg as a single dose or 30 mg q 6 hr p.r.n. *Maximum:* 120 mg daily for no longer than 5 days.

DOSAGE ADJUSTMENT For patients weighing less than 50 kg, elderly patients, and patients with impaired renal function, initial dose reduced to 15 mg, followed by oral ketorolac if needed; or 15 mg q 6 hr p.r.n., up to maximum of 60 mg daily for no longer than 5 days.

Route	Onset	Peak	Duration
I.V.	30 to 60 min	1 to 2 hr	4 to 6 hr

Mechanism of Action

Blocks the activity of cyclooxygenase, the enzyme needed to synthesize prostaglandins. Prostaglandins mediate the inflammatory response and cause local vasodilation, swelling, and pain. They also promote pain transmission from the periphery to the spinal cord. By blocking cyclooxygenase and inhibiting prostaglandins, this NSAID reduces inflammatory symptoms and relieves pain.

Contraindications

Advanced renal impairment or risk of renal impairment due to volume depletion; before or during surgery if hemostasis is critical; breast-feeding; cerebrovascular bleeding; concurrent use of aspirin or other salicylates, other NSAIDs, or probenecid; hemophilia or other bleeding problems, including coagulation or platelet function disorders; hemorrhagic diathesis; history of GI bleeding, GI perforation, or peptic ulcer disease; hypersensitivity to ketorolac tromethamine, aspirin, other NSAIDs, or their components; incomplete hemostasis; labor and delivery

Interactions

DRUGS

ACE inhibitors: Increased risk of renal function impairment
acetaminophen, gold compounds: Increased risk of adverse renal effects
amphotericin, penicillamine, and other nephrotoxic drugs: Increased risk or severity of adverse renal effects
antihypertensives, diuretics: Possibly reduced effects of these drugs
aspirin and other salicylates, other NSAIDs: Additive toxicity
cefamandole, cefoperazone, cefotetan: Possibly hypoprothrombinemia
corticosteroids, potassium supplements: Increased risk of gastric ulceration or hemorrhage
furosemide: Decreased effects of furosemide
heparin, oral anticoagulants, platelet aggregation inhibitors, thrombolytics: Increased risk of GI bleeding
lithium: Possibly increased blood lithium level and increased risk of lithium toxicity
methotrexate: Possibly methotrexate toxicity
plicamycin, valproic acid: Possibly hypoprothrombinemia and increased risk of bleeding
probenecid: Decreased elimination of ketorolac, increased risk of adverse effects

ACTIVITIES

alcohol use: Increased risk of adverse GI effects

Adverse Reactions

CNS: Dizziness, drowsiness, headache
CV: Edema, fluid retention, hypertension
EENT: Stomatitis
GI: Abdominal pain; bloating; constipation; diarrhea; flatulence; GI bleeding, perforation, or ulceration; hepatic failure; indigestion; nausea; vomiting
SKIN: Diaphoresis, pruritus, rash
Other: Anaphylaxis, injection site pain, unusual weight gain

Nursing Considerations

- Read ketorolac label carefully. Don't use I.M. form for I.V. administration. Be aware that ketorolac is not for intrathecal or epidural use.
- Administer drug over at least 15 seconds.

- Notify prescriber if pain relief is inadequate or if breakthrough pain occurs between doses because supplemental doses of an opioid analgesic may be required.
- **WARNING** Monitor liver function test results for possible elevations. If elevated levels persist or worsen, notify prescriber and expect to discontinue drug, as ordered, to prevent hepatic impairment.
- **WARNING** Monitor patients with a history of peripheral edema, heart failure, or hypertension for adequate fluid balance because drug can promote fluid retention and exacerbate these conditions. Assess for dyspnea, edema, unexplained rapid weight gain, and decreased activity tolerance. Notify prescriber if such symptoms develop.
- Be aware that maximum duration of ketorolac therapy (including oral and I.M. forms) is 5 days.
- Store drug at 15° to 30° C (59° to 86° F), and protect from light.

PATIENT TEACHING

- Advise patient to avoid taking acetaminophen, aspirin, other salicylates, and other NSAIDs while receiving ketorolac unless prescriber approves.
- Caution patient to avoid potentially hazardous activities until drug's CNS effects are known.
- Urge patient to avoid alcohol during ketorolac therapy because of increased risk of adverse GI effects.
- Encourage patient to have dental procedures performed before starting drug therapy because of increased risk of bleeding.
- Teach patient proper oral hygiene measures, and encourage him to use a soft-bristled toothbrush during ketorolac therapy.

labetalol hydrochloride

Normodyne, Trandate

Class and Category

Chemical: Benzamine derivative
Therapeutic: Antihypertensive
Pregnancy category: C

Indications and Dosages

▶ *To manage severe hypertension and treat hypertensive emergencies*

I. V. INFUSION

Adults. 200 mg diluted in 160 ml of D_5W and infused at 2 mg/min until desired response occurs.

I.V. INJECTION

Adults. 20 mg given over 2 min; additional doses given in increments of 40 to 80 mg q 10 min as indicated until desired response occurs. *Maximum:* 300 mg.

Route	Onset	Peak	Duration
I.V.	2 to 5 min	5 to 15 min	2 to 4 hr

Mechanism of Action

Selectively blocks $alpha_1$ and $beta_2$ receptors in vascular smooth muscle and $beta_1$ receptors in the heart. These actions reduce peripheral vascular resistance and blood pressure. Potent beta blockade prevents reflex tachycardia, which commonly occurs when alpha blockers reduce the resting heart rate, cardiac output, or stroke volume.

Incompatibilities

Don't dilute labetalol in sodium bicarbonate solution or administer through same I.V. line as alkaline drugs, such as furosemide; doing so may cause a white precipitate to form.

Contraindications

Asthma, cardiogenic shock, heart failure, hypersensitivity to labetalol or its components, second- or third-degree heart block, severe bradycardia

Interactions

DRUGS

allergen immunotherapy, allergenic extracts for skin testing: Increased risk of serious systemic reaction or anaphylaxis
calcium channel blockers, clonidine, diazoxide, guanabenz, reserpine: Possibly hypotension
cimetidine: Possibly increased labetalol effects
estrogens, NSAIDs: Possibly reduced antihypertensive effect of labetalol
general anesthetics: Increased risk of hypotension and myocardial depression
insulin, oral antidiabetic drugs: Increased risk of hyperglycemia
nitroglycerin: Possibly hypertension
phenoxybenzamine, phentolamine: Possibly additive $alpha_1$-blocking effects
sympathomimetics with alpha- and beta-adrenergic effects (such as pseu-

doephedrine): Possibly hypertension, excessive bradycardia, or heart block
xanthines (aminophylline and theophylline): Possibly decreased therapeutic effects of both drugs
FOODS
all food: Increased blood labetalol level
ACTIVITIES
alcohol use: Increased labetalol effects

Adverse Reactions

CNS: Anxiety, confusion, depression, dizziness, drowsiness, fatigue, paresthesia, syncope, vertigo, weakness, yawning
CV: Bradycardia, chest pain, edema, heart block, heart failure, hypotension, orthostatic hypotension, ventricular arrhythmias
EENT: Nasal congestion, taste perversion
GI: Elevated liver function test results, hepatic necrosis, hepatitis, indigestion, nausea, vomiting
GU: Ejaculation failure, impotence
RESP: Dyspnea, wheezing
SKIN: Jaundice, pruritus, rash, scalp tingling

Nursing Considerations

- Dilute labetalol to a final concentration of 1 or 3 mg/ml. Administer infusion by infusion pump or another method that allows precise measurement.
- During labetalol administration, monitor blood pressure according to facility policy, usually every 5 minutes for 30 minutes, then every 30 minutes for 2 hours, and then every hour for 6 hours. Monitor ECG as ordered.
- Keep patient in supine position for 3 hours after I.V. administration.
- **WARNING** Be aware that labetalol masks common signs of shock.
- Monitor blood glucose level in diabetic patient because labetalol may conceal symptoms of hypoglycemia such as tachycardia.
- Expect to discontinue drug if patient's liver function test results are elevated. Monitor closely for signs of hepatotoxicity, such as jaundice and flulike symptoms.
- Monitor for signs of heart failure, such as dyspnea and crackles. Expect to administer a digitalis glycoside, a diuretic, or both at first sign of heart failure. If heart failure continues, expect to discontinue labetalol gradually, if possible.
- Monitor patients who are receiving other drugs with antihypertensive effects. Expect labetalol dosage to be adjusted if patient

experiences adverse reactions, such as hypotension or bradycardia, or if prescriber adds or discontinues another drug.
- Store drug at 2° to 30° C (36° to 86° F); protect from freezing and light.

PATIENT TEACHING
- Advise patient to report confusion, difficulty breathing, rash, slow pulse, and swelling in arms or legs during labetalol therapy.
- Suggest that patient rise slowly and avoid sudden position changes to minimize effects of orthostatic hypotension.
- Inform diabetic patient that her blood glucose level will be monitored often; instruct her to report signs of hypoglycemia.
- Inform patient that transient scalp tingling may occur during early phase of treatment.

lansoprazole
Prevacid, Prevacid I.V., Prevacid SoluTab

Class and Category
Chemical: Substituted benzimidazole
Therapeutic: Antisecretory, antiulcer
Pregnancy category: B

Indications and Dosages
▶ *To treat erosive esophagitis short-term (up to 7 days) in patients unable to take oral medication*

I.V. INFUSION
Adults. 30 mg daily infused over 30 min for up to 7 days.

Route	Onset	Peak	Duration
P.O.	1 to 3 hr	Unknown	More than 24 hr

Mechanism of Action
Binds to and inactivates the hydrogen-potassium adenosine triphosphate enzyme system (also called the proton pump) in gastric parietal cells. This action blocks the final step of gastric acid production.

Incompatibilities
Don't give any other drugs with parenteral lansoprazole, and dilute only with solutions recommended by manufacturer (sterile water for initial reconstitution and normal saline solution, lactated Ringer's solution, or D_5W for further dilution).

Contraindications
Hypersensitivity to lansoprazole or its components

Interactions
DRUGS
ampicillin, digoxin, iron salts, ketoconazole, other drugs that depend on low gastric pH for bioavailability: Inhibited absorption of these drugs
sucralfate: Delayed lansoprazole absorption
theophylline: Slightly decreased blood theophylline level

Adverse Reactions
CNS: Dizziness, headache
GI: Abdominal pain, anorexia, diarrhea, hepatotoxicity, increased appetite, nausea, pancreatitis, pseudomembranous colitis, vomiting
GU: Urine retention
HEME: Agranulocytosis, aplastic anemia, hemolytic anemia, leukopenia, neutropenia, pancytopenia, thrombocytopenia, thrombotic thrombocytopenic purpura
MS: Arthralgia
SKIN: Erythema multiforme, pruritus, rash, Stevens-Johnson syndrome, toxic epidermal necrolysis
Other: Anaphylaxis, injection site reaction

Nursing Considerations
- Reconstitute parenteral form by injecting 5 ml of sterile water into 30-mg vial of drug. Mix gently until powder dissolves. Use within 1 hour. After reconstitution, dilute with 50 ml of normal saline solution, lactated Ringer's solution, or D_5W. Give within 12 hours if mixed with D_5W or 24 hours if mixed with normal saline solution or lactated Ringer's solution.
- Give parenteral drug with a filter following manufacturer's guidelines. Change filter every 24 hours. Give as an I.V. infusion over 30 minutes. Flush the line with normal saline solution, lactated Ringer's solution, or D_5W before and after giving lansoprazole.
- Expect to use lansoprazole with antibiotics because decreased gastric acid secretion helps antibiotics eradicate *Helicobacter pylori.*
- If given with antibiotics, watch for diarrhea from possible pseudomembranous colitis.

PATIENT TEACHING
- Advise patient to report diarrhea, severe headache, or worsening of symptoms immediately to prescriber.

lepirudin

Refludan

Class and Category

Chemical: Yeast-derived recombinant form of hirudin
Therapeutic: Anticoagulant
Pregnancy category: B

Indications and Dosages

▶ *To prevent thromboembolic complications in patients with heparin-induced thrombocytopenia and associated thromboembolic disease*

I.V. INFUSION AND INJECTION

Adults. *Initial:* 0.4 mg/kg, but no more than 44 mg, given by bolus over 15 to 20 sec, followed by continuous infusion of 0.15 mg/kg/ hr for 2 to 10 days or longer, as indicated. *Maximum:* 0.21 mg/kg/hr.

DOSAGE ADJUSTMENT For patients with renal insufficiency, bolus dose decreased to 0.2 mg/kg and infusion rate adjusted as follows: for creatinine clearance of 45 to 60 ml/min/1.73 m^2, 50% of standard infusion rate; for creatinine clearance of 30 to 44 ml/min/1.73 m^2, 30% of standard infusion rate; for creatinine clearance of 15 to 29 ml/min/1.73 m^2, 15% of standard infusion rate; for clearance of less than 15 ml/min/1.73 m^2, expect drug to be stopped.

Route	Onset	Peak	Duration
I.V.	Immediate	Unknown	Unknown

Mechanism of Action

Forms a tight bond with thrombin, neutralizing this enzyme's actions, even when the enzyme is trapped within clots. One molecule of lepirudin binds with one molecule of thrombin. Thrombin causes fibrinogen to convert to fibrin, which is essential for clot formation.

Incompatibilities

Don't mix lepirudin in same I.V. line with other drugs.

Contraindications

Hypersensitivity to lepirudin or other hirudins

Interactions

oral anticoagulants, platelet aggregation inhibitors, thrombolytics: Increased risk of bleeding complications and enhanced effects of lepirudin

Adverse Reactions

CNS: Chills, fever, intracranial hemorrhage
CV: Heart failure
EENT: Epistaxis
GI: GI or rectal bleeding, hepatic dysfunction
GU: Hematuria, vaginal bleeding
HEME: Anemia, easy bruising, hematoma
RESP: Hemoptysis, pneumonia
SKIN: Excessive bleeding from wounds, rash, pruritus, urticaria
Other: Anaphylaxis, injection site bleeding, sepsis

Nursing Considerations

- Be aware that patients with heparin-induced thrombocytopenia have low platelet counts, which can lead to severe bleeding and even death. Lepirudin prevents clotting without further reducing platelet count.
- To reconstitute, mix drug with normal saline solution or sterile water for injection. Warm solution to room temperature before administering.
- For I.V. bolus, reconstitute 50 mg with 1 ml of sterile water for injection or sodium chloride for injection. Then further dilute by withdrawing reconstituted solution into a 10-ml syringe and adding enough sterile water for injection, sodium chloride for injection, or D_5W to produce a total volume of 10 ml, or 5 mg of lepirudin/ml. Administer prescribed dose over 15 to 20 seconds.
- For I.V. infusion, reconstitute 2 vials of drug and transfer to infusion bag that contains 250 or 500 ml of normal saline solution or D_5W. Concentration will be 0.4 or 0.2 mg/ml.
- Adjust infusion rate as prescribed, according to patient's APTT ratio, which is APTT divided by a control value. Target APTT ratio during treatment is 1.5 to 2.5.
- Expect to obtain first APTT 4 hours after starting infusion and to obtain follow-up APTT daily (more often for patients with hepatic or renal impairment).
- Stop infusion for 2 hours, as ordered, if APTT is above target range. Expect to decrease infusion rate by one-half when restarting. If APTT is below target range, expect to increase rate in 20% increments and recheck APTT in 4 hours.
- Avoid I.M. injections or needle sticks during therapy to minimize risk of hematoma.

- Observe I.M. injection sites, I.V. infusion sites, and wounds for bleeding.
- Monitor for ecchymoses on arms and legs, epistaxis, hematemesis, hematuria, melena, and vaginal bleeding.

PATIENT TEACHING
- Tell patient to report unexpected bleeding, such as blood in urine, easy bruising, nosebleeds, tarry stools, and vaginal bleeding.
- Advise patient to avoid bumping arms and legs because of the risk of bruising.
- Encourage patient to use an electric razor and a soft toothbrush to reduce the risk of bleeding.

levetiracetam

Keppra

Class and Category

Chemical: Pyrrolidine derivative
Therapeutic: Anticonvulsant
Pregnancy category: C

Indications and Dosages

▶ *As adjunct to treat partial seizures in patients with epilepsy who are temporarily unable to take oral form*

I.V. INFUSION

Adults and adolescents over age 16. *Initial:* 500 mg b.i.d., over 15 min, increased by 1,000 mg daily q 2 wk if needed. *Maximum:* 3,000 mg daily.

DOSAGE ADJUSTMENT Maximum dosage reduced to 2,000 mg/day if creatinine clearance is 50 to 80 ml/min/1.73 m^2; reduced to 1,500 mg/day if clearance is 30 to 49 ml/min/1.73 m^2; and reduced to 1,000 mg/day if clearance is less than 30 ml/min/1.73 m^2. For patients with end-stage renal disease who are receiving dialysis, expect to give another 250 to 500 mg/dose, as prescribed, after each session.

Mechanism of Action

May protect against secondary generalized seizure activity by preventing coordination of epileptiform burst firing. Levetiracetam doesn't seem to involve inhibitory and excitatory neurotransmission.

Contraindications

Hypersensitivity to levetiracetam or its components

Adverse Reactions

CNS: Aggression, agitation, anger, anxiety, apathy, asthenia, ataxia, confusion, depresson, dizziness, emotional lability, fatigue, headache, hostility, increased reflexes, irritability, mental or mood changes, nervousness, neurosis, paresthesia, personality disorder, somnolence, vertigo
EENT: Amblyopia, conjunctivitis, diplopia, ear pain, pharyngitis, rhinitis, sinusitis
GI: Anorexia, constipation, diarrhea, gastroenteritis, pancreatitis, vomiting
GU: Albuminuria
HEME: Leukopenia, neutropenia, pancytopenia, thrombocytopenia
MS: Neck pain
RESP: Asthma, cough
SKIN: Alopecia, ecchymosis, pruritus, skin discoloration, vesiculobullous rash
Other: Dehydration, facial edema, infection

Nursing Considerations

- Dilute levetiracetam (500 mg/5 ml) solution in 100 ml of normal saline solution, lactated Ringer's solution, or 5% dextrose before administration
- Assess compliance during first 4 weeks of therapy, when adverse reactions are most common.
- Monitor patient for seizure activity during levetiracetam therapy. As appropriate, implement seizure precautions according to facility policy.
- Stopping drug may increase seizure activity. Expect to taper dosage gradually.

PATIENT TEACHING

- Caution patient that levetiracetam may cause dizziness and drowsiness, especially during first 4 weeks of therapy.
- Advise patient to avoid hazardous activities until drug's full CNS effects are known.
- Caution patient not to stop taking levetiracetam abruptly; inform her that drug dosage should be tapered under prescriber's direction to reduce the risk of breakthrough seizures.
- Advise patient to keep taking other anticonvulsants, as ordered, while taking levetiracetam.

- Encourage patient to avoid alcohol during therapy because alcohol can increase incidence of drowsiness and dizziness.
- Instruct patient to see prescriber regularly so that her progress can be monitored.

levofloxacin

Levaquin

Class and Category

Chemical: Fluoroquinolone
Therapeutic: Antibiotic
Pregnancy category: C

Indications and Dosages

▶ *To treat acute maxillary sinusitis caused by* Haemophilus influenzae, Moraxella catarrhalis, *or* Streptococcus pneumoniae

I.V. INFUSION

Adults. 500 mg daily (over 60 to 90 min) for 10 to 14 days.

▶ *To treat acute exacerbations of chronic bacterial bronchitis caused by* H. influenzae, Haemophilus parainfluenzae, M. catarrhalis, S. pneumoniae, *or* Staphylococcus aureus

I.V. INFUSION

Adults. 500 mg daily (over 60 to 90 min) for 7 days.

▶ *To treat community-acquired pneumonia caused by* Chlamydia pneumoniae, H. influenzae, H. parainfluenzae, Klebsiella pneumoniae, Legionella pneumophila, M. catarrhalis, Mycoplasma pneumoniae, S. aureus, *or* S. pneumoniae

I.V. INFUSION

Adults. 500 mg daily (over 60 to 90 min) for 7 to 14 days. Alternatively, for infection caused by *C. pneumoniae, H. influenzae, H. parainfluenzae, M. pneumoniae, or S. pneumoniae,* 750 mg daily (over 60 to 90 min) for 5 days.

▶ *To treat uncomplicated UTI caused by* Escherichia coli, K. pneumoniae, *or* Staphylococcus saprophyticus

I.V. INFUSION

Adults. 250 mg daily (over 60 to 90 min) for 3 days.

▶ *To treat complicated UTI and acute pyelonephritis caused by* E. coli

I.V. INFUSION

Adults. 250 mg daily (over 60 to 90 min) for 10 days.

▶ *To treat mild to moderate skin and soft-tissue infections caused by* S. aureus *or* Streptococcus pyogenes

I.V. INFUSION

Adults. 500 mg daily (over 60 to 90 min) for 7 to 10 days.

▶ *To treat complicated skin and soft-tissue infections caused by methicillin-sensitive* Enterococcus faecalis, Proteus mirabilis, S. aureus, *or* S. pyogenes; *to treat nosocomial pneumonia caused by* S. aureus, Pseudomonas aeruginosa, Serratia marcescens, E. coli, K. pneumoniae, H. influenzae, *or* S. pneumoniae

I.V. INFUSION

Adults. 750 mg daily (over 60 to 90 min) for 7 to 14 days.

▶ *To treat chronic bacterial prostatitis caused by* E. coli, E. faecalis, *or* S. epidermidis

I.V. INFUSION

Adults. 500 mg daily (over 60 to 90 min for I.V. infusion) for 28 days.

DOSAGE ADJUSTMENT For complicated UTI in patient with creatinine clearance of 10 to 19 ml/min/1.73 m^2, 250 mg initially and then maintenance dosage of 250 mg q 48 hr. For complicated skin and soft-tissue infection or nosocomial pneumonia when creatinine clearance is 19 ml/min/1.73 m^2 or less, 750 mg initially and then maintenance dosage of 500 mg q 48 hr; when creatinine clearance is 20 to 49 ml/min/1.73 m^2, 750 mg initially and then maintenance dosage of 750 mg q 48 hr. For all other indications, when creatinine clearance is 19 ml/ min/1.73 m^2 or less, 500 mg initially and then maintenance dosage of 250 mg q 48 hr; when creatinine clearance is 20 to 49 ml/ min/1.73 m^2, 500 mg initially and then maintenance dosage of 250 mg q 24 hr.

Mechanism of Action

Interferes with bacterial cell replication by inhibiting the bacterial enzyme DNA gyrase, which is essential for replication and repair of bacterial DNA.

Contraindications

Hypersensitivity to levofloxacin, other fluoroquinolones, or their components

Interactions

DRUGS

aluminum-, calcium-, or magnesium-containing antacids; didanosine; iron; sucralfate; zinc: Reduced GI absorption of levofloxacin

antineoplastics: Decreased blood levofloxacin level
cimetidine: Increased blood levofloxacin level
cyclosporine: Increased risk of nephrotoxicity
NSAIDs: Possibly increased CNS stimulation and risk of seizures
oral anticoagulants: Increased anticoagulant effect and risk of bleeding
oral antidiabetic drugs: Possibly hyperglycemia or hypoglycemia
theophylline: Increased blood theophylline level and risk of toxicity

ACTIVITIES

sun exposure: Increased risk of photosensitivity

Adverse Reactions

CNS: Anxiety, CNS stimulation, dizziness, headache, increased ICP, light-headedness, nervousness, peripheral neuropathy, psychosis, seizures, sleep disturbance
CV: Arrhythmias, prolonged QT interval
EENT: Taste perversion
ENDO: Hyperglycemia, hypoglycemia
GI: Abdominal pain, anorexia, constipation, diarrhea, flatulence, indigestion, nausea, pseudomembranous colitis, vomiting
GU: Crystalluria, vaginal candidiasis
HEME: Eosinophilia, hemolytic anemia
MS: Back pain, rhabdomyolysis, tendon rupture
SKIN: Photosensitivity, pruritus, rash, urticaria
Other: Anaphylaxis

Nursing Considerations

- Use levofloxacin cautiously in patients with renal insufficiency. Monitor renal function as appropriate during treatment.
- Use drug cautiously in patients with CNS disorders that may lower the seizure threshold, such as epilepsy.
- Expect to obtain culture and sensitivity tests before levofloxacin treatment begins.
- Avoid giving drug within 2 hours of antacids.
- Give parenteral form over 60 to 90 minutes, depending on dosage, because bolus or rapid I.V. delivery may cause hypotension.
- **WARNING** Stop levofloxacin at the first sign of hypersensitivity, including rash, because it may lead to anaphylaxis. Reaction may occur after the first dose. Expect to give epinephrine, and provide supportive care.
- Monitor blood glucose level, especially in diabetic patient who takes an oral antidiabetic or insulin, because levfloxacin may al-

ter blood glucose levels. If so, notify prescriber, stop drug immediately for hypoglycemia, and provide prescribed treatment.
- Monitor QT interval if needed. If it lengthens, notify prescriber immediately and stop drug. Patients with hypokalemia, significant bradycardia, or cardiomyopathy and those receiving a class Ia or III antiarrhythmic shouldn't receive levofloxacin.
- Notify prescriber if patient has symptoms of peripheral neuropathy (pain, burning, tingling, numbness, weakness, or altered sensations of light touch, pain, temperature, position sense, or vibration sense), which could be permanent; tendon rupture, which requires immediate rest; or CNS abnormalities (seizures, psychosis, increased ICP or CNS stimulation), which may lead to more serious adverse reactions, such as suicidal thoughts. In each case, expect to stop levofloxacin.
- Monitor patient's bowel elimination. If diarrhea develops, obtain stool culture to check for pseudomembranous colitis. If confirmed, expect to stop drug and give fluid, electrolytes, and antibiotics effective against Clostridium difficile.

PATIENT TEACHING
- Advise patient to increase fluid intake during levofloxacin therapy to prevent crystalluria.
- Advise patient to avoid excessive exposure to sunlight and to wear sunscreen because of increased risk of photosensitivity. Tell patient to notify prescriber at first sign of photosensitivity.
- Caution patient to avoid hazardous activities until drug's CNS effects are known.
- Tell patient to stop drug and notify prescriber if he develops tendon pain or inflammation or abnormal changes in motor or sensory function.
- Urge patient to stop drug and tell prescriber if a rash or other allergic reaction develops.
- Advise diabetic patient to monitor blood glucose level and notify prescriber about changes.

levorphanol tartrate

Levo-Dromoran

Class, Category, and Schedule

Chemical: Morphinan derivative
Therapeutic: Opioid analgesic
Pregnancy category: Not rated
Controlled substance: Schedule II

Indications and Dosages

▶ *To relieve moderate to severe pain*

I.V. INJECTION

Adults. Up to 1 mg q 3 to 6 hr, p.r.n. *Maximum:* 8 mg daily for non–opioid-dependent patients.

Route	Onset	Peak	Duration
I.V.	Unknown	In 20 min	4 to 5 hr

Mechanism of Action

Decreases intracellular cAMP level by inhibiting adenylate cyclase, which regulates the release of pain neurotransmitters, such as substance P, gamma-aminobutyric acid, dopamine, acetylcholine, and noradrenaline. Levorphanol also stimulates mu and kappa opioid receptors, altering the perception of pain and, possibly, the emotional response to it.

Incompatibilities

Don't mix levorphanol tartrate with solutions that contain aminophylline, ammonium chloride, amobarbital sodium, chlorothiazide sodium, heparin sodium, methicillin sodium, nitrofurantoin sodium, novobiacin sodium, pentobarbital sodium, perphenazine, phenobarbital sodium, phenytoin, secobarbital sodium, sodium bicarbonate, sodium iodide, sulfadiazine sodium, sulfisoxazole diethanolamine, or thiopental sodium.

Contraindications

Acute alcoholism, acute or severe asthma, anoxia, hypersensitivity to levorphanol tartrate or its components, increased ICP, respiratory depression, upper airway obstruction

Interactions

DRUGS

alfentanil, CNS depressants, fentanyl, sufentanil: Possibly increased CNS and respiratory depression and hypotension

anticholinergics: Increased risk of severe constipation

antidiarrheals (such as difenoxin and atropine, kaolin, and loperamide): Possibly severe constipation and increased CNS depression

antihypertensives: Increased risk of hypotension

buprenorphine: Possibly decreased therapeutic effects of levorphanol and increased risk of respiratory depression

hydroxyzine: Increased risk of CNS depression and hypotension

metoclopramide: Possibly antagonized effects of metoclopramide
naloxone, naltrexone: Decreased therapeutic effects of levorphanol
neuromuscular blockers: Increased risk of prolonged CNS and respiratory depression

ACTIVITIES

alcohol use: Possibly increased CNS and respiratory depression and hypotension

Adverse Reactions

CNS: Amnesia, coma, confusion, delusions, depression, dizziness, drowsiness, dyskinesia, hypokinesia, insomnia, nervousness, personality disorder, seizures
CV: Bradycardia, cardiac arrest, hypotension, orthostatic hypotension, palpitations, shock, tachycardia
EENT: Abnormal vision, diplopia, dry mouth
GI: Abdominal pain, biliary tract spasm, constipation, hepatic failure, indigestion, nausea, vomiting
GU: Dysuria, urine retention
RESP: Apnea, hyperventilation
SKIN: Cyanosis, pruritus, rash, urticaria
Other: Injection site pain, redness, and swelling; physical and psychological dependence

Nursing Considerations

- **WARNING** Be aware that levorphanol may be habit-forming and that patients with a history of drug abuse (including acute alcoholism), emotional instability, or suicidal ideation or attempts are at increased risk for opioid abuse.
- **WARNING** Give levorphanol slowly, over several minutes, because rapid administration of other opioid analgesics has caused anaphylaxis, severe respiratory depression, hypotension, peripheral circulatory collapse, and cardiac arrest. Keep emergency equipment and drugs nearby.
- Assess patient's respiratory status closely, especially in patients having an acute asthma attack and those with adrenal insufficiency, chronic respiratory disease, hypothyroidism, myxedema, severe hepatic or renal impairment, or conditions that increase CSF pressure, because drug causes respiratory depression. Elderly, extremely ill, or debilitated patients and patients who have recently taken, or are currently taking, drugs with respiratory depressant effects are also more sensitive to levorphanol's effects.

- Monitor supine and standing blood pressure periodically, and notify prescriber of orthostatic hypotension.
- Watch carefully for adverse reactions in elderly patients because they're especially sensitive to levorphanol and at increased risk for constipation.
- Monitor for signs of drug-induced CNS depression or increased CSF pressure, such as altered LOC, restlessness, and irritability, in patients with a coma, head injury, intracranial lesions, or other conditions that could cause these effects. Patients who are taking, or have recently taken, drugs that depress the CNS are also more susceptible to these effects.
- Be aware that opioids such as levorphanol may induce or worsen arrhythmias or seizures in patients who have a history of these conditions. It also may mask acute abdominal conditions.
- Because levorphanol is metabolized in the liver, be aware of need to monitor patients with hepatic impairment and those taking drugs that decrease hepatic clearance for signs of increased sedation.
- Monitor patients with prostatic hypertrophy, renal function impairment, or urethral stricture and those who have recently undergone urinary tract surgery for signs of urine retention, such as difficulty voiding or feeling that bladder isn't empty after voiding, peripheral edema, or weight gain. Impaired renal function can affect excretion of levorphanol, causing increased effects.
- Monitor patients with biliary tract disease for biliary colic (pain in upper midline area that may radiate to the back and right shoulder), which may be caused by drug-induced increase in intracholedochal pressure.
- Because levorphanol's effects on the heart aren't known, expect limited use of this drug in patients with acute MI, ventricular dysfunction, or coronary insufficiency.
- Store drug between 15° and 30° C (59° and 86° F); don't freeze.

PATIENT TEACHING

- Instruct patient to lie down during levorphanol administration and for a period afterward to lessen drug's hypotensive effects (dizziness, light-headedness) and other adverse effects, such as nausea and vomiting.
- Advise patient to avoid potentially hazardous activities until drug's CNS effects are known.

- Instruct patient to avoid alcoholic beverages while taking levorphanol.
- Direct patient to change position slowly to minimize effects of orthostatic hypotension.
- Advise patient to report constipation, nausea, or vomiting to prescriber.
- Suggest that patient relieve dry mouth with sugarless candy or gum or ice chips.

levothyroxine sodium

(L-thyroxine sodium, T_4, thyroxine sodium)

Levothroid, Synthroid

Class and Category

Chemical: Synthetic thyroxine (T_4)
Therapeutic: Thyroid hormone replacement
Pregnancy category: A

Indications and Dosages

▶ *To treat severe hypothyroidism*

I.V. INJECTION

Adults. 50 to 100 mcg daily until therapeutic blood level is reached.

Children. 75% of usual P.O. dose daily until therapeutic blood level is reached.

▶ *To treat myxedema coma*

I.V. INJECTION

Adults. 200 to 500 mcg on day 1. If no significant improvement occurs, 100 to 300 mcg on day 2. Daily dose continued as prescribed until therapeutic blood level is reached and P.O. route is tolerated.

Children. 75% of usual P.O. dose daily until therapeutic blood level is reached and P.O. route is tolerated.

Route	Onset	Peak	Duration
I.V.	6 to 8 hr	24 hr	Unknown

Contraindications

Acute MI (unless caused or complicated by hyperthyroidism), hypersensitivity to levothyroxine or its components, uncorrected adrenal insufficiency, untreated thyrotoxicosis

Mechanism of Action

Replaces endogenous thyroid hormone, which may exert its physiologic effects by controlling DNA transcription and protein synthesis. Levothyroxine exhibits all of the following actions of endogenous thyroid hormone. The drug:

- increases energy expenditure
- accelerates the rate of cellular oxidation, which stimulates body tissue growth, maturation, and metabolism
- regulates differentiation and proliferation of stem cells
- aids in myelination of nerves and development of synaptic processes in the nervous system
- regulates growth
- decreases blood and hepatic cholesterol concentrations
- enhances carbohydrate and protein metabolism, increasing gluconeogenesis and protein synthesis.

Interactions

DRUGS

adrenocorticoids: Possibly adrenocorticoid dosage adjustments as thyroid status changes
aluminum- and magnesium-containing antacids, bile acid sequestrants, calcium carbonate, cation exchange resins, cholestyramine, colestipol, ferrous sulfate, kayexalate, sucralfate: Possibly reduced effects of levothyroxine
amiodarone, iodide: Possibly hyperthyroidism
beta blockers: Possibly impaired action of beta blockers and decreased conversion of T_4 to triiodothyronine (T_3)
cholestyramine, colestipol: Delayed or inhibited levothyroxine absorption
digoxin: Reduced therapeutic effects of digoxin
estrogen, phenylbutazone, phenytoin: Reduced binding of levothyroxine to protein, possibly requiring increased levothyroxine dosage
insulin, oral antidiabetic drugs: Possibly uncontrolled diabetes mellitus, requiring increased dosage of insulin or oral antidiabetic drug
ketamine: Possibly hypertension and tachycardia
maprotiline: Increased risk of arrhythmias
oral anticoagulants: Altered anticoagulant activity, possibly need for anticoagulant dosage adjustment
selective serotonin reuptake inhibitors, tricyclic and tetracyclic antidepressants: Increased therapeutic and toxic effects of both drugs

sympathomimetics: Increased risk of coronary insufficiency in patients with coronary artery disease
theophylline: Decreased theophylline clearance
FOODS
dietary fiber, soybean flour (infant formula), walnuts: Possibly decreased absorption of levothyroxine from GI tract

Adverse Reactions

CNS: Fatigue, headache, insomnia, somnolence
ENDO: Hyperthyroidism (with overdose)
GI: Dysphagia
MS: Muscle weakness, myalgia, slipped capital femoral epiphysis
SKIN: Alopecia (transient), rash, urticaria
Other: Weight gain

Nursing Considerations

- Expect to give drug I.V. if patient can't take tablets. Be aware that drug shouldn't be given S.C.
- For I.V. use, reconstitute drug by adding 5 ml of normal saline solution.
- Monitor PT of patient who is receiving anticoagulants; she may require a dosage adjustment.
- Monitor blood glucose level of diabetic patient. Prescriber may reduce antidiabetic drug dosage as thyroid hormone level enters therapeutic range.
- Expect patient to undergo regular thyroid function tests during levothyroxine therapy.

PATIENT TEACHING

- Inform patient that levothyroxine replaces a hormone that is normally produced by the thyroid gland and that she'll probably need to take drug for life.
- Inform patient that drug may require a few weeks to take effect.
- Instruct patient to report signs of hyperthyroidism, such as diarrhea, excessive sweating, heat intolerance, insomnia, palpitations, weight loss, chest pain, shortness of breath, leg cramps, headache, nervousness, irritability, tremors, changes in appetite, vomiting, fever, and changes in menstrual periods.
- Tell patient to notify prescriber if rash or hives develop during drug use.
- Inform patient that transient hair loss may occur during first few months of therapy.

- Instruct female patient of childbearing age to notify prescriber immediately if she becomes pregnant because levothyroxine dosage may need to be increased.

lidocaine hydrochloride
(lignocaine hydrochloride)

Xylocaine, Xylocard (CAN)

Class and Category

Chemical: Aminoacyamide
Therapeutic: Class IB antiarrhythmic
Pregnancy category: B

Indications and Dosages

▶ *To treat ventricular tachycardia or ventricular fibrillation*

I.V. INFUSION AND INJECTION

Adults. *Loading:* 50 to 100 mg (or 1 to 1.5 mg/kg), administered at 25 to 50 mg/min. If desired response isn't achieved after 5 to 10 min, second dose of 25 to 50 mg (or 0.5 to 0.75 mg/kg) is given q 5 to 10 min until maximum loading dose (300 mg in 1 hr) has been given. *Maintenance:* 20 to 50 mcg/kg/min (1 to 4 mg/min) by continuous infusion. Smaller bolus dose repeated 15 to 20 min after start of infusion if needed to maintain therapeutic blood level. *Maximum:* 300 mg (or 3 mg/kg) over 1 hr.
Children. *Loading:* 1 mg/kg. *Maintenance:* 30 mcg/kg/min by continuous infusion. *Maximum:* 3 mg/kg.

DOSAGE ADJUSTMENT For elderly patients receiving lidocaine to treat arrhythmias and for patients with acute hepatitis or decompensated cirrhosis, loading dose and continuous infusion rate reduced by 50%.

Route	Onset	Peak	Duration
I.V.	45 to 90 sec	Immediate	10 to 20 min

Mechanism of Action

Combines with fast sodium channels in myocardial cell membranes, which inhibits sodium influx into cells and decreases ventricular depolarization, automaticity, and excitability during diastole.

Contraindications

Adams-Stokes syndrome; hypersensitivity to lidocaine, amide

anesthetics, or their components; severe heart block (without artificial pacemaker); Wolff-Parkinson-White syndrome

Interactions

DRUGS

beta blockers, cimetidine: Increased blood lidocaine level and risk of toxicity
MAO inhibitors, tricyclic antidepressants: Risk of severe, prolonged hypertension
mexiletine, tocainide: Additive cardiac effects
neuromuscular blockers: Possibly increased neuromuscular blockade
phenytoin, procainamide: Increased cardiac depression

Adverse Reactions

CNS: Anxiety, confusion, difficulty speaking, dizziness, hallucinations, lethargy, paresthesia, seizures
CV: Bradycardia, cardiac arrest, hypotension, new or worsening arrhythmias
EENT: Blurred vision, diplopia, tinnitus
GI: Nausea
MS: Muscle twitching
RESP: Respiratory arrest or depression
Other: Allergic reaction; injection site burning, irritation, stinging, swelling, or tenderness

Nursing Considerations

- Carefully check prefilled lidocaine syringes before using. Use only syringes labeled "FOR CARDIAC ARRHYTHMIAS."
- Check label to verify that you're using a lidocaine preparation that does *not* contain preservatives or other drugs. Dilute drug with D_5W, typically to a final concentration of 1 or 2 mg/ml. Consult manufacturer's guidelines for alternative dilution information. Include final concentration on label. Administer drug using an infusion pump or another device that allows precise measurement.
- Observe for respiratory depression after bolus injection and during I.V. infusion of lidocaine.
- Keep life-support equipment and vasopressors nearby during administration in case respiratory depression or other reactions occur.
- Titrate dosage, as prescribed, to minimum amount needed to prevent arrhythmias.
- During administration, place patient on cardiac monitor, as ordered, and closely observe her at all times. Monitor for worsen-

ing arrhythmias, widening QRS complex, and prolonged PR interval—possible signs of drug toxicity.
- Monitor blood lidocaine level, as ordered. Check for therapeutic level of 2 to 5 mcg/ml.
- If signs of toxicity, such as dizziness, occur, notify prescriber and expect to discontinue or slow infusion.
- Monitor vital signs as well as BUN and serum creatinine and electrolyte levels during and after therapy.
- Store drug at 15° to 30° C (59° to 86° F).

PATIENT TEACHING
- Advise patient who receives lidocaine to report difficulty speaking, dizziness, injection site pain, nausea, numbness or tingling, or vision changes.

lincomycin hydrochloride

Lincocin

Class and Category

Chemical: Lincosamide
Therapeutic: Bacteriostatic or bactericidal antibiotic
Pregnancy category: C

Indications and Dosages

▶ *To treat serious respiratory, skin, and soft-tissue infections caused by susceptible strains of streptococci, pneumococci, and staphylococci*

I.V. INFUSION

Adults. 600 mg to 1 g q 8 to 12 hr. *Maximum:* 8 g daily in divided doses for life-threatening infection.
Children over age 1 month. 10 to 20 mg/kg daily in divided doses q 8 to 12 hr, depending on severity of infection.
DOSAGE ADJUSTMENT Dosage reduced by 25% to 30% in patients with severely impaired renal function.

Mechanism of Action

Inhibits protein synthesis in susceptible bacteria by binding to the 50S subunit of bacterial ribosomes and preventing peptide bond formation, thus causing bacterial cells to die.

Incompatibilities

Don't administer lincomycin with novobiocin or kanamycin.

Contraindications

Hypersensitivity to lincomycin or clindamycin

Interactions

DRUGS

antimyasthenic drugs: Possibly antagonized effects of antimyasthenic drug

chloramphenicol, clindamycin, erythromycin: Possibly blocked access of lincomycin to its site of action

hydrocarbon inhalation anesthetics, neuromuscular blockers: Increased neuromuscular blockade, possibly severe respiratory depression

opioid analgesics: Increased risk of prolonged or increased respiratory depression

Adverse Reactions

CNS: Fever, vertigo

CV: Cardiac arrest and hypotension (with rapid administration)

EENT: Glossitis, stomatitis, tinnitus

GI: Abdominal cramps, colitis, diarrhea, nausea, pseudomembranous colitis, rectal candidiasis, vomiting

GU: Vaginal candidiasis

HEME: Agranulocytosis, eosinophilia, leukopenia, neutropenia, thrombocytopenic purpura

SKIN: Erythema multiforme, rash, Stevens-Johnson syndrome, urticaria

Other: Anaphylaxis, angioedema, superinfection

Nursing Considerations

- Expect to obtain a specimen for culture and sensitivity testing before administering first dose of lincomycin.
- **WARNING** Be aware that some preparations of lincomycin contain benzyl alcohol, which can cause a fatal toxic syndrome in neonates or premature infants, characterized by CNS, respiratory, circulatory, and renal impairment and metabolic acidosis. Because lincomycin has appeared in breast milk, breast-feeding patient may be required to discontinue drug or stop breast-feeding.
- Dilute 600-mg dose in at least 100 ml of D_5W, $D_{10}W$, normal saline solution, dextrose 5% in normal saline solution, or other compatible diluent identified on manufacturer's insert. Dilute higher doses with 100 ml of a compatible diluent for each gram being administered—for example, you'd dilute a 3-g dose in at least 300 ml of diluent. Use diluted solution within 24 hours if stored at room temperature.

- **WARNING** Administer lincomycin over at least 1 hour for each gram being administered. For example, you'd infuse 1 g over 1 hour and 3 g over 3 hours. Too-rapid infusion may result in cardiac arrest or hypotension.
- **WARNING** Monitor for a hypersensitivity reaction, such as rash, pruritus, wheezing, and dysphagia due to laryngeal edema. If such reactions occur, discontinue infusion and notify prescriber immediately. If anaphylaxis occurs, administer epinephrine, antihistamines, oxygen, and corticosteroids, as prescribed. Be aware that patients with a history of asthma or significant allergies are at increased risk for a hypersensitivity reaction.
- Observe patient for signs of superinfection, such as vaginal itching and sore mouth.
- Monitor patient for signs of pseudomembranous colitis, such as watery, loose stools. Patients with a history of GI disease, particularly colitis or regional enteritis, are at increased risk for colitis. Be aware that antibiotic-related diarrhea may be more severe and less well tolerated in elderly patients. Expect to discontinue lincomycin if diarrhea occurs.
- Monitor results of liver and renal function tests, CBC, and platelet counts periodically during lincomycin therapy.
- Before diluting drug, store it at a controlled room temperature of 20° to 25° C (68° to 77° F).

PATIENT TEACHING

- Review with patient possibly serious adverse reactions associated with lincomycin use, such as difficulty breathing, rash, and chest tightness, and tell him to report any that occur.
- Inform him that yogurt or buttermilk can help maintain intestinal flora and may decrease the risk of diarrhea.
- Stress the importance of following dosage regimen and keeping follow-up medical appointments and appointments for laboratory tests.

linezolid

Zyvox

Class and Category

Chemical: Oxazolidinone
Therapeutic: Antibiotic
Pregnancy category: C

Indications and Dosages

▶ *To treat vancomycin-resistant* Enterococcus faecium *infections, including bacteremia*
I.V. INFUSION
Adults and adolescents. 600 mg q 12 hr for 14 to 28 days.
Infants and children. 10 mg/kg q 8 hr for 14 to 28 days.

▶ *To treat nosocomial pneumonia caused by* Staphylococcus aureus *(methicillin-susceptible and -resistant strains) or* Streptococcus pneumoniae *(penicillin-susceptible strains only) and community-acquired pneumonia, including accompanying bacteremia, caused by* S. aureus *(methicillin-susceptible strains only) or* S. pneumoniae *(penicillin-susceptible strains only); to treat complicated skin and soft-tissue infections, including diabetic foot infections without concomitant osteomyelitis, caused by* S. aureus *(methicillin-susceptible and -resistant strains),* Streptococcus pyogenes, *or* Streptococcus agalactiae
I.V. INFUSION
Adults and adolescents. 600 mg q 12 hr for 10 to 14 days.
Infants and children. 10 mg/kg q 8 hr for 10 to 14 days.

Incompatibilities

Don't add other drugs to linezolid solution. Don't infuse linezolid in the same I.V. line as amphotericin B, chlorpromazine hydrochloride, co-trimoxazole, diazepam, erythromycin lactobionate, pentamidine isethionate, or phenytoin sodium because these drugs are physically incompatible. Don't infuse linezolid with ceftriaxone sodium because these two drugs are chemically incompatible.

Contraindications

Hypersensitivity to linezolid or its components; phenylketonuria (oral suspension)

Interactions

DRUGS
adrenergics, including pseudoephedrine and phenylpropanolamine: Enhanced vasopressor response of adrenergics, resulting in increased blood pressure
serotonergics: Possibly serotonin syndrome
FOODS
tyramine-containing foods and beverages: Possibly hypertension

Adverse Reactions

CNS: Dizziness, fever, headache, insomnia, optic and peripheral neuropathy, serotonin syndrome
CV: Hypertension

Mechanism of Action

Inhibits bacterial protein synthesis by interfering with translation of ribonucleic acid (RNA) to protein. In bacteria, protein synthesis begins with binding of a 30S ribosomal subunit and a 50S ribosomal subunit to a messenger RNA (mRNA) molecule to form a 70S initiation complex, as shown in the top illustration. The 50S ribosomal subunit consists of 23S ribosomal RNA (rRNA) and other ribosomal subunits. Then translation begins. Transfer RNA (tRNA) attaches to the 50S subunit and brings specific amino acids into place. As the tRNA and amino acids fall into place, they are joined together by peptide bonds and elongate to form a polypeptide chain. This chain eventually combines with other polypeptide chains to form a complete protein molecule. After translation is complete, the ribosomal subunits fall away and are ready to combine with more mRNA to start the translation process over again.

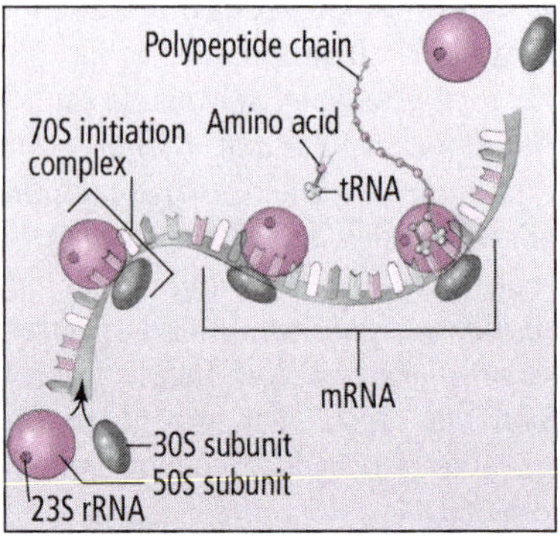

Linezolid binds to a site on the bacterial 23S rRNA of the 50S subunit, as shown in the bottom illustration. This action prevents formation of a functional 70S initiation complex, an essential component of the bacterial translation. Without proper protein production, susceptible bacteria can't multiply. Linezolid is bacteriostatic against staphylococci and enterococci and bactericidal against most streptococci.

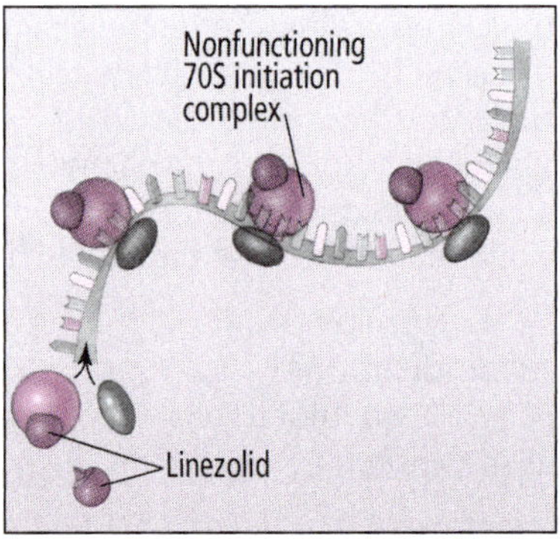

EENT: Oral candidiasis, tongue discoloration
GI: Abdominal pain, constipation, diarrhea, indigestion, nausea, pseudomembranous colitis, vomiting
GU: Vaginal candidiasis
HEME: Anemia, leukopenia, pancytopenia, thrombocytopenia

SKIN: Pruritus, rash
Other: Lactic acidosis

Nursing Considerations

- Obtain body tissue and fluid specimens for culture and sensitivity tests, as ordered, before giving first dose of linezolid. Expect to begin drug before test results are known.
- Infuse I.V. solution over 30 to 120 minutes with D_5W, normal saline solution, or lactated Ringer's solution.
- **WARNING** Monitor CBC weekly, as ordered, to detect or track worsening myelosuppression in patients who need more than 2 weeks of therapy, who have preexisting myelosuppression and are receiving drugs that produce bone marrow suppression, or who have chronic infection and are receiving or have received antibiotic therapy.
- Notify prescriber if patient develops visual impairment that suggests optic neuropathy, such as changes in visual acuity or color vision, blurred vision, lost vision, or visual field defect. If optic or peripheral neuropathy develops, the drug may need to be stopped.
- Monitor bowel pattern daily. Assess patient for secondary infection, including oral candidiasis and profuse, watery diarrhea.

PATIENT TEACHING

- Advise patient not to take OTC cold remedies without consulting prescriber because medications that contain pseudoephedrine or propanolamine may cause or worsen hypertension.
- Instruct patient to avoid foods and beverages that contain large amounts of tyramine, including aged cheese, fermented or air-dried meats, sauerkraut, soy sauce, tap beers, red wines, and protein-rich foods that have been stored for long periods or poorly refrigerated.
- Instruct patient to notify prescriber immediately about severe diarrhea, vision changes, or changes in limb sensation (such as pins and needles, numbness, or tingling) because drug may need to be stopped.

liothyronine sodium

(L-triiodothyronine, sodium L-triiodothyronine, T_3, thyronine sodium)

Triostat

Class and Category

Chemical: Synthetic triiodothyronine (T_3)
Therapeutic: Thyroid hormone replacement
Pregnancy category: A

Indications and Dosages

▶ *To treat myxedema coma or premyxedema coma (severe hypothyroidism)*

I.V. INJECTION

Adults. *Initial:* 25 to 50 mcg; repeated q 4 to 12 hr, depending on patient's response.

DOSAGE ADJUSTMENT Initial dose decreased to 10 to 20 mcg for patients with known or suspected cardiovascular disease who are being treated for myxedema coma.

Route	Onset	Peak	Duration
I.V.	2 to 4 hr	2 days	Unknown

Mechanism of Action

Replaces endogenous thyroid hormone, which may exert its physiologic effects by controlling DNA transcription and protein synthesis. Liothyronine exhibits all of the following actions of endogenous thyroid hormone:

- increases energy expenditure
- accelerates the rate of cellular oxidation, which stimulates body tissue growth, maturation, and metabolism
- regulates differentiation and proliferation of stem cells
- aids in myelination of nerves and development of synaptic processes in the nervous system
- regulates growth
- decreases blood and hepatic cholesterol concentrations
- enhances carbohydrate and protein metabolism, increasing gluconeogenesis and protein synthesis.

Contraindications

Acute MI (unless caused or complicated by hypothyroidism), hypersensitivity to liothyronine or its components, uncorrected adrenal insufficiency, untreated thyrotoxicosis

Interactions

DRUGS

adrenocorticoids: Possibly need for adrenocorticoid dosage adjustments as thyroid status changes

beta blockers: Possibly impaired action of beta blockers
cholestyramine, colestipol: Decreased liothyronine absorption
digoxin: Reduced therapeutic effects of digoxin
estrogen, phenylbutazone, phenytoin: Reduced binding of liothyronine to protein, possibly requiring increased liothyronine dosage
insulin, oral antidiabetic drugs: Possibly uncontrolled diabetes mellitus, requiring increased dosage of insulin or oral antidiabetic drug
ketamine: Possibly hypertension and tachycardia
maprotiline: Increased risk of arrhythmias
oral anticoagulants: Altered anticoagulant activity, possibly need for anticoagulant dosage adjustment
sympathomimetics: Increased risk of coronary insufficiency in patients with coronary artery disease
theophylline: Decreased theophylline clearance
tricyclic antidepressants: Increased therapeutic and toxic effects of both drugs

Adverse Reactions

CNS: Insomnia
ENDO: Hyperthyroidism (with overdose)
SKIN: Alopecia (transient), rash, urticaria

Nursing Considerations

- Be aware that liothyronine is used most often when rapid-onset or rapidly reversible thyroid hormone replacement is needed.
- Give I.V. injections more than 4 hours but less than 12 hours apart.
- Evaluate response to therapy by monitoring pulse rate and blood pressure.
- Expect patient to undergo regular thyroid function tests during liothyronine therapy.
- Monitor PT of patient receiving anticoagulants; she may require a dosage adjustment.
- Monitor patients with a history of cardiovascular disease for signs of ischemia or tachyarrhythmias. If such signs occur, notify prescriber and expect to adjust liothyronine dosage.
- Frequently monitor blood glucose level of diabetic patient. Prescriber may reduce antidiabetic drug dosage as thyroid hormone level enters therapeutic range.
- Expect oral thyroid hormone replacement therapy to be initiated or resumed as soon as possible. Expect to discontinue infusion gradually if patient is switched to levothyroxine tablets because of levothyroxine's delayed onset of action.

- Be aware that patients with myxedema coma may also be prescribed corticosteroids; those with pituitary myxedema may also receive adrenocortical hormone replacement before or at beginning of liothyronine therapy; and those with primary myxedema may receive adrenocortical hormone replacement to prevent adrenocortical insufficiency and shock.
- Store drug at 2° to 8° C (36° to 46° F).

PATIENT TEACHING

- Advise patient receiving liothyronine to report signs or symptoms of hyperthyroidism, such as chest pain, excessive sweating, heat intolerance, increased pulse rate, nervousness, and palpitations.
- Tell diabetic patient that her blood glucose level will be tested often because antidiabetic dosage may need to be reduced.
- Inform patient of need for periodic blood tests to monitor drug's effectiveness.

lorazepam

Ativan

Class, Category, and Schedule

Chemical: Benzodiazepine
Therapeutic: Amnestic, antianxiety, anticonvulsant, sedative
Pregnancy category: D
Controlled substance: Schedule IV

Indications and Dosages

▶ *To provide preoperative sedation*

I.V. INJECTION

Adults and adolescents. 0.044 mg/kg or 2 mg, whichever is less, given 2 hr before procedure. *Maximum:* 0.05 mg/kg or total of 4 mg.

▶ *To treat status epilepticus*

I.V. INJECTION

Adults and adolescents. *Initial:* 4 mg at 2 mg/min; if seizures don't subside, repeat in 10 to 15 min . *Maximum:* 8 mg/24 hr.

Route	Onset	Peak	Duration
I.V.	5 min	Unknown	12 to 24 hr

Incompatibilities

Don't mix I.V. lorazepam in same syringe as buprenorphine.

Mechanism of Action

May potentiate the effects of gamma-aminobutyric acid (GABA) and other inhibitory neurotransmitters by binding to specific benzodiazepine receptors in the limbic and cortical areas of the CNS. GABA inhibits excitatory stimulation, which helps control emotional behavior. The limbic system contains a highly dense area of benzodiazepine receptors, which may explain the drug's antianxiety effects. Also, lorazepam hyperpolarizes neuronal cells, thereby interfering with their ability to generate seizures.

Contraindications

Acute angle-closure glaucoma, hypersensitivity to lorazepam or its components, intra-arterial administration, psychosis

Interactions

DRUGS

CNS depressants: Additive CNS depression
digoxin: Possibly increased blood digoxin level and risk of digitalis toxicity
fentanyl: Possibly decreased therapeutic effects of fentanyl
probenecid: Possibly increased therapeutic and adverse effects of lorazepam

ACTIVITIES

alcohol use: Increased CNS depression

Adverse Reactions

CNS: Amnesia, anxiety, ataxia, confusion, delusions, depression, dizziness, drowsiness, euphoria, headache, hypokinesia, irritability, malaise, nervousness, slurred speech, tremor
CV: Chest pain, palpitations, tachycardia
EENT: Blurred vision, dry mouth, increased salivation, photophobia
GI: Abdominal pain, constipation, diarrhea, nausea, thirst, vomiting
GU: Libido changes
SKIN: Diaphoresis
Other: Injection site phlebitis, physical and psychological dependence, withdrawal symptoms

Nursing Considerations

- Use extreme caution when giving lorazepam to elderly patients because it can cause hypoventilation.

- Dilute drug with equal amount of sterile water for injection, sodium chloride for injection, or D_5W. Discard solution if you observe particles or discoloration. Give diluted drug slowly, at no more than 2 mg/minute.
- Monitor respirations every 5 to 15 minutes, and keep emergency resuscitation equipment readily available.
- Because abrupt drug discontinuation increases the risk of withdrawal symptoms, expect to taper dosage gradually, especially in epileptic patients.
- Store drug at 2° to 8° C (36° to 46° F); protect from freezing and light.

PATIENT TEACHING

- Instruct patient to report excessive drowsiness and nausea during lorazepam therapy.
- Advise patient to avoid potentially hazardous activities until drug's CNS effects are known.
- Urge patient to avoid alcohol because it increases drug's CNS depressant effects.

M

magnesium chloride

(contains 200 mg of elemental magnesium per 1 ml of injection)
Chloromag

magnesium sulfate

(contains 100 to 500 mg of elemental magnesium per 1 ml of injection and 1 to 5 g of elemental magnesium per 10 ml of injection)

Class and Category

Chemical: Cation, electrolyte
Therapeutic: Antiarrhythmic, anticonvulsant, electrolyte replacement
Pregnancy category: A

Indications and Dosages

▶ *To treat severe hypomagnesemia*

I.V. INFUSION (MAGNESIUM CHLORIDE)

Adults. 4 g diluted in 250 ml of D_5W and infused at no more than 3 ml/min. *Maximum:* 40 g daily.

I.V. INFUSION (MAGNESIUM SULFATE)

Adults and adolescents. 5 g diluted in 1 L of I.V. solution and infused over 3 hr.

▶ *To provide supplemental magnesium in total parenteral nutrition*

I.V. INFUSION (MAGNESIUM SULFATE)

Adults. 1 to 3 g daily.
Children. 0.25 to 1.25 g daily.
DOSAGE ADJUSTMENT Adult dosage may be increased to 6 g daily for certain conditions, such as short-bowel syndrome.

▶ *To prevent and control seizures in preeclampsia or eclampsia as well as seizures caused by epilepsy, glomerulonephritis, or hypothyroidism*

I.V. INFUSION OR INJECTION (MAGNESIUM SULFATE)

Adults. *Loading:* 4 g diluted in 250 ml of compatible solution and infused over 30 min. *Maintenance:* 1 to 2 g/hr by continuous infusion.

Route	Onset	Peak	Duration
I.V. *	Immediate	Unknown	About 30 min

*For anticonvulsant effect.

Mechanism of Action

Assists all enzymes involved in phosphate transfer reactions that use ATP. Magnesium is required for normal function of the ATP-dependent sodium-potassium pump in muscle membranes. It may effectively treat digitalis glycoside–induced arrhythmias because correction of hypomagnesemia improves the sodium-potassium pump's ability to distribute potassium into intracellular spaces and because magnesium decreases calcium uptake and potassium outflow through myocardial cell membranes.

As an anticonvulsant, magnesium depresses the CNS and blocks peripheral neuromuscular impulse transmission by decreasing the amount of available acetylcholine.

Incompatibilities

Don't combine magnesium sulfate with alkali carbonates or bicarbonates, alkali hydroxides, arsenates, calcium, clindamycin phosphate, dobutamine, fat emulsions, heavy metals, hydrocortisone sodium succinate, phosphates, polymyxin B, procaine hydrochloride, salicylates, sodium bicarbonate, strontium, and tartrates.

Contraindications

Hypersensitivity to magnesium salts or any component of magnesium-containing preparations
Magnesium chloride: Coma, heart disease, renal impairment
Magnesium sulfate: Heart block, MI, preeclampsia 2 hours or less before delivery

Interactions

DRUGS

amphotericin B, cisplatin, cyclosporine, gentamicin: Possibly magnesium wasting and need for magnesium dosage adjustment
calcium salts (I.V.): Possibly neutralization of magnesium sulfate's effects
CNS depressants: Possibly increased CNS depression
digoxin: Possibly heart block and conduction changes, especially when calcium salts are also administered
diuretics (loop or thiazide): Possibly hypomagnesemia
misoprostol: Increased misoprostol-induced diarrhea
neuromuscular blockers: Possibly increased neuromuscular blockade
nifedipine: Possibly increased hypotensive effects when taken with magnesium sulfate
potassium-sparing diuretics: Increased risk of hypermagnesemia

streptomycin, tetracycline, tobramycin: Possibly decreased therapeutic effectiveness of these drugs

FOODS

high-glucose intake: Increased urinary excretion of magnesium

ACTIVITIES

alcohol use: Increased urinary excretion of magnesium

Adverse Reactions

CNS: Decreased reflexes, dizziness, syncope
CV: Arrhythmias, hypotension
GI: Vomiting
MS: Muscle cramps
RESP: Dyspnea, respiratory depression or paralysis
SKIN: Diaphoresis
Other: Allergic reaction, hypermagnesemia, magnesium toxicity

Nursing Considerations

- **WARNING** Observe for early signs of hypermagnesemia: bradycardia, diminished deep tendon reflexes, diplopia, dyspnea, flushing, hypotension, nausea, slurred speech, vomiting, and weakness. Notify prescriber immediately if patient displays any of these signs.
- **WARNING** Be aware that magnesium may precipitate myasthenic crisis by decreasing patient's sensitivity to acetylcholine.
- Frequently assess cardiac status of patient taking drugs that lower heart rate, such as beta blockers, because magnesium may aggravate symptoms of heart block.
- **WARNING** Be aware that magnesium chloride for injection contains the preservative benzyl alcohol, which may cause a fatal toxic syndrome in neonates and premature infants, characterized by CNS, respiratory, circulatory, and renal impairment and metabolic acidosis.
- Monitor serum electrolyte levels in patients with renal insufficiency because they're at risk for magnesium toxicity.
- Be aware that magnesium salts aren't intended for long-term use.
- Store drug at 15° to 30° C (59° to 86° F); don't freeze.

PATIENT TEACHING

- Instruct patient to report signs of hypermagnesemia, such as shortness of breath, flushing, dizziness, and nausea.
- Inform patient that magnesium supplements used to replace electrolytes can cause diarrhea.

mannitol

Osmitrol, Resectisol

Class and Category

Chemical: Hexahydroxy alcohol
Therapeutic: Antiglaucoma, diagnostic agent, osmotic diuretic, urinary irrigant
Pregnancy category: B

Indications and Dosages

▶ *To reduce intracranial or intraocular pressure*

I.V. INFUSION

Adults and adolescents. 0.25 to 2 g/kg as 15% to 25% solution given over 30 to 60 min. If used before eye surgery, 1.5 to 2 g/kg 60 to 90 min before procedure. *Maximum:* 6 g/kg daily.
DOSAGE ADJUSTMENT For small or debilitated patients, dosage reduced to 0.5 g/kg.

▶ *To diagnose oliguria or inadequate renal function*

I.V. INFUSION

Adults and adolescents. 200 mg/kg or 12.5 g as 15% to 20% solution given over 3 to 5 min. Second dose given only if patient fails to excrete 30 to 50 ml of urine in 2 to 3 hr. Drug discontinued if no response after second dose. Or, 100 ml of 20% solution diluted in 180 ml of normal saline solution (forming 280 ml of 7.2% solution) and infused at 20 ml/min; followed by measurement of urine output. *Maximum:* 6 g/kg daily.

▶ *To prevent oliguria or acute renal failure*

I.V. INFUSION

Adults and adolescents. 50 to 100 g as 5% to 25% solution. *Maximum:* 6 g/kg daily.

▶ *To treat oliguria*

I.V. INFUSION

Adults and adolescents. 50 to 100 g as 15% to 25% solution given over 90 min to several hr. *Maximum:* 6 g/kg daily.

▶ *To promote diuresis in drug toxicity*

I.V. INFUSION

Adults and adolescents. *Loading:* 25 g. *Maintenance:* Up to 200 g as 5% to 25% solution given continuously to maintain urine output of 100 to 500 ml/hr with positive fluid balance of 1 to 2 L. *Maximum:* 6 g/kg daily.

▶ *To promote diuresis in hemolytic transfusion reaction*

I.V. INFUSION

Adults. 20 g over 5 min. Repeat if needed. *Maximum:* 6 g/kg daily.

Route	Onset	Peak	Duration
I.V.*	1 to 3 hr	Unknown	Up to 8 hr
I.V.†	30 to 60 min	Unknown	4 to 8 hr
I.V.‡	In 15 min	Unknown	3 to 8 hr

Mechanism of Action

Elevates plasma osmolality, causing water to flow from tissues, such as the brain and eyes, and from CSF, into extracellular fluid, thereby decreasing intracranial and intraocular pressure.

As an osmotic diuretic, mannitol increases the osmolarity of glomerular filtrate, which decreases water reabsorption. This leads to increased excretion of water, sodium, chloride, and toxic substances.

As an irrigant, mannitol minimizes hemolytic effects of water as an irrigant and reduces movement of hemolyzed blood from the urethra to the systemic circulation, preventing hemoglobinemia and serious renal complications.

Incompatibilities

Don't administer mannitol through same I.V. line as blood or blood products.

Contraindications

Active intracranial bleeding (except during craniotomy), anuria, hepatic failure, hypersensitivity to mannitol or its components, pulmonary edema, severe dehydration, severe heart failure, severe pulmonary congestion, severe renal insufficiency

Interactions

DRUGS

digoxin: Increased risk of digitalis toxicity from hypokalemia
diuretics: Possibly increased therapeutic effects of mannitol

Adverse Reactions

CNS: Chills, dizziness, fever, headache, seizures
CV: Chest pain, heart failure, hypertension, tachycardia, thrombophlebitis
EENT: Blurred vision, dry mouth, rhinitis
GI: Diarrhea, nausea, thirst, vomiting
GU: Polyuria, urine retention

* To produce diuresis.
† To decrease intraocular pressure.
‡ To decrease ICP.

RESP: Pulmonary edema
SKIN: Extravasation with edema and tissue necrosis, rash, urticaria
Other: Dehydration, hyperkalemia, hypernatremia, hypervolemia, hypokalemia, hyponatremia (dilutional), metabolic acidosis, water intoxication

Nursing Considerations

- If crystals form in mannitol solution exposed to low temperature, place solution in hot-water bath to redissolve crystals.
- Use a 5-micron in-line filter when administering drug solution of 15% or greater.
- Do not piggyback connections, pressurize intravenous mannitol solutions contained in flexible plastic containers, or use a vented intravenous administration set with the vent in the open position when administering drug solution because air embolism may occur because of residual air being drawn from one container before administration of the fluid from a secondary container is finished.
- Be aware that electrolyte-free mannitol should not be given simultaneously with blood without adding at least 20 mEq of sodium chloride to each liter of mannitol solution, as prescribed, to prevent pseudoagglutination.
- During I.V. infusion of mannitol, monitor vital signs, central venous pressure, and fluid intake and output every hour. Measure urine output with indwelling urinary catheter, as appropriate.
- Check weight and monitor BUN and serum creatinine electrolyte levels daily.
- Provide frequent mouth care to relieve thirst and dry mouth.

PATIENT TEACHING

- Inform patient that he may experience dry mouth and thirst during mannitol therapy.
- Instruct patient to report chest pain, difficulty breathing, or pain at I.V. site.

meperidine hydrochloride
(pethidine hydrochloride)

Demerol

Class, Category, and Schedule

Chemical: Phenylpiperidine derivative opioid
Therapeutic: Analgesic
Pregnancy category: C

Controlled substance: Schedule II

Indications and Dosages

▶ *To provide preoperative sedation*

I.V. INJECTION

Adults. 15 to 35 mg/hr, p.r.n.

▶ *As adjunct to anesthesia*

I.V. INFUSION OR INJECTION

Adults. Individualized. Repeated slow injections of 10 mg/ml solution or continuous infusion of dilute solution (1 mg/ml) titrated as needed.

DOSAGE ADJUSTMENT For patients with creatinine clearance of 10 to 50 ml/min/1.73 m^2, 75% of usual dose is used; with creatinine clearance of less than 10 ml/min/1.73 m^2, 50% of usual dose is used.

Route	Onset	Peak	Duration
I.V.	1 min	5 to 7 min	2 to 4 hr

Mechanism of Action

Binds with opiate receptors in the spinal cord and higher levels of the CNS. In this way, meperidine stimulates mu and kappa receptors, which alters the perception of and emotional response to pain.

Incompatibilities

Don't mix meperidine in same syringe with aminophylline, barbiturates, heparin, iodides, methicillin, morphine sulfate, phenytoin, sodium bicarbonate, sulfadiazine, or sulfisoxazole.

Contraindications

Acute asthma; hypersensitivity to meperidine, narcotics, or their components; increased intracranial pressure; severe respiratory depression; upper respiratory tract obstruction; use within 14 days of MAO inhibitor therapy

Interactions

DRUGS

acyclovir, ritonavir: Possibly increased blood meperidine level

alfentanil, CNS depressants, fentanyl, sufentanil: Increased risk of CNS and respiratory depression and hypotension

amphetamines, MAO inhibitors: Risk of increased CNS excitation or depression with possibly fatal reactions

anticholinergics: Increased risk of severe constipation
antidiarrheals (such as loperamide and difenoxin and atropine): Increased risk of severe constipation and increased CNS depression
antihypertensives: Increased risk of hypotension
buprenorphine: Possibly decreased therapeutic effects of meperidine and increased risk of respiratory depression
cimetidine: Reduced clearance and volume of distribution of meperidine
hydroxyzine: Increased risk of CNS depression and hypotension
metoclopramide: Possibly decreased effects of metoclopramide
naloxone, naltrexone: Decreased pharmacologic effects of meperidine
neuromuscular blockers: Increased risk of prolonged respiratory and CNS depression
oral anticoagulants: Possibly increased anticoagulant effect and risk of bleeding
phenytoin: Possibly enhanced hepatic metabolism of meperidine
ACTIVITIES
alcohol use: Possibly increased CNS and respiratory depression and hypotension

Adverse Reactions

CNS: Confusion, depression, dizziness, drowsiness, euphoria, headache, increased intracranial pressure, lack of coordination, malaise, nervousness, nightmares, restlessness, seizures, syncope, tremor
CV: Hypotension, orthostatic hypotension, tachycardia
EENT: Blurred vision, diplopia, dry mouth
GI: Abdominal cramps or pain, anorexia, constipation, ileus, nausea, vomiting
GU: Dysuria, urinary frequency, urine retention
RESP: Dyspnea, respiratory arrest or depression, wheezing
SKIN: Diaphoresis, flushing, pruritus, rash, urticaria
Other: Injection site pain, redness, and swelling; physical and psychological dependence

Nursing Considerations

- Use meperidine with extreme caution in patients with acute abdominal conditions, hepatic or renal disorders, hypothyroidism, prostatic hyperplasia, seizures, or supraventricular tachycardia.
- To minimize local anesthetic effect, dilute syrup with water before administration.

- Give I.V. dose slowly by direct injection or as a slow continuous infusion. Mix with D_5W, normal saline solution, or Ringer's or lactated Ringer's solution.
- Keep naloxone available when giving I.V. meperidine.
- Monitor patient's respiratory and cardiovascular status during treatment. Notify prescriber immediately and expect to discontinue drug if respiratory rate falls to less than 12 breaths/minute or if respiratory depth decreases.
- Monitor bowel function to detect constipation, and assess the need for stool softeners.
- Assess for signs of physical dependence and abuse.
- Expect withdrawal symptoms to occur if drug is abruptly withdrawn after long-term use.

PATIENT TEACHING

- Inform patient that meperidine is a controlled substance and that he'll need identification to purchase it.
- Advise patient to take drug exactly as prescribed.
- Instruct patient to report constipation, severe nausea, and shortness or breath.
- Advise patient to avoid potentially hazardous activities until drug's CNS effects are known.
- Instruct patient to prevent postoperative atelectasis by turning, coughing, and deep-breathing.
- Urge patient to avoid alcohol, sedatives, and tranquilizers during meperidine therapy.

mephentermine sulfate

Wyamine

Class and Category

Chemical: Sympathomimetic amine
Therapeutic: Vasopressor
Pregnancy category: C

Indications and Dosages

▶ *To treat hypotension secondary to spinal anesthesia*

I.V. INJECTION

Adults. 30 to 45 mg (15 mg for obstetrical patients); may be repeated as needed to maintain blood pressure.

I.V. INFUSION

Adults. Dosage individualized based on patient response to therapy. Average dose is 1 to 5 mg/min.

Route	Onset	Peak	Duration
I.V.	Almost immediate	Unknown	15 to 30 min

Mechanism of Action

Stimulates alpha-adrenergic receptors directly and indirectly, resulting in positive inotropic and chronotropic effects. Indirect stimulation occurs by the release of norepinephrine from its storage sites in the heart and other tissues. By enhancing cardiac contraction, mephentermine improves cardiac output, thereby increasing blood pressure. Increased peripheral resistance from peripheral vasoconstriction may also contribute to increased blood pressure. Mephentermine can affect the heart rate but the change is variable, based on vagal tone. It may also stimulate beta-adrenergic receptors.

Contraindications

Hypersensitivity to mephentermine, phenothiazine-induced hypotension, use within 14 days of MAO inhibitor therapy

Interactions

DRUGS

alpha blockers, other drugs with alpha-blocking effects: Possibly decreased peripheral vasoconstrictive and hypertensive effects of mephentermine

beta blockers (ophthalmic): Decreased effects of mephentermine; increased risk of bronchospasm, wheezing, decreased pulmonary function, and respiratory failure

beta blockers (systemic): Increased risk of bronchospasm, decreased effects of both drugs

diuretics and other antihypertensives: Possibly reduced effectiveness of these drugs

doxapram: Possibly increased vasopressor effects of either drug

ergot alkaloids: Increased vasopressor effects

guanadrel, guanethidine, mecamylamine, methyldopa, reserpine: Possibly decreased effects of these drugs and increased risk of adverse effects

hydrocarbon inhalation anesthetics: Increased risk of atrial and ventricular arrhythmias

MAO inhibitors: Intensified and extended cardiac stimulation and vasopressor effects, possibly severe headache and hypertensive crisis

maprotiline, tricyclic antidepressants: Increased vasopressor response;

increased risk of prolonged QTc interval, arrhythmias, hypertension, and hyperpyrexia
methylphenidate: Possibly increased vasopressor effect of mephentermine
nitrates: Possibly reduced antianginal effects of nitrates and decreased vasopressor effect
other sympathomimetics (such as dopamine): Possibly increased cardiac effects and adverse reactions
oxytocin: Possibly severe hypertension
thyroid hormones: Increased effects of both drugs, increased risk of coronary insufficiency in patients with coronary artery disease

Adverse Reactions

CNS: Anxiety, dizziness, drowsiness, euphoria, headache, incoherence, nervousness, psychosis, restlessness, seizures, weakness
CV: Angina, arrhythmias (including bradycardia, tachycardia, and ventricular arrhythmias), hypertension, hypotension, palpitations, peripheral vasoconstriction
GI: Nausea, vomiting
RESP: Dyspnea
SKIN: Peripheral necrosis

Nursing Considerations

- Before administering mephentermine, expect to intervene, as ordered, to correct hemorrhage, hypovolemia, metabolic acidosis, or hypoxia.
- Discard vial if you observe discoloration or precipitate.
- Using D_5W or normal saline solution, prepare a 1-mg/ml solution for infusion.
- Administer drug using an infusion pump to provide a controlled rate.
- Monitor blood pressure, cardiac rate and rhythm, central venous pressure (if appropriate), and urine output during administration. Adjust infusion rate according to patient response, as ordered. Be aware that patients with a history of cardiovascular disease (including hypertension) or hyperthyroidism and chronically ill patients are at increased risk for mephentermine's adverse cardiovascular effects.
- Assess patients with angle-closure glaucoma for signs of an exacerbation, such as eye pain or blurred vision.
- Assess circulation in patients with a history of occlusive vascular disease, such as atherosclerosis and Raynaud's disease, because mephentermine may cause decreased circulation and

increase the risk of necrosis or gangrene. Inspect I.V. site periodically for signs of extravasation.

- **WARNING** Be aware that weeping, excitability, seizures, and hallucinations are some of the symptoms of mephentermine overdose. Contact prescriber immediately if patient experiences such symptoms, and expect to provide supportive treatment.
- Be aware that mephentermine can increase contractions in pregnant women, especially during the third trimester. Expect drug to be prescribed only when benefits outweigh potential adverse effects.
- Store drug at 15° to 30° C (59° to 86° F); don't freeze.

PATIENT TEACHING

- Instruct patient receiving mephentermine to report adverse reactions, including chest pain, difficulty breathing, dizziness, irregular heartbeat, headache, and weakness.

meropenem

Merrem I.V.

Class and Category

Chemical: Carbapenem
Therapeutic: Antibiotic
Pregnancy category: B

Indications and Dosages

▶ *To treat complicated appendicitis and peritonitis caused by susceptible strains of alpha-hemolytic streptococci,* Bacteroides fragilis, Bacteroides thetaiotaomicron, Escherichia coli, Klebsiella pneumoniae, Peptostreptococcus *sp., or* Pseudomonas aeruginosa

I.V. INFUSION OR INJECTION

Adults and children weighing more than 50 kg (110 lb). 1 g q 8 hr infused over 15 to 30 min or given as a bolus over 3 to 5 min.

Children over age 3 months weighing less than 50 kg. 20 mg/kg q 8 hr infused over 15 to 30 min or given as a bolus over 3 to 5 min. *Maximum:* 1 g q 8 hr.

DOSAGE ADJUSTMENT For patients with creatinine clearance of 26 to 50 ml/min/1.73 m^2, dosage reduced to 1 g q 12 hr. For those with creatinine clearance of 10 to 25 ml/min/1.73 m^2, dosage reduced to 500 mg q 12 hr. For those with creatinine clearance of less than 10 ml/min/1.73 m^2, dosage reduced to 500 mg q 24 hr.

▶ *To treat complicated skin and skin structure infections caused by* Staphylococcus aureus, Streptococcus agalactiae, Streptococcus pyogenes, *viridans group streptococci,* Enterococcus faecalis *(excluding vancomycin-resistant isolates),* Pseudomonas aeruginosa, Escherichia coli, Proteus mirabilis, Bacteroides fragilis, *and* Peptostreptococcus *sp.*

I.V. INFUSION

Adults and children weighing more than 50 kg (110 lb). 500 mg q 8 hr infused over 15 to 30 min.

Children older than age 3 months weighing less than 50 kg. 10 mg/kg q 8 hr infused over 15 to 30 min. *Maximum:* 500 mg q 8 hr.

DOSAGE ADJUSTMENT For patients with creatinine clearance of 26 to 50 ml/min/1.73 m^2, dosage reduced to 500 mg q 12 hr. For those with creatinine clearance of 10 to 25 ml/min/1.73 m^2, dosage reduced to 250 mg q 12 hr. For those with creatinine clearance of less than 10 ml/min/1.73 m^2, dosage reduced to 250 mg q 24 hr.

▶ *To treat bacterial meningitis caused by* Haemophilus influenzae, Neisseria meningitidis, *or* Streptococcus pneumoniae *in children*

I.V. INFUSION OR INJECTION

Children weighing more than 50 kg. 2 g q 8 hr infused over 15 to 30 min or given as a bolus over 3 to 5 min.

Children over age 3 months weighing less than 50 kg. 40 mg/kg q 8 hr infused over 15 to 30 min or given as a bolus over 3 to 5 min. *Maximum:* 2 g q 8 hr.

Mechanism of Action

Penetrates cell walls of most gram-negative and gram-positive bacteria, inactivating penicillin-binding proteins. This action inhibits bacterial cell wall synthesis and causes cell death.

Incompatibilities

Don't mix meropenem in same solution with other drugs.

Contraindications

Hypersensitivity to meropenem, other carbapenem drugs, beta lactams, or their components

Interactions

DRUGS

probenecid: Inhibited renal excretion of meropenem

valproic acid: Possibly reduced blood level of valproic acid to subtherapeutic level

Adverse Reactions

CNS: Headache, seizures
CV: Shock
EENT: Epistaxis, glossitis, oral candidiasis
GI: Anorexia, constipation, diarrhea, elevated liver function test results, nausea, pseudomembranous colitis, vomiting
GU: Elevated BUN and serum creatinine levels, hematuria, renal failure
HEME: Agranulocytosis, leukopenia, neutropenia
RESP: Apnea, dyspnea
SKIN: Diaper rash from candidiasis (children), erythema multiforme, pruritus, rash, Stevens-Johnson syndrome, toxic epidermal necrolysis
Other: Anaphylaxis; angioedema; injection site inflammation, pain, phlebitis, or thrombophlebitis; sepsis

Nursing Considerations

- Obtain body fluid and tissue samples, as ordered, for culture and sensitivity testing. Expect to review test results, if possible, before giving first dose of meropenem.
- For I.V. bolus, add 10 ml sterile water for injection to 500 mg/20-ml vial, or 20 ml of diluent to 1 g/30-ml vial of drug. Shake to dissolve.
- **WARNING** Be aware that fatal hypersensitivity reactions have occurred with meropenem administration. Determine whether patient has had previous reactions to antibiotics or other allergens.
- Be prepared to administer emergency treatment for anaphylaxis.
- Institute seizure precautions, according to facility policy, for patients with bacterial meningitis or CNS or renal disorders because these patients are at increased risk of seizures with meropenem.
- Monitor patient with creatinine clearance of 10 to 26 ml/min/1.73 m^2 for signs and symptoms of seizures, heart failure, renal failure, or shock.

PATIENT TEACHING

- Tell patient to report trouble breathing, diarrhea, injection site pain, or mouth soreness.

metaraminol bitartrate

Aramine

Class and Category

Chemical: Sympathomimetic amine
Therapeutic: Vasopressor
Pregnancy category: C

Indications and Dosages

▶ *To treat hypotension secondary to spinal anesthesia or as adjunct to treat hypotension caused by hemorrhage, adverse drug reactions, surgical complications, or shock resulting from brain damage secondary to trauma or tumor*

I.V. INFUSION

Adults. 15 to 100 mg (base) mixed in 500 ml of normal saline solution or D_5W; dosage individualized to maintain desired blood pressure.

▶ *To treat severe shock*

I.V. INJECTION

Adults. 500 mcg (0.5 mg) to 5 mg (base), followed by I.V. infusion individualized to maintain desired blood pressure.

Route	Onset	Peak	Duration
I.V.	1 to 2 min	Unknown	20 to 60 min

Mechanism of Action

May directly stimulate alpha-adrenergic receptors and inhibit activity of the intracellular enzyme adenyl cyclase, which then inhibits production of cAMP. Inhibition of cAMP causes arterial and venous constriction and increases peripheral vascular resistance and systolic blood pressure. Metaraminol also directly stimulates beta-adrenergic receptors in the myocardium and increases adenyl cyclase activity, producing positive inotropic and chronotropic effects.

Incompatibilities

Don't mix metaraminol with barbiturates, penicillins, phenytoin, sodium salts, or other drugs that have poor solubility in acidic solutions.

Contraindications

Hypersensitivity to metaraminol or its components, including sulfites; use with cyclopropane or halothane anesthesia unless clinically warranted

Interactions

DRUGS

alpha blockers, other drugs with alpha-blocking effects: Possibly decreased peripheral vasoconstrictive and hypertensive effects of metaraminol
beta blockers (ophthalmic): Decreased effects of metaraminol; increased risk of bronchospasm, wheezing, decreased pulmonary function, and respiratory failure
beta blockers (systemic): Increased risk of bronchospasm, decreased effects of both drugs
digoxin: Increased risk of arrhythmias
diuretics and other antihypertensives: Possibly reduced effectiveness of these drugs
doxapram: Possibly increased vasopressor effects of both drugs
ergot alkaloids: Increased vasopressor effects
guanadrel, guanethidine, mecamylamine, methyldopa: Possibly decreased effects of these drugs and increased risk of adverse effects
hydrocarbon inhalation anesthetics: Increased risk of atrial and ventricular arrhythmias
MAO inhibitors: Intensified and extended cardiac stimulation and vasopressor effects; possibly severe hypertension
maprotiline, tricyclic antidepressants: Increased vasopressor response; increased risk of prolonged QTc interval, arrhythmias, hypertension, and hyperpyrexia
methylphenidate: Possibly increased vasopressor effect of metaraminol
nitrates: Possibly reduced antianginal effects of nitrates, decreased vasopressor effect
other sympathomimetics (such as dopamine): Possibly increased cardiac effects and adverse reactions
oxytocin: Possibly severe hypertension
thyroid hormones: Increased effects of both drugs, increased risk of coronary insufficiency in patients with coronary artery disease

Adverse Reactions

CNS: Anxiety, dizziness, headache, nervousness, seizures, weakness
CV: Angina, arrhythmias (including bradycardia, tachycardia, and ventricular arrhythmias), hypertension, hypotension, palpitations, peripheral vasoconstriction
GI: Nausea, vomiting
RESP: Dyspnea
SKIN: Extravasation with tissue necrosis and sloughing
Other: Injection site abscess

Nursing Considerations

- Before starting metaraminol therapy, expect to administer blood, plasma volume expanders, I.V. fluids, and electrolyte replacement therapy, as ordered, to correct conditions that caused hypotension, such as hemorrhage or hypovolemia.
- Discard vial if you observe discoloration or precipitates.
- To prepare an I.V. infusion, add 15 to 100 mg of metaraminol to 500 ml of appropriate solution, such as normal saline soluion or D_5W. (You may use a smaller or larger amount of solution, depending on patient's fluid needs.) Use within 24 hours.
- Expect to use large veins for I.V. administration, such as antecubital fossa or a vein in the thigh. Administer infusion using an infusion pump to provide a controlled rate.
- Monitor blood pressure, cardiac rate and rhythm, central venous pressure, and urine output during administration. Be aware that vasoconstrictive effects of prolonged metaraminol administration may prevent volume expansion and prolong shock state. If this occurs, expect to administer blood and plasma volume expanders, as ordered.
- Allow at least 10 minutes to pass between dosage adjustments to let dose achieve maximum effect. Adjust infusion rate to patient response, as ordered.
- **WARNING** Assess for allergic reactions—including anaphylaxis and, possibly, life-threatening asthmatic episodes—because drug contains sodium bisulfite.
- Expect to discontinue metaraminol infusion gradually. Continue to monitor patient's blood pressure after infusion has stopped; elevated blood pressure may persist from drug's cumulative effects. Expect to restart metaraminol, as prescribed, if hypotension recurs.
- Be aware that patients with a history of cardiovascular disease (including hypertension) or hyperthyroidism and chronically ill patients are at increased risk for drug's adverse cardiovascular effects. Monitor patients with acute MI for worsening of condition because metaraminol can intensify or prolong myocardial ischemia.
- Monitor patients with cirrhosis for arrhythmias and diuresis. Expect to administer electrolytes, as prescribed, if diuresis occurs.
- Assess patients with angle-closure glaucoma for signs of an exacerbation, such as eye pain or blurred vision.
- Assess circulation in patients with a history of occlusive vascular disease, such as atherosclerosis, diabetic endarteritis, and

Raynaud's disease, because metaraminol may cause decreased circulation and increase the risk of necrosis or gangrene. Inspect I.V. site periodically for signs of extravasation.
- **WARNING** Be aware that metaraminol overdose may cause headache, euphoria, arrhythmias, severe hypertension, and MI. Contact prescriber immediately if patient experiences such symptoms, and expect to provide supportive treatment.
- Monitor patients with a history of malaria for evidence of a metaraminol-induced relapse, such as fever, chills, or muscle aches.
- Store drug at 15° to 30° C (59° to 86° F); protect from freezing and light.

PATIENT TEACHING
- Advise patient to immediately report any discomfort at metaraminol infusion site, such as pain, swelling, or redness.
- Instruct patient to report adverse reactions, including chest pain, difficulty breathing, dizziness, irregular heartbeat, headache, and weakness.

methicillin sodium

Staphcillin

Class and Category

Chemical: Penicillinase-resistant penicillin
Therapeutic: Antibiotic
Pregnancy category: B

Indications and Dosages

▶ *To treat general infections, such as sepsis, sinusitis, and skin and soft-tissue infections, caused by susceptible organisms (including penicillinase-producing and non–penicillinase-producing strains of* Staphylococcus epidermidis, Staphylococcus saprophyticus, *and* Streptococcus pneumoniae*)*

I.V. INFUSION

Adults and children weighing 40 kg (88 lb) or more. 1 g q 6 hr. *Maximum:* 24 g daily.

Children weighing less than 40 kg. 25 mg/kg q 6 hr.

DOSAGE ADJUSTMENT For adults and children with cystic fibrosis, dosage decreased to 50 mg/kg q 6 hr.

▶ *To treat bacterial meningitis*

I.V. INFUSION

Neonates weighing 2 kg (4.4 lb) or more. 50 mg/kg q 8 hr for first wk after birth and then 50 mg/kg q 6 hr.

Neonates weighing less than 2 kg. 25 to 50 mg/kg q 12 hr for first wk after birth and then 50 mg/kg q 8 hr.

Mechanism of Action

Kills bacterial cells by inhibiting bacterial cell wall synthesis. In susceptible bacteria, the rigid, cross-linked cell wall is assembled in several steps. In the final stage of cross-linking, methicillin binds with and inactivates penicillin-binding proteins (enzymes responsible for linking cell wall strands), resulting in bacterial cell lysis and death. *Staphylococcus aureus* has developed resistance to methicillin by altering its penicillin-binding proteins.

Incompatibilities

Don't mix methicillin in same syringe or I.V. solution with other drugs. Don't mix methicillin with dextrose solutions because their low acidity may damage drug. Administer methicillin at least 1 hour before or after aminoglycosides and at different sites to prevent mutual inactivation.

Contraindications

Hypersensitivity to methicillin sodium, other penicillins, or their components

Interactions

DRUGS

aminoglycosides: Substantial aminoglycoside inactivation
chloramphenicol, erythromycins, sulfonamides, tetracyclines: Possibly decreased therapeutic effects of methicillin
methotrexate: Increased risk of methotrexate toxicity
probenecid: Possibly decreased renal clearance, increased blood level, and increased risk of toxicity of methicillin

Adverse Reactions

CNS: Aggressiveness, agitation, anxiety, confusion, depression, headache, seizures
EENT: Oral candidiasis
GI: Abdominal pain, diarrhea, hepatotoxicity, nausea, pseudomembranous colitis, vomiting
GU: Interstitial nephritis, vaginitis
HEME: Leukopenia, neutropenia, thrombocytopenia
SKIN: Exfoliative dermatitis, pruritus, rash, urticaria
Other: Anaphylaxis; infusion site redness, swelling, and tenderness; serum-sicknesslike reaction

Nursing Considerations

- **WARNING** Be aware that methicillin is not a first-line treatment for the indications listed previously because of the prevalence of methicillin-resistant *Staphylococcus aureus.*
- Before giving first dose, obtain appropriate body fluid or tissue specimens for culture and sensitivity tests, as ordered, and review test results if available.
- Add 1.5 ml, 5.7 ml, or 8.6 ml of sterile water for injection or 0.9% sodium chloride injection to 1-g, 4-g, or 6-g vial, respectively, to yield a concentration of 500 mg/ml. Dilute further with 25 ml of normal saline solution for each 500 mg (1 ml) of drug. Use concentrations of 2 to 20 mg/ml within 8 hours if stored at room temperature.
- Observe infusion site closely during administration for redness, swelling, and tenderness.
- Monitor fluid intake and output and renal function test results during methicillin therapy.
- Observe for signs of superinfection, such as diarrhea, vaginal itching, and white patches or sores in mouth or on tongue. Notify prescriber if they occur.
- Closely monitor renal function test results, including serum creatinine level; about one-third of patients experience interstitial nephritis after 10 days of methicillin therapy.
- Monitor liver function test results, and observe for signs of hepatotoxicity, such as fever and nausea. Notify prescriber if such signs occur.
- When calculating sodium intake for patients on a sodium-restricted diet, keep in mind that each gram of methicillin contains approximately 2.24 mEq of sodium.
- Store drug at 15° to 30° C (59° to 86° F).

PATIENT TEACHING

- Unless contraindicated, instruct patient to drink extra fluids during methicillin therapy.
- Advise patient to report diarrhea, infusion site pain, mouth sores, or rash.

methocarbamol

Carbacot, Robaxin, Skelex

Class and Category

Chemical: Carbamate derivative of guaifenesin
Therapeutic: Skeletal muscle relaxant

Pregnancy category: C

Indications and Dosages

▶ *To relieve discomfort caused by acute, painful musculoskeletal conditions*

I.V. INJECTION (100 MG/ML)

Adults and adolescents. Up to 3,000 mg daily given at 8-hr intervals for 3 consecutive days. Regimen repeated as prescribed after patient is drug-free for 48 hr.

▶ *To provide supportive therapy for tetanus*

I.V. INFUSION OR INJECTION (100 MG/ML)

Adults and adolescents. 1,000 to 3,000 mg by infusion or 1,000 to 2,000 mg by direct injection q 6 hr. *Maximum:* 300 mg (3 ml)/min.

Children. 15 mg/kg q 6 hr.

Route	Onset	Peak	Duration
I.V.	Immediate	Unknown	Unknown

Mechanism of Action

May depress the CNS, which leads to sedation and reduced skeletal muscle spasms. Methocarbamol also alters the perception of pain.

Contraindications

Hypersensitivity to methocarbamol or its components, renal disease (injectable form)

Interactions

DRUGS

CNS depressants: Increased CNS depression

ACTIVITIES

alcohol use: Increased CNS depression

Adverse Reactions

CNS: Dizziness, drowsiness, fever, headache, light-headedness, seizures (I.V.), syncope, vertigo, weakness

CV: Bradycardia, hypotension, and thrombophlebitis (parenteral)

EENT: Blurred vision, conjunctivitis, diplopia, metallic taste, nasal congestion, nystagmus

GI: Nausea

GU: Black, brown, or green urine

SKIN: Flushing, pruritus, rash, urticaria

Other: Anaphylaxis, angioedema, injection site sloughing

Nursing Considerations

- Administer I.V. form directly through infusion line at 3 ml/min. To prepare solution, add 10 ml to no more than 250 ml of D_5W or normal saline solution. Infuse at no more than 300 mg (3 ml)/minute to avoid hypotension and seizures.
- Keep patient recumbent during I.V. administration and for at least 15 minutes afterward. Then have him rise slowly.
- Monitor I.V. site regularly for signs of phlebitis.
- Keep epinephrine, antihistamines, and corticosteroids available in case patient experiences anaphylactic reaction.
- Be aware that the parenteral dosage form shouldn't be used in patients with renal dysfunction because the polyethylene glycol 300 vehicle is nephrotoxic.

PATIENT TEACHING

- Inform patient that urine may turn green, black, or brown until drug is discontinued.
- Advise patient to avoid potentially hazardous activities until drug's CNS effects are known.
- Instruct patient to avoid alcohol and other CNS depressants during therapy.

methotrexate (amethopterin)

Rheumatrex

methotrexate sodium

Folex, Folex PFS, Mexate, Mexate-AQ

Class and Category

Chemical: Folic acid analogue
Therapeutic: Antipsoriatic, antirheumatic
Pregnancy category: X

Indications and Dosages

▶ *To treat severe psoriasis unresponsive to other therapy*
I.V. (methotrexate sodium)
Adults. 10 mg/wk. *Maximum:* 25 mg/wk.

Route	Onset	Peak	Duration
I.V.	3 to 6 wk	Unknown	Unknown

Contraindications

Breast-feeding, hypersensitivity to methotrexate or its components, pregnancy

Mechanism of Action

May exert immunosuppressive effects by inhibiting replication and function of T and possibly B lymphocytes. Methotrexate also slows the growth of rapidly proliferating cells, such as epithelial skin cells associated with psoriasis. This action may result from the drug's ability to inhibit dihydrofolate reductase, the enzyme that reduces folic acid to tetrahydrofolic acid. Inhibition of tetrahydrofolic acid interferes with DNA synthesis and cell reproduction in rapidly proliferating cells.

Interactions

DRUGS

bone marrow depressants: Possibly increased bone marrow depression
co-trimoxazole: Possibly increased bone marrow suppression
folic acid: Possibly decreased effectiveness of methotrexate
hepatotoxic drugs: Increased risk of hepatotoxicity
chloramphenicol, neomycin, tetracycline: Possibly decreased absorption of methotrexate
NSAIDs, penicillins, phenylbutazone, phenytoin, probenecid, salicylates, sulfonamides: Increased risk of methotrexate toxicity
oral anticoagulants: Increased risk of bleeding
sulfonamides: Increased risk of hepatotoxicity
theophylline: Possibly increased risk of theophylline toxicity
trimethoprim and sulfamethoxazole: Possibly increased bone marrow suppression
vaccines: Risk of disseminated infection with live-virus vaccines, risk of suppressed response to killed-virus vaccines

ACTIVITIES

alcohol use: Increased risk of hepatotoxicity

Adverse Reactions

CNS: Aphasia, cerebral thrombosis, chills, dizziness, drowsiness, fatigue, fever, headache, hemiparesis, leukoencephalopathy, malaise, paresis, seizures
CV: Chest pain, deep vein thrombosis, hypotension, pericardial effusion, pericarditis, thromboembolism
ENDO: Gynecomastia
EENT: Blurred vision, conjunctivitis, gingivitis, glossitis, pharyngitis, stomatitis, transient blindness, tinnitus
GI: Abdominal pain, anorexia, cirrhosis, diarrhea, elevated liver function test results, enteritis, GI bleeding and ulceration, hepatitis, hepatotoxicity, nausea, pancreatitis, vomiting

GU: Cystitis, hematuria, infertility, menstrual dysfunction, nephropathy, renal failure, tubular necrosis, vaginal discharge
HEME: Anemia, aplastic anemia, leukopenia, neutropenia, pancytopenia, thrombocytopenia
MS: Arthralgia, dysarthia, myalgia, stress fracture
RESP: Dry nonproductive cough, dyspnea, interstitial pneumonitis, pneumonia, pulmonary fibrosis or failure, pulmonary infiltrates
SKIN: Acne, alopecia, altered skin pigmentation, ecchymosis, erythema multiforme, exfoliative dermatitis, furunculosis, necrosis, photosensitivity, pruritus, psoriatic lesions, rash, Stevens-Johnson syndrome, telangiectasia, toxic epidermal necrolysis, ulceration, urticaria
Other: Anaphylaxis, increased risk of infection, lymphadenopathy, lymphoproliferative disease

Nursing Considerations

- Follow facility policy for preparing and handling drug; parenteral form poses a risk of carcinogenicity, mutagenicity, and teratogenicity. Avoid skin contact.
- Monitor results of CBC, chest X-ray, liver and renal function tests, and urinalysis before and during treatment.
- Unless contraindicated, increase patient's fluid intake to 2 to 3 L daily to reduce the risk of adverse GU reactions.
- Assess patient for signs of bleeding and infection.
- **WARNING** Expect renal impairment to severely alter drug elimination.
- Be aware that high doses of methotrexate can impair renal elimination by forming crystals that obstruct urine flow. To prevent drug precipitation, alkalinize patient's urine with sodium bicarbonate tablets, as ordered.
- Follow standard precautions because drug can cause immunosuppression.
- If patient becomes dehydrated from vomiting, notify prescriber and expect to withhold drug until patient recovers.
- If patient receives high doses of drug, keep leucovorin readily available to use as antidote.
- Be aware that methotrexate resistance may develop with prolonged use.

PATIENT TEACHING

- Instruct patient to avoid alcohol during methotrexate therapy.
- Encourage frequent mouth care to reduce the risk of mouth sores.

- Instruct patient to use sunblock when exposed to sunlight.
- Advise patient to notify prescriber about bruising, chills, cough, fever, dark or bloody urine, mouth sores, shortness of breath, sore throat, and yellow skin or eyes.
- Urge women of childbearing age to use contraception during methotrexate therapy.

methyldopate hydrochloride

Aldomet

Class and Category

Chemical: 3,4-dihydroxyphenylalanine (DOPA) analogue
Therapeutic: Antihypertensive
Pregnancy category: C

Indications and Dosages

▶ *To manage hypertension, to treat hypertensive crisis*

I.V. INFUSION

Adults. 250 to 500 mg diluted in D_5W and infused over 30 to 60 min q 6 hr. *Maximum:* 1,000 mg q 6 hr.
Children. 20 to 40 mg/kg infused over 30 to 60 min q 6 hr. *Maximum:* 65 mg/kg or 3,000 mg daily.

Route	Onset	Peak	Duration
I.V.	Unknown	4 to 6 hr	10 to 16 hr

Mechanism of Action

Is decarboxylated in the body to produce alpha-methylnorepinephrine, a metabolite that stimulates central inhibitory alpha-adrenergic receptors. This action may reduce blood pressure by decreasing sympathetic stimulation of the heart and peripheral vascular system.

Incompatibilities

Don't administer methyldopate through same I.V. line as barbiturates or sulfonamides.

Contraindications

Active hepatic disease; hypersensitivity to methyldopa, methyldopate, or their components; impaired hepatic function from previous methyldopa or methyldopate therapy; use within 14 days of MAO inhibitor therapy

Interactions

DRUGS

antihypertensives: Increased hypotension
appetite suppressants, NSAIDs, tricyclic antidepressants: Possibly decreased therapeutic effects of methyldopate
central anesthetics: Possibly need for reduced anesthetic dosage
CNS depressants: Possibly increased CNS depression
haloperidol: Increased risk of adverse CNS effects
levodopa: Possibly decreased therapeutic effects of levodopa and increased risk of adverse CNS effects
lithium: Increased risk of lithium toxicity
MAO inhibitors: Possibly hallucinations, headaches, hyperexcitability, and severe hypertension
oral anticoagulants: Possibly increased therapeutic effects of anticoagulants
sympathomimetics: Possibly decreased therapeutic effects of methyldopate and increased vasopressor effects of sympathomimetics

ACTIVITIES

alcohol use: Possibly increased CNS depression

Adverse Reactions

CNS: Decreased concentration, depression, dizziness, drowsiness, fever, headache, involuntary motor activity, memory loss (transient), nightmares, paresthesia, parkinsonism, sedation, vertigo, weakness
CV: Angina, bradycardia, edema, heart failure, myocarditis, orthostatic hypotension
EENT: Black or sore tongue, dry mouth, nasal congestion
ENDO: Gynecomastia
GI: Constipation, diarrhea, flatulence, hepatic necrosis, hepatitis, nausea, pancreatitis, vomiting
GU: Decreased libido, impotence
HEME: Agranulocytosis, hemolytic anemia, leukopenia, positive Coombs' test, positive tests for ANA and rheumatoid factor, thrombocytopenia
SKIN: Eczema, rash, urticaria
Other: Weight gain

Nursing Considerations

- Expect to monitor CBC and differential results before and periodically during methyldopate therapy.
- Add methyldopate to 100 ml of D_5W, and administer over 30 to 60 minutes.

- Monitor blood pressure regularly during therapy.
- Monitor results of Coombs' test; a positive result after several months of treatment indicates that patient has hemolytic anemia. Expect prescriber to discontinue drug.
- Assess for weight gain and edema. If they occur, administer a diuretic, as prescribed.
- Notify prescriber if patient experiences abnormal liver function test results, signs of heart failure (dyspnea, edema, hypertension), jaundice, fever, or involuntary jerky movements.
- Be aware that hypertension may return within 48 hours after drug is discontinued. Expect prescriber to convert patient to oral methyldopa, typically at same dosage as parenteral form. Maximum adult oral dosage is 3,000 mg daily.
- Store drug at 15° to 30° C (59° to 86° F); don't freeze.

PATIENT TEACHING

- Instruct patient to avoid potentially hazardous activities until methyldopate's CNS effects are known.
- Advise patient to change position slowly to minimize effects of orthostatic hypotension.
- Direct patient to report bruising, chest pain, fever, involuntary jerky movements, prolonged dizziness, rash, or yellow eyes or skin.

methylprednisolone sodium succinate

A-methaPred, Solu-Medrol

Class and Category

Chemical: Synthetic glucocorticoid
Therapeutic: Anti-inflammatory, immunosuppressant
Pregnancy category: Not rated

Indications and Dosages

▶ *To treat ulcerative colitis*

I.V. INFUSION

Adults. 40 to 120 mg 3 to 7 times/wk for 2 or more wk. Later doses based on patient's condition and response.
Children. 0.14 to 0.84 mg/kg daily in divided doses q 12 to 24 hr.

▶ *To treat a wide range of immune and inflammatory disorders, including allergic rhinitis, asthma, Crohn's disease, and systemic lupus erythematosus*

I.V. INFUSION

Adults. *Initial:* 10 to 40 mg infused over several min. Later doses based on patient's condition and response.

Children. 0.14 to 0.84 mg/kg q 12 to 24 hr.

▶ *To treat acute exacerbations of multiple sclerosis*

I.V. INJECTION

Adults. 160 mg daily for 1 wk, followed by 64 mg q other day for 1 mo.

Route	Onset	Peak	Duration
I.V.	Rapid	30 min	Unknown

Mechanism of Action

Binds to intracellular glucocorticoid receptors and suppresses inflammatory and immune responses by:

- inhibiting the accumulation of neutrophils and monocytes at inflammation sites
- stabilizing lysosomal membranes
- suppressing the antigen response of macrophages and helper T cells
- inhibiting the synthesis of inflammatory response mediators, such as cytokines, interleukins, and prostaglandins.

Incompatibilities

Don't mix methylprednisolone with any drug without first consulting pharmacist.

Contraindications

Fungal infection, hypersensitivity to methylprednisolone or its components

Interactions

DRUGS

acetaminophen: Increased risk of hepatotoxicity

amphotericin B, carbonic anhydrase inhibitors: Possibly severe hypokalemia

anabolic steroids, androgens: Increased risk of edema and worsening of acne

anticholinergics: Possibly increased intraocular pressure

asparaginase: Increased risk of hyperglycemia and toxicity

aspirin, NSAIDs: Increased risk of adverse GI effects and bleeding

cyclosporine: Increased risk of seizures

digoxin: Possibly hypokalemia-induced arrhythmias and digitalis toxicity
ephedrine, phenobarbital, phenytoin, rifampin: Decreased blood methylprednisolone level
estrogens, oral contraceptives: Possibly increased therapeutic and toxic effects of methylprednisolone
isoniazid: Possibly decreased therapeutic effects of isoniazid
mexiletine: Possibly decreased blood mexiletine level
neuromuscular blockers: Possibly increased neuromuscular blockade, causing respiratory depression or apnea
oral anticoagulants, thrombolytics: Increased risk of GI ulceration and hemorrhage, possibly decreased therapeutic effects of these drugs
potassium-depleting drugs (such as thiazide diuretics): Possibly severe hypokalemia
potassium supplements: Possibly decreased effects of these supplements
somatrem, somatropin: Possibly decreased therapeutic effects of these drugs
streptozocin: Increased risk of hyperglycemia
troleandomycin: Increased blood methylprednisolone level
vaccines: Decreased antibody response and increased risk of neurologic complications
ACTIVITIES
alcohol use: Increased risk of adverse GI effects and bleeding

Adverse Reactions

CNS: Ataxia, behavioral changes, depression, dizziness, euphoria, fatigue, headache, increased ICP with papilledema, insomnia, malaise, mood changes, paresthesia, restlessness, seizures, steroid psychosis, syncope, vertigo
CV: Arrhythmias (from hypokalemia), edema, fat embolism, heart failure, hypertension, hypotension, thromboembolism, thrombophlebitis
EENT: Exophthalmos, glaucoma, increased intraocular pressure, nystagmus, posterior subcapsular cataracts
ENDO: Adrenal insufficiency, cushingoid symptoms (moon face, buffalo hump, central obesity, supraclavicular fat pad enlargement), diabetes mellitus, growth suppression in children, hyperglycemia, negative nitrogen balance from protein catabolism
GI: Abdominal distention, hiccups, increased appetite, melena, nausea, pancreatitis, peptic ulcer, ulcerative esophagitis, vomiting
GU: Amenorrhea, glycosuria, menstrual irregularities, perineal burning or tingling

HEME: Easy bruising, leukocytosis
MS: Arthralgia; aseptic necrosis of femoral and humeral heads; compression fractures; muscle atrophy, twitching, or weakness; myalgia; osteoporosis; spontaneous fractures; steroid myopathy; tendon rupture
SKIN: Acne; altered skin pigmentation; diaphoresis; erythema; hirsutism; necrotizing vasculitis; petechiae; purpura; rash; scarring; sterile abscess; striae; subcutaneous fat atrophy; thin, fragile skin; urticaria
Other: Anaphylaxis, hypocalcemia, hypokalemia, hypokalemic alkalosis, impaired wound healing, masking of infection, metabolic alkalosis, suppressed skin test reaction, weight gain

Nursing Considerations

- **WARNING** Don't administer methylprednisolone preparations that contain benzyl alcohol to neonates or premature infants because this preservative has been linked to a fatal toxic syndrome characterized by CNS, respiratory, circulatory, and renal impairment and metabolic acidosis.
- Don't give acetate injectable form by I.V. route; it's used for intra-articular, intralesional, I.M., and soft-tissue injections.
- After reconstituting drug according to manufacturer's directions, use it within 48 hours.
- Discard parenteral products if you observe discoloration or particles.
- Provide a low-sodium diet with added potassium, as prescribed.
- Protect patient from falling, especially elderly patient at risk for fractures from osteoporosis.
- Closely monitor patient for signs of infection because drug may mask them.
- Assess for possible depression or psychotic episodes during therapy.
- Monitor blood glucose level; dosage of insulin or oral antidiabetic drug may need to be adjusted for diabetic patient.
- **WARNING** To avoid possibly fatal acute adrenocortical insufficiency, expect to taper long-term therapy when it must be discontinued.
- Store drug at a controlled room temperature of 20° to 25° C (68° to 77° F), and protect from light.

PATIENT TEACHING

- Urge patient receiving methylprednisolone to immediately report dark or tarry stools; signs of impending adrenocortical insufficiency, such as anorexia, dizziness, fainting, fatigue, fever, joint pain, muscle weakness, or nausea; and sudden weight gain or swelling.

- Inform patient with diabetes that his blood glucose level will be checked frequently during therapy because methylprednisolone may affect glucose level.
- Advise patient to notify prescriber if he develops another illness or requires surgery during therapy or if his condition recurs or worsens after dosage is reduced or therapy is discontinued.
- Instruct patient not to obtain vaccinations unless approved by prescriber.
- Urge patient to take vitamin D, calcium supplements, or both if recommended by prescriber.
- Instruct patient on long-term therapy to follow a low-sodium, high-potassium, high-protein diet, if prescribed, to help minimize weight gain. Advise him to inform prescriber if he's on a special diet.
- Inform patient that insomnia and restlessness usually resolve after 1 to 3 weeks of therapy.
- Caution patient to avoid people with contagious diseases, such as chicken pox or measles.
- Discuss the need for regular exercise or physical therapy to maintain muscle mass.
- Urge patient to avoid alcoholic beverages during therapy because alcohol increases the risk of GI bleeding.
- Encourage patient to keep regularly scheduled follow-up medical appointments, even after therapy stops.
- Instruct patient to undergo periodic ophthalmic examinations.
- Advise patient to carry medical identification that documents his need for long-term corticosteroid therapy.

metoclopramide hydrochloride

Reglan

Class and Category

Chemical: Benzamide
Therapeutic: Antiemetic, upper GI stimulant
Pregnancy category: B

Indications and Dosages

▶ *To treat diabetic gastroparesis*

I.V. INJECTION

Adults and adolescents. 10 mg t.i.d. or q.i.d. for severe symptoms; dosage adjusted as needed.

▶ *To prevent chemotherapy-induced vomiting*
I.V. INFUSION
Adults and adolescents. 3 mg/kg before chemotherapy and then 0.5 mg/kg/hr for 8 hr.
I.V. INJECTION
Adults and adolescents. 1 to 2 mg/kg 30 min before chemotherapy and then repeated q 2 to 3 hr, as needed.
Children. 1 mg/kg as a single dose, repeated in 1 hr. *Maximum:* 2 mg/kg.

Route	Onset	Peak	Duration
I.V.	1 to 3 min	Unknown	1 to 2 hr

Mechanism of Action
May enhance gastric motility by antagonizing the inhibitory neurotransmitter effect of dopamine on GI smooth muscle. This results in gastric contraction, which promotes gastric emptying and peristalsis, thereby reducing gastroesophageal reflux. Metoclopramide also blocks dopaminergic receptors in the chemoreceptor trigger zone, preventing nausea and vomiting.

Incompatibilities
Don't administer metoclopramide through same I.V. line as calcium gluconate, cephalothin sodium, chloramphenicol sodium, cisplatin, erythromycin lactobionate, furosemide, methotrexate, penicillin G potassium, or sodium bicarbonate.

Contraindications
Concurrent use of butyrophenones, phenothiazines, or other drugs that may cause extrapyramidal reactions; GI hemorrhage, mechanical obstruction, or perforation; hypersensitivity to metoclopramide or its components; pheochromocytoma; seizure disorders

Interactions
DRUGS
anticholinergics, opioid analgesics: Possibly decreased therapeutic effects of metoclopramide
apomorphine: Possibly decreased antiemetic effect of apomorphine, possibly increased CNS depression
bromocriptine, pergolide: Possibly decreased therapeutic effects of these drugs
cimetidine: Possibly decreased cimetidine absorption and effects

CNS depressants: Possibly increased CNS depression
cyclosporine: Increased blood cyclosporine level
digoxin: Decreased gastric absorption of digoxin
levodopa: Possibly decreased levodopa effectiveness
MAO inhibitors: Increased risk of severe hypertension if patient has essential hypertension
mexiletine: Possibly faster mexiletene absorption
succinylcholine: Possibly prolonged therapeutic action of succinylcholine
ACTIVITIES
alcohol use: Increased risk of excessive sedation

Adverse Reactions

CNS: Agitation, anxiety, depression, dizziness, drowsiness, extrapyramidal reactions (motor restlessness, parkinsonism, tardive dyskinesia), fatigue, headache, insomnia, irritability, lassitude, neuroleptic malignant syndrome, panic reaction, restlessness
CV: AV block, fluid retention, heart failure, hypertension, hypotension, supraventricular tachycardia
EENT: Dry mouth
ENDO: Galactorrhea, gynecomastia
GI: Constipation, diarrhea, nausea
GU: Menstrual irregularities
HEME: Agranulocytosis
SKIN: Rash
Other: Restless leg syndrome

Nursing Considerations

- Use metoclopramide cautiously in patients with hypertension because it may increase catecholamine levels.
- Use drug cautiously in elderly patients because they have an increased risk of tardive dyskinesia and parkinsonian effects. Expect to stop drug if these symptoms develop.
- Monitor patient with NADH-cytochrome b5 reductase deficiency because metoclopramide increases the risk of methemoglobinemia and sulfhemoglobinemia and patient can't receive methylene blue.
- Assess patient for signs of intestinal obstruction, such as abnormal bowel sounds, diarrhea, nausea, and vomiting, before administering metoclopramide. Notify prescriber if you detect them.
- For I.V. administration, you needn't dilute doses of 10 mg or less. Give drug over 1 to 2 minutes. For doses larger than 10 mg, dilute in 50 ml of normal saline solution, half-normal

(0.45) saline solution, D_5W, or lactated Ringer's solution and infuse over at least 15 minutes.
- Avoid rapid I.V. delivery because it may cause anxiety, restlessness, and drowsiness.
- **WARNING** Notify prescriber if patient displays signs of toxicity, such as disorientation, drowsiness, and extrapyramidal reactions.
- Monitor patient, especially one with heart failure or cirrhosis, for possible signs of fluid retention or volume overload due to transient increase in plasma aldosterone level.
- Monitor patient closely for neuroleptic malignant syndrome, a rare but potentially fatal disorder characterized by hyperthermia, muscle rigidity, altered level of consciousness, irregular pulse or blood pressure, tachycardia, diaphoresis, and arrhythmias.
- Store drug in a light-resistant container; discard if discolored or contains particulate.

PATIENT TEACHING
- Advise against activities that require alertness for about 2 hours after each dose.
- Urge patient to avoid alcohol and CNS depressants while taking metoclopramide because they may increase CNS depression.
- Tell patient to immediately report involuntary movements of face, eyes, tongue, or hands.
- Alert patient that a withdrawal period may occur after metoclopramide is discontinued that may include dizziness, nervousness and/or headaches.

metoprolol succinate

Toprol-XL

metoprolol tartrate

Apo-Metoprolol (CAN), Betaloc (CAN), Lopresor (CAN), Lopressor, Novometoprol (CAN)

Class and Category

Chemical: $Beta_1$-adrenergic antagonist
Therapeutic: Antianginal, antihypertensive, MI prophylaxis and treatment
Pregnancy category: C

Indications and Dosages

▶ *To treat acute MI or evolving acute MI*

I.V. INJECTION (METOPROLOL TARTRATE)

Adults. *Initial:* 5 mg by I.V. bolus q 2 min for 3 doses followed by 50 mg P.O. for patients who tolerate total I.V. dose (or 25 to 50 mg P.O. for patients who can't tolerate total I.V. dose) q 6 hr for 48 hr, starting 15 min after final I.V. dose; after 48 hr, 100 mg b.i.d. followed by maintenance dosage. *Maintenance:* 100 mg P.O. b.i.d. for at least 3 mo.

Route	Onset	Peak	Duration
I.V.	Unknown	20 min	Unknown

Mechanism of Action

Inhibits stimulation of $beta_1$-receptor sites, located mainly in the heart, resulting in decreased cardiac excitability, cardiac output, and myocardial oxygen demand. These effects help relieve angina. Metoprolol also helps reduce blood pressure by decreasing renal release of renin.

Contraindications

Acute heart failure, bradycardia of less than 45 beats/minute, cardiogenic shock, hypersensitivity to metoprolol, or its components, hypersensitivity to other beta blockers, pheochromocytoma, second- or third-degree AV block, severe peripheral arterial circulatory disorder, sick sinus syndrome

Interactions

DRUGS

aluminum salts, barbiturates, calcium salts, cholestyramine, colestipol, NSAIDs, rifampin, salicylates, sulfinpyrazone: Decreased therapeutic effects of metoprolol

amiodarone, digoxin, diltiazem, verapamil: Increased risk of complete AV block

calcium channel blockers: Increased risk of heart failure, increased effects of both drugs

cimetidine: Increased blood metoprolol level

clonidine, diazoxide, guanabenz: Increased risk of hypotension

CYP2D6 inhibitors: May increase plasma metoprolol levels

estrogens: Possibly decreased antihypertensive effect of metoprolol

general anesthetics: Increased risk of hypotension and heart failure

insulin, oral antidiabetic drugs: Decreased blood glucose control, possibly masking of signs and symptoms of hypoglycemia (by metoprolol)

lidocaine: Increased risk of lidocaine toxicity
MAO inhibitors: Increased risk of hypertension
neuromuscular blockers: Possibly enhanced and prolonged neuromuscular blockade
other antihypertensives: Additive hypotensive effect
phenothiazines: Possibly increased blood levels of both drugs
propafenone: Increased blood level and half-life of metoprolol
sympathomimetics, xanthines: Possibly decreased therapeutic effects of these drugs or metoprolol
FOODS
all foods: Increased bioavailability of metoprolol

Adverse Reactions

CNS: Anxiety, confusion, depression, dizziness, drowsiness, fatigue, hallucinations, headache, insomnia, weakness
CV: Angina, arrhythmias (including AV block and bradycardia), chest pain, heart failure, hypertension, orthostatic hypotension
EENT: Nasal congestion, taste disturbance
GI: Constipation, diarrhea, hepatitis, nausea, vomiting
GU: Impotence
HEME: Leukopenia, thrombocytopenia
MS: Arthralgia, back pain, gangrene of extremity, myalgia
RESP: Bronchospasm, dyspnea
SKIN: Diaphoresis, photosensitivity, rash, urticaria

Nursing Considerations

- For patient with acute MI who can't tolerate initial dosage or who delays treatment, start with maintenance dosage, as prescribed and tolerated.
- **WARNING** If dosage exceeds 400 mg daily, monitor patient for bronchospasm and dyspnea because metoprolol competitively blocks $beta_2$-adrenergic receptors in bronchial and vascular smooth muscles.
- **WARNING** When substituting metoprolol for clonidine, expect to gradually reduce clonidine dosage and increase metoprolol dosage over several days. Giving these drugs together causes additive hypotensive effects.
- Be aware that patients who take metoprolol may be at risk for AV block. If AV block results from depressed AV node conduction, prepare to administer appropriate drug, as prescribed, or assist with insertion of temporary pacemaker.
- Check for signs of poor glucose control in patient with diabetes mellitus. Metoprolol may interfere with therapeutic effects of

insulin and oral antidiabetic drugs. It also may mask evidence of hypoglycemia, such as palpitations, tachycardia, and tremor.
- Monitor patient with peripheral vascular disease for signs and symptoms of arterial insufficiency (pain, pallor, and coldness in affected extremity) because metoprolol can precipitate or aggravate peripheral vascular disease.
- Be aware that abrupt withdrawal of drug can precipitate thyroid storm in patient with hyperthyroidism or thyrotoxicosis.
- **WARNING** Expect to taper metoprolol dosage when drug is discontinued; abrupt discontinuation can cause myocardial ischemia, MI, ventricular arrhythmias, or severe hypertension, especially in patients with cardiac disease.

PATIENT TEACHING
- Advise patient to notify prescriber if pulse rate falls below 60 beats/minute or is significantly lower than usual.
- Urge diabetic patient to check blood glucose level frequently during metoprolol therapy.

metronidazole

Flagyl, Flagyl I.V. RTU, Metro I.V.

metronidazole hydrochloride

Flagyl I.V.

Class and Category

Chemical: Nitroimidazole derivative
Therapeutic: Antibiotic, antiprotozoal
Pregnancy category: B

Indications and Dosages

▶ *To treat systemic anaerobic infections caused by* Bacteroides fragilis, Clostridium difficile, Clostridium perfringens, Eubacterium, Fusobacterium, Peptococcus, Peptostreptococcus, *and* Veillonella *sp.*

I.V. INFUSION

Adults and adolescents. *Initial:* 15 mg/kg and then 7.5 mg/kg up to 1,000 mg q 6 hr for 7 days or longer. *Maximum:* 4,000 mg daily.

Children. 7.5 mg/kg q 6 hr or 10 mg/kg q 8 hr.

▶ *To prevent perioperative bowel infection*

I.V. INFUSION

Adults and adolescents. 15 mg/kg 1 hr before surgery and then 7.5 mg/kg 6 and 12 hr after initial dose.

Incompatibilities
Don't administer I.V. metronidazole with aluminum needles or hubs or through same I.V. line as other drugs.

> **Mechanism of Action**
> Undergoes intracellular chemical reduction during anaerobic metabolism. After metronidazole is reduced, it damages DNA's helical structure and breaks its strands, which inhibits bacterial nucleic acid synthesis and causes cell death.

Contraindications
Breast-feeding, hypersensitivity to metronidazole or its components, trichomoniasis during first trimester of pregnancy

Interactions
DRUGS
cimetidine: Possibly delayed elimination and increased blood level of metronidazole
disulfiram: Possibly combined toxicity, resulting in confusion and psychotic reactions
neurotoxic drugs: Increased risk of neurotoxicity
oral anticoagulants: Possibly increased anticoagulant effect
phenobarbital: Increased metabolism and decreased blood level and half-life of metronidazole
phenytoin: Decreased phenytoin clearance
ACTIVITIES
alcohol use: Possibly disulfiram-like effects

Adverse Reactions
CNS: Ataxia, dizziness, encephalopathy, fever, headache, lightheadedness, peripheral neuropathy, seizures (high doses)
EENT: Dry mouth, lacrimation (topical form), metallic taste, pharyngitis
GI: Abdominal cramps or pain, anorexia, diarrhea, nausea, pancreatitis, vomiting
GU: Darkened urine, vaginal candidiasis (oral, parenteral, and topical forms); burning or irritation of sexual partner's penis, candidal cervicitis or vaginitis, dysuria, urinary frequency, vulvitis (vaginal form)
HEME: Leukopenia
MS: Back pain
SKIN: Burning sensation, stinging sensation, dry skin (topical

form); erythema, pruritus, rash, urticaria (oral and parenteral forms)
Other: Injection site edema, pain, or tenderness

Nursing Considerations

- Give I.V. drug by slow infusion over 1 hour; don't give by direct I.V. injection.
- Discontinue primary I.V. infusion during metronidazole infusion.
- **WARNING** If patient has adverse CNS reactions, such as seizures or peripheral neuropathy, tell prescriber and stop drug immediately.
- Monitor patient with severe liver disease because slowed metronidazole metabolism may cause drug to accumulate in body and increase the risk of adverse effects.
- Monitor CBC and culture and sensitivity tests if therapy lasts longer than 10 days or if second course of treatment is needed.

PATIENT TEACHING

- Instruct female patient to notify prescriber if she is pregnant, intends to get pregnant, or is breast-feeding.
- Caution patient to avoid alcohol during therapy and for at least 1 day afterward.
- Advise patient to avoid hazardous activities until drug's CNS effects are known.
- If patient reports dry mouth, suggest ice chips or sugarless hard candy or gum; suggest a dental visit if dryness lasts longer than 2 weeks.
- Instruct patient to notify prescriber if no improvement occurs within a few days of taking tablets or capsules.
- Urge patient to follow up with prescriber to make sure infection is gone.

mezlocillin sodium

Mezlin

Class and Category

Chemical: Acyclaminopenicillin
Therapeutic: Antibiotic
Pregnancy category: B

Indications and Dosages

▶ *To treat moderate to severe infections, including bacteremia, bone and joint infections, gynecologic infections (such as endometritis, pelvic cellu-*

litis, and pelvic inflammatory disease), intra-abdominal infections (such as cholangitis, cholecystitis, hepatic abscess, intra-abdominal abscess, and peritonitis), lower respiratory tract infections (such as pneumonia and lung abscess), meningitis, septicemia caused by susceptible bacteria, or skin and soft-tissue infections (such as cellulitis and diabetic foot ulcer); to manage febrile neutropenia

I.V. INFUSION

Adults and adolescents. 3 g q 4 hr or 4 g q 6 hr.

▶ *To treat life-threatening infections of the types listed above*

I.V. INFUSION

Adults and adolescents. Up to 350 mg/kg daily. *Maximum:* 24,000 mg daily.

Children and infants. 50 mg/kg q 4 hr.

Neonates over age 7 days weighing 2,000 g (4 lb, 6 oz) or less. 75 mg/kg q 8 hr.

Neonates age 7 days or less weighing 2,000 g or less. 75 mg/kg q 12 hr.

Neonates age 7 days or less weighing more than 2,000 g. 75 mg/kg q 6 hr.

▶ *To treat uncomplicated UTI*

I.V. INFUSION

Adults. 1.5 to 2 g q 6 hr.

▶ *To treat complicated UTI*

I.V. INFUSION

Adults. 3 g q 6 hr.

DOSAGE ADJUSTMENT Dosing interval extended to q 6 to 8 hr, if needed, for patients with creatinine clearance of 10 to 30 ml/min/1.73 m^2. Dosing interval extended and dosage reduced to 1.5 to 2 g for patients with creatinine clearance of less than 10 ml/min/1.73 m^2.

▶ *To treat uncomplicated gonorrhea caused by susceptible strains of* Neisseria gonorrhoeae

I.V. INFUSION

Adults. 1 to 2 g as a single dose given with 1 g of probenecid P.O. (or probenecid given up to 30 min before mezlocillin).

▶ *To prevent infection from potentially contaminated surgical procedures*

I.V. INFUSION

Adults. 4 g 30 min before surgery and then 4 g q 6 hr for 2 more doses.

▶ *To prevent infection in cesarean section*

I.V. INFUSION

Adults. 4 g as soon as umbilical cord is clamped; then 4 g q 4 hr for 2 more doses, starting 4 hr after initial dose.

Mechanism of Action
Inhibits bacterial cell wall synthesis. In susceptible bacteria, the rigid, cross-linked cell wall is assembled in several steps. Mezlocillin exerts its effects in the final stage of the cross-linking process by binding with and inactivating penicillin-binding proteins (enzymes responsible for linking cell wall strands). This action causes bacterial cell lysis and death.

Incompatibilities
Administer mezlocillin at separate sites and at least 1 hour before or after aminoglycosides. Don't mix mezlocillin in same I.V. bag, bottle, or tubing as other drugs.

Contraindications
Hypersensitivity to mezlocillin, other penicillins, or their components

Interactions
DRUGS
aminoglycosides: Substantial aminoglycoside inactivation
chloramphenicol, erythromycins, sulfonamides, tetracyclines: Possibly decreased therapeutic effects of mezlocillin
methotrexate: Increased risk of methotrexate toxicity
probenecid: Increased blood level and prolonged half-life of mezlocillin

Adverse Reactions
CNS: Depression, headache, seizures
EENT: Oral candidiasis
GI: Abdominal pain, diarrhea, pseudomembranous colitis, nausea, vomiting
GU: Vaginitis
HEME: Leukopenia, neutropenia
SKIN: Exfoliative dermatitis, pruritus, rash, urticaria
Other: Anaphylaxis; hypokalemia; injection site pain, redness, and swelling; serum sickness–like reaction

Nursing Considerations
- **WARNING** Before administering first dose of mezlocillin, make sure patient has had no previous hypersensitivity reactions to penicillins.
- Expect mezlocillin therapy to continue for at least 2 days after signs and symptoms have resolved—typically 7 to 10 days, depending on severity of infection. Complicated infections may need longer treatment. Group A beta-hemolytic streptococcal

infections usually are treated for at least 10 days to reduce the risk of rheumatic fever or glomerulonephritis.
- Reconstitute each gram of mezlocillin with 10 ml of sterile water for injection, D_5W, or sodium chloride for injection and shake vigorously. Don't exceed a concentration of 100 mg/ml (10%). Be aware that stability of reconstituted solution varies, depending on type of diluent used, concentration, and storage temperature. Consult manufacturer's insert for specific storage guidelines. If a precipitate forms during refrigeration, warm solution to 37° C (98.6° F) using a water bath for 20 minutes. Shake well. Inject slowly, directly into I.V. tubing, over 3 to 5 minutes.
- For intermittent infusion, further dilute to desired volume (50 to 100 ml) with an appropriate I.V. solution and administer over 30 minutes. Discontinue other infusions during mezlocillin administration.
- Be aware that mezlocillin powder and reconstituted solution may darken slightly but that potency isn't affected.
- Periodically monitor serum potassium level of patients receiving long-term therapy, as appropriate.
- When calculating sodium intake for patients on a sodium-restricted diet, keep in mind that each gram of mezlocillin contains approximately 1.9 mEq of sodium.
- During long-term therapy, monitor for signs and symptoms of superinfection, such as oral candidiasis and vaginitis.
- Before reconstituting drug, store it at less than 30° (86° F).

PATIENT TEACHING
- Instruct patient receiving mezlocillin to immediately report increased bruising or other bleeding tendencies.
- Advise patient to report diarrhea and to check with prescriber before taking an antidiarrheal because it may mask symptoms of pseudomembranous colitis.

micafungin sodium

Mycamine

Class and Category

Chemical: Semisynthetic lipopeptide echinocandin
Therapeutic: Antifungal
Pregnancy category: C

Indications and Dosages

▶ *To treat esophageal candidiasis*

I.V. INFUSION

Adults. 150 mg infused over 1 hr daily.

▶ *To prevent* Candida *infection in patients undergoing hematopoietic stem cell transplantation*

I.V. INFUSION

Adults. 50 mg infused over 1 hr daily.

Route	Onset	Peak	Duration
I.V.	Unknown	Unknown	Unknown

Mechanism of Action

Inhibits synthesis of 1,3-beta-D-glucan, which is an essential component of the *Candida* fungal cell wall. Without 1,3-beta-D-glucan, the fungal cell dies.

Contraindications

Hypersensitivity to micafungin or its components

Incompatibilities

Mixing or infusing with other drugs may cause micafungin to precipitate.

Interactions

DRUGS

immunosuppressants: Possibly additive adverse hematologic effects

nifedipine, sirolimus: Increased plasma nifedipine and sirolimus levels

Adverse Reactions

CNS: Delirium, dizziness, dysgeusia, fatigue, fever, headache, rigors, somnolence

CV: Hypertension, hypotension, shock, vasodilation

EENT: Mucosal inflammation

GI: Abdominal pain, anorexia, constipation, diarrhea, dyspepsia, elevated liver enzyme levels, hepatic dysfunction, hiccups, hyperbilirubinemia, nausea, vomiting

GU: Acute renal failure, elevated serum creatinine and blood urea levels

HEME: Anemia, eosinophilia, hemolytic anemia, leukopenia, lymphopenia, neutropenia, thrombocytopenia

SKIN: Flushing, pruritus, rash, urticaria

Other: Anaphylaxis, angioedema, hypocalcemia, hypokalemia, hypomagnesemia, hypophosphatemia, injection site reactions including phlebitis and thrombophlebitis

Nursing Considerations

- Use cautiously in patients with hepatic or renal insufficiency.
- Reconstitute micafungin by adding 5 ml of normal saline solution to each 50-mg vial, yielding 10 mg micafungin/ml. Swirl vial gently to minimize excessive foaming. Add reconstituted solution to 100 ml of normal saline solution, and administer over 1 hour. Protect diluted solution from light, although you need not cover the infusion drip chamber or tubing.
- Always flush an existing intravenous line with normal saline solution before administering micafungin through that line.
- Monitor infusion rate carefully because infusions that took less than 1 hour to infuse have been associated with more frequent hypersensitivity reactions.
- **WARNING Monitor patient closely for hypersensitivity reactions including anaphylaxis and angioedema. Discontinue micafungin infusion immediately if present, notify prescriber, and provide supportive care, as prescribed.**
- Monitor patient's liver and renal function closely throughout therapy because liver and renal abnormalities may occur in patients receiving micafungin.
- Monitor patient's hematologic status closely because a variety of hematologic abnormalities may occur. If abnormalities are detected, monitor patient closely. If condition worsens, expect micafungin to be discontinued.

PATIENT TEACHING

- Instruct patient to report any infusion site discomfort immediately.
- Tell patient to report any unusual or persistent signs and symptoms to prescriber.

midazolam hydrochloride

Versed

Class, Category, and Schedule

Chemical: Benzodiazepine
Therapeutic: Sedative-hypnotic
Pregnancy category: D
Controlled substance: Schedule IV

Indications and Dosages

▶ *To induce preoperative sedation or amnesia, to control preoperative anxiety*

I.V. INJECTION

Adults age 60 and over. 1.5 mg over 2 min given immediately before procedure. After 2-min waiting period, dosage adjusted to desired level in 25% increments, as ordered. *Maximum:* 1 mg in 2 min.

Adults under age 60 and adolescents. Up to 2.5 mg over 2 min immediately before procedure. After 2-min waiting period, dosage adjusted to desired level in 25% increments, as ordered. *Maximum:* 5 mg.

Children ages 6 to 12. *Initial:* 0.025 to 0.05 mg/kg, up to 0.4 mg/kg, if needed. *Maximum:* 10 mg.

Children ages 6 months to 5 years. *Initial:* 0.05 to 0.1 mg/kg, up to 0.6 mg/kg, if needed. *Maximum:* 6 mg.

▶ *To relieve agitation and anxiety in mechanically ventilated patients*

I.V. INFUSION

Adults. *Initial:* 0.01 to 0.05 mg/kg infused over several min, repeated at 10- to 15-min intervals until adequate sedation occurs. *Maintenance:* 0.02 to 0.1 mg/kg/hr initially, adjusted to desired level in 25% to 50% increments, as ordered. After achieving desired level of sedation, infusion rate decreased by 10% to 25% every few hr, as ordered, until minimum effective infusion rate is determined.

Children. *Initial:* 50 to 200 mcg/kg over 2 to 3 min followed by 1 to 2 mcg/kg/min by continuous infusion. *Maintenance:* 0.4 to 6 mcg/kg/min.

Infants age 32 weeks or over. 1 mcg/kg/min by continuous infusion.

Infants under age 32 weeks. 0.5 mcg/kg/min by continuous infusion.

Route	Onset	Peak	Duration
I.V.*	1.5 to 5 min	Rapid	2 to 6 hr

Mechanism of Action

May exert its sedating effect by increasing the activity of gamma-aminobutyric acid, a major inhibitory neurotransmitter in the brain. As a result, midazolam produces a calming effect, relaxes skeletal muscles, and—at high doses—induces sleep.

* For sedation.

Contraindications

Acute angle-closure glaucoma; alcohol intoxication; coma; hypersensitivity to midazolam, other benzodiazepines, or their components; shock

Interactions

DRUGS

antihypertensives: Increased risk of hypotension
cimetidine, diltiazem, erythromycin, fluconazole, indinavir, itraconazole, ketoconazole, ranitidine, ritonavir, roxithromycin, saquinavir, verapamil: Prolonged sedation caused by reduced midazolam metabolism
CNS depressants: Possibly increased CNS and respiratory depression and hypotension
rifampin: Decreased blood midazolam level

FOODS

grapefruit, grapefruit juice: Possibly increased blood midazolam level and risk of toxicity

ACTIVITIES

alcohol use: Possibly increased CNS and respiratory depression and hypotension

Adverse Reactions

CNS: Agitation, delirium, or dreaming during emergence from anesthesia; anxiety; ataxia; chills; combativeness; confusion; dizziness; drowsiness; euphoria; excessive sedation; headache; insomnia; lethargy; nervousness; nightmares; paresthesia; prolonged emergence from anesthesia; restlessness; retrograde amnesia; sleep disturbance; slurred speech; weakness; yawning
CV: Cardiac arrest, hypotension, nodal rhythm, PVCs, tachycardia, vasovagal episodes
EENT: Blurred vision, diplopia, or other vision changes; increased salivation; laryngospasm; miosis; nystagmus; toothache
GI: Hiccups, nausea, retching, vomiting
RESP: Airway obstruction, bradypnea, bronchospasm, coughing, decreased tidal volume, dyspnea, hyperventilation, respiratory arrest, shallow breathing, tachypnea, wheezing
SKIN: Pruritus, rash, urticaria
Other: Infusion site burning, edema, induration, pain, redness, and tenderness

Nursing Considerations

- **WARNING** Be aware that I.V. midazolam is given only in hospitals or ambulatory care settings that allow continuous

monitoring of respiratory and cardiac function. Keep resuscitative drugs and equipment readily available.
- As needed, combine midazolam injection with D_5W, normal saline solution, or lactated Ringer's solution. Solutions mixed with D_5W or normal saline solution are stable 24 hours; those mixed with lactated Ringer's solution are stable 4 hours.
- As needed, mix injection in same syringe with atropine sulfate, meperidine hydrochloride, morphine sulfate, or scopolamine hydrobromide. The resulting solution is stable for 30 minutes.
- Expect child's dosage to be based on ideal body weight. This is especially important for an obese child.
- **WARNING** Be aware that midazolam contains the preservative benzyl alcohol, which may cause a fatal toxic syndrome in neonates and premature infants, characterized by CNS, respiratory, circulatory, and renal impairment and metabolic acidosis. Because the 5-mg/ml and 1-mg/ml vials contain the same amount of benzyl alcohol, using the 5-mg/ml vial to prepare neonatal doses may decrease the amount of benzyl alcohol the patient receives.
- Be aware that neonates have a higher risk of respiratory depression than other pediatric or adult patients.
- Assess LOC frequently because the range between sedation and unconsciousness or disorientation is narrower with midazolam than with other benzodiazepines.
- Be aware that recovery time is usually 2 hours but may take up to 6 hours.
- Store drug at 15° to 30° C (59° to 86° F); don't freeze.

PATIENT TEACHING
- Inform patient that he may not remember procedure because midazolam produces amnesia.
- Advise patient to avoid hazardous activities until drug's adverse CNS effects, such as dizziness and drowsiness, have worn off.
- Instruct patient to avoid alcohol and other CNS depressants for 24 hours after receiving drug unless prescriber directs otherwise.

milrinone lactate
Primacor

Class and Category
Chemical: Bipyridine derivative
Therapeutic: Inotropic, vasodilator
Pregnancy category: C

Indications and Dosages

▶ *To provide short-term treatment of acute heart failure*

I.V. INFUSION

Adults. *Loading:* 50 mcg/kg over 10 min (at least 0.375 mcg/kg/min). *Usual:* 0.375 to 0.75 mcg/kg/min. *Maximum:* 1.13 mg/kg daily.

DOSAGE ADJUSTMENT Dosage adjusted according to cardiac output, pulmonary artery wedge pressure, and clinical response. For patients with creatinine clearance of 30 to 39 ml/min/1.73 m^2, infusion rate reduced to 0.33 mcg/kg/min; of 20 to 29 ml/min/1.73 m^2, to 0.28 mcg/kg/min; of 10 to 19 ml/min/1.73 m^2, to 0.23 mcg/kg/min; and of less than 9 ml/min/1.73 m^2, to 0.20 mcg/kg/min.

Route	Onset	Peak	Duration
I.V.	5 to 15 min	Unknown	3 to 6 hr

Mechanism of Action

An inotropic drug, milrinone increases the force of myocardial contraction—and cardiac output—by blocking the enzyme phosphodiesterase. Normally, this enzyme is activated by hormones binding to cell membrane receptors. As shown at top, phosphodiesterase degrades intracellular cAMP, which restricts calcium movement into myocardial cells. By inhibiting phosphodiesterase, as shown at bottom, milrinone slows cAMP degradation, increasing intracellular cAMP and the amount of calcium that enters myocardial cells. In blood vessels, increased cAMP causes smooth-muscle relaxation, which improves cardiac output by reducing preload and afterload.

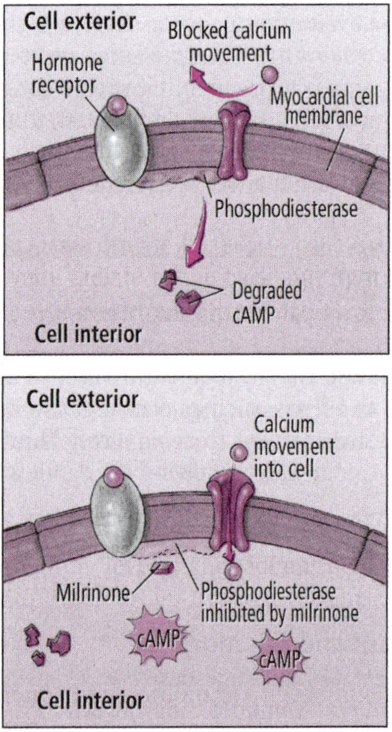

Incompatibilities

Don't administer milrinone through same I.V. line as furosemide because precipitate will form. Don't add other drugs to premixed milrinone flexible containers.

Contraindications

Hypersensitivity to milrinone or its components

Interactions

DRUGS

antihypertensives: Possibly hypotension

Adverse Reactions

CNS: Headache, tremor

CV: Angina, hypotension, supraventricular arrhythmias, ventricular ectopic activity, ventricular fibrillation, ventricular tachycardia, torsades de pointes

GI: Liver function test abnormalities

HEME: Thrombocytopenia

RESP: Bronchospasm

SKIN: Rash

Other: Anaphylactic shock, hypokalemia

Nursing Considerations

- Make sure ECG equipment is available for continuous monitoring during milrinone therapy.
- Discard drug if it's discolored or contains particles.
- For loading dose, directly infuse undiluted drug into I.V. line with a compatible infusing solution. For continuous infusion, dilute drug with half-normal (0.45) saline solution, normal saline solution, or D_5W. Dilution isn't needed when using premixed milrinone flexible containers.
- Check platelet count before and during infusion, as ordered. Expect to stop drug if platelet count falls below 150,000/mm^3.
- Give loading dose using a controlled-rate infusion device. For continuous infusion, use a calibrated electronic infusion device.
- Monitor cardiac output, pulmonary artery wedge pressure, blood pressure, heart rate, weight, and fluid status during therapy to determine drug effectiveness.
- Monitor renal and liver function test results and serum electrolyte levels. Notify prescriber of abnormalities.
- If severe hypotension develops, notify prescriber immediately and expect to stop drug.
- Expect patient to receive digoxin before starting milrinone, which can increase ventricular response rate.

PATIENT TEACHING
- Reassure patient that you'll be present and he'll be monitored constantly during therapy.

minocycline
Minocin
minocycline hydrochloride
Alti-Minocycline (CAN), Apo-Minocycline (CAN), Dynacin, Gen-Minocycline (CAN), Minocin, Novo-Minocycline (CAN), Vectrin

Class and Category
Chemical: Tetracycline
Therapeutic: Antibiotic, antiprotozoal
Pregnancy category: D

Indications and Dosages
▶ *To treat bartonellosis, brucellosis, chancroid, granuloma inguinale, inclusion conjunctivitis, lymphogranuloma venereum, nongonococcal urethritis, plague, psittacosis, Q fever, relapsing fever, respiratory tract infections (including pneumonia), rickettsial pox, Rocky Mountain spotted fever, tularemia, typhus, and UTI caused by gram-negative organisms (including* **Bartonella bacilliformis, Brucella** *sp.,* Haemophilus ducreyi, Haemophilus influenzae, Vibrio cholerae, *and* Yersinia pestis*), susceptible gram-positive organisms (including certain strains of* Streptococcus pneumoniae*), and other organisms (including* Actinomyces *sp.,* Bacillus anthracis, Borrelia recurrentis, Chlamydia *sp.,* Mycoplasma pneumoniae, *and* Rickettsiae*); adjunct to treat intestinal amebiasis; alternative to treat listeriosis caused by* Listeria monocytogenes, *syphilis caused by* Treponema pallidum, *and yaws caused by* Treponema pertenue *for nonpregnant patients allergic to penicillin*
I.V. INJECTION
Adults and adolescents. *Initial:* 200 mg. *Maintenance:* 100 mg q 12 hr. *Maximum:* 400 mg daily.
Children over age 8. *Initial:* 4 mg/kg. *Maintenance:* 2 mg/kg q 12 hr.
DOSAGE ADJUSTMENT If patient has renal impairment, don't exceed 200 mg daily.

Route	Onset	Peak	Duration
I.V.	Unknown	Unknown	6 to 12 hr

Incompatibilities
Don't mix minocycline in same syringe with solution that contains calcium because precipitate will form.

Mechanism of Action

Inhibits bacterial protein synthesis by competitively binding to the 30S ribosomal subunit of the mRNA-ribosome complex of certain organisms.

Contraindications

Hypersensitivity to minocycline, other tetracyclines, or their components

Interactions

DRUGS

aluminum-, calcium-, or magnesium-containing antacids; calcium supplements; choline and magnesium salicylates; iron-containing preparations; magnesium-containing laxatives; sodium bicarbonate: Possibly formation of nonabsorbable complex, impaired minocycline absorption
cholestyramine, colestipol: Possibly impaired cholestyramine or colestipol absorption
cimetidine: Possibly decreased GI absorption and effectiveness of minocycline
digoxin: Possibly increased blood digoxin level and risk of digitalis toxicity
ergot alkaloids and derivatives: Increased risk of ergotism
insulin: Possibly decreased need for insulin
iron salts: Possibly decreased GI absorption and antimicrobial effect of minocycline
lithium: Possibly altered blood lithium level
methoxyflurane: Increased risk of nephrotoxicity
oral anticoagulants: Possibly potentiated anticoagulant effects
oral contraceptives containing estrogen: Decreased contraceptive effectiveness, increased risk of breakthrough bleeding
penicillin: Interference with bactericidal action of penicillin
vitamin A: Possibly benign intracranial hypertension

Adverse Reactions

CNS: Dizziness, fever, headache, light-headedness, unsteadiness, vertigo
CV: Pericarditis
EENT: Blurred vision, darkened or discolored tongue, glossitis, papilledema, tooth discoloration, vision changes
GI: Abdominal cramps or pain, anorexia, diarrhea, dysphagia, enterocolitis, esophageal irritation and ulceration, hepatitis, hepatotoxicity, indigestion, nausea, pancreatitis, vomiting
GU: Genital candidiasis, nephrotoxicity

HEME: Eosinophilia, hemolytic anemia, neutropenia, thrombocytopenia, thrombocytopenic purpura
MS: Arthralgia, myopathy (transient)
RESP: Pulmonary infiltrates (with eosinophilia)
SKIN: Erythema multiforme, exfoliative dermatitis, brown pigmentation of skin and mucous membranes, erythematous and maculopapular rash, jaundice, onycholysis, photosensitivity, pruritus, purpura (anaphylactoid), Stevens-Johnson syndrome, urticaria
Other: Anaphylaxis, angioedema, serum sickness-like reaction, systemic lupus erythematosus exacerbation

Nursing Considerations

- Administer minocycline cautiously in patients who have renal or hepatic dysfunction and in patients who take other hepatotoxic drugs because minocycline may cause nephrotoxicity or hepatotoxicity.
- **WARNING** Notify prescriber if patient is breast-feeding because minocycline appears in breast milk and may have toxic effects.
- Monitor blood, renal, and hepatic tests before and during long-term therapy.
- To prepare drug for I.V. use, reconstitute each 100-mg vial with 5 to 10 ml of sterile water for injection. Further dilute in 500 to 1,000 ml of normal saline solution, D_5W, dextrose 5% in normal saline solution, or Ringer's or lactated Ringer's solution. Give final dilution immediately, but avoid giving it rapidly.
- Store reconstituted drug at room temperature and use within 24 hours.
- Assess patient for signs of superinfection; if they appear, notify prescriber, discontinue minocycline, and start appropriate therapy, as ordered.
- Monitor PT in patient who also takes an anticoagulant during minocycline therapy.

PATIENT TEACHING

- Instruct patient to notify prescriber if no improvement occurs in a few days.
- Advise patient to avoid prolonged exposure to sun or sunlamps during therapy.
- Counsel female patient to avoid becoming pregnant because minocycline should be avoided, if possible, during tooth development (last half of gestation up to age 8). Drug may permanently turn teeth yellow, gray, or brown and cause enamel hy-

poplasia. It also may slow skeletal growth and cause congenital anomalies, including limb reduction.

- Encourage patient who takes an oral contraceptive to use an additional method of contracepton during therapy with minocycline.
- Instruct patient to notify prescriber immediately about blurred vision, dizziness, headache, known or suspected pregnancy, and unsteadiness.

mitoxantrone hydrochloride

Novantrone

Class and Category

Chemical: Anthracenedione
Therapeutic: Antineoplastic
Pregnancy category: D

Indications and Dosages

▶ *To reduce neurologic disability and frequency of relapses in patients with secondary (chronic) progressive, progressive relapsing, or worsening relapsing-remitting multiple sclerosis (patients whose neurologic status is significantly abnormal between relapses)*

I.V. INFUSION

Adults. 12 mg/m^2 over 5 to 15 min q 3 mo. *Maximum:* Cumulative dose of 140 mg/m^2.

▶ *As adjunct to treat pain related to advanced hormone-refractory prostate cancer*

I.V. INFUSION

Adults. 12 to 14 mg/m^2 over 5 to 15 min q 21 days.

▶ *As adjunct to treat acute nonlymphocytic leukemia (ANLL)*

I.V. INFUSION

Adults. *Initial:* 12 mg/m^2 over at least 3 min on days 1 to 3 with 100 mg/m^2 of cytarabine as a continuous 24-hr infusion on days 1 to 7. If patient's antileukemic response is inadequate or incomplete, a second induction course is given at the same dosage. *Maintenance:* 6 wk after induction, 12 mg/m^2 over at least 3 min on days 1 and 2 with 100 mg/m^2 of cytarabine as a continuous 24-hr infusion on days 1 to 5. A second maintenance course is given 4 wk after the first if needed and tolerated.

Incompatibilities

Don't mix mitoxantrone in the same infusion as heparin (because a precipitate may form); don't mix with any other drugs.

Mechanism of Action

Binds to DNA, causing cross-linkage and strand breakage, interfering with RNA synthesis, and inhibiting topoisomerase II, an enzyme that uncoils and repairs damaged DNA. Mitoxantrone produces a cytocidal effect on proliferating and nonproliferating cells and doesn't appear to be cell-cycle specific. It's known to inhibit B-cell, T-cell, and macrophage proliferation and impair antigen function.

Contraindications

Hypersensitivity to mitoxantrone or its components

Interactions

DRUGS

allopurinol, colchicine, probenecid, sulfinpyrazone: Possibly interference with antihyperuricemic action of these drugs
blood-dyscrasia–causing drugs, such as cephalosporins and sulfasalazine: Increased risk of leukopenia and thrombocytopenia
bone marrow depressants, such as carboplatin and lomustine: Possibly additive bone marrow depression
daunorubicin, doxorubicin: Increased risk of cardiotoxicity
methotrexate and other antineoplastics: Risk of developing leukemia
vaccines, killed virus: Decreased antibody response to vaccine
vaccines, live virus: Increased risk of replication of and adverse effects of vaccine virus, decreased antibody response to vaccine

Adverse Reactions

CNS: Headache, seizures
CV: Arrhythmias, chest pain, congestive heart failure, decreased left ventricular ejection fraction, ECG changes
EENT: Blue-colored cornea, conjunctivitis, mucositis, stomatitis
GI: Abdominal pain, diarrhea, GI bleeding, nausea, vomiting
GU: Blue-green urine, renal failure
HEME: Acute myelogenous leukemia, leu-kopenia, other leukemias, thrombocytopenia
MS: Myelodysplasia
RESP: Cough, dyspnea
SKIN: Alopecia, extravasation, jaundice
Other: Allergic reaction, anaphylaxis, hyperuricemia, infection, infusion site pain or redness

Nursing Considerations

- Before and during therapy, expect patient to have an echocardiogram, ECG, and radionuclide angiography to evaluate cardiac status. Expect to obtain hematocrit, hemoglobin level, and CBC with platelet count.

- Be aware that drug shouldn't be given to patient with multiple sclerosis whose neutrophil count is less than $1{,}500/mm^3$.
- Obtain liver function test results, as ordered, before each course of therapy. Expect that drug won't be given to patient with multiple sclerosis and abnormal liver function.
- Anticipate obtaining pregnancy test before each course of therapy for women of childbearing age who have multiple sclerosis.
- Follow facility policy for handling antineoplastics. Be aware that manufacturer recommends goggles, gloves, and a gown during drug preparation and administration.
- Before infusing drug, dilute it in at least 50 ml of normal saline solution or D_5W.
- **WARNING** Be aware that drug shouldn't be given intrathecally because paralysis may occur.
- If mitoxantrone solution contacts your skin or mucosa, wash thoroughly with warm water. If it contacts your eyes, irrigate them thoroughly with water or normal saline solution.
- Discard unused diluted solution because it contains no preservatives. After penetration of the stopper, store undiluted drug for up to 7 days at room temperature or 14 days under refrigeration. Avoid freezing drug.
- If extravasation occurs, stop the infusion immediately and notify prescriber. Reinsert the I.V. line in another vein and resume the infusion. Although mitoxantrone is a nonvesicant, observe the extravasation site for signs of necrosis or phlebitis.
- Monitor patients with chickenpox or recent exposure to it and patients with herpes zoster for severe, generalized disease.
- Watch for evidence of cardiotoxicity, such as arrhythmias and chest pain, in patient with heart disease. Risk increases when cumulative dose reaches $140\ mg/m^2$ in cancer patient, $100\ mg/m^2$ in multiple sclerosis patient.
- Monitor blood uric acid level for hyperuricemia in patients with a history of gout or renal calculi. Expect to give allopurinol, as prescribed, to patients with leukemia or lymphoma who have elevated blood uric acid level to prevent uric acid nephropathy.
- **WARNING** If severe or life-threatening nonhematologic or hematologic toxicity occurs during the first induction course, expect to withhold the second course until it resolves.
- If patient develops thrombocytopenia, take precautions according to facility policy.

- Assess patient for evidence of infection, such as fever, if leukopenia occurs. Expect to obtain appropriate specimens for culture and sensitivity testing.
- Be aware that patients receiving mitoxantrone in combination with other antineoplastics or radiation therapy are at risk for developing secondary leukemia, including acute myelogenous leukemia.

PATIENT TEACHING

- Advise patient to complete dental work, if possible, before treatment begins or defer it until blood counts return to normal; drug may delay healing and cause gingival bleeding. Teach proper oral hygiene, and advise using a soft toothbrush.
- Urge patient to drink plenty of fluid to increase urine output and uric acid excretion.
- Advise patient to contact prescriber immediately if GI upset occurs, but to continue taking drug unless otherwise directed.
- Stress the importance of complying with the dosage regimen and keeping follow-up medical and laboratory appointments.
- Explain that urine may appear blue-green for 24 hours after treatment and that the whites of the eyes may appear blue. Stress that these effects are temporary and harmless. Explain that hair loss is possible, but that hair should return after therapy ends.
- Caution patient not to receive immunizations unless approved by prescriber. Also, advise persons who live in same household as patient to avoid receiving immunization with oral polio vaccine. Tell patient to avoid persons who recently received the oral polio vaccine or to wear a mask over his nose and mouth.
- Instruct patient to avoid persons with infections if bone marrow depression occurs. Advise patient to contact prescriber if fever, chills, cough, hoarseness, lower back or side pain, or painful or difficult urination occurs; these changes may signal an infection.
- Tell patient to contact prescriber immediately if he notices unusual bleeding or bruising, black or tarry stools, blood in urine or stool, or pinpoint red spots on his skin.
- Urge patient not to touch his eyes or inside his nose unless he has just washed his hands.
- Stress the need to avoid accidental cuts, as from a razor or fingernail clippers, because they may cause excessive bleeding or infection.
- Caution patient to avoid contact sports or activities that may cause bruising or injury.

morphine sulfate

Astramorph PF, Duramorph, Epimorph (CAN), Morphine Extra-Forte (CAN), Morphine Forte (CAN), Morphine H.P. (CAN)

Class, Category, and Schedule

Chemical: Phenanthrene derivative
Therapeutic: Analgesic
Pregnancy category: C
Controlled substance: Schedule II

Indications and Dosages

▶ *To relieve acute or chronic moderate to severe pain; as adjunct to treat pulmonary edema caused by left-sided heart failure; to supplement general, local, or regional anesthesia*

I.V. INFUSION

Adults. *Initial:* 15 mg (or more) followed by 0.8 to 10 mg/hr, increased as needed for effectiveness. *Maintenance:* 0.8 to 80 mg/hr.
Children. 0.01 to 0.04 mg/kg/hr postoperatively, 0.025 to 2.6 mg/kg/hr for severe chronic cancer pain, or 0.03 to 0.15 mg/kg/hr for sickle cell crisis.
Neonates. *Initial:* 0.010 mg/kg/hr (10 mcg/kg/hr) postoperatively. *Maintenance:* 0.015 to 0.02 mg/kg/hr (15 to 20 mcg/kg/hr).

I.V. INJECTION

Adults. 2.5 to 15 mg injected slowly.
Children. 0.5 to 0.1 mg/kg administered slowly.

▶ *To relieve MI pain*

I.V. INJECTION

Adults. 1 to 4 mg by slow I.V. injection. Repeated up to q 5 min, if needed. *Maximum:* 2 to 15 mg.

Route	Onset	Peak	Duration
I.V.	Unknown	20 min	4 to 5 hr

Mechanism of Action

Binds with and activates opioid receptors (mainly mu receptors) in brain and spinal cord to produce analgesia and euphoria.

Contraindications

Acute alcoholism, alcohol withdrawal syndrome, arrhythmias, asthma, brain tumor, heart failure caused by chronic lung disease, hypersensitivity to morphine or its components, labor (premature delivery), prematurity (in infants), respiratory depression, seizure disorders, upper airway obstruction.

Interactions

DRUGS

amitriptyline, clomipramine, nortriptyline: Increased CNS and respiratory depression
anticholinergics: Possibly severe constipation leading to ileus, urine retention
antidiarrheals, such as loperamide and paregoric: CNS depression, possibly severe constipation
antihistamines, chloral hydrate, glutethimide, MAO inhibitors, methocarbamol: Increased CNS and respiratory depressant effects of morphine
antihypertensives, hypotension-producing drugs: Increased hypotension, risk of orthostatic hypotension
buprenorphine: Decreased therapeutic effects of morphine, increased respiratory depression, possibly withdrawal symptoms
cimetidine: Increased analgesic and CNS and respiratory depressant effects of morphine
CNS depressants (antiemetics, general anesthetics, hypnotics, phenothiazines, sedatives, tranquilizers): Possibly coma, hypotension, respiratory depression, severe sedation
diuretics: Decreased diuretic efficacy
hydroxyzine: Increased analgesic, CNS depressant, and hypotensive effects of morphine
metoclopramide: Possibly antagonized metoclopramide effect on GI motility
mixed agonist-antagonist analgesics: Possibly withdrawal symptoms
naloxone: Antagonized analgesic and CNS and respiratory depressant effects of morphine, possibly withdrawal symptoms
naltrexone: Possibly induction or worsening of withdrawal symptoms if morphine given within 7 to 10 days before naltrexone
neuromuscular blockers: Increased or prolonged respiratory depression
opioid analgesics, such as alfentanil and sufentanil: Increased CNS and respiratory depression, increased hypotension
OTC preparations containing alcohol: Increased CNS and respiratory depression and hypotension
zidovudine: Decreased zidovudine clearance

ACTIVITIES

alcohol use: Increased CNS and respiratory depression, increased hypotension

Adverse Reactions

CNS: Amnesia, anxiety, coma, confusion, decreased concentration, delirium, delusions, depression, dizziness, drowsiness, euphoria, fever, hallucinations, headache, insomnia, lethargy, lightheadedness, malaise, psychosis, restlessness, sedation, seizures, syncope, tremor

CV: Bradycardia, cardiac arrest, hypotension, orthostatic hypotension, palpitations, shock, tachycardia

EENT: Blurred vision, diplopia, dry mouth, laryngeal edema or laryngospasm (allergic), miosis, nystagmus, rhinitis

GI: Abdominal cramps or pain, anorexia, biliary tract spasm, constipation, diarrhea, dysphagia, elevated liver function test results, gastroesophageal reflux, hiccups, ileus and toxic megacolon (in patients with inflammatory bowel disease), intestinal obstruction, indigestion, nausea, vomiting

GU: Decreased ejaculate potency, decreased libido, difficult ejaculation, impotence, menstrual irregularities, oliguria, prolonged labor, urinary hesitancy, urine retention

HEME: Anemia, leukopenia, thrombocytopenia

MS: Arthralgia

RESP: Apnea, asthma exacerbation, atelectasis, bronchospasm, depressed cough reflex, hypoventilation, pulmonary edema, respiratory arrest and depression, wheezing

SKIN: Diaphoresis, flushing, pallor, pruritus, urticaria

Other: Allergic reaction; anaphylaxis; facial edema; injection site edema, pain, rash, or redness; physical and psychological dependence; withdrawal symptoms

Nursing Considerations

- Store morphine sulfate at room temperature.
- Before giving morphine, make sure opioid antagonist and equipment for giving oxygen and controlling respiration are available.
- Before therapy, assess patient's drug use, including all prescription and OTC drugs.
- Discard injection solution that is discolored or darker than pale yellow or that contains precipitates that don't dissolve with shaking.
- **WARNING** Don't use highly concentrated morphine solutions (such as 10 to 25 mg/ml) for single-dose I.V. administration. These solutions are intended for use in continuous, controlled microinfusion devices.

- For direct I.V. injection, dilute appropriate dose with 4 to 5 ml of sterile water for injection. Inject 2.5 to 15 mg directly into tubing of free-flowing I.V. solution over 4 to 5 minutes. Rapid I.V. injection may increase adverse reactions.
- For continuous I.V. infusion, dilute drug in D_5W and administer with infusion-control device. Adjust dose and rate based on patient response, as prescribed.
- **WARNING** Monitor respiratory and cardiovascular status carefully and frequently during morphine therapy. Be alert for respiratory depression and hypotension.
- Monitor patient for excessive or persistent sedation; dosage may need to be adjusted.
- If patient is receiving a continuous morphine infusion, watch for and notify prescriber about new neurologic signs or symptoms. Inflammatory masses (such as granulomas) have caused serious neurologic reactions, including paralysis.
- Expect morphine to cause physical and psychological dependence; watch for drug tolerance and withdrawal symptoms, such as body aches, diaphoresis, diarrhea, fever, piloerection, rhinorrhea, sneezing, and yawning.
- If tolerance to morphine develops, expect prescriber to increase dosage.
- Morphine may have a prolonged duration and cumulative effect in patients with impaired hepatic or renal function. It also may prolong labor by reducing strength, duration, and frequency of uterine contractions.
- When discontinuing morphine in patients receiving more than 30 mg daily, expect prescriber to reduce daily dose by about one-half for 2 days and then by 25% every 2 days thereafter until total dose reaches initial amount recommended for patients who haven't received opioids (15 to 30 mg daily). This regimen minimizes the risk of withdrawal symptoms.

PATIENT TEACHING

- Urge patient to avoid alcohol including OTC preparations containing alcohol and other CNS depressants during morphine therapy.
- Advise patient to avoid potentially hazardous activities during morphine therapy.
- Tell patient to change positions slowly to minimize the effects of orthostatic hypotension.
- Instruct patient to notify prescriber about worsening or breakthrough pain.

- Inform patient that morphine may be habit-forming. Urge him to notify prescriber if he experiences anxiety, decreased appetite, excessive tearing, irritability, muscle aches or twitching, rapid heart rate, or yawning.
- Advise female patient to notify prescriber if she becomes pregnant. Regular morphine use during pregnancy may cause physical dependence in fetus and withdrawal in neonate.

moxifloxacin hydrochloride

Avelox, Avelox IV

Class and Category

Chemical: Fluoroquinolone
Therapeutic: Antibiotic
Pregnancy category: C

Indications and Dosages

▶ *To treat acute sinusitis caused by* Haemophilus influenzae, Moraxella catarrhalis, *or* Streptococcus pneumoniae; *to treat mild to moderate community-acquired pneumonia caused by* Chlamydia pneumoniae, H. influenzae, M. catarrhalis, Mycoplasma pneumoniae, *or* S. pneumoniae *(including penicillin- or multi-drug–resistant strains)*

I.V. INFUSION

Adults. 400 mg q 24 hr for 10 days.

▶ *To treat acute exacerbation of chronic bronchitis caused by* H. influenzae, H. parainfluenzae, Klebsiella pneumoniae, M. catarrhalis, S. pneumoniae, *or* Staphylococcus aureus

I.V. INFUSION

Adults. 400 mg q 24 hr for 5 days.

▶ *To treat uncomplicated skin and soft-tissue infections caused by* S. aureus *or* Streptococcus pyogenes

I.V. INFUSION

Adults. 400 mg q 24 hr for 7 days.

▶ *To treat complicated skin and skin structure infections caused by* S. aureus, E. coli, K. pneumoniae, *or* Enterobacter cloacae

I.V. INFUSION

Adults. 400 mg q 24 hr for 7 to 21 days.

▶ *To treat complicated intra-abdominal infections, including polymicrobial infections such as abscesses caused by* E. coli, Bacteroides fragilis, Streptococcus anginosus, Streptococcus constellatus, Enterococcus faecalis, Proteus mirabilis, Clostridium perfringens,

Bacteroides thetaiotaomicron, *or* Peptostreptococcus *sp.*
I.V. INFUSION
Adults. 400 mg q 24 hr for 5 to 14 days with initial dosage given as I.V. infusion.

Mechanism of Action

Inhibits synthesis of the bacterial enzyme DNA gyrase by counteracting the excessive supercoiling of DNA during replication or transcription. Inhibition of DNA gyrase causes rapid- and slow-growing bacterial cells to die.

Incompatibilities

Do not infuse I.V. form of moxifloxacin simultaneously through the same I.V. line with other I.V. substances, additives, or drugs.

Contraindications

Hypersensitivity to moxifloxacin, other fluoroquinolones, or their components

Interactions

DRUGS

aluminum- or magnesium-containing antacids; drug formulations with divalent or trivalent cations, such as didanosine chewable buffered tablets or powder for oral solution; metal cations, such as iron; multivitamins containing iron or zinc; sucralfate: Possibly substantial interference with moxifloxacin absorption, causing low blood moxifloxacin level

class Ia antiarrhythmics, such as quinidine; class III antiarrhythmics, such as sotalol; other drugs known to prolong QTc interval, such as disopyramide and pentamidine: Possibly prolonged QTc interval

corticosteroids: Increased risk of Achilles and other tendon ruptures

NSAIDs: Increased risk of CNS stimulation and seizures

warfarin: Possibly increased anticoagulation

Adverse Reactions

CNS: Dizziness, headache, psychosis, psychotic reaction, seizures, syncope

CV: Hypertension, hypotension, palpitations, peripheral edema, tachycardia, vasodilation, ventricular tachyarrhythmias

EENT: Altered taste

GI: Abdominal pain, abnormal liver function test results,

cholestatic hepatitis, diarrhea, dyspepsia, hepatitis, nausea, pseudomembranous colitis, vomiting
HEME: Anemia, eosinophilia, leukopenia, prolonged PT, thrombocytopenia
MS: Tendon inflammation, pain, or rupture
Skin: Stevens-Johnson syndrome
Other: Anaphylaxis, anaphylactic shock, angioedema

Nursing Considerations

- Obtain a fluid or tissue specimen for culture and sensitivity, as ordered. Expect to begin therapy before results are available.
- **WARNING** Before starting therapy, determine if patient receives a class Ia antiarrhythmic, such as quinidine; a class III antiarrhythmic, such as sotalol; or other drugs that prolong the QTc interval. Be aware that these drugs should be avoided in patients taking moxifloxacin because they may prolong the QTc interval and lead to life-threatening ventricular tachycardia or torsades de pointes.
- Infuse over 60 minutes with ready-to-use flexible bags with 400 mg of moxifloxacin in 250 ml of 0.8% saline. Don't dilute further.
- If giving through Y-type tubing or piggyback method, stop other solutions during moxifloxacin infusion, and flush the line before and after infusion with a compatible solution, such as normal saline solution, 1M sodium chloride, 5% dextrose, sterile water for injection, 10% dextrose, or lactated Ringer's. Also flush line before and after giving other drugs in the same I.V. line.
- Don't refrigerate I.V. moxifloxacin ready-to-use bags because precipitation will occur. Discard any unused portion; premixed bags are for single-use only.
- Expect to obtain a 12-lead ECG to assess patient for a prolonged QTc interval. Ask patient if he or a blood relative has a history of prolonged QTc interval.
- If patient has hypokalemia, expect to correct it before beginning moxifloxacin therapy to prevent arrhythmias.
- Determine if patient has a history of a CNS disorder, such as cerebral arteriosclerosis or epilepsy, because drug may lower the seizure threshold. Notify prescriber before therapy starts, and take seizure precautions.
- If profuse, watery diarrhea develops, contact prescriber and expect to obtain a stool specimen to rule out pseudomembranous colitis.

- Monitor serum potassium level, as ordered, during therapy to assess for hypokalemia.
- Keep emergency resuscitation equipment readily available, and observe for evidence of hypersensitivity, such as angioedema, dyspnea, and urticaria. If you suspect anaphylaxis, prepare to give epinephrine, corticosteroids, and diphenhydramine, as prescribed.

PATIENT TEACHING

- Advise patient to notify prescriber immediately about palpitations or fainting because they may indicate a serious arrhythmia.
- Urge patient to drink plenty of fluids while receiving moxifloxacin.
- Caution patient to stop taking drug and notify prescriber if he experiences difficulty breathing, a rash, or other signs of an allergic reaction.
- Urge patient to stop any exercise and contact prescriber immediately if he develops tendon inflammation, pain, or rupture.
- Caution patient to avoid activities of mental alertness until adverse CNS effects are known.
- Urge patient to tell prescriber about diarrhea.
- Caution patient to complete the prescribed course of therapy even if he feels better.

N·O

nafcillin sodium

Nafcil, Nallpen, Unipen

Class and Category

Chemical: Penicillin
Therapeutic: Antibiotic
Pregnancy category: B

Indications and Dosages

▶ *To treat infections caused by penicillinase-producing* Staphylococcus aureus

I.V. INFUSION

Adults and adolescents. 500 to 1,500 mg q 4 hr. *Maximum:* 20,000 mg daily.

Children from birth to age 12. 10 to 20 mg/kg q 4 hr, or 20 to 40 mg/kg q 8 hr.

▶ *To treat bone and joint infections, endocarditis, meningitis, and pericarditis caused by susceptible organisms*

I.V. INFUSION

Adults and adolescents. 1,500 to 2,000 mg q 4 to 6 hr. *Maximum:* 20,000 mg daily.

I.V. INFUSION

Children from birth to age 12. 10 to 20 mg/kg q 4 hr or 20 to 40 mg/kg q 8 hr. For meningitis in neonates weighing up to 2 kg (4.4 lb), 25 to 50 mg/kg q 12 hr for first week after birth and then 50 mg/kg q 8 hr. For neonates weighing 2 kg or more, 50 mg/kg q 8 hr during first week after birth and then 50 mg/kg q 6 hr.

Incompatibilities

Don't mix nafcillin in same I.V. bag as aminoglycosides; they're chemically incompatible.

Contraindications

Hypersensitivity to nafcillin, other penicillins, their components, or to corn or corn-containing products

Mechanism of Action

Binds to certain penicillin-binding proteins in bacterial cell walls, thereby inhibiting the final stage of bacterial cell wall synthesis. The result is cell lysis. Nafcillin's action is bolstered by its chemical composition; its unique side chain resists destruction by beta-lactamases.

Interactions

DRUGS

aminoglycosides: Substantial mutual inactivation
chloramphenicol, erythromycins, sulfonamides, tetracyclines: Possibly decreased therapeutic effects of nafcillin
hepatotoxic drugs: Increased risk of hepatotoxicity
methotrexate: Increased risk of methotrexate toxicity
probenecid: Increased blood nafcillin level

FOODS

all foods: Decreased nafcillin absorption

Adverse Reactions

CNS: Depression, headache, seizures
EENT: Oral candidiasis
GI: Abdominal pain, diarrhea, nausea, pseudomembranous colitis, vomiting
GU: Vaginitis
HEME: Leukopenia, neutropenia
SKIN: Exfoliative dermatitis, pruritus, rash, urticaria
Other: Anaphylaxis; hypokalemia; injection site pain, redness, and swelling; serum sickness–like reaction

Nursing Considerations

- Obtain body fluid or tissue samples for culture and sensitivity testing, as prescribed, and obtain test results, if possible, before giving nafcillin, as ordered.
- For intermittent I.V. infusion, infuse over 30 to 60 minutes.
- Give nafcillin at least 1 hour before or after aminoglycosides, especially if patient has renal disease.
- When giving nafcillin to patient at risk for hypertension or fluid overload, be aware that each gram contains 2.5 mEq of sodium.
- **WARNING** Avoid giving nafcillin to premature neonate if drug was reconstituted with bacteriostatic water that contains benzyl alcohol. Doing so can cause potentially fatal metabolic

acidosis and circulatory, CNS, renal, and respiratory dysfunction.
- Monitor serum nafcillin levels closely in children, as ordered, because the liver and biliary tract, principal routes of nafcillin elimination, function immaturely in children.
- Monitor for signs of superinfection, such as oral candidiasis and pseudomembranous colitis, especially in elderly, immunocompromised, or debilitated patients who receive large doses of nafcillin.

PATIENT TEACHING
- Advise patient to notify prescriber if she experiences chills, fever, GI distress, or rash.

nalbuphine hydrochloride

Nubain

Class and Category

Chemical: Phenanthrene derivative
Therapeutic: Analgesic, anesthesia adjunct
Pregnancy category: B

Indications and Dosages

▶ *To relieve moderate to severe pain*

I.V. INJECTION

Adults weighing 70 kg (154 lb). 10 mg q 3 to 6 hr, p.r.n. Dosage adjusted for patients weighing more or less.

▶ *As adjunct to anesthesia*

I.V. INJECTION

Adults. 0.3 to 3 mg/kg over 10 to 15 min followed by 0.25 to 0.5 mg/kg, as needed.

DOSAGE ADJUSTMENT For patients who have repeatedly received an opioid agonist, initial dose possibly reduced to 25% of usual dosage. For patients in whom tolerance to drug's effects hasn't developed, maximum usually is 20 mg/dose or 160 mg daily.

Route	Onset	Peak	Duration
I.V.	2 to 3 min	30 min	3 to 4 hr

Incompatibilities

Don't administer nalbuphine with diazepam or pentobarbital. Use separate I.V. line or flush line well before and after administration.

Mechanism of Action

Binds with and stimulates mu and kappa opiate receptors in the spinal cord and higher levels in the CNS. In this way, nalbuphine alters the perception of and emotional response to pain.

Contraindications

Hypersensitivity to nalbuphine or its components

Interactions

DRUGS

alfentanil, CNS depressants, fentanyl, sufentanil: Increased risk of hypotension and CNS and respiratory depression
anticholinergics: Increased risk of severe constipation and urine retention
antidiarrheals, such as difenoxin and atropine, loperamide, and paregoric: Increased risk of severe constipation and increased CNS depression
antihypertensives: Increased risk of hypotension
buprenorphine: Possibly decreased therapeutic effects of nalbuphine and increased risk of respiratory depression
hydroxyzine: Increased risk of CNS depression and hypotension
MAO inhibitors: Risk of possibly fatal increased CNS excitation or depression
metoclopramide: Possibly antagonized effects of metoclopramide
naloxone, naltrexone: Decreased pharmacologic effects of nalbuphine
neuromuscular blockers: Increased risk of prolonged CNS and respiratory depression

ACTIVITIES

alcohol use: Increased risk of coma, hypotension, profound sedation, and respiratory depression

Adverse Reactions

CNS: Anxiety, confusion, decreased or loss of consciousness, depression, dizziness, euphoria, fatigue, fever, hallucinations, headache, nervousness, restlessness, seizures, somnolence, syncope, tiredness, tremor, weakness
CV: Bradycardia, cardiac arrest, edema, hypertension, hypotension, tachycardia

EENT: Blurred vision, diplopia, dry mouth, laryngeal edema, stridor
GI: Abdominal cramps, anorexia, constipation, nausea, vomiting
GU: Decreased urine output, ureteral spasm
RESP: Dyspnea, pulmonary edema, respiratory depression, wheezing
SKIN: Diaphoresis, flushing, pruritus, rash, sensation of warmth, urticaria
Other: Anaphylaxis, injection site burning, pain, redness, swelling, and warmth

Nursing Considerations

- Use nalbuphine cautiously in patients taking other drugs that can cause respiratory depression.
- Be aware that nalbuphine is not recommended for use during labor and delivery because placental transfer of nalbuphine is high, increasing risk of fetal mortality or permanent fetal neurological damage.
- Keep resuscitation equipment and naloxone readily available to reverse nalbuphine's effects, if needed.
- For direct I.V. injection through an I.V. line with a compatible infusing solution, give drug slowly—no more than 10 mg over 3 to 5 minutes. Inject into free-flowing normal saline solution, D_5W, or lactated Ringer's solution.
- During prolonged use, expect to give a stool softener to minimize constipation.
- If patient is opioid-dependent, expect drug to cause withdrawal symptoms, such as abdominal cramps, anorexia, anxiety, backache, bone or joint pain, confusion, depression, diaphoresis, dysphoria, erythema, fear, fever, irritability, labile blood pressure and pulse, lacrimation, muscle spasms, myalgia, mydriasis, nasal congestion, nausea, opioid craving, piloerection, restlessness, rhinorrhea, sensation of crawling skin, sleep disturbances, tremor, uneasiness, vomiting, and yawning.
- **WARNING** Be aware that drug may obscure neurologic assessment findings if patient has a cerebral aneurysm, head injury, or increased intracranial pressure.

PATIENT TEACHING

- Advise patient to avoid potentially hazardous activities until nalbuphine's CNS effects are known.
- Counsel patient against making important decisions while receiving drug because it may cloud her judgment.

nalmefene hydrochloride

Revex

Class and Category

Chemical: 6-Methylene analogue of naltrexone
Therapeutic: Opioid antagonist
Pregnancy category: B

Indications and Dosages

▶ *To treat known or suspected opioid overdose*

I.V. INJECTION

Adults. 500 mcg/70 kg (154 lb) of body weight, followed by second dose of 1,000 mcg/70 kg in 2 to 5 min, as indicated. *Maximum:* 1,500 mcg/70 kg.

▶ *To treat postoperative opioid-induced respiratory depression*

I.V. INJECTION

Adults. *Initial:* 0.25 mcg/kg q 2 to 5 min until desired degree of reversal is achieved. *Maximum:* 1 mcg/kg.

DOSAGE ADJUSTMENT Initial and subsequent doses possibly reduced to 0.1 mcg/kg for patients at increased risk for CV complications.

Route	Onset	Peak	Duration
I.V.	2 to 5 min	Unknown	30 to 60 min*

Mechanism of Action

Antagonizes mu, kappa, and sigma opioid receptors in the CNS, thus reversing the analgesia, hypotension, respiratory depression, and sedation caused by most opioids. Mu receptors are responsible for analgesia, euphoria, miosis, and respiratory depression. Kappa receptors are responsible for analgesia and sedation. Sigma receptors control dysphoria and other delusional states.

Contraindications

Hypersensitivity to nalmefene or its components

Interactions

DRUGS

opioid analgesics (including alfentanil, fentanyl, and sufentanil): Reversal of these drugs' analgesic and adverse effects, possibly withdrawal symptoms in opioid-dependent patients

* For partial reversal of opioid effects; up to several hr for full reversal.

Adverse Reactions

CNS: Agitation, chills, confusion, depression, dizziness, fever, hallucinations, headache, nervousness, somnolence, tremor
CV: Arrhythmias, hypertension, hypotension, tachycardia, vasodilation
EENT: Dry mouth, pharyngitis
GI: Diarrhea, nausea, vomiting
GU: Urine retention
SKIN: Pruritus
Other: Withdrawal symptoms

Nursing Considerations

- **WARNING** Read the label carefully before administering nalmefene because drug comes in concentrations of 100 mcg/ml and 1 mg/ml.
- Monitor patients with hepatic or renal dysfunction for signs of increased nalmefene effects because drug is metabolized by liver and excreted by kidneys.
- Monitor heart rate, respiratory rate, and blood pressure to detect CV complications. Patients who have received a cardiotoxic drug and those with cardiac disease are at increased risk.
- Continue to monitor patient after nalmefene administration because symptoms of opioid toxicity may return if opioid's duration of action is longer than that of nalmefene.
- **WARNING** Monitor for withdrawal symptoms, especially in opioid-dependent patients. Symptoms include abdominal cramps, anorexia, anxiety, backache, bone or joint pain, confusion, depression, diaphoresis, dysphoria, erythema, fear, fever, irritability, labile blood pressure and pulse, lacrimation, muscle spasms, myalgia, mydriasis, nasal congestion, nausea, opioid craving, piloerection, restlessness, rhinorrhea, sensation of crawling skin, sleep disturbances, tremor, uneasiness, vomiting, and yawning.
- Be prepared to provide mechanical or assisted ventilation if reversal of opioid-induced respiratory depression is incomplete.
- Store drug at 15° to 30° C (59° to 86° F).

PATIENT TEACHING

- Inform patient or family members that nalmefene is administered to reverse opioid-induced adverse reactions.
- Urge opioid-dependent patient to seek drug rehabilitation.

naloxone hydrochloride

Narcan

Class and Category

Chemical: Thebaine derivative
Therapeutic: Opioid antagonist
Pregnancy category: B

Indications and Dosages

▶ *To treat known or suspected opioid overdose*

I.V. INJECTION

Adults, children age 5 and over, and children under age 5 weighing more than 20 kg (44 lb). 0.4 to 2 mg repeated q 2 to 3 min, p.r.n. If no response after 10 mg, patient may not have narcotic-induced respiratory depression.

Infants and children under age 5 weighing less than 20 kg. 0.01 mg/kg as a single dose; if no improvement, another 0.1 mg/kg, as prescribed. Alternatively, 0.1 mg/kg repeated q 2 to 3 min, as needed.

I.V. INJECTION

Neonates. 0.01 mg/kg repeated q 2 to 3 min, as prescribed, until desired response occurs. Alternatively, initial dose of 0.1 mg/kg.

▶ *To treat postoperative opioid-induced respiratory depression*

I.V. INJECTION

Adults and adolescents. *Initial:* 0.1 to 0.2 mg q 2 to 3 min until desired response occurs. Additional doses given q 1 to 2 hr, if needed, based on patient response.

Children. *Initial:* 0.005 to 0.01 mg q 2 to 3 min until desired response occurs. Additional doses given q 1 to 2 hr, if needed, based on patient response.

▶ *To reverse opioid-induced asphyxia*

I.V. INJECTION

Neonates. *Initial:* 0.01 mg/kg q 2 to 3 min until desired response occurs. Additional doses given q 1 to 2 hr, if needed, based on patient response.

▶ *As adjunct to treat hypotension caused by septic shock*

I.V. INFUSION OR INJECTION

Adults. 0.03 to 0.2 mg/kg over 5 min, followed by continuous infusion of 0.03 to 0.3 mg/kg/hr for 1 to 24 hr, as needed, based on patient response.

Route	Onset	Peak	Duration
I.V.	1 to 2 min	5 to 15 min	45 min or longer

Mechanism of Action

Briefly and competitively antagonizes mu, kappa, and sigma opioid receptors in the CNS, thus reversing the analgesia, hypotension, respiratory depression, and sedation caused by most opioids. Mu receptors are responsible for analgesia, euphoria, miosis, and respiratory depression. Kappa receptors are responsible for analgesia and sedation. Sigma receptors control dysphoria and other delusional states.

Incompatibilities

Don't mix naloxone with any other solution unless you verify that drugs are compatible; drug is incompatible with alkaline, bisulfite, and metabisulfite solutions.

Contraindications

Hypersensitivity to naloxone or its components

Interactions

DRUGS

butorphanol, nalbuphine, pentazocine: Reversal of these drugs' analgesic and adverse effects
opioid analgesics: Reversal of these drugs' analgesic and adverse effects, possibly withdrawal symptoms in opioid-dependent patients

Adverse Reactions

CNS: Excitement, irritability, nervousness, restlessness, seizures, tremor, violent behavior
CV: Hypertension (severe), hypotension, ventricular fibrillation, ventricular tachycardia
GI: Nausea, vomiting
RESP: Pulmonary edema
SKIN: Diaphoresis
Other: Withdrawal symptoms

Nursing Considerations

- Keep resuscitation equipment readily available during naloxone administration.
- If needed, dilute naloxone with sterile water before administering I.V. injection. To prepare a continuous infusion, add 2 mg of naloxone to 500 ml of normal saline solution or D_5W to yield 4 mcg/ml. Use within 24 hours.
- Give repeat doses as prescribed, depending on patient's response. Continue to monitor patient after naloxone administra-

tion because symptoms of opioid toxicity may return if opioid's duration of action is longer than that of naloxone.
- Be aware that rapid reversal of opioid effects can cause diaphoresis, nausea, and vomiting.
- **WARNING** Monitor for withdrawal symptoms, especially in opioid-dependent patients. Symptoms may include abdominal cramps, anorexia, anxiety, backache, bone or joint pain, confusion, depression, diaphoresis, dysphoria, erythema, fear, fever, irritability, labile blood pressure and pulse, lacrimation, muscle spasms, myalgia, mydriasis, nasal congestion, nausea, opioid craving, piloerection, restlessness, rhinorrhea, sensation of crawling skin, sleep disturbances, tremor, uneasiness, vomiting, and yawning.
- Monitor cardiac and respiratory status of patients with a history of CV or pulmonary disease for signs of exacerbation.
- Expect patient with hepatic or renal dysfunction to have increased circulating blood naloxone level.
- Store naloxone at 15° to 30° C (59° to 86° F); protect from freezing and light.

PATIENT TEACHING
- Inform patient or family that naloxone is administered to reverse opioid-induced adverse reactions.
- Urge opioid-dependent patient to seek drug rehabilitation services.

natalizumab

Tysabri

Class and Category

Chemical: Recombinant humanized IgG4k monoclonal antibody
Therapeutic: Immune modulator
Pregnancy category: C

Indications and Dosages

▶ *To delay physical disability and reduce the frequency of exacerbations in relapsing forms of multiple sclerosis*

I.V. INFUSION
Adults. 300 mg q 4 wk.

Route	Onset	Peak	Duration
I.V.	Unknown	24 wk	Unknown

Mechanism of Action

Inhibits migration of leukocytes out of the vascular space, increasing the number of circulating leukocytes, by binding to select integrins on the surface of all leukocytes except neutrophils. Also inhibits adhesion of leukocytes to their counter-receptors. In multiple sclerosis, lesions are believed to occur when activated inflammatory cells, including T-lymphocytes, cross the blood-brain barrier.

Contraindications

History or presence of progressive multifocal leukoencephalopathy (PML), hypersensitivity to natalizumab or its components

Interactions

DRUGS

immunosuppressants, immunomodulating agents, other antineoplastics: Increased risk of infection

Adverse Reactions

CNS: Depression, dizziness, fatigue, headache, PML, rigors, somnolence, suicidal ideation, vertigo
CV: Chest discomfort, peripheral edema
EENT: Tonsillitis, tooth infections
GI: Abdominal discomfort, abnormal liver function test results, cholelithiasis, diarrhea, gastroenteritis
GU: Amenorrhea, dysmenorrhea, irregular menstruation, ovarian cyst, UTI, urinary incontinence, urinary frequency or urgency, vaginitis
MS: Arthralgia, extremity pain, joint swelling, muscle cramps
RESP: Pneumonia
SKIN: Dermatitis, night sweats, pruritus, rash, urticaria
Other: Acute hypersensitivity reaction, anaphylaxis, antibody formation, herpes, weight gain or loss

Nursing Considerations

- Determine that patient has enrolled in the TOUCH Prescribing Program before administering natalizumab. Once patient's signature and initials have been obtained on the TOUCH program enrollment form, place the original signed form in the patient's medical record, send a copy to Biogen Idec, and give a copy to the patient.

- Be aware that all serious opportunistic and atypical infections need to be reported to Biogen Idec at 1-800-456-2255 and to the FDA MedWatch Program at 1-800-FDA-1088.
- Make sure that patient has had a brain MRI before starting natalizumab therapy to help distinguish evidence of multiple sclerosis from PML if they arise after therapy has begun.
- Dilute natalizumab concentrate 300 mg/15 ml in 100 ml of normal saline solution. Gently invert the solution to mix completely. Do not shake.
- Following dilution, infuse drug immediately over 1 hour. After infusion, flush line with normal saline solution injection.
- Do not administer as an I.V. push or bolus injection.
- If administration is delayed after dilution, refrigerate drug and use within 8 hours.
- Observe patient during and for 1 hour after infusion for evidence of a hypersensitivity reaction. If present, notify prescriber, expect to withhold drug, and provide supportive care.
- **WARNING** Monitor patient closely for evidence of PML because natalizumab increases the risk of this opportunistic viral brain infection. PML can lead to severe disability or death. If any unexplained neurological signs and symptoms occur, notify prescriber, withhold natalizumab, and prepare patient for a gadolinium-enhanced MRI of the brain and possible cerebrospinal fluid analysis, as ordered.
- Know that the patient should be reevaluated 3 months after the first infusion, 6 months after the first infusion, and every 6 months thereafter.
- Assess patient for signs of infection, such as fever, if leukopenia develops. Expect to obtain appropriate specimens for culture and sensitivity testing.

PATIENT TEACHING

- Explain the benefits and risks of natalizumab therapy, and provide patient with medication guide.
- Encourage patient to ask questions before signing the enrollment form.
- Emphasize importance of reporting any symptoms that persist or worsen over several days to the prescriber.
- Tell patient to inform all physicians that he is receiving natalizumab therapy.
- Stress importance of follow-up visits 3 months after the first infusion, 6 months after the first infusion, and at least every 6 months thereafter.

- Instruct patient to report signs and symptoms of an allergic reaction, such as urticaria, dizziness, fever, rash, rigors, pruritus, nausea, flushing, hypotension, dyspnea, and chest pain.
- Instruct patient to avoid people with infections. Advise him to report fever, cough, lower back or side pain, or other unexplained signs and symptoms. They may indicate infection.

neostigmine methylsulfate

Prostigmin

Class and Category

Chemical: Quaternary ammonium compound
Therapeutic: Anticholinesterase, curare antidote
Pregnancy category: C

Indications and Dosages

▶ *To reverse nondepolarizing neuromuscular blockade*

I.V. INJECTION

Adults. 0.5 to 2 mg by slow push, repeated as needed up to 5 mg; 0.6 to 1.2 mg of atropine or 0.2 to 0.6 mg of glycopyrrolate is given with or a few minutes before neostigmine, as ordered.
Children. 0.04 mg/kg by slow push; 0.02 mg/kg of atropine is given I.M. or S.C. with each dose or with alternate doses.

Route	Onset	Peak	Duration
I.V.	4 to 8 min	30 min	2 to 4 hr

Mechanism of Action

Inhibits the action of cholinesterase, an enzyme that destroys acetylcholine at myoneuronal junctions, thereby increasing acetylcholine accumulation at myoneuronal junctions and facilitating nerve impulse transmission. This action reverses the effects of nondepolarizing neuromuscular blockers.

Contraindications

Hypersensitivity to neostigmine, other anticholinesterases, bromides, or their components; mechanical obstruction of intestinal or urinary tract; peritonitis

Interactions

DRUGS

aminoglycosides, anesthetics, capreomycin, colistimethate, colistin, lido-

caine, lincomycins, polymyxin B, quinine: Increased risk of neuromuscular blockade
anticholinergics: Possibly masked signs of cholinergic crisis
guanadrel, guanethidine, mecamylamine, trimethaphan: Possibly antagonized effects of neostigmine, possibly decreased antihypertensive effects
neuromuscular blockers: Possibly prolonged action of depolarizing—and antagonized action of nondepolarizing—neuromuscular blockers
procainamide, quinidine: Possibly antagonized effects of neostigmine
quinine: Decreased neostigmine effectiveness

Adverse Reactions

CNS: Dizziness, drowsiness, headache, seizures, syncope, weakness
CV: Arrhythmias (AV block, bradycardia, nodal rhythm, tachycardia), cardiac arrest, ECG changes, hypotension
EENT: Increased salivation, lacrimation, miosis, vision changes
GI: Abdominal cramps, diarrhea, flatulence, increased peristalsis, nausea, vomiting
GU: Urinary frequency
MS: Arthralgia, dysarthria, muscle spasms
RESP: Bronchospasm, dyspnea, increased bronchial secretions, respiratory arrest or depression
SKIN: Flushing, diaphoresis, rash, urticaria

Nursing Considerations

- If also giving atropine, be sure to administer it with or before neostigmine, as prescribed.
- Make sure patient is well ventilated and airway remains patent until normal respiration is assured.
- **WARNING Monitor for signs of neostigmine overdose, which can cause life-threatening cholinergic crisis (increased muscle weakness, including respiratory muscles). Expect to stop neostigmine and atropine, as ordered.**
- Be aware that patients with postoperative atelectasis, pneumonia, UTI, or asthma may experience an exacerbation of their condition if given neostigmine.
- Store drug at 15° to 30° C (59° to 86° F); protect from freezing and light.

PATIENT TEACHING

- Instruct patient to report muscle weakness, excessive salivation, dizziness, urinary frequency, or other adverse reactions after receiving neostigmine.

nesiritide

Natrecor

Class and Category

Chemical: Human B-type natriuretic peptide
Therapeutic: Arterial and venous smooth-muscle cell relaxant
Pregnancy category: C

Indications and Dosages

▶ *To reduce dyspnea at rest or with minimal activity in patients with acute decompensated heart failure*

I.V. INJECTION, I.V. INFUSION

Adults. 2-mcg/kg bolus, followed by a continuous infusion of 0.01 mcg/kg/min for up to 48 hr.

Route	Onset	Peak	Duration
I.V.	In 15 min	1 hr	3 hr

Mechanism of Action

Binds to the guanylate cyclase receptor of vascular smooth-muscle and endothelial cells. This action increases intracellular levels of cGMP, which leads to arterial and venous smooth-muscle cell relaxation. Ultimately, nesiritide reduces pulmonary artery wedge pressure and systemic arterial pressure in patients with heart failure, thereby decreasing the heart's workload and subsequently relieving dyspnea.

Incompatibilities

Don't infuse nesiritide through the same I.V. line as bumetanide, enalaprilat, ethacrynate sodium, furosemide, heparin, hydralazine, or insulin because these drugs are chemically and physically incompatible with nesiritide. Don't infuse drugs that contain the preservative sodium metabisulfite through the same I.V. line as nesiritide because they're incompatible.

Contraindications

Hypersensitivity to nesiritide or its components, patients with a systolic blood pressure less than 90 mm Hg, primary therapy for cardiogenic shock

Interactions

DRUGS

ACE inhibitors: Increased risk of symptomatic hypotension

Adverse Reactions

CNS: Anxiety, dizziness, headache, insomnia
CV: Angina, bradycardia, hypotension, PVCs, ventricular tachycardia
GI: Abdominal pain, nausea, vomiting
GU: Elevated serum creatinine level
MS: Back pain

Nursing Considerations

- **WARNING** Be aware that nesiritide is not recommended for patients for whom vasodilating drugs are inappropriate, such as those with significant valvular stenosis, restrictive or obstructive cardiomyopathy, constrictive pericarditis, pericardial tamponade, or other conditions in which cardiac output is dependent upon venous return, or for patients suspected of having low cardiac filling pressures.
- Reconstitute 1.5-mg vial by adding 5 ml of diluent from a 250-ml plastic I.V. bag containing preservative-free D_5W, normal saline solution, dextrose 5% half-normal (0.45) saline solution, or dextrose 5% in quarter-normal (0.2) saline solution.
- Don't shake vial. To ensure complete reconstitution, rock vial gently so that all surfaces, including the stopper, come in contact with diluent. Inspect drug for particles and discoloration; if present, discard drug.
- Withdraw entire contents of reconstituted solution and add it to the same 250-ml plastic I.V. bag used to withdraw the diluent to yield a solution of approximately 6 mcg/ml. Invert I.V. bag several times to ensure that solution is completely mixed.
- After preparing infusion bag, withdraw bolus volume from infusion bag and give over approximately 60 seconds. Immediately after giving bolus, infuse drug at a flow rate of 0.1 ml/kg/hour, which will deliver a dose of 0.01 mcg/kg/minute.
- Prime I.V. tubing with 25 ml of solution before connecting to I.V. line and before administering bolus dose or starting infusion.
- Flush I.V. line between administering nesiritide and incompatible drugs.
- Because nesiritide binds to heparin and could bind to heparin lining of a heparin-coated catheter, don't administer drug through a central heparin-coated catheter.
- Store reconstituted vials at room temperature (20° to 25° C [68° to 77° F]) or refrigerate (2° to 8° C [36° to 46° F]) for up to 24 hours.

- Because nesiritide contains no antimicrobial preservatives, discard reconstituted solution after 24 hours.
- Monitor blood pressure and heart rate and rhythm frequently during drug therapy. If hypotension occurs, notify prescriber and expect dosage to be reduced or drug to be discontinued. Implement measures to support blood pressure, as prescribed.
- Assess breath sounds and respiratory rate, rhythm, depth, and quality frequently during nesiritide therapy.
- Monitor serum creatinine level during therapy and notify prescriber of abnormal results.
- Store unopened drug at controlled room temperature or refrigerate. Keep in carton until time of use.

PATIENT TEACHING

- Instruct patient to report dizziness during nesiritide therapy because this may indicate hypotension.
- Reassure patient that her blood pressure, heart rate, and breathing will be monitored frequently.

netilmicin sulfate

Netromycin

Class and Category

Chemical: Aminoglycoside
Therapeutic: Antibiotic
Pregnancy category: D

Indications and Dosages

▶ *To treat serious systemic infections, such as intra-abdominal infections, lower respiratory tract infections, septicemia, and skin and soft-tissue infections, caused by* Enterobacter aerogenes, Escherichia coli, Klebsiella pneumoniae, Proteus mirabilis, Pseudomonas aeruginosa, Serratia *sp., and* Staphylococcus aureus

I.V. INFUSION

Adults and children age 12 and over. 1.3 to 2.2 mg/kg q 8 hr or 2 to 3.25 mg/kg q 12 hr for 7 to 14 days. *Maximum:* 7.5 mg/kg daily.

Children ages 6 weeks to 12 years. 1.8 to 2.7 mg/kg q 8 hr or 2.7 to 4 mg/kg q 12 hr for 7 to 14 days.

Infants up to age 6 weeks. 2 to 3.25 mg/kg q 12 hr for 7 to 14 days.

▶ *To treat complicated UTI caused by* Citrobacter *sp.,* Enterobacter *sp.,* E. coli, K. pneumoniae, P. mirabilis, P. aeruginosa, Serratia *sp., and* Staphylococcus *sp.*

I.V. INFUSION
Adults and adolescents. 1.5 to 2 mg/kg q 12 hr for 7 to 14 days. *Maximum:* 7.5 mg/kg daily.

Mechanism of Action
Is transported into bacterial cells, where it competes with messenger RNA to bind with a specific receptor protein on the 30S ribosomal subunit of DNA. This action causes abnormal, nonfunctioning proteins to form. A lack of functional proteins causes bacterial cell death.

Incompatibilities
Don't mix netilmicin with beta-lactam antibiotics (penicillins and cephalosporins) because substantial mutual inactivation may result. If these drugs are prescribed concurrently, administer them at separate sites.

Contraindications
Hypersensitivity to netilmicin, other aminoglycosides, or their components

Interactions
DRUGS
capreomycin, other aminoglycosides: Increased risk of nephrotoxicity, neuromuscular blockade, and ototoxicity
cephalosporins, nephrotoxic drugs: Increased risk of nephrotoxicity
loop diuretics, ototoxic drugs: Increased risk of ototoxicity
methoxyflurane, polymyxins (parenteral): Increased risk of nephrotoxicity and neuromuscular blockade
neuromuscular blockers: Increased neuromuscular blockade

Adverse Reactions
CNS: Disorientation, dizziness, encephalopathy, headache, myasthenia gravis–like syndrome, neuromuscular blockade (acute muscle paralysis and apnea), paresthesia, peripheral neuropathy, seizures, vertigo, weakness
CV: Hypotension, palpitations
EENT: Blurred vision, hearing loss, nystagmus, tinnitus
GI: Diarrhea, elevated liver function tests results, nausea, vomiting
GU: Elevated BUN and serum creatinine levels, nephrotoxicity, oliguria, proteinuria
HEME: Anemia, eosinophilia, leukopenia, prolonged PT, thrombocytopenia, thrombocytosis

MS: Muscle twitching
RESP: Apnea
SKIN: Allergic dermatitis, erythema, pruritus, rash
Other: Angioedema; hyperkalemia; injection site hematoma, induration, and pain

Nursing Considerations

- To prepare netilmicin for I.V. use, dilute each dose in 50 to 200 ml of suitable diluent, such as normal saline solution, D_5W, or lactated Ringer's solution, and administer slowly over 30 to 60 minutes. When giving drug to children, adjust amount of diluent proportionately, as required. Prepared solution typically may be stored for up to 72 hours at room temperature; however, storage times vary, depending on type of diluent used, type of container, concentration, and storage method. Consult manufacturer's insert for specific stability and storage information.
- Ensure adequate hydration during therapy to maintain adequate renal function.
- Monitor blood netilmicin level; optimum peak level is 6 to 10 mcg/ml and trough level is 0.5 to 2 mcg/ml.
- Check BUN and serum creatinine levels, urine specific gravity, and creatinine clearance during netilmicin therapy, as ordered.
- Anticipate higher risk of nephrotoxicity in infants, elderly patients, those with impaired renal function or dehydration, and those receiving high-dose or prolonged netilmicin therapy.
- Decrease dosage or discontinue drug, as ordered, if signs of drug-induced ototoxicity or vestibular toxicity occur, to reduce the risk of permanent damage. Patients with cranial nerve VIII impairment are at increased risk for both types of toxicity.
- Be aware that infants with botulism and patients with myasthenia gravis or Parkinson's disease may experience increased muscle weakness.
- Store drug at 15° to 30° C (59° to 86° F); don't freeze.

PATIENT TEACHING

- Urge patient to drink plenty of fluids during netilmicin therapy.
- Instruct patient to immediately report dizziness, hearing loss, muscle twitching, nausea, numbness and tingling, ringing or buzzing in ears, seizures, significant changes in amount of urine or frequency of urination, and vomiting.
- Urge patient to keep follow-up appointments—for example, for audiometric and renal function tests—to monitor progress.

niacin
niacinamide
(nicotinic acid, vitamin B_3)

Class and Category

Chemical: B complex vitamin
Therapeutic: Antihyperlipidemic (niacin), nutritional supplement
Pregnancy category: C (for doses above the RDA)

Indications and Dosages

▶ *To prevent niacin deficiency based on U.S. and Canadian recommended daily allowances*

I.V. INFUSION

Adults and children. Dosage individualized based on severity of deficiency, as prescribed, and given as part of total parenteral nutrition solution.

▶ *To treat niacin deficiency*

I.V. INJECTION

Adults and children age 11 and over. 25 to 100 mg at least b.i.d.

Children. Up to 300 mg daily.

Mechanism of Action

Acts as dietary supplement for vitamin B_3. After conversion to niacinamide, niacin becomes a compound of two coenzymes needed for tissue respiration, glycogenolysis, and metabolism of lipids, amino acids, proteins, and purines. Niacin also lowers serum cholesterol and triglyceride levels by inhibiting synthesis of very-low-density lipoproteins, which are needed to form low-density lipoproteins, the primary carrier of blood cholesterol.

Contraindications

Active peptic ulcer disease; arterial bleeding; hepatic impairment (significant or unexplained); hypersensitivity to niacin, niacinamide, or their components

Interactions

DRUGS

chenodiol, ursodiol: Decreased antihyperlipidemic effects of niacin
HMG-CoA reductase inhibitors: Increased risk of rhabdomyolysis and acute renal failure

Adverse Reactions

CNS: Asthenia, chills, dizziness, headache (niacin), insomnia, nervousness, paresthesia, syncope
CV: Arrhythmias, hypotension, palpitations, peripheral edema, peripheral vasodilation (niacin), syncope, tachycardia
EENT: Dry eyes, macular edema, rhinitis, toxic amblyopia
ENDO: Hyperglycemia
GI: Abdominal pain, cholestasis (E.R. niacin), diarrhea, dyspepsia, epigastric pain, eructation, flatulence, hepatotoxicity (E.R. niacin), jaundice, nausea, peptic ulceration, vomiting
GU: Hyperuricemia
MS: Leg cramps, myalgia, myasthenia
RESP: Dyspnea
SKIN: Acanthosis nigricans, dry skin, flushing (niacin), hyperpigmentation, maculopapular rash, pruritus, rash, sensation of warmth (niacin), urticaria
Other: Anaphylaxis (injection), angioedema, facial edema, gout

Nursing Considerations

- Dilute injection solution to a concentration of 2 mg/ml for direct I.V. injection and administer at a rate not exceeding 2 mg/min.
- For intermittent or continuous infusion, dilute appropriate dose in 500 ml of normal saline solution or other compatible solution and administer at no more than 2 mg/minute.
- Monitor patient for "niacin flush," a reaction caused by dilation of peripheral cutaneous blood vessels, which increases blood flow and causes redness, mainly in the face, neck, and chest. Expect patient to develop tolerance to this effect after 2 weeks of therapy. Notify prescriber of persistent flushing; effects may be controlled with aspirin, as prescribed, taken before each niacin dose.
- Expect to monitor liver function tests every 6 months during therapy or as clinically indicated. Expect niacin to be discontinued if serum transaminase levels rise to 3 times the upper limit of normal or if patient exhibits clinical symptoms of hepatic dysfunction.
- Monitor patients with peptic ulcer disease for possible worsened symptoms because nicotinic acid can stimulate histamine release, leading to increased gastric acid production.
- Monitor patients with or predisposed to gout for worsening of symptoms because drug can cause hyperuricemia at high doses.

- In patients taking statins and niacin for hyperlipidemia, watch for rhabdomyolysis (muscle pain, tenderness, or weakness), especially early in therapy or when dosage of either drug increases. Be prepared to stop therapy if rhabdomyolysis occurs.
- Monitor patients with diabetes mellitus for altered glucose control because high doses of niacin may cause hyperglycemia.
- Monitor complete blood count, especially if patient has thrombocytopenia or coagulopathy or takes an anticoagulant, because niacin may cause slight decrease in platelet count or increased prothrombin time.

PATIENT TEACHING

- Instruct patient to avoid activities requiring mental alertness, such as driving or operating machinery, until full effects of drug are known because vasodilatory response to niacin may be dramatic at start of treatment.
- Inform patient that she may experience skin flushing, mainly in the face, neck, and chest, but that she may develop a tolerance to this effect after 2 weeks of therapy. Advise her to notify prescriber of persistent or intolerable flushing because prescriber may adjust drug dosage or recommend that patient take aspirin before each niacin dose to control flushing.

nicardipine hydrochloride

Cardene, Cardene I.V., Cardene SR

Class and Category

Chemical: Dihydropyridine derivative
Therapeutic: Antianginal, antihypertensive
Pregnancy category: C

Indications and Dosages

▶ *To manage angina pectoris and Prinzmetal's angina, to manage hypertension*

I.V. INFUSION

Adults. 0.5 to 2.2 mg/hr by continuous infusion.

▶ *To control acute hypertension*

I.V. INFUSION

Adults. *Initial:* 5 mg/hr by continuous infusion; increased by 2.5 mg/hr q 5 to 15 min, as prescribed. *Maximum:* 15 mg/hr.

Route	Onset	Peak	Duration
I.V.	Immediate	Unknown	Unknown

Mechanism of Action

May slow extracellular calcium movement into myocardial and vascular smooth-muscle cells by deforming calcium channels in cell membranes, inhibiting ion-controlled gating mechanisms, and interfering with calcium release from the sarcoplasmic reticulum. By decreasing the intracellular calcium level, nicardipine inhibits smooth-muscle–cell contraction and dilates coronary and systemic arteries. As with other calcium channel blockers, these actions lead to decreased myocardial oxygen requirements and reduced peripheral resistance, blood pressure, and afterload.

Incompatibilities

Don't mix nicardipine with, or administer through same I.V. line as, sodium bicarbonate or LR solution.

Contraindications

Advanced aortic stenosis, hypersensitivity to any calcium channel blocker, second- or third-degree AV block in patient without artificial pacemaker

Interactions

DRUGS

anesthetics (hydrocarbon inhalation): Possibly hypotension
beta blockers, other antihypertensives, prazosin: Increased risk of hypotension
calcium supplements: Possibly impaired action of nicardipine
cimetidine: Increased nicardipine bioavailability
digoxin: Transiently increased blood digoxin level, increased risk of digitalis toxicity
disopyramide, flecainide: Increased risk of bradycardia, conduction defects, and heart failure
estrogens: Possibly increased fluid retention and decreased therapeutic effects of nicardipine
lithium: Increased risk of neurotoxicity
NSAIDs, sympathomimetics: Possibly decreased therapeutic effects of nicardipine
procainamide, quinidine: Possibly prolonged QT interval

FOODS

grapefruit, grapefruit juice: Possibly increased drug bioavailability
high-fat meals: Decreased blood nicardipine level

ACTIVITIES

alcohol use: Increased hypotensive effect

Adverse Reactions

CNS: Anxiety, asthenia, ataxia, confusion, dizziness, drowsiness, headache, nervousness, paresthesia, psychiatric disturbance, syncope, tremor, weakness
CV: Bradycardia, chest pain, heart failure, hypotension, orthostatic hypotension, palpitations, peripheral edema, tachycardia
EENT: Altered taste, blurred vision, dry mouth, epistaxis, gingival hyperplasia, pharyngitis, rhinitis, tinnitus
ENDO: Gynecomastia, hyperglycemia
GI: Anorexia, constipation, diarrhea, elevated liver function test results, indigestion, nausea, thirst, vomiting
GU: Dysuria, nocturia, polyuria, sexual dysfunction, urinary frequency
HEME: Anemia, leukopenia, thrombocytopenia
MS: Joint stiffness, muscle spasms
RESP: Bronchitis, cough, upper respiratory tract infection
SKIN: Dermatitis, diaphoresis, erythema multiforme, flushing, photosensitivity, pruritus, rash, Stevens-Johnson syndrome, urticaria
Other: Hypokalemia, weight gain

Nursing Considerations

- Check blood pressure and pulse rate before nicardipine therapy begins, during dosage changes, and periodically throughout therapy. During prolonged therapy, periodically assess ECG tracings for arrhythmias and other changes.
- Dilute each 25-mg ampule of nicardipine with 240 ml of compatible solution to yield 0.1 mg/ml. Mixture is stable at room temperature for 24 hours when prepared with D_5W, dextrose 5% in normal saline solution, dextrose 5% in half-normal (0.45) saline solution, half-normal saline solution, or normal saline solution.
- Administer continuous infusion by I.V. pump or controller, and adjust according to patient's blood pressure, as prescribed.
- Change peripheral I.V. site every 12 hours, if feasible.
- Give first dose of oral nicardipine 1 hour before stopping I.V. infusion, as prescribed.
- Monitor fluid intake and output and daily weight for signs of fluid retention, which may precipitate heart failure. Also assess for signs of heart failure, such as crackles, dyspnea, jugular vein distention, peripheral edema, and weight gain.
- Monitor liver and renal function test results periodically during long-term therapy. Patients with impaired hepatic or renal func-

tion may require dosage adjustment. Expect elevated liver function test results to return to normal after drug is discontinued.
- Monitor serum potassium level during prolonged therapy. Hypokalemia increases the risk of arrhythmias.
- Because of drug's negative inotropic effect on some patients, closely monitor patients who take a beta blocker or have heart failure or significant left ventricular dysfunction.
- **WARNING** Expect to taper dosage gradually before discontinuing drug to prevent angina or dangerously high blood pressure.
- Store drug at 20° to 25° C (68° to 77° F); protect from light and elevated temperatures.

PATIENT TEACHING
- Advise patient to change position slowly during nicardipine therapy to minimize effects of orthostatic hypotension.
- Urge patient to avoid potentially hazardous activities until drug's CNS effects are known.
- Advise patient to immediately report chest pain that is not relieved by rest or nitroglycerin, constipation, irregular heartbeat, nausea, pronounced dizziness, severe or persistent headache, and swelling of hands or feet.
- Urge patient to take oral nicardipine as prescribed, even if she feels well.
- Instruct patient to swallow E.R. capsules whole, not to chew, crush, cut, or open them.
- Advise patient not to take drug within 1 hour of eating a high-fat meal or grapefruit product. Urge her not to alter the amount of grapefruit products in her diet without consulting prescriber.
- **WARNING** Caution patient against stopping nicardipine abruptly because angina or dangerously high blood pressure could result.
- Teach patient how to take her pulse, and urge her to notify prescriber immediately if it falls below 50 beats/minute.
- Teach patient how to measure her blood pressure, and advise her to do so weekly if nicardipine was prescribed for hypertension. Suggest that she keep a log of blood pressure readings to take to follow-up appointments with her doctor.
- Encourage patient to comply with suggested lifestyle changes, such as alcohol moderation, low-sodium or low-fat diet, regular exercise, smoking cessation, stress management, and weight loss.
- Inform patient that saunas, hot tubs, and prolonged hot showers may cause dizziness or fainting.

- Instruct patient to avoid prolonged sun exposure and to use sunscreen when going outdoors.

nitroglycerin
(glyceryl trinitrate)

Deponit, Minitran, Nitro-Bid, Nitrocot, Nitro-Dur, Nitrogard, Nitroglyn E-R, Nitroject, Nitrol, Nitrolingual, Nitrong SR, Nitropar, Nitrostat, Nitro-time, Transderm-Nitro, Tridil

Class and Category

Chemical: Nitrate
Therapeutic: Antianginal, antihypertensive, vasodilator
Pregnancy category: C

Indications and Dosages

▶ *To prevent or treat angina, to manage hypertension or heart failure*

I.V. INFUSION

Adults. 5 mcg/min, increased by 5 mcg/min q 3 to 5 min to 20 mcg/min, as prescribed, and then by 10 to 20 mcg/min q 3 to 5 min until desired effect occurs.

Route	Onset	Peak	Duration
I.V.	1 to 2 min	Unknown	3 to 5 min

Incompatibilities

Don't administer I.V. nitroglycerin through I.V. bags or tubing made of polyvinyl chloride. Don't mix drug with other solutions.

Contraindications

Acute MI (S.L.), angle-closure glaucoma, cerebral hemorrhage, concurrent use of phosphodiesterase inhibitors, constrictive pericarditis (I.V.), head trauma, hypersensitivity to adhesive in transdermal form, hypersensitivity to nitrates, hypotension (I.V.), hypovolemia (I.V.), inadequate cerebral circulation (I.V.), increased intracranial pressure, orthostatic hypotension, pericardial tamponade, severe anemia

Interactions

DRUGS

acetylcholine, norepinephrine: Possibly decreased therapeutic effects of these drugs
heparin: Possibly decreased anticoagulant effect of heparin (I.V. nitroglycerin)

Mechanism of Action

May interact with nitrate receptors in vascular smooth-muscle cell membranes. This interaction reduces nitroglycerin to nitric oxide, as shown, which activates the enzyme guanylate cyclase, increasing intracellular formation of cGMP. The increased cGMP level may relax vascular smooth muscle by forcing calcium out of muscle cells, causing vasodilation. Venous dilation decreases venous return to the heart, reducing left ventricular end-diastolic pressure and pulmonary artery wedge pressure. Arterial dilation decreases systemic vascular resistance, systolic arterial pressure, and mean arterial pressure. Thus, nitroglycerin reduces preload and afterload, decreasing myocardial workload and oxygen demand. It also dilates coronary arteries, increasing blood flow to ischemic myocardial tissue.

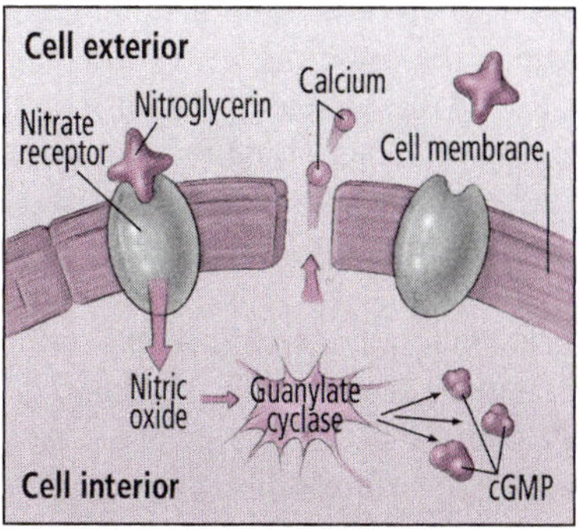

opioid analgesics, other antihypertensives, vasodilators: Possibly increased orthostatic hypotension
phosphodiesterase inhibitors, such as sildenafil: Possibly severe hypotensive effect of nitroglycerin
sympathomimetics: Possibly decreased antianginal effect of nitroglycerin and increased risk of hypotension
ACTIVITIES
alcohol use: Possibly increased orthostatic hypotension

Adverse Reactions

CNS: Agitation, anxiety, dizziness, headache, insomnia, restlessness, syncope, weakness
CV: Arrhythmias (including tachycardia), edema, hypotension, orthostatic hypotension, palpitations
EENT: Blurred vision, burning or tingling in mouth (buccal, S.L. forms), dry mouth
GI: Abdominal pain, diarrhea, indigestion, nausea, vomiting
GU: Dysuria, impotence, urinary frequency
HEME: Methemoglobinemia
MS: Arthralgia

RESP: Bronchitis, pneumonia
SKIN: Contact dermatitis (transdermal forms), flushing of face and neck, rash

Nursing Considerations

- Use nitroglycerin cautiously in elderly patients, especially those who are volume depleted or taking several medications, because of the increased risk of hypotension and falls. Hypotension may be accompanied by angina and paradoxical slowing of the heart rate. Notify prescriber if these occur, and provide appropriate treatment, as ordered.
- Be aware that I.V. nitroglycerin should be diluted only in D_5W or normal saline solution and shouldn't be mixed with other infusions. The pharmacist should add drug to a glass bottle, not a container made of polyvinyl chloride. Don't use a filter because plastic absorbs drug. Administer with infusion pump.
- Check vital signs before every dosage adjustment and frequently during therapy.
- Monitor heart and breath sounds, level of consciousness, fluid intake and output, and pulmonary artery wedge pressure closely.
- Store premixed containers in the dark; don't freeze them.
- **WARNING** Assess for signs of overdose, such as confusion, diaphoresis, dyspnea, flushing, headache, hypotension, nausea, palpitations, tachycardia, vertigo, vision changes, and vomiting. Treat as prescribed by removing nitroglycerin source, if possible; elevating the legs above heart level; and administering an alpha-adrenergic agonist, such as phenylephrine, as prescribed, to treat severe hypotension.

PATIENT TEACHING

- Teach patient to recognize signs and symptoms of angina pectoris, including chest fullness, pain, and pressure, which may be accompanied by sweating and nausea. Pain may radiate down left arm or into neck or jaw. Inform female patients and those with diabetes mellitus or hypertension that they may experience only fatigue and shortness of breath.
- Advise patient to notify prescriber immediately about blurred vision, dizziness, and severe headache.
- Suggest that patient change positions slowly to minimize effects of orthostatic hypotension.
- Advise patient to avoid potentially hazardous activities until drug's CNS effects are known.
- Urge patient to avoid alcohol and erectile dysfunction drugs during therapy.

nitroprusside sodium

Nipride, Nitropress

Class and Category

Chemical: Cyanonitrosylferrate
Therapeutic: Antihypertensive, vasodilator
Pregnancy category: C

Indications and Dosages

▶ *To treat hypertensive crisis and manage severe heart failure*

I.V. INFUSION

Adults and children. *Initial:* 0.25 to 0.3 mcg/kg/min, increased gradually q few minutes until blood pressure reaches desired level. *Maintenance:* 3 mcg/kg/min (range, 0.25 to 10 mcg/kg/min). *Maximum:* 10 mcg/kg/min for 10 min.

Route	Onset	Peak	Duration
I.V.	1 to 2 min	Immediate	1 to 10 min

Mechanism of Action

May interact with nitrate receptors in vascular smooth-muscle–cell membranes. This interaction reduces nitroprusside to nitric oxide, which activates the enzyme guanylate cyclase, increasing intracellular formation of cGMP. The increased cGMP level may relax vascular smooth muscle by forcing calcium out of muscle cells. Smooth-muscle relaxation causes arteries and veins to dilate, which reduces peripheral vascular resistance and blood pressure.

Incompatibilities

Don't mix nitroprusside with any other drug.

Contraindications

Acute heart failure with decreased peripheral vascular resistance, congenital optic atrophy, decreased cerebral perfusion, hypersensitivity to nitroprusside or its components, hypertension from aortic coarctation or AV shunting, tobacco-induced amblyopia

Interactions

DRUGS

dobutamine: Increased cardiac output, decreased pulmonary artery wedge pressure

ganglionic blockers, general anesthetics, hypotension-producing drugs: Increased hypotensive effect

sympathomimetics: Decreased antihypertensive effect of nitroprusside

Adverse Reactions

CNS: Anxiety, dizziness, headache, increased ICP, nervousness, restlessness
CV: Hypotension, tachycardia
ENDO: Hypothyroidism
GI: Abdominal pain, ileus, nausea, vomiting
HEME: Methemoglobinemia
MS: Muscle twitching
SKIN: Diaphoresis, flushing, rash
Other: Infusion site phlebitis

Nursing Considerations

- Obtain baseline vital signs before administering nitroprusside.
- **WARNING** Don't infuse drug undiluted. Reconstitute with 2 ml of D_5W, and add solution to 250 to 500 ml of D_5W to produce 200 mcg/ml or 100 mcg/ml, respectively.
- Be aware that solution is stable at room temperature for 24 hours when protected from light. Don't use reconstituted solution if it contains particles or is blue, green, red, or darker than faint brown.
- Use an infusion pump. Place opaque covering over infusion container because drug is metabolized by light. I.V. tubing doesn't need to be covered.
- Keep patient supine when starting drug or titrating dose up or down.
- Monitor blood pressure continuously with intra-arterial pressure monitor. Record blood pressure every 5 minutes at start of infusion and every 15 minutes thereafter.
- If patient has severe heart failure, expect to administer an inotropic drug, such as dopamine or dobutamine, as prescribed.
- Monitor level of serum thiocyanate (which forms during nitroprusside metabolism) at least every 72 hours; levels exceeding 100 mcg/ml are associated with toxicity.
- **WARNING** Monitor patients receiving prolonged or high-dose nitroprusside therapy for signs of thiocyanate toxicity (ataxia, blurred vision, delirium, dizziness, dyspnea, headache, hyperreflexia, loss of consciousness, nausea, tinnitus, vomiting). Toxicity can cause arrhythmias, metabolic acidosis, severe hypotension, and death.
- **WARNING** Assess for signs of cyanide toxicity (absence of reflexes, coma, distant heart sounds, hypotension, metabolic acidosis, mydriasis, pink skin, shallow respirations, and weak pulse). If you detect such signs, discontinue nitroprus-

side, as ordered, and give 4 to 6 mg/kg of sodium nitrite over 2 to 4 minutes to convert hemoglobin to methemoglobin. Follow with 150 to 200 mg/kg of sodium thiosulfate. Repeat this regimen at one-half the original doses after 2 hours, as ordered.

- Monitor infusion site for redness, swelling, and pain.
- Store nitroprusside at 15° to 30° C (59° to 86° F), and protect it from light.

PATIENT TEACHING

- Advise patient to change position slowly during nitroprusside therapy to minimize dizziness from sudden, severe hypotension.
- Instruct patient to report adverse reactions, such as rash, dizziness, headache, and abdominal pain.

norepinephrine bitartrate
(levarterenol bitartrate)

Levophed

Class and Category

Chemical: Catecholamine
Therapeutic: Cardiac stimulant, vasopressor
Pregnancy category: C

Indications and Dosages

▶ *To treat acute hypotension, cardiogenic shock, and septic shock*

I.V. INFUSION

Adults. *Initial:* 0.5 to 1 mcg/min; increased, as ordered, until systolic blood pressure reaches desired level. *Maintenance:* 2 to 12 mcg/min.

Children. 0.1 mcg/kg/min. *Maximum:* 1 mcg/kg/min.

▶ *To treat refractory shock*

I.V. INFUSION

Adults. Up to 30 mcg/min.

Route	Onset	Peak	Duration
I.V.	Rapid	Unknown	1 to 2 min

Incompatibilities

Don't mix norepinephrine with iron salts, alkalies, or oxidizing solutions. Don't mix norepinephrine with normal saline solution alone.

Mechanism of Action

At high doses (more than 4 mcg/min), directly stimulates alpha-adrenergic receptors and inhibits activity of the intracellular enzyme adenyl cyclase, which then inhibits cAMP production. Inhibition of cAMP causes arterial and venous constriction and increases peripheral vascular resistance and systolic blood pressure. At low doses (less than 2 mcg/min), norepinephrine directly stimulates beta-adrenergic receptors in the myocardium and increases adenyl cyclase activity, producing positive inotropic and chronotropic effects.

Contraindications

Concurrent use of hydrocarbon inhalation anesthetics, hypersensitivity to norepinephrine or its components, hypovolemia, mesenteric or peripheral vascular thrombosis

Interactions

DRUGS

alpha blockers: Decreased vasopressor effects of norepinephrine
beta blockers: Decreased cardiac-stimulating effect of norepinephrine, possibly decreased therapeutic effects of both drugs
digoxin: Increased risk of arrhythmias, possibly potentiated inotropic effect
doxapram: Possibly increased vasopressor effects of both drugs
ergonovine, ergotamine, methylergonovine, methysergide, oxytocin: Possibly increased vasoconstriction
general anesthetics: Increased risk of arrhythmias
guanadrel, guanethidine: Increased vasopressor response to norepinephrine, possibly severe hypertension
MAO inhibitors: Possibly life-threatening adverse effects, including arrhythmias, hyperpyrexia, severe headache, severe hypertension, and vomiting
maprotiline, tricyclic antidepressants: Possibly potentiated cardiovascular and pressor effects of norepinephrine, including arrhythmias, severe hypertension, and hyperpyrexia
methylphenidate: Possibly potentiated vasopressor effects
nitrates: Possibly decreased therapeutic effects of both drugs
phenoxybenzamine: Possibly arrhythmias or hypotension
sympathomimetics: Increased risk of adverse cardiovascular effects
thyroid hormones: Increased risk of coronary insufficiency

Adverse Reactions

CNS: Anxiety, dizziness, headache, insomnia, nervousness, tremor, weakness

CV: Angina, bradycardia, ECG changes, edema, hypertension, hypotension, palpitations, peripheral vascular insufficiency (including gangrene), PVCs, sinus tachycardia
GI: Nausea, vomiting
GU: Decreased renal perfusion
RESP: Apnea, dyspnea
SKIN: Pallor
Other: Infusion site sloughing and tissue necrosis, metabolic acidosis

Nursing Considerations

- Dilute norepinephrine concentrate for infusion in D_5W or D_5 in normal saline solution before administering. Concentrations typically range from 16 to 32 mcg/ml. Discard any unused portion of prepared solution.
- Make sure solution contains no particles and isn't discolored before administering.
- Administer drug with infusion pump or other flow-control device.
- Check blood pressure every 2 to 3 minutes, preferably by direct intra-arterial monitoring, until stabilized and then every 5 minutes.
- **WARNING** Because extravasation can cause severe tissue damage and necrosis, expect prescriber to give multiple S.C. injections of phentolamine (5 to 10 mg diluted in 10 to 15 ml of normal saline solution) around extravasated infusion site.
- If blanching occurs along vein, change infusion site and notify prescriber immediately.
- Monitor ECG tracing continuously during drug administration.
- Store drug in light-resistant container at 15° to 30° C (59° to 86° F); don't freeze.

PATIENT TEACHING

- Urge patient receiving norepinephrine to immediately report burning, leaking, or tingling around I.V. site.

octreotide acetate

Sandostatin

Class and Category

Chemical: Cyclic octapeptide, somatostatin analogue
Therapeutic: Antidiarrheal, hormone suppressant
Pregnancy category: B

Indications and Dosages

▶ *To treat symptoms of acromegaly, to suppress the release of growth hormone from pituitary tumors*

I.V. INJECTION

Adults. *Initial:* 50 mcg t.i.d. *Usual:* 100 mcg t.i.d. *Maximum:* 1,500 mcg daily.

Mechanism of Action

Controls many types of secretory diarrhea by inhibiting secretion of serotonin and pituitary and GI hormones (including insulin, glucagon, growth hormone, thyrotropin, and, possibly, thyroid-stimulating hormone) as well as vasoactive intestinal peptides and pancreatic polypeptides (including gastrin, secretin, and motilin). Inhibition of serotonin and peptides increases intestinal absorption of water and electrolytes, decreases pancreatic and gastric acid secretions, and increases intestinal transit time by slowing gastric motility.

By inhibiting hormones involved in vasodilation, octreotide increases splanchnic arterial resistance and decreases GI blood flow, hepatic vein wedge pressure, hepatic blood flow, portal vein pressure, and intravariceal pressure, thus raising seated and standing blood pressures. By inhibiting serotonin secretion, the drug decreases symptoms of acromegaly, including diarrhea, flushing, wheezing, and urinary excretion of 5-hydroxyindoleacetic acid.

Incompatibilities

Don't mix octreotide in same syringe with fat emulsions or total parenteral nutrition solutions.

Contraindications

Hypersensitivity to octreotide or its components

Interactions

DRUGS

beta blockers, calcium channel blockers: Additive cardiovascular effects of these drugs

bromocriptine: Increased blood bromocriptine level

cisapride: Decreased effectiveness of both drugs

cyclosporine: Decreased blood cyclosporine level

CYP3A4 metabolizers such as quinidine, terfenadine: Decreased metabolic clearance and increased blood levels of these drugs

diuretics: Increased risk of fluid and electrolyte imbalances

insulin, oral antidiabetic drugs: Increased risk of hypoglycemia

vitamin B_{12}: Decreased blood levels of vitamin B_{12}

Adverse Reactions

CNS: Dizziness, drowsiness, fatigue, headache
CV: Arrhythmias (including conduction abnormalities), edema, hypotension, orthostatic hypotension
EENT: Vision changes
ENDO: Hyperglycemia, hypoglycemia
GI: Abdominal distention, guarding, pain, or tenderness; acute cholecystitis; ascending cholangitis; biliary obstruction; cholelithiasis; cholestatic hepatitis; constipation; diarrhea; epigastric pain; flatulence; nausea; pancreatitis; vomiting
GU: Increased urine output
Other: Dehydration, electrolyte imbalances, injection site irritation

Nursing Considerations

- Give octreotide by I.V. injection only in an emergency, as ordered.
- Be aware that octreotide increases risk of acute cholecystitis, ascending cholangitis, biliary obstruction, cholestatic hepatitis, and pancreatitis.
- Monitor vital signs, bowels sounds, and stool consistency. Assess for abdominal pain and signs of gallbladder disease. Although rare, GI side effects such as progressive abdominal distension, severe epigastric pain, and abdominal distension, severe epigastric pain, and abdominal tenderness and guarding may occur together, giving the appearance of acute intestinal obstruction.
- Monitor serum liver enzyme levels, as appropriate.
- Monitor patient for electrolyte imbalances and dehydration.
- Carefully monitor diabetic patient for altered glucose control.
- If patient has periodic flare-ups of symptoms, expect to give additional S.C. octreotide temporarily, as prescribed.

PATIENT TEACHING

- Advise patient to change position slowly to minimize effects of orthostatic hypotension.
- Instruct patient to notify prescriber about adverse reactions, especially abdominal pain, which may indicate pancreatitis.
- Urge diabetic patient to monitor blood glucose level often.

ofloxacin

Floxin

Class and Category

Chemical: Fluoroquinolone
Therapeutic: Antibiotic
Pregnancy category: C

Indications and Dosages

▶ *To treat acute, uncomplicated cystitis caused by* Escherichia coli *or* Klebsiella pneumoniae

I.V. INFUSION

Adults. 200 mg q 12 hr for 3 days.

▶ *To treat uncomplicated cystitis caused by* Citrobacter diversus, Enterobacter aerogenes, Proteus mirabilis, *or* Pseudomonas aeruginosa

I.V. INFUSION

Adults. 200 mg q 12 hr for 7 days.

▶ *To treat complicated UTI caused by* C. diversus, E. coli, K. pneumoniae, P. mirabilis, *or* P. aeruginosa

I.V. INFUSION

Adults. 200 mg q 12 hr for 10 days.

▶ *To treat uncomplicated gonorrhea*

I.V. INFUSION

Adults and adolescents. 400 mg as single dose.

▶ *To treat urethritis or cervicitis caused by* Chlamydia trachomatis *or* Neisseria gonorrhoeae

I.V. INFUSION

Adults and adolescents. 300 mg b.i.d. for 7 days as an alternative to doxycycline or azithromycin.

▶ *To treat pelvic inflammatory disease caused by susceptible organisms*

I.V. INFUSION

Adults and adolescents. 400 mg q 12 hr with metronidazole I.V. and then switched to oral therapy, as prescribed, after 24 hr. Complete course of therapy lasts 14 days.

▶ *To treat prostatitis caused by* E. coli

I.V. INFUSION

Adults. 300 mg q 12 hr for 6 wk.

▶ *To treat lower respiratory tract infections caused by* Haemophilus influenzae *or* Streptococcus pneumoniae *and skin and soft-tissue infections caused by* Staphylococcus aureus *or* Streptococcus pyogenes

I.V. INFUSION

Adults. 400 mg q 12 hr for 10 days.

DOSAGE ADJUSTMENT If creatinine clearance is 20 to 50 ml/min/1.73 m^2, dosing interval possibly reduced to q 24 hr; if clearance is less than 10 ml/min/1.73 m^2, dosage possibly reduced by 50% and given q 24 hr.

Incompatibilities

Don't mix ofloxacin with other I.V. drugs or additives.

Mechanism of Action

Normally, the enzyme DNA gyrase is responsible for unwinding and supercoiling of bacterial DNA before it replicates, as shown top right. Ofloxacin inhibits synthesis of this enzyme, as shown bottom right, by counteracting the excessive supercoiling of DNA during replication and transcription. In this way, ofloxacin causes the death of both rapidly growing and slow-growing bacterial cells.

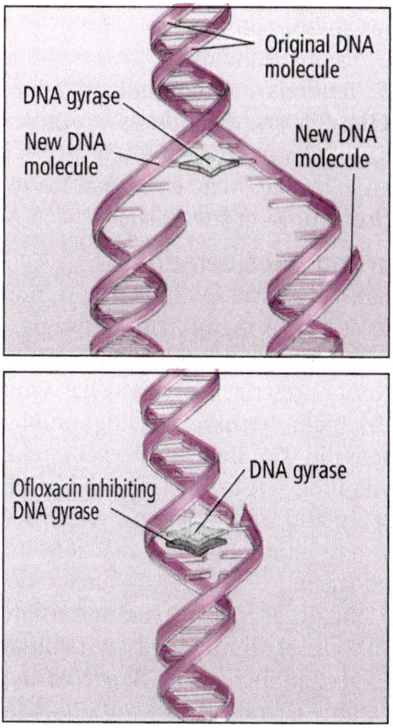

Contraindications

Hypersensitivity to ofloxacin, other fluoroquinolones, or their components

Interactions

DRUGS

aluminum-, calcium-, or magnesium-containing antacids; didanosine; ferrous sulfate; magnesium-containing laxatives; multivitamins; sevelamer; sucralfate; zinc: Decreased absorption of oral ofloxacin
probenecid: Decreased ofloxacin excretion, increased risk of toxicity
procainamide: Decreased renal clearance of procainamide
warfarin: Possibly increased anticoagulant activity and risk of bleeding

Adverse Reactions

CNS: Dizziness, drowsiness, headache, insomnia, peripheral neuropathy
CV: Arrhythmias, prolonged QT interval

GI: Abdominal cramps or pain, diarrhea, nausea, pseudomembranous colitis, vomiting
GU: Vaginal candidiasis
MS: Tendinitis; tendon inflammation, pain, or rupture
SKIN: Blisters, diaphoresis, erythema, erythema multiforme, exfoliative dermatitis, photosensitivity, pruritus, rash, Stevens-Johnson syndrome, toxic epidermal necrolysis, urticaria
Other: Infusion site phlebitis

Nursing Considerations

- For I.V. infusion, dilute drug in normal saline solution or D_5W to at least 4 mg/ml, and infuse over 60 minutes to minimize the risk of hypotension. Discard unused portion.
- Notify prescriber if patient has symptoms of peripheral neuropathy (pain, burning, tingling, numbness, weakness, or altered sensations of light touch, pain, temperature, position sense, or vibration sense), which could be permanent; tendon rupture (pain and inflammation), which requires immediate rest; or a severe photosensitivity reaction. In each case, expect to stop ofloxacin.
- Maintain adequate hydration to prevent development of highly concentrated urine and crystalluria.
- Expect an increased risk of toxicity in severe hepatic disease, including cirrhosis.
- Be aware that ofloxacin may stimulate the CNS and aggravate seizure disorders.
- If diarrhea develops, consider the possibility of pseudomembranous colitis.
- Be alert for secondary fungal infection.

PATIENT TEACHING

- Advise patient to avoid hazardous activities until CNS effects of drug are known.
- Tell patient to limit exposure to sun and ultraviolet light to prevent phototoxicity.
- Advise patient to notify prescriber immediately about burning skin, hives, itching, rash, rapid heart rate, abnormal motor or sensory function, and tendon pain.
- Encourage patient to seek medical attention immediately for trouble breathing or swallowing, which may signal an allergic reaction.
- Instruct a diabetic patient who takes insulin or an antidiabetic to notify prescriber immediately if he develops a hypoglycemic reaction; ofloxacin will have to be stopped.

ondansetron hydrochloride

Zofran

Class and Category

Chemical: Carbazole
Therapeutic: Antiemetic
Pregnancy category: B

Indications and Dosages

▶ *To prevent chemotherapy-induced nausea and vomiting*

I.V. INFUSION

Adults. 32 mg infused over 15 min starting 30 min before chemotherapy; or three 0.15-mg/kg doses, each infused over 15 min, starting with the first dose given 30 min before chemotherapy and second and third doses given 4 and 8 hr after first dose.
Children ages 6 months to 18 years. Three 0.15-mg/kg doses, each infused over 15 min, starting with first dose given 30 min before chemotherapy and second and third doses given 4 and 8 hr after first dose.

▶ *To prevent postoperative nausea and vomiting*

I.V. INJECTION

Adults and children age 12 and over. 4 mg as a single dose over 2 to 5 min just before anesthesia induction or if nausea or vomiting develops shortly after surgery.
Children ages 2 to 12 weighing more than 40 kg (88 lb). 4 mg as a single dose over 2 to 5 min just before anesthesia induction or if nausea or vomiting develops shortly after surgery.
Children ages 1 month to 12 years weighing less than 40 kg. 0.1 mg/kg as a single dose over 2 to 5 min just before or immediately after anesthesia induction or if nausea or vomiting develops shortly after surgery.
DOSAGE ADJUSTMENT For patients with hepatic impairment, maximum dosage limited to 8 mg daily.

Incompatibilities

Don't give ondansetron in same I.V. line as acyclovir, allopurinol, aminophylline, amphotericin B, ampicillin, ampicillin and sulbactam, amsacrine, cefepime, cefoperazone, furosemide, ganciclovir, lorazepam, methylprednisolone, mezlocillin, piperacillin, or sargramostim. Alkaline solutions and highly concentrated fluorouracil solutions are physically incompatible.

Contraindications

Hypersensitivity to ondansetron or its components

Mechanism of Action

Blocks serotonin receptors centrally in the chemoreceptor trigger zone and peripherally at vagal nerve terminals in the intestine. This action reduces nausea and vomiting by preventing serotonin release in the small intestine (the probable cause of chemotherapy- and radiation-induced nausea and vomiting) and by blocking signals to the CNS. Ondansetron may also bind to other serotonin receptors and to mu-opioid receptors.

Interactions

DRUGS

cisplatin, cyclophosphamide: Possibly altered blood levels of these drugs

ACTIVITIES

alcohol use: Increased stimulant and sedative effects, including mood and physical sensations

Adverse Reactions

CNS: Agitation, akathisia, anxiety, ataxia, dizziness, drowsiness, fever, headache, hypotension, restlessness, seizures, syncope, somnolence, weakness

CV: Arrythmias, chest pain, hypotension, prolonged QT interval, pulmonary embolism, shock, tachycardia

EENT: Accommodation disturbances, altered taste, blurred vision, dry mouth, laryngeal edema, laryngospasm, transient blindness

GI: Abdominal pain, anorexia, constipation, diarrhea, elevated liver function test results, flatulence, indigestion, intestinal obstruction, thirst

RESP: Bronchospasm, shortness of breath

SKIN: Flushing, hyperpigmentation, maculopapular rash, pruritus

Other: Anaphylaxis, angioedema, injection site burning, pain, and redness

Nursing Considerations

- Give up to 4 mg I.V. diluted in 50 ml of D_5W or normal saline solution.
- **WARNING** Be aware that drug may mask symptoms of adynamic ileus or gastric distention after abdominal surgery.

PATIENT TEACHING

- Advise patient to notify prescriber immediately about signs of hypersensitivity reaction, such as rash.

- Reassure patient who has transient blindness after administration of ondansetron that vision returns within a few minutes to 48 hours.

orphenadrine citrate

Aniflex, Banflex, Flexoject, Miolin, Mio-Rel, Myotrol, Norflex, Orfro, Orphenate

Class and Category

Chemical: Tertiary amine
Therapeutic: Skeletal muscle relaxant
Pregnancy category: C

Indications and Dosages

▶ *To relieve muscle spasms in painful musculoskeletal conditions*

I.V. INJECTION

Adults and adolescents. 60 mg q 12 hr, p.r.n.

Route	Onset	Peak	Duration
I.V.	Immediate	Unknown	4 to 6 hr

Mechanism of Action

May reduce muscle spasms by acting on the cerebral motor centers or the medulla. Postganglionic anticholinergic effects and some antihistaminic and local anesthetic action contribute to skeletal muscle relaxation.

Contraindications

Angle-closure glaucoma; hypersensitivity to orphenadrine or its components; myasthenia gravis; obstruction of bladder neck, duodenum, or pylorus; prostatic hypertrophy; stenosing peptic ulcers

Interactions

DRUGS

amantadine, amitriptyline, amoxapine, antimuscarinics, atropine, bupropion, carbinoxamine, chlorpromazine, clemastine, clomipramine, clozapine, cyclobenzaprine, diphenhydramine, disopyramide, doxepin, imipramine, maprotiline, mesoridazine, methdilazine, nortriptyline, phenothiazines, procainamide, promazine, promethazine, protriptyline, thioridazine, triflupromazine, trimeprazine, trimipramine: Possibly additive anticholinergic effects

CNS depressants: Increased CNS depression

haloperidol: Increased schizophrenic symptoms, possibly tardive dyskinesia
propoxyphene: Increased risk of anxiety, confusion, and tremor
ACTIVITIES
alcohol use: Increased CNS depression

Adverse Reactions

CNS: Agitation, confusion, dizziness, drowsiness, light-headedness, syncope, tremor
CV: Palpitations, tachycardia
EENT: Blurred vision, dry eyes and mouth, increased contact lens awareness
GI: Abdominal distention, constipation, nausea, vomiting
GU: Urine retention

Nursing Considerations

- Be aware that orphenadrine shouldn't be given to patients with tachycardia or cardiac insufficiency.
- Administer drug over 5 minutes with patient in supine position. Have patient remain in this position for 5 to 10 minutes to minimize adverse reactions. Then help him to a sitting position.
- Be aware that drug can aggravate myasthenia gravis and cause tachycardia.
- Anticipate that drug's anticholinergic effects may cause blurred vision, dry eyes, and increased contact lens awareness.
- Be aware that elderly patients may be at increased risk for adverse CNS effects, such as confusion and syncope.
- Monitor blood count and liver and renal function test results periodically for patients receiving long-term orphenadrine therapy.
- Before using drug, store it at 15° to 30° C (59° to 86° F); protect from freezing and light.

PATIENT TEACHING

- Advise patient to avoid potentially hazardous activities until orphenadrine's CNS effects are known.
- Inform patient that dry mouth can be relieved by ice chips, sugarless candy or gum, and increased intake of fluid.
- Suggest that patient use artificial tears during orphenadrine therapy (especially if he wears contact lenses) to reduce discomfort from dry eyes.
- Instruct patient to avoid alcohol and other CNS depressants during orphenadrine therapy.

oxacillin sodium

Bactocill, Prostaphlin

Class and Category

Chemical: Penicillin
Therapeutic class: Antibiotic
Pregnancy category: B

Indications and Dosages

▶ *To treat mild to moderate infections caused by penicillinase-producing strains of* Staphylococcus *or other susceptible organisms*

I.V. INFUSION

Adults and children weighing 40 kg or more. 250 to 500 mg q 4 to 6 hr.

Infants and children weighing less than 40 kg. 50 mg/kg daily in divided doses q 4 to 6 hr.

Neonates over age 7 days weighing more than 2,000 g. 25 to 50 mg/kg q 6 hr.

Neonates over age 7 days weighing less than 2,000 g. 25 to 50 mg/kg q 8 hr.

Neonates age 7 days and younger weighing more than 2,000 g. 25 to 50 mg/kg q 8 hr.

Neonates age 7 days and younger weighing 2,000 g or less. 25 to 50 mg/kg q 12 hr.

▶ *To treat severe infections caused by penicillinase-producing strains of* Staphylococcus *or other susceptible organisms*

I.V. INFUSION

Adults and children weighing 40 kg or more. 1,000 mg q 4 to 6 hr.

Infants and children weighing less than 40 kg. 100 to 200 mg/kg daily in divided doses q 4 to 6 hr.

Neonates over age 7 days weighing more than 2,000 g. 25 to 50 mg/kg q 6 hr.

Neonates over age 7 days weighing less than 2,000 g. 25 to 50 mg/kg q 8 hr.

Neonates age 7 days and younger weighing more than 2,000 g. 25 to 50 mg/kg q 8 hr.

Neonates age 7 days and younger weighing 2,000 g or less. 25 to 50 mg/kg q 12 hr.

▶ *To treat endocarditis caused by methicillin-susceptible* Staphylococcus aureus *in patients without a prosthetic valve*

I.V. INFUSION

Adults. 2 g q 4 hr for 4 to 6 wk.

▶ *To treat endocarditis caused by methicillin-susceptible* S. aureus *in patients with a prosthetic valve*

I.V. INFUSION

Adults. 2 g q 4 hr for at least 6 wk.

Mechanism of Action

Inhibits bacterial cell wall synthesis. In susceptible bacteria, the rigid, cross-linked cell wall is assembled in several steps. Oxacillin exerts its effects in the final stage of the cross-linking process by binding with and inactivating penicillin-binding proteins (enzymes responsible for linking the cell wall strands). This action causes bacterial cell lysis and death.

Incompatibilities

Don't give oxacillin at same time or in same admixture as aminoglycosides because they are chemically and physically incompatible and will inactivate each other.

Contraindications

Hypersensitivity to oxacillin, penicillins, or their components

Interactions

DRUGS

aminoglycosides: Inactivation of both drugs

chloramphenicol, erythromycins, sulfonamides, tetracyclines: Decreased therapeutic effects of oxacillin

oral contraceptives: Decreased contraceptive efficacy

probenecid: Increased blood oxacillin level

FOODS

all foods: Altered absorption of oxacillin

Adverse Reactions

CNS: Anxiety, depression, fatigue, hallucinations, headache, seizures

EENT: Oral candidiasis

GI: Diarrhea, nausea, pseudomembranous colitis, vomiting

GU: Interstitial nephritis, vaginal candidiasis

HEME: Agranulocytosis, anemia, granulocytopenia, neutropenia

SKIN: Exfoliative dermatitis, pruritus, rash, urticaria

Other: Anaphylaxis

Nursing Considerations

- Administer oxacillin at least 1 hour before other antibiotics.

- Before reconstitution, tap bottle several times to loosen powder. For I.M. injection, reconstitute with sterile water for injection, 0.45 normal saline solution, or normal saline solution. Shake until solution is clear.
- For I.V. infusion, reconstitute only with normal saline solution or D_5W.
- When giving drug to patient at risk for hypertension or fluid overload, be aware that each gram of oxacillin contains 4.02 mEq of sodium.

PATIENT TEACHING

- Instruct patient to notify prescriber immediately if rash develops.
- Advise female patient who uses an oral contraceptive to use an additional contraceptive method during oxacillin therapy.

oxymorphone hydrochloride

Numorphan

Class, Category, and Schedule

Chemical: Phenanthrene derivative
Therapeutic: Analgesic
Pregnancy category: Not rated
Controlled substance: Schedule II

Indications and Dosages

▶ *To relieve moderate to severe pain; to relieve anxiety in patients with dyspnea from pulmonary edema caused by acute left ventricular dysfunction*

I.V. INJECTION

Adults. *Initial:* 0.5 mg, repeated q 3 to 6 hr, p.r.n.

DOSAGE ADJUSTMENT For patients with creatinine clearance rate less than 50 ml/min, dosage reduced; for patients concurrently receiving other CNS depressants, dosage reduced to ⅓ to ½ usual dosage.

Route	Onset	Peak	Duration
I.V.	5 to 10 min	15 to 30 min	3 to 4 hr

Mechanism of Action

Alters the perception of and emotional response to pain at the spinal cord and higher levels of the CNS by blocking the release of inhibitory neurotransmitters, such as gamma-aminobutyric acid and acetylcholine.

Contraindications

Acute or severe asthma; hypersensitivity to oxymorphone, other morphine analogues, or their components; ileus; moderate to severe hepatic impairment; pulmonary edema from a chemical respiratory irritant; severe respiratory depression; upper airway obstruction

Interactions

DRUGS

agonist and antagonist analgesics such as butorphanol, buprenorphine, nalbuphine, or pentazocine: Possibly reduced analgesic effect of oxymorphone and increased risk of precipitating withdrawal symptoms
anticholingerics: Increased risk of urine retention, severe constipation
antidiarrheals, antiperistaltics: Increased risk of severe constipation, CNS depression
antihypertensives, diuretics, hypotension-producing drugs: Increased hypotensive effects
cimetidine: Increased risk of CNS and respiratory adverse reactions
CNS depressants: Additive CNS depressant effects, increased risk of habituation
hydroxyzine, other opioid analgesics: Increased analgesia, CNS depression, and hypotensive effects
MAO inhibitors: Increased risk of unpredictable, severe, sometimes fatal adverse reactions
metoclopramide: Antagonized effects of metoclopramide on GI motility
naloxone: Antagonized analgesic, CNS, and respiratory depressant effects of oxymorphone
naltrexone: Withdrawal symptoms in oxymorphone-dependent patients
neuromuscular blockers: Additive respiratory depression
propofol: Increased incidence of bradycardia

ACTIVITIES

alcohol use: Additive CNS depressant effects, increased risk of habituation

Adverse Reactions

CNS: Asthenia, confusion, delusions, depersonalization, dizziness, drowsiness, euphoria, fatigue, headache, insomnia, light-headedness, nervousness, nightmares, restlessness, seizures, somnolence, tiredness, tremor, weakness

CV: Bradycardia, hypertension, hypotension, palpitations, tachycardia
EENT: Blurred vision, diplopia, dry mouth, laryngeal edema, laryngospasm, miosis, tinnitus
GI: Abdominal cramps or pain, anorexia, biliary colic, constipation, hepatotoxicity, nausea, paralytic ileus, vomiting
GU: Decreased urine output; dysuria; urinary frequency, hesitation or retention
MS: Muscle rigidity (with large doses), uncontrolled muscle movements
RESP: Apnea, atelectasis, bradypnea, bronchospasm, dyspnea, irregular breathing, respiratory depression, wheezing
SKIN: Allergic dermatitis, diaphoresis, erythema, flushing or swelling of face, pruritus, urticaria
Other: Injection site burning, pain, redness, and swelling

Nursing Considerations

- Use with extreme caution in patients with conditions accompanied by hypoxia, hypercapnia, or decreased respiratory reserve such as asthma, chronic obstructive pulmonary disease or cor pulmonale, severe obesity, sleep apnea syndrome, myxedema, kyphoscoliosis, CNS depression or coma.
- Use cautiously in patients with circulatory shock because vasodilation produced by oxymorphone may further reduce cardiac output and blood pressure.
- Use oxymorphone cautiously in patients with mild hepatic function because of potential for greater plasma oxymophone concentrations to occur which increases the patient's risk for serious adverse reactions such as hypotension and respiratory depression.
- Use oxymorphone cautiously in elderly or debilitated patients and in patients with underlying medical conditions such as acute alcoholism, adrenocortical insufficiency, biliary tract disease, CNS depression or coma, delirium tremens, kyphoscoliosis associated with respiratory depression, myxedema or hypothyroidism, prostatic hypertrophy or urethral stricture, severe pulmonary or renal function, or toxic pyschosis.
- Monitor vital signs during oxymorphone therapy to detect respiratory depression and hypotension.
- **WARNING** Be aware that oxymophone may obscure neurologic signs of increased intracranial pressure or in the presence of head injury, intracranial lesions or a preexisting increase in intracranial pressure, cause an exaggerated response

to respiratory depression and elevated cerebrospinal fluid pressure. Monitor the patient closely and notify prescriber immediately if significant alterations occur in the patient's vital signs or neurologic status.

- **WARNING** Know that oxymorphone therapy may obscure the clinical presentation of acute abdominal conditions or aggravate seizures in patients with seizure disorders. Provide protective measures such as seizure precautions and assess patients GI function regularly throughout the course of oxymorphone therapy.
- Monitor patient closely for withdrawal symptoms following abrupt discontinuation of oxymorphone such as irritability, abdominal cramps, vomiting, diarrhea, restlessness, rhinorrhea, yawning, perspiration, chills, myalgia and mydriasis, and changes in vital signs. If present, alert prescriber.
- Monitor urinary and bowel status; constipation may become so severe that it causes ileus.
- Offer fluids to relieve dry mouth.

PATIENT TEACHING

- Warn patient that drug can cause physical dependence.
- Encourage patient to increase fluid and fiber intake to prevent constipation.
- Urge patient not to drink alcohol or use CNS depressants during therapy without first consulting prescriber.
- Caution patient to avoid potentially hazardous activities until drug's CNS effects are known.
- Advise female patient to stop drug and notify prescriber about known or suspected pregnancy.

P

paclitaxel

Taxol

Class and Category

Chemical: Diterpenoid taxane
Therapeutic: Antimicrotubule antineoplastic
Pregnancy category: D

Indications and Dosages

▶ *To treat ovarian cancer*

I.V. INFUSION

Previously untreated adults. 135 mg/m^2 infused over 24 hr, followed by 75 mg/m^2 of cisplatin; repeated q 21 days. Alternatively, 175 mg/m^2 over 3 hr, followed by 75 mg/m^2 of cisplatin; repeated q 21 days.

Previously treated adults. 135 mg/m^2 or 175 mg/m^2 over 3 hr q 21 days.

▶ *To treat metastatic breast cancer, as a single agent or in combination with other drugs, as first-line treatment; to treat metastatic breast cancer if initial chemotherapy regimen fails or if relapse occurs within 6 months of adjuvant chemotherapy that included an anthracycline antineoplastic*

I.V. INFUSION

Adults. 175 mg/m^2 over 3 hr q 21 days.

▶ *To treat node-positive breast cancer sequentially with doxorubicin-containing combination therapy*

I.V. INFUSION

Adults. 175 mg/m^2 over 3 hr q 21 days for four courses, administered sequentially with doxorubicin-containing combination chemotherapy

▶ *To treat non–small-cell lung cancer*

I.V. INFUSION

Adults. 135 mg/m^2 over 24 hr, followed by 75 mg/m^2 of cisplatin.

▶ *To treat AIDS-related Kaposi's sarcoma*

I.V. INFUSION

Adults. 135 mg/m^2 over 3 hr q 21 days. Or, 100 mg/m^2 over 3 hr q 14 days.

DOSAGE ADJUSTMENT Subsequent dosage reduced by 20% if peripheral neuropathy occurs or if patient's neutrophil count falls below 500/mm^3 for 1 week or longer during paclitaxel therapy.

Mechanism of Action

Stabilizes microtubules, which normally contribute to cell structure and movement, and promotes microtubule assembly. In this way, paclitaxel inhibits the normal reorganization of the microtubule network, which is active during interphase and mitotic cellular functions. Paclitaxel also causes abnormal groups of microtubules to form throughout the cell cycle and multiple asters of microtubules to form during mitosis, when cell division normally occurs.

Incompatibilities

Don't let paclitaxel come in contact with plasticized polyvinyl chloride (PVC) equipment or devices, such as infusion bags or sets, to avoid exposing patient to plasticizer DEHP, which can be leached from these materials.

Contraindications

Hypersensitivity to paclitaxel or its components; hypersensitivity to other drugs formulated in polyoxyethylated castor oil, such as cyclosporine or teniposide; patients with solid tumors whose baseline neutrophil count is less than 1,500/mm^3; patients with AIDS-related Kaposi's sarcoma whose baseline neutrophil count is less than 1,000/mm^3

Interactions

DRUGS

blood-dyscrasia–causing drugs (such as cephalosporins and sulfasalazine): Increased risk of leukopenia and thrombocytopenia

bone marrow depressants (such as carboplatin and lomustine): Possibly additive bone marrow depression

vaccines, killed virus: Possibly decreased antibody response to vaccine

vaccines, live virus: Possibly decreased antibody response to vaccine, increased adverse effects of vaccine, and severe infection

Adverse Reactions

CNS: Motor dysfunction, paresthesia, peripheral neuropathy, seizures

CV: Arrhythmias (including bradycardia and ventricular tachycardia), AV block, chest pain, ECG changes, hypotension, MI

EENT: Mucositis

GI: Anorexia, diarrhea, elevated liver function test results, esophageal necrosis and ulceration, nausea, vomiting
GU: Nephrotoxicity
HEME: Anemia, leukopenia, neutropenia, thrombocytopenia
MS: Arthralgia, myalgia
RESP: Dyspnea
SKIN: Alopecia, extravasation with phlebitis or cellulitis, rash, urticaria
Other: Anaphylaxis, angioedema, hypersensitivity reaction, infection

Nursing Considerations

- Follow facility protocols for preparation and handling of antineoplastic drugs and for appropriate disposal of used equipment.
- Monitor CBC, including hematocrit, platelet count, and WBC with differential, before and frequently during paclitaxel therapy, as ordered.
- **WARNING** Don't administer paclitaxel to patients with AIDS-related Kaposi's sarcoma whose neutrophil count is below 1,000/mm^3. For all other indications, don't administer paclitaxel if neutrophil count falls below 1,500/mm^3.
- If paclitaxel solution comes in contact with your skin or mucosa, wash it off thoroughly with warm water. If drug comes in contact with your eye, irrigate it thoroughly with water or normal saline solution.
- Dilute and store drug in glass or polypropylene bottles or in plastic bags made of polypropylene or polyolefin, and administer it through polyethylene-line administration sets to avoid exposing patient to plasticizer DEHP, which can be leached from PVC supplies.
- Dilute paclitaxel with normal saline solution, D_5W, dextrose 5% in normal saline solution, or dextrose 5% in lactated Ringer's solution to a final concentration of 0.3 to 1.2 mg/ml. Use solution within 27 hours if stored at controlled room temperature and in ambient lighting.
- Use an in-line filter no greater than 0.22 micron when administering paclitaxel. Be aware that filter may need to be changed periodically if clogging occurs during infusion.
- To prevent a hypersensitivity reaction, expect to premedicate patient, as ordered, with 20 mg P.O. of dexamethasone (10 mg P.O. for treatment of AIDS-associated Kaposi's sarcoma) about 12 and 6 hours before paclitaxel administration; 50 mg of

diphenhydramine I.V. 30 to 60 minutes before paclitaxel administration; and 300 mg of cimetidine or 50 mg of ranitidine 30 to 60 minutes before paclitaxel administration.

- Observe patient continuously for first 30 minutes of each paclitaxel infusion and frequently thereafter. If anaphylaxis occurs, administer epinephrine, antihistamines, corticosteroids, or oxygen, as prescribed.
- Monitor vital signs during paclitaxel therapy, especially during the first hour of administration, assessing for signs of bradycardia or hypotension. Patients with a history of angina, cardiac conduction abnormalities, MI within past 6 months, or heart failure may be at increased risk for adverse cardiac effects.
- Maintain continuous cardiac monitoring, as prescribed, of patients with a history of cardiac conduction abnormalities.
- Be aware that adverse reactions can vary when paclitaxel is administered in combination therapy. Review information for all drugs administered as part of a specific regimen, including drug interactions and adverse effects.
- If extravasation occurs, stop the infusion immediately and notify prescriber. Then resume the infusion in another vein.
- Monitor patients who have, or have recently been exposed to, chicken pox and those who have herpes zoster for signs and symptoms of severe generalized disease.
- Be aware that patients who have previously received cytotoxic therapy and those who are receiving concurrent or consecutive radiation therapy are at risk for additive bone marrow depression.
- If patient develops thrombocytopenia, implement protective precautions according to facility policy.
- Assess for signs of infection, such as fever, if patient develops leukopenia. Expect to obtain appropriate specimens for culture and sensitivity testing.
- Before diluting paclitaxel, store it at controlled room temperature of 20° to 25° C (68° to 77° F). Protect from light.

PATIENT TEACHING

- Advise patient to have dental work completed before beginning paclitaxel treatment, if possible, or to defer such work until blood counts return to normal because drug can delay healing and cause gingival bleeding. Teach patient proper oral hygiene, and advise her to use a soft-bristled toothbrush.
- Advise patient to immediately report burning at injection site or other signs of extravasation.

- Also instruct patient to immediately report unusual bleeding or bruising, black or tarry stools, blood in urine or stools, or red pinpoint spots on skin.
- Stress the importance of avoiding accidental cuts from sharp objects, such as razor blades and fingernail clippers, because excessive bleeding or infection may occur.
- Caution patient to avoid contact sports and other activities that put her at risk for bruising or injury.
- Suggest that patient with mucositis eat bland, soft foods served cold or at room temperature to decrease irritation.
- Instruct patient who develops bone marrow depression to avoid people with infections. Advise her to report fever, chills, cough, hoarseness, lower back or side pain, and painful or difficult urination because these signs and symptoms may signal an infection.
- Instruct patient to wash her hands immediately before touching her eyes or inside of her nose.
- Caution patient to avoid receiving immunizations unless approved by prescriber. Instruct her to avoid people who have recently received vaccines or to wear a protective mask that covers her nose and mouth when in their presence.
- Stress the importance of complying with the dosage regimen and of keeping follow-up medical appointments and appointments for laboratory tests.
- Inform patient that her hair should grow back after paclitaxel therapy has been completed.
- Advise patient to use contraception because of the risk of fetal harm from paclitaxel therapy. Instruct her to notify prescriber immediately if she becomes pregnant.

palonosetron hydrochloride

Aloxi

Class and Category

Chemical: Selective serotonin subtype 3 (5-HT_3) receptor antagonist
Therapeutic: Antiemetic
Pregnancy category: B

Indications and Dosages

▶ *To prevent acute and delayed nausea and vomiting from chemotherapy*

I.V. INJECTION
Adults. 0.25 mg over 30 sec approximately 30 min before start of chemotherapy.

Mechanism of Action

Chemotherapy-induced nausea and vomiting may occur when a chemotherapeutic drug irritates the small intestine's mucosa, causing enterochromaffin cells within the mucosa to release serotonin ($5\text{-}HT_3$). Then, $5\text{-}HT_3$ stimulates sympathetic receptors on afferent vagal nerve endings and the vagus nerve initiates the vomiting reflex.

Palonosetron selectively blocks $5\text{-}HT_3$ receptors in afferent vagal nerve endings, preventing the vagus nerve from inducing the vomiting reflex and thereby averting or reducing the nausea and vomiting associated with chemotherapy. Palonosetron may also block $5\text{-}HT_3$ receptors centrally, in the chemoreceptor trigger zone of the brain's area postrema.

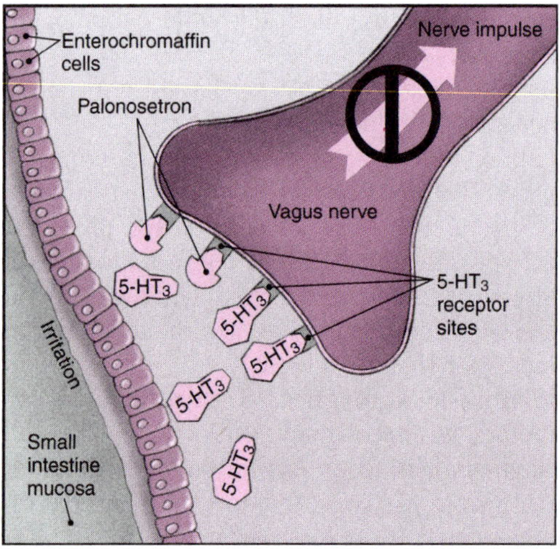

Incompatibilities

Palonosetron should not be mixed with any other drug.

Contraindications

Hypersensitivity to palonosetron or its components

Interactions

DRUGS
None reported.

Adverse Reactions

CNS: Anxiety, dizziness, drowsiness, fatigue, headache, insomnia, weakness

CV: Bradycardia, hypotension, prolonged QT interval, tachycardia
GI: Abdominal pain, constipation, diarrhea
SKIN: Dermatitis, pruritus, rash
Other: Hyperkalemia, hypersensitivity reactions, injection site reactions (burning, induration, pain)

Nursing Considerations

- Use palonosetron cautiously in patients who have or may develop prolonged cardiac conduction intervals—especially QT interval—such as those with congenital QT syndrome, hypokalemia, or hypomagnesemia; those taking a diuretic known to induce electrolyte abnormalities, an antiarrhythmic, or another drug that may prolong QT interval; and those who have received cumulative high-dose anthracycline therapy. With these patients, obtain a baseline ECG before giving palonosetron; repeat the ECG 15 minutes or 24 hours after giving drug, as ordered. Notify prescriber of any delayed conduction.
- Flush I.V. line before and after palonosetron administration with normal saline solution.
- Closely monitor any patient hypersensitive to other selective serotonin receptor antagonists for a similar reaction. If a reaction occurs, notify prescriber immediately.

PATIENT TEACHING

- Advise patient to avoid hazardous activities until drug's CNS effects are known.
- Instruct patient to notify prescriber of any hypersensitivity reaction, such as rash or allergic dermatitis.

pamidronate disodium

Aredia

Class and Category

Chemical: Bisphosphonate
Therapeutic: Antihypercalcemic, bone resorption inhibitor
Pregnancy category: D

Indications and Dosages

▶ *To treat cancer-induced hypercalcemia that's inadequately managed by oral hydration alone*

I.V. INFUSION

Adults. 60 to 90 mg over 2 to 24 hr as a single dose when corrected serum calcium level is 12 to 13.5 mg/dl; 90 mg over 2 to 24 hr when corrected serum calcium level is greater than

13.5 mg/dl. May be repeated as prescribed after 7 days if hypercalcemia recurs.

DOSAGE ADJUSTMENT For patients with renal failure, dosage is limited to 30 mg over 4 to 24 hr, as prescribed. For patients with cardiac or renal failure, drug is given in a smaller volume of fluid or at a slower rate, as prescribed.

▶ *To treat moderate to severe Paget's disease of bone*

I.V. INFUSION

Adults. 30 mg daily over 4 hr on 3 consecutive days for a total dose of 90 mg. Repeated as needed and tolerated.

▶ *To treat osteolytic bone metastases of breast cancer*

I.V. INFUSION

Adults. 90 mg over 2 hr q 3 to 4 wk.

▶ *To treat osteolytic bone metastases of multiple myeloma*

I.V. INFUSION

Adults. 90 mg over 4 hr q mo.

Mechanism of Action

Inhibits bone resorption, possibly by impairing attachment of osteoclast precursors to mineralized bone matrix, thus reducing the rate of bone turnover in Paget's disease and osteolytic metastases. Pamidronate also reduces the flow of calcium from resorbing bone into the bloodstream.

Incompatibilities

Don't mix pamidronate with calcium-containing infusion solutions, such as Ringer's solution.

Contraindications

Hypersensitivity to pamidronate, other bisphosphonates, or their components

Interactions

DRUGS

calcium-containing preparations; vitamin D preparations, such as calcifediol and calcitriol: Antagonized pamidronate effects when used to treat hypercalcemia

Adverse Reactions

CNS: Confusion, fever, psychosis

CV: Hypotension

GI: Abdominal cramps, anorexia, GI bleeding, indigestion, nausea, vomiting

GU: Azotemia

HEME: Leukopenia, lymphopenia
MS: Bone pain, muscle spasms or stiffness, osteonecrosis (mainly of jaw)
RESP: Dyspnea
Other: Anaphylaxis, angioedema, hypocalcemia, hypokalemia, hypomagnesemia, hypophosphatemia, injection site pain and swelling

Nursing Considerations

- Make sure patient has had a dental checkup before invasive dental procedures during pamidronate therapy, especially if patient has cancer; is receiving chemotherapy, head or neck radiation, or a corticosteroid; or has poor oral hygiene because the risk of osteonecrosis is increased in these patients.
- Stay alert for fever during the first 3 days of pamidronate therapy, especially in patients receiving high doses. If fever develops, obtain the patient's CBC with differential, as ordered.
- Obtain serum creatinine level before each treatment. Notify prescriber of abnormal results because drug may need to be held or dosage adjusted until creatinine level returns to normal.
- Assess patient with anemia, leukopenia, or thrombocytopenia for worsening of the condition during first 2 weeks of therapy.

PATIENT TEACHING

- Stress the importance of complying with prescribed administration schedule for pamidronate.
- Advise patient to avoid calcium and vitamin D supplements during pamidronate therapy.
- Instruct patient on proper oral hygiene and on need to notify prescriber about invasive dental procedures.

pantoprazole sodium

Pantoloc (CAN), Protonix I.V.

Class and Category

Chemical: Substituted benzimidazole
Therapeutic: Antiulcer, gastric acid proton pump inhibitor
Pregnancy category: B

Indications and Dosages

▶ *To treat gastroesophageal reflux disease (GERD)*

I.V. INFUSION

Adults. 40 mg daily infused over 2 min or 15 min for 7 to 10 days, followed by oral doses.

▶ *To treat pathological hypersecretion associated with Zollinger-Ellison syndrome or other neoplastic conditions*

I.V. INFUSION

Adults. 80 mg q 12 hr infused over 2 min or 15 min; adjusted based on patient's acid output measurements up to 80 mg q 8 hr.

Route	Onset	Peak	Duration
I.V.	1 day	Unknown	1 wk

Mechanism of Action

Interferes with gastric acid secretion by inhibiting the hydrogen-potassium-adenosine triphosphatase (H^+-K^+-ATPase) enzyme system, or proton pump, in gastric parietal cells. Normally, the proton pump uses energy from the hydrolysis of ATPase to drive H^+ and chloride (Cl^-) out of parietal cells and into the stomach lumen in exchange for potassium (K^+), which leaves the stomach lumen and enters parietal cells. After this exchange, H^+ and Cl^- combine in the stomach to form hydrochloric acid (HCl). Pantoprazole irreversibly inhibits the final step in gastric acid production by blocking the exchange of intracellular H^+ and extracellular K^+, thus preventing H^+ from entering the stomach and additional HCl from forming.

Incompatibilities

Midazolam and products containing zinc may cause precipitation or discoloration.

Contraindications

Hypersensitivity to pantoprazole, substituted benzimidazoles (omeprazole, lansoprazole, rabeprazole sodium), or their components

Interactions

DRUGS

ampicillin, cyanocobalamin, digoxin, iron salts, ketoconazole: Possibly impaired absorption of these drugs

warfarin: Increased INR, PT, and bleeding risk

Adverse Reactions

CNS: Anxiety, asthenia, confusion, dizziness, headache, hypertonia, hypokinesia, insomnia, malaise, migraine, speech disorder vertigo

CV: Chest pain, hypercholesterolemia, hyperlipidemia

EENT: Anterior ischemic optic neuropathy, blurred vision, in-

creased salivation, pharyngitis, rhinitis, sinusitis, tinnitus
ENDO: Hyperglycemia
GI: Abdominal pain, constipation, diarrhea, elevated liver function tests results, flatulence, gastroenteritis, hepatotoxicity, indigestion, nausea, pancreatitis, vomiting
GU: Elevated serum creatinine level, interstitial nephritis
HEME: Pancytopenia
MS: Arthralgia, back or neck pain, rhabdomyolysis
RESP: Bronchitis, dyspnea, increased cough, upper respiratory tract infection
SKIN: Erythema multiforme, rash, Stevens-Johnson syndrome, toxic epidermal necrolysis
Other: Anaphylaxis, angioedema, elevated creatine kinase and phosphokinase levels, flulike symptoms, generalized pain, hyperuricemia, infection, injection site reaction

Nursing Considerations

- Ensure the continuity of gastric acid suppression during transition from oral to I.V. pantoprazole (or vice versa) because even a brief interruption of effective suppression can lead to serious complications.
- Don't give pantoprazole within 4 weeks of testing for *Helicobacter pylori* because antibiotics, proton pump inhibitors, and bismuth preparations suppress *H. pylori* and may lead to false-negative results. Be aware that drug may cause false-positive results in urine screening tests for tetrahydrocannabinol. Obtain guidelines regarding pantoprazole use from prescriber before testing.
- Flush I.V. line with D_5W, normal saline solution, or lactated Ringer's injection before and after giving drug.
- When giving I.V. over 2 minutes, reconstitute with 10 ml of normal saline solution injection. Solution may be stored up to 2 hours at room temperature.
- When giving I.V. over 15 minutes, reconstitute with 10 ml normal saline solution injection. Then, further reconstitute with 100 ml (for GERD) or 80 ml (for pathological hypersecretion in Zollinger-Ellison syndrome) of D_5W, normal saline injection, or lactated Ringer's injection. Solution may be stored up to 2 hours before further dilution and up to 22 hours before use.
- Monitor PT or INR during therapy, as ordered, if patient takes an oral anticoagulant.
- Be aware that, if drug is given for more than 3 years, patient may not be able to absorb vitamin B_{12} because of hypochlorhy-

dria or achlorhydria. Treatment for cyanocobalamin deficiency may be needed.

PATIENT TEACHING

- Advise patient to expect relief of symptoms within 2 weeks of starting therapy.
- Advise patient who takes warfarin to follow bleeding precautions and to notify prescriber immediately if bleeding occurs.

paricalcitol

Zemplar

Class and Category

Chemical: Sterol derivative, vitamin D analogue
Therapeutic: Antihyperparathyroid
Pregnancy category: Not rated

Indications and Dosages

▶ *To prevent and treat secondary hyperparathyroidism in patients with chronic renal failure stage 3 or 4*

I.V. INJECTION

Adults. *Initial:* 0.04 to 0.1 mcg/kg (2.8 to 7 mcg) no more than q other day at any time during dialysis. *Maintenance:* If initial dosage doesn't produce a satisfactory response, 2 to 4 mcg given q 2 to 4 wk. *Maximum:* 0.24 mcg/kg/dose or up to 16.8 mcg/dose.
Children age 5 and older. *Initial:* 0.04 mcg/kg three times weekly if baseline intact parathyroid hormone (iPTH) level is less than 500 pg/ml. Give 0.08 mcg/kg three times weekly if baseline iPTH level is 500 pg/ml or more. *Maintenance:* If initial dosage isn't adequate, adjust it in 0.04-mcg/kg increments as needed and ordered.

DOSAGE ADJUSTMENT If serum PTH level remains the same or increases, dosage is increased. If serum PTH level decreases by less than 30%, dosage is increased. If serum PTH level decreases by 30% to 60%, dosage is maintained. If serum PTH level decreases by more than 60%, dosage is decreased. If serum PTH level is 1.5 to 3 times the upper limit of normal, dosage is maintained.

DOSAGE ADJUSTMENT Dosage is immediately reduced or stopped if serum calcium level is elevated or serum calcium-phosphorus product exceeds 75. Dosage restarted at a lower dose when these levels return to normal.

Route	Onset	Peak	Duration
I.V.	Unknown	Unknown	15 hr

Mechanism of Action

Reduces serum PTH level by an unknown mechanism. In chronic renal failure, decreased renal synthesis of vitamin D leads to chronic hypocalcemia. In response, parathyroid glands secrete PTH to stimulate vitamin D synthesis, but serum calcium levels can't normalize because of renal failure.

Contraindications

Evidence of vitamin D toxicity, hypercalcemia, hypersensitivity to paricalcitol or components

Interactions

DRUGS

atazanavir, clarithromycin, indinavir, itraconazole, ketoconazole, nefazodone, nelfinavir, ritonavir, saquinavir, telithromycin, voriconazole: Increased effects of oral paricalcitol
digoxin: Possibly increased risk of digitalis toxicity
drugs, such as cholestyramine, that impair absorption of fat-soluble vitamins: Possibly impaired absorption of oral paricalcitol

Adverse Reactions

CNS: Arthritis, asthenia, chills, depression, dizziness, fever, headache, insomnia, light-headedness, malaise, neuropathy, syncope, vertigo
CV: Cardiomyopathy, chest pain, congestive heart failure, edema, hypertension, hypotension, MI, orthostatic hypotension, palpitations
EENT: Amblopia, dry mouth, epistaxis, pharyngitis, retinal abnormality, rhinitis, sinusitis, taste perversion
ENDO: Hypoglycemia
GI: Abdominal pain, constipation, diarrhea, dyspepsia, gastritis, gastroenteritis, GI bleeding, nausea, vomiting
GU: Abnormal kidney function, uremia, UTI
MS: Back pain, leg cramps, myalgia
RESP: Bronchitis, increased cough, pneumonia
SKIN: Ecchymosis, hypertrophy, pruritus, rash (including vesiculobullous), ulceration, urticaria
Other: Acidosis; allergic reaction; dehydration; facial, oral or generalized edema; gout; hyperkalemia; hyperphosphatemia; hypervolemia; hypokalemia; infections; influenza; sepsis

Nursing Considerations

- Before giving paricalcitol, look for particles and discoloration; if present, discard drug.
- Give as I.V. bolus; discard unused portion.
- Monitor serum calcium and phosphorus levels, as ordered, twice weekly to guide dosage adjustments and then monthly.
- **WARNING** Drug may lead to vitamin D toxicity and hypercalcemia. Look for early evidence, including arthralgia, constipation, dry mouth, headache, metallic taste, myalgia, nausea, somnolence, vomiting, and weakness. Also look for late evidence, including albuminuria, anorexia, arrhythmias, azotemia, conjunctivitis (calcific), decreased libido, elevated BUN and serum ALT and AST levels, vascular calcification, hypercholesterolemia, hypertension, hyperthermia, irritability, mild acidosis, nephrocalcinosis, nocturia, pancreatitis, photophobia, polydipsia, polyuria, pruritus, rhinorrhea, and weight loss.
- If toxicity occurs, notify prescriber immediately and expect to decrease or stop drug. Place patient on bed rest and give fluids, low-calcium diet, and laxative, as prescribed. For hypercalcemic crisis and dehydration, expect to infuse normal saline solution and a loop diuretic to prompt renal calcium excretion.
- Expect to check patient's serum PTH level every 3 months.
- If patient also takes digoxin, monitor her for evidence of digitalis glycoside toxicity, which is potentiated by hypercalcemia.
- Store drug at 25° C (77° F).

PATIENT TEACHING

- Advise patient to follow high-calcium, low-phosphorus diet.
- Explain that patient may need phosphate binders to control serum phosphorus level.
- Review early evidence of hypercalcemia and vitamin D toxicity. Tell patient to contact prescriber immediately if it develops.
- Urge patient to avoid hazardous activities until drug's adverse CNS effects are known.
- If patient takes digoxin, explain evidence of toxicity and the need to contact prescriber immediately if it develops.

penicillin G potassium

Megacillin (CAN), Pentids, Pfizerpen

penicillin G sodium

Class and Category

Chemical: Penicillin

Therapeutic: Antibiotic
Pregnancy category: B

Indications and Dosages

▶ *To treat systemic infections caused by gram-positive organisms (including* Bacillus anthracis, Corynebacterium diphtheriae, *enterococci,* Listeria monocytogenes, Staphylococcus aureus, *and* Staphylococcus epidermidis*), gram-negative organisms (including* Neisseria gonorrhoeae, Neisseria meningitidis, Pasteurella multocida, *and* Streptobacillus moniliformis *[rat-bite fever]), and gram-positive anaerobes (including* Actinomyces israelii *[actinomycosis],* Clostridium perfringens, Clostridium tetani, Peptococcus *sp.,* Peptostreptococcus *sp., and spirochetes, especially* Treponema carateum *[pinta],* Treponema pallidum, *and* Treponema pertenue *[yaws])*

I.V. INFUSION

Adults and adolescents. 1 to 5 million units q 4 to 6 hr. *Maximum:* 80 million units daily.

Children. 8,333 to 16,667 units/kg q 4 hr or 12,500 to 25,000 units/kg q 6 hr.

▶ *To treat bacterial meningitis*

I.V. INFUSION

Adults. 50,000 units/kg q 4 hr or 24 million units daily in divided doses q 2 to 4 hr.

Mechanism of Action

Inhibits the final stage of bacterial cell wall synthesis by competitively binding to penicillin-binding proteins inside the cell wall. Penicillin-binding proteins are responsible for various steps in bacterial cell wall synthesis. By binding to these proteins, penicillin leads to cell wall lysis.

Contraindications

Hypersensitivity to penicillin or its components

Incompatibilities

Don't mix any penicillin in the same syringe or container with aminoglycosides because aminoglycosides will be inactivated. Don't mix penicillin G with drugs that may result in a pH below 5.5 or above 8.

Interactions

DRUGS

ACE inhibitors, potassium-containing drugs, potassium-sparing diuretics:

Increased risk of hyperkalemia (penicillin G potassium)
chloramphenicol, erythromycin, sulfonamides, tetracycline, thrombolytics: Possibly interference with penicillin's bactericidal effect
cholestyramine, colestipol: Possibly impaired absorption of oral penicillin G
methotrexate: Decreased methotrexate clearance, increased risk of toxicity
oral contraceptives: Decreased contraceptive effectiveness (with penicillin V)
probenecid: Increased blood penicillin level
FOODS
acidic beverages, such as fruit juices: Possibly altered effects of oral penicillin G

Adverse Reactions

CNS: Confusion, dizziness, dysphasia, hallucinations, headache, lethargy, sciatic nerve irritation, seizures
CV: Labile blood pressure, palpitations
EENT: Black "hairy" tongue, oral candidiasis, stomatitis, taste perversion
GI: Abdominal pain, diarrhea, elevated liver function test results (transient), indigestion, nausea, pseudomembranous colitis
GU: Interstitial nephritis (acute), vaginal candidiasis
MS: Muscle twitching
SKIN: Rash
Other: Electrolyte imbalances; injection site necrosis, pain, or redness

Nursing Considerations

- Obtain body tissue and fluid samples for culture and sensitivity tests as ordered before giving first dose. Expect to begin drug therapy before test results are known.
- Reconstitute vials of penicillin for injection with sterile water for injection, D_5W, or sodium chloride for injection.
- Give penicillin at least 1 hour before giving other antibiotics.
- Assess patient for signs of secondary infection, such as profuse, watery diarrhea.
- Monitor serum sodium level and assess patiebt for early signs of heart failure in patients receiving high doses of penicillin G sodium.
- When giving penicillin G potassium to patient at risk for hypertension or fluid overload, be aware that each gram of pencillin G potassium also contains 1.02 mEq of sodium.
- Monitor patients with renal impairment closely throughout

drug therapy because these patients are at increased risk for toxic reactions as penicillin G is primarily excreted primarily by the kidneys.

PATIENT TEACHING

- Instruct patient to report previous allergies to penicillins and to immediately report adverse reactions, including fever.

pentamidine isethionate

Pentacarinat (CAN), Pentam 300

Class and Category

Chemical: Diamidine derivative
Therapeutic: Antiprotozoal
Pregnancy category: C

Indications and Dosages

▶ *To treat* Pneumocystis jiroveci (carinii) *pneumonia*

I.V. INFUSION

Adults and children. 4 mg/kg daily infused over 1 to 2 hr for 14 to 21 days.

DOSAGE ADJUSTMENT Dosage possibly reduced or I.V. infusion time or dosing interval extended for patients with renal failure.

Mechanism of Action

May bind to DNA and inhibit DNA replication in *Pneumocystis jiroveci* (formerly *carinii*). Pentamidine also may inhibit dihydrofolate reductase, an enzyme needed to convert dihydrofolic acid to tetrahydrofolic acid in this organism. This action inhibits the formation of coenzymes that are essential to the growth and replication of *P. jiroveci.*

Incompatibilities

Don't mix pentamidine with other drugs or with saline solutions because precipitation may occur.

Contraindications

History of anaphylactic reaction to pentamidine or its components, hypersensitivity to pentamidine or its components

Interactions

DRUGS

blood-dyscrasia–causing drugs, bone marrow depressants: Increased risk

of adverse hematologic effects
didanosine: Increased risk of pancreatitis
erythromycin: Increased risk of torsades de pointes
foscarnet: Increased risk of severe but reversible hypocalcemia, hypomagnesemia, and nephrotoxicity
nephrotoxic drugs: Increased risk of nephrotoxicity

Adverse Reactions

CNS: Chills, confusion, dizziness, fatigue, fever, hallucinations, headache
CV: Arrhythmias, edema, hypotension, prolonged QT interval, torsades de pointes, ventricular tachycardia
EENT: Bitter or metallic taste
ENDO: Diabetes mellitus, hyperglycemia, hypoglycemia
GI: Abdominal pain, anorexia, diarrhea, elevated liver function test results, nausea, vomiting, pancreatitis
GU: Elevated serum creatinine level
HEME: Anemia, leukopenia, thrombocytopenia, unusual bleeding or bruising
MS: Myalgia
SKIN: Night sweats, rash
Other: Hyperchloremic acidosis, hyperkalemia, hypocalcemia, hypomagnesemia, infusion site phlebitis

Nursing Considerations

- To prepare initial dilution, add 3 to 5 ml of sterile water for injection or D_5W to 300-mg vial of pentamidine. Use drug prepared with D_5W within 24 hours of reconstitution, and protect from light until ready to use. Further dilute in 50 to 250 ml of D_5W, and infuse over 1 to 2 hours.
- Keep patient supine during infusion, and monitor blood pressure frequently during and after administration. Keep emergency resuscitation equipment readily available.
- Assess for hypoglycemia and arrhythmias. Although uncommon, these adverse reactions can be severe.
- Monitor CBC; platelet count; liver function test results; BUN, serum creatinine and calcium, and blood glucose levels; and ECG tracing throughout therapy, as ordered.
- Monitor blood glucose level because pentamidine use can induce insulin release from pancreas, causing severe hypoglycemia that can last from 1 day to several weeks.
- Be aware that hyperglycemia and diabetes mellitus can occur up to several months after parenteral pentamidine therapy stops.

- Before reconstituting pentamidine, store it at 2° to 8° C (36° to 46° F) and protect from light.

PATIENT TEACHING

- Advise patient to avoid potentially hazardous activities until pentamidine's CNS effects are known.
- Instruct patient to report unusual bleeding or bruising and to take precautions to avoid bleeding, such as using a soft-bristled toothbrush and an electric shaver.
- Caution patient about possible hypoglycemic effects of pentamidine therapy.
- Advise patient to undergo follow-up testing for diabetes mellitus, which can occur up to several months after pentamidine therapy is completed.

pentazocine lactate

Talwin

Class, Category, and Schedule

Chemical: Synthetic opioid
Therapeutic: Analgesic
Pregnancy category: C
Controlled substance: Schedule IV

Indications and Dosages

▶ *To relieve moderate to severe pain*

I.V. INJECTION

Adults. *Initial:* 30 mg q 3 to 4 hr, p.r.n. *Maximum:* 30 mg/single dose I.V., 360 mg/24 hr

▶ *To relieve obstetric pain*

I.V. INJECTION

Adults. 20 mg when contractions become regular; repeated 2 or 3 times q 2 to 3 hr, as prescribed.

Route	Onset	Peak	Duration
I.V.	2 to 3 min	15 to 30 min	2 to 3 hr

Mechanism of Action

Binds with opioid receptors, primarily kappa and sigma receptors, at many CNS sites to alter the perception of and emotional response to pain.

Incompatibilities

Don't mix pentazocine in same syringe with a soluble barbiturate because precipitation will occur.

Contraindications

Hypersensitivity to pentazocine or its components

Interactions

DRUGS

anticholinergics: Increased risk of urine retention and severe constipation

antidiarrheals, antiperistaltics: Increased risk of severe constipation and CNS depression

antihypertensives, diuretics, other hypotension-producing drugs: Additive hypotensive effects

buprenorphine: Decreased pentazocine effectiveness, increased respiratory depression

CNS depressants: Increased CNS depression, increased risk of habituation

hydroxyzine, other opioid analgesics: Increased analgesia, CNS depression, and hypotensive effects

MAO inhibitors: Increased risk of unpredictable, severe, and sometimes fatal adverse reactions

metoclopramide: Antagonized metoclopramide effects on GI motility

naloxone: Antagonized analgesic, CNS, and respiratory depressant effects of pentazocine

naltrexone: Withdrawal symptoms in patients physically dependent on pentazocine

neuromuscular blockers: Increased respiratory depression

ACTIVITIES

alcohol use: Additive CNS depression and increased risk of habituation

Adverse Reactions

CNS: Chills, dizziness, drowsiness, euphoria, fatigue, headache, insomnia, light-headedness, nervousness, nightmares, paresthesia, restlessness, weakness

CV: Hypotension, tachycardia

EENT: Blurred vision, diplopia, dry mouth, laryngeal edema, laryngospasm

GI: Constipation, hepatotoxicity, nausea, vomiting

GU: Decreased urine output, dysuria, urinary frequency, urine retention

MS: Muscle rigidity (with large doses)

RESP: Atelectasis, bronchospasm, dyspnea, hypoventilation, wheezing
SKIN: Diaphoresis, erythema multiforme, facial flushing, pruritus, rash, Stevens-Johnson syndrome, toxic epidermal necrolysis, urticaria
Other: Facial edema; injection site burning, pain, redness, or swelling; physical and psychological dependence

Nursing Considerations

- Use pentazocine with extreme caution in patients who have head injury, intracranial lesion, or increased intracranial pressure because drug may mask neurologic signs and symptoms.
- Use drug cautiously in patients who are physically dependent on opioid agonists because drug may prompt withdrawal symptoms; in patients with acute MI because drug's cardiovascular effects can increase cardiac workload; in patients with renal or hepatic dysfunction because drug is metabolized in the liver and excreted in urine; and in patients with respiratory conditions because drug depresses the respiratory system.
- After giving parenteral form, expect to taper dosage gradually, as prescribed, to reduce the risk of withdrawal symptoms.

PATIENT TEACHING

- Caution patient that prolonged use of pentazocine may result in drug dependence.
- Advise patient to avoid potentially hazardous activities until drug's CNS effects are known.
- Caution patient not to use alcohol or OTC drugs without consulting prescriber.
- Advise patient to notify prescriber if she notices signs of an allergic reaction, such as a rash or itching.

pentobarbital sodium

Nembutal

Class, Category, and Schedule

Chemical: Barbiturate
Therapeutic: Anticonvulsant, sedative-hypnotic
Pregnancy category: D
Controlled substance: Schedule II

Indications and Dosages

▶ *To provide short-term treatment of insomnia*

I.V. INJECTION

Adults. *Initial:* 100 mg, with additional small doses at 1-min intervals, as prescribed. *Maximum:* 500 mg.

▶ *To provide emergency treatment of seizures associated with eclampsia, meningitis, status epilepticus, tetanus, or toxic reactions to local anesthetics or strychnine*

I.V. INJECTION

Adults. 100 mg, with additional small doses at 1-min intervals, as prescribed. *Maximum:* 500 mg.

Children. 50 mg, with additional small doses at 1-min intervals, as prescribed, until desired effect occurs.

DOSAGE ADJUSTMENT Dosage possibly reduced for elderly or debilitated patients and those with hepatic dysfunction.

Route	Onset	Peak	Duration
I.V.	In 1 min	Unknown	15 min

Mechanism of Action

Inhibits ascending conduction of impulses in the reticular formation, which controls CNS arousal to produce drowsiness, hypnosis, and sedation. Pentobarbital also decreases the spread of seizure activity in the cortex, thalamus, and limbic system. It promotes an increased threshold for electrical stimulation in the motor cortex, which may contribute to its anticonvulsant properties.

Contraindications

Hepatic disease; history of addiction to hypnotics or sedatives; hypersensitivity to pentobarbital, other barbiturates, or their components; nephritis; porphyria; severe respiratory disease with airway obstruction or dyspnea

Interactions

DRUGS

acetaminophen: Possibly decreased effects of acetaminophen (with long-term pentobarbital use)

carbamazepine, chloramphenicol, corticosteroids, cyclosporine, dacarbazine, digoxin, disopyramide, doxycycline, griseofulvin, metronidazole, oral contraceptives, phenylbutazone, quinidine, theophyllines, vitamin D: Decreased effectiveness of these drugs

CNS depressants: Increased CNS depression and risk of habituation

divalproex sodium, valproic acid: Increased risk of CNS toxicity and neurotoxicity

guanadrel, guanethidine: Possibly increased risk of orthostatic hypotension
halogenated hydrocarbon anesthetics: Increased risk of hepatotoxicity (with long-term pentobarbital use)
haloperidol: Possibly decreased blood haloperidol level, possibly altered seizure pattern or frequency
hydantoins: Possibly interference with hydantoin metabolism
leucovorin: Possibly decreased anticonvulsant effect of pentobarbital
maprotiline: Possibly enhanced CNS depression and decreased therapeutic effects of pentobarbital
mexiletine: Possibly decreased blood mexiletine level
oral anticoagulants: Possibly decreased therapeutic effects of these drugs, possibly increased risk of bleeding when pentobarbital is discontinued
tricyclic antidepressants: Possibly decreased therapeutic effects of these drugs
ACTIVITIES
alcohol use: Increased CNS depression

Adverse Reactions

CNS: Agitation, anxiety, ataxia, confusion, delusions, depression, dizziness, drowsiness, fever, hallucinations, headache, insomnia, irritability, nervousness, nightmares, paradoxical stimulation, seizures, syncope, tremor
CV: Orthostatic hypotension
EENT: Vision changes
GI: Anorexia, constipation, hepatic dysfunction, nausea, vomiting
HEME: Agranulocytosis
MS: Arthralgia, bone pain, muscle twitching or weakness
RESP: Respiratory depression
SKIN: Exfoliative dermatitis, rash, Stevens-Johnson syndrome
Other: Physical and psychological dependence, weight loss

Nursing Considerations

- Inject pentobarbital at 50 mg or less/minute to prevent adverse respiratory and circulatory reactions.
- Be aware that pentobarbital shouldn't be given during third trimester of pregnancy because repeated use can cause dependence in neonate. It also shouldn't be given to breast-feeding women because it may cause CNS depression in infants.
- Closely monitor blood pressure, pulse, and respirations during administration. Keep emergency equipment and drugs nearby in case respiratory depression or adverse hemodynamic effects

occur. Be aware that patients with cardiovascular disease are at increased risk for adverse circulatory reactions, particularly if drug is administered too fast, and that those with pulmonary diseases associated with obstruction or dyspnea are at increased risk for ventilatory depression. Anticipate the risk of hypotension, even when giving drug at recommended rate.

- Monitor patient for hypersensitivity reactions, such as bronchospasm, difficulty breathing, facial edema, and urticaria, especially in patients with a history of asthma, angioedema, or urticaria.
- Anticipate that pentobarbital's CNS effects may exacerbate major depression, suicidal tendencies, or other mental disorders.
- Be aware that pentobarbital may cause paradoxical stimulation (excitement, euphoria, restlessness) in patients with acute pain, children, and elderly or debilitated patients. Elderly or debilitated patients are also more likely to experience such adverse CNS reactions as confusion and depression; monitor these patients closely and take safety precautions.
- Assess hyperthyroid patients for worsened symptoms, such as increased nervousness and palpitations.
- Be aware that barbiturate-induced respiratory depression may cause complications in patients with severe anemia.
- Be aware that drug may trigger signs and symptoms in patients with acute intermittent porphyria.
- If patient shows premonitory signs of hepatic coma, withhold drug and notify prescriber immediately.
- Monitor I.V. site closely and be careful to avoid extravasation. Drug is highly alkaline and may cause local tissue damage and necrosis.
- Store drug at 2° to 15° (36° to 59° F) in a tightly closed container.

PATIENT TEACHING

- Inform patient that pentobarbital is habit-forming.
- Advise patient to avoid potentially hazardous activities until pentobarbital's CNS effects are known.
- Urge patient to avoid alcohol and other CNS depressants because they may increase drug's adverse CNS effects.

perphenazine

Apo-Perphenazine (CAN), PMS Perphenazine (CAN), Trilafon, Trilafon Concentrate

Class and Category

Chemical: Piperazine phenothiazine
Therapeutic: Antiemetic
Pregnancy category: Not rated

Indications and Dosages

▶ *To treat severe nausea and vomiting*

I.V. INFUSION OR INJECTION

Adults and adolescents. 1 mg q 1 to 2 min, up to total of 5 mg.
DOSAGE ADJUSTMENT Initial dose possibly reduced and gradually increased for elderly, emaciated, or debilitated patients. Lower end of adult dosage range possibly needed for adolescents.

Mechanism of Action

Prevents nausea and vomiting by inhibiting or blocking dopamine receptors in the medullary chemoreceptor trigger zone and peripherally by blocking the vagus nerve in the GI tract.

Contraindications

Blood dyscrasias; bone marrow depression; cerebral arteriosclerosis; coma; concurrent use of CNS depressants (large doses); coronary artery disease; hepatic impairment; hypersensitivity to perphenazine, other phenothiazines, or their components; myeloproliferative disorders; severe CNS depression; severe hypertension or hypotension; subcortical brain damage

Interactions

DRUGS

amantadine, anticholinergics, antidyskinetics, antihistamines: Increased adverse anticholinergic effects
amphetamines: Decreased therapeutic effects of both drugs
anticonvulsants: Decreased seizure threshold, inhibited metabolism and toxicity of anticonvulsant
antithyroid drugs: Increased risk of agranulocytosis
apomorphine: Additive CNS depression, decreased emetic response to apomorphine if perphenazine is given first
appetite suppressants (except phenmetrazine): Antagonized anorectic effect of appetite suppressants
beta blockers: Increased blood levels of both drugs and risk of arrhythmias, hypotension, irreversible retinopathy, and tardive dyskinesia

bromocriptine: Possibly interference with bromocriptine's effects
CNS depressants: Increased CNS and respiratory depression, increased hypotensive effects
dopamine: Antagonized peripheral vasoconstriction with high doses of dopamine
ephedrine: Decreased vasopressor response to ephedrine
epinephrine: Blocked alpha-adrenergic effects of epinephrine, possibly causing severe hypotension and tachycardia
hepatotoxic drugs: Increased risk of hepatotoxicity
hypotension-causing drugs: Increased risk of severe orthostatic hypotension
levodopa: Inhibited antidyskinetic effects of levodopa
lithium: Possibly neurotoxicity (disorientation, extrapyramidal symptoms, unconsciousness)
maprotiline, tricyclic antidepressants: Prolonged and intensified sedative and anticholinergic effects of these drugs or perphenazine
metrizamide: Decreased seizure threshold
opioid analgesics: Increased CNS and respiratory depression, increased risk of orthostatic hypotension and severe constipation
ototoxic drugs (especially antibiotics): Possibly masking of some symptoms of ototoxicity, such as dizziness, tinnitus, and vertigo
probucol, other drugs that prolong QT interval: Prolonged QT interval, which may increase risk of ventricular tachycardia
thiazide diuretics: Possibly hyponatremia and water intoxication
ACTIVITIES
alcohol use: Increased CNS and respiratory depression, hypotensive effects, and risk of heatstroke

Adverse Reactions

CNS: Behavioral changes, cerebral edema, dizziness, drowsiness, extrapyramidal reactions (such as akathisia, dystonia, pseudoparkinsonism), fever, headache, neuroleptic malignant syndrome, seizures, syncope, tardive dyskinesia (persistent)
CV: Bradycardia, cardiac arrest, hypertension, hypotension, orthostatic hypotension, tachycardia
EENT: Blurred vision, dry mouth, glaucoma, laryngeal edema, miosis, mydriasis, nasal congestion, ocular changes (corneal opacification, retinopathy)
ENDO: Decreased libido, galactorrhea, gynecomastia, syndrome of inappropriate ADH secretion
GI: Anorexia, constipation, diarrhea, fecal impaction, nausea, vomiting
GU: Bladder paralysis, ejaculation failure, menstrual irregularities,

polyuria, urinary frequency, urinary incontinence, urine retention
HEME: Agranulocytosis, eosinophilia, hemolytic anemia, leukopenia, pancytopenia, thrombocytopenic purpura
RESP: Asthma
SKIN: Diaphoresis, eczema, erythema, exfoliative dermatitis, hyperpigmentation, jaundice, pallor, photosensitivity, pruritus, urticaria
Other: Anaphylaxis, angioedema

Nursing Considerations

- Wear gloves when working with perphenazine because the parenteral solution may cause contact dermatitis.
- Dilute drug to 0.5 mg/ml with sodium chloride for injection. Protect solution from light. Slight yellowing is acceptable, but discard solution if it is markedly discolored or contains precipitate.
- Be aware that some perphenazine solutions contain sulfites. Patients with a history of sulfite sensitivity may be at increased risk for a hypersensitivity reaction.
- Obtain blood samples for CBC and liver and renal function tests, as ordered, to detect adverse reactions.
- Monitor temperature frequently, and notify prescriber if it rises; a significant increase suggests drug intolerance.
- Monitor blood pressure of patient who takes large doses of perphenazine, especially if surgery is indicated, because of the increased risk of hypotension.
- **WARNING** Be alert for possible suppressed cough reflex, which increases patient's risk of aspirating vomitus.
- Monitor patients (especially children) with chronic respiratory disorders (such as severe asthma or emphysema) or acute respiratory tract infections for exacerbations of these conditions caused by perphenazine's CNS depressant effects. Be aware that patients with cardiovascular or renal disease are at increased risk for developing hypotension, heart failure, and arrhythmias.
- **WARNING** If patient develops neuroleptic malignant syndrome (hyperpyrexia, muscle rigidity, altered mental status, autonomic instability), notify prescriber immediately and expect to stop drug and start intensive medical treatment. Watch carefully for recurrence if patient resumes perphenazine therapy.
- Be aware that patient with impaired hepatic function is at risk for decreased perphenazine metabolism or further hepatic dysfunction. If patient has history of hepatic encephalopathy from cirrhosis, watch for increased sensitivity to drug's CNS effects.

- Because of perphenazine's anticholinergic effects, monitor patients with a history of, or predisposition to, glaucoma for signs and symptoms of this disorder, such as eye pain, vision changes, or nausea and vomiting from increased intraocular pressure.
- Be aware that drug should be used cautiously in those who are exposed to organophosphorus insecticides.
- Monitor patients who have been exposed to extreme heat for heatstroke due to drug-induced suppression of temperature regulation. Symptoms include tachycardia, fever, and confusion.
- Be aware that children and elderly patients are at increased risk for developing hypotension amd extrapyramidal reactions, especially if they're acutely ill or debilitated.
- Store drug at 15° to 30° C (59 to 86° F); protect from freezing and light.

PATIENT TEACHING

- Stress the importance of reporting persistent or severe adverse reactions resulting from perphenazine therapy.
- Urge patient to avoid alcohol and other CNS depressants during perphenazine therapy and to avoid potentially hazardous activities until drug's CNS effects are known.
- Advise patient to avoid excessive sun exposure and to protect skin when outdoors.
- Advise patient, especially if elderly, to rise slowly from a supine or seated position to avoid feeling dizzy or faint.
- Inform patient that drug may reduce body's response to heat and cold; advise her to avoid temperature extremes, as in very cold or hot showers.
- Suggest sugarless chewing gum, hard candy, and fluids to relieve dry mouth.
- Urge patient to report sore throat or other signs of infection.

phenobarbital sodium

Luminal

Class, Category, and Schedule

Chemical: Barbiturate
Therapeutic: Anticonvulsant, sedative-hypnotic
Pregnancy category: D
Controlled substance: Schedule IV

Indications and Dosages

▶ *To treat seizures*

I.V. INJECTION
Adults. 100 to 320 mg, repeated as needed and as prescribed. *Maximum:* 600 mg daily.
Children. *Initial:* 10 to 20 mg/kg as a single dose. *Maintenance:* 1 to 6 mg/kg daily.

▶ *To treat status epilepticus*
I.V. INFUSION, I.V. INJECTION
Adults. 10 to 20 mg/kg given slowly and repeated as needed and as prescribed.
Children. 15 to 20 mg/kg over 10 to 15 min.

▶ *To provide short-term treatment of insomnia*
I.V. INJECTION
Adults. 100 to 325 mg h.s.

▶ *To provide daytime sedation*
I.V. INJECTION
Adults. 30 to 120 mg daily in divided doses b.i.d. or t.i.d.

▶ *To provide preoperative sedation*
I.V. INJECTION
Children. 1 to 3 mg/kg 60 to 90 min before surgery.

DOSAGE ADJUSTMENT Possibly reduced for elderly or debilitated patients to reduce confusion, depression, and excitement.

Route	Onset	Peak	Duration
I.V.	5 min	30 min	4 to 6 hr

Mechanism of Action

Inhibits ascending conduction of impulses in the reticular formation, which controls CNS arousal to produce drowsiness, hypnosis, and sedation. Phenobarbital also decreases the spread of seizure activity in the cortex, thalamus, and limbic system. It promotes an increased threshold for electrical stimulation in the motor cortex, which may contribute to its anticonvulsant properties.

Contraindications

Hepatic disease; history of addiction to hypnotics or sedatives; hypersensitivity to phenobarbital, other barbiturates, or their components; nephritis; porphyria; severe respiratory disease with airway obstruction or dyspnea

Interactions

DRUGS
acetaminophen: Decreased acetaminophen effectiveness with long-

term phenobarbital therapy
anticonvulsants (hydantoin): Unpredictable effects on metabolism of anticonvulsant
anticonvulsants (succinimide, including carbamazepine): Decreased blood levels and elimination half-lives of these drugs
calcium channel blockers: Possibly excessive hypotension
carbonic anhydrase inhibitors: Enhanced osteopenia induced by phenobarbital
chloramphenicol, corticosteroids, cyclosporine, dacarbazine, digoxin, metronidazole, quinidine: Decreased effectiveness of these drugs from enhanced metabolism
CNS depressants: Additive CNS depression
cyclophosphamide: Possibly reduced half-life and increased leukopenic activity of cyclophosphamide
disopyramide: Possibly ineffectiveness of disopyramide
doxycycline, fenoprofen: Shortened half-life of these drugs
griseofulvin: Possibly decreased absorption and effectiveness of griseofulvin
guanadrel, guanethidine: Possibly increased orthostatic hypotension
halogenated hydrocarbon anesthetics: Possibly hepatotoxicity
haloperidol: Decreased seizure threshold, decreased blood haloperidol level
ketamine (high doses): Increased risk of hypotension and respiratory depression
leucovorin: Interference with phenobarbital's anticonvulsant effect
levothyroxine, oral contraceptives, phenylbutazone, tricyclic antidepressants: Decreased effectiveness of these drugs
loxapine, phenothiazines, thioxanthenes: Decreased seizure threshold
MAO inhibitors: Prolonged phenobarbital effects, possibly altered pattern of seizure activity
maprotiline: Increased CNS depression, decreased seizure threshold at high doses, decreased phenobarbital effectiveness
methoxyflurane: Possibly hepatotoxicity and nephrotoxicity
methylphenidate: Increased risk of phenobarbital toxicity
mexiletine: Decreased blood mexiletine level
oral anticoagulants: Decreased anticoagulant activity, increased risk of bleeding when phenobarbital is discontinued
pituitary hormones (posterior): Increased risk of arrhythmias and coronary insufficiency
primidone: Altered pattern of seizures, increased CNS effects of both drugs

valproate, valproic acid: Decreased phenobarbital metabolism, increased risk of barbiturate toxicity
vitamin D: Decreased phenobarbital effectiveness
xanthines: Increased xanthine metabolism, antagonized hypnotic effect of phenobarbital
ACTIVITIES
alcohol use: Additive CNS depression

Adverse Reactions

CNS: Anxiety, depression, dizziness, drowsiness, headache, irritability, lethargy, mood changes, paradoxical stimulation, sedation, vertigo
CV: Hypotension, sinus bradycardia
EENT: Miosis, ptosis
GI: Constipation, diarrhea, nausea, vomiting
GU: Decreased libido, impotence, sexual dysfunction
MS: Arthralgia, bone tenderness
RESP: Bronchospasm, respiratory depression
SKIN: Dermatitis, photosensitivity, rash, urticaria
Other: Injection site phlebitis, physical and psychological dependence

Nursing Considerations

- Be aware that phenobarbital shouldn't be given during third trimester of pregnancy because repeated use can cause dependence in neonate. The drug also shouldn't be given to breast-feeding women because it may cause CNS depression in infants.
- Because drug can cause respiratory depression, assess respiratory rate and depth before use, especially in patient with bronchopneumonia, pulmonary disease, respiratory tract infection, or status asthmaticus.
- Be aware that phenobarbital is available as a solution and as a powder that can be reconstituted. Reconstitute sterile powder with the recommended amount of sterile water for injection. Don't use reconstituted solution if it fails to clear within 5 minutes. Use within 30 minutes. Further dilute prescribed dose with normal saline solution or D_5W, and infuse over 30 to 60 minutes.
- Don't give I.V. injection at more than 60 mg/minute to prevent respiratory depression.
- Monitor blood pressure, respiratory rate, and heart rate and rhythm during drug administration. Anticipate an increased risk of hypotension, even when giving drug at recommended rate.

Keep resuscitation equipment readily available. Patients with cardiovascular disease are at increased risk for adverse circulatory reactions, particularly if drug is administered too rapidly. Patients with pulmonary diseases associated with obstruction or dyspnea are at increased risk for ventilatory depression.

- Watch for hypersensitivity reactions, such as bronchospasm, difficulty breathing, facial edema, and urticaria, especially in patients with a history of asthma, angioedema, or urticaria.
- Be aware that I.V. phenobarbital may not reach peak effects for up to 30 minutes. Expect to wait for drug to take effect before a second dose is ordered.
- Be aware that drug may cause physical and psychological dependence.
- Anticipate that phenobarbital's CNS effects may worsen major depression, suicidal tendencies, and other mental disorders.
- Take safety precautions for elderly patients, as appropriate, because they're more likely to experience confusion, depression, and excitement as adverse CNS reactions.
- Be aware that phenobarbital may cause paradoxical stimulation (excitement, euphoria, restlessness) in patients with acute pain, children, and elderly or debilitated patients. Elderly or debilitated patients are also more likely to experience such adverse CNS reactions as confusion and depression; monitor these patients closely and take safety precautions.
- Be aware that drug may trigger signs and symptoms in patients with acute intermittent porphyria.
- Assess hyperthyroid patients for exacerbated symptoms resulting from phenobarbital use, such as increased nervousness and palpitations.
- Be aware that barbiturate-induced respiratory depression may cause complications in patients with severe anemia.
- Store phenobarbital at 15° to 30° C (59° to 86° F), and don't freeze it.

PATIENT TEACHING

- Caution patient about possible drowsiness and reduced alertness. Advise her to avoid potentially hazardous activities until phenobarbital's CNS effects are known.
- Urge patient to avoid alcohol during therapy.
- Inform parents that child may react to phenobarbital with paradoxical excitement. Tell them to notify prescriber if it occurs.
- Instruct female patient to report suspected, known, or intended pregnancy. Advise against breast-feeding during therapy.

phentolamine mesylate

Regitine, Rogitine (CAN)

Class and Category

Chemical: Imidazoline
Therapeutic: Antihypertensive, diagnostic aid, vasodilator
Pregnancy category: Not rated

Indications and Dosages

▶ *To diagnose pheochromocytoma*

I.V. INJECTION

Adults. 2.5 mg as a single dose. After negative result, repeat test with 5-mg dose, as prescribed.

Children. 1 mg as a single dose. After negative result, repeat test with 0.1-mg/kg dose, as prescribed.

▶ *To manage hypertension before or during pheochromocytomectomy*

I.V. INJECTION

Adults. 5 mg 1 to 2 hr before surgery, repeated as needed and as prescribed. During surgery, 5 mg, as ordered.

Children. 1 mg 1 to 2 hr before surgery, repeated as needed and as prescribed. During surgery, 1 mg, as ordered.

▶ *To prevent dermal necrosis or sloughing after extravasation of I.V. norepinephrine*

I.V. INJECTION

Adults, children, and infants. 10 mg/L of I.V. fluid that contains norepinephrine at rate determined by patient response.

Mechanism of Action

Blocks the actions of circulating epinephrine and norepinephrine by antagonizing $alpha_1$ and $alpha_2$ receptors. Phentolamine causes peripheral vasodilation through direct relaxation of vascular smooth muscle and alpha blockade. Positive inotropic and chronotropic effects increase cardiac output. A positive inotropic effect primarily raises blood pressure, but in larger doses, phentolamine causes peripheral vasodilation and can reduce blood pressure.

In patients with pheochromocytoma, phentolamine causes systolic and diastolic blood pressures to fall dramatically. In those without pheochromocytoma, it causes blood pressure to fall or rise slightly or remain the same.

Contraindications

Angina, hypersensitivity to phentolamine or its components, MI

Interactions

DRUGS

antihypertensives: Additive hypotensive effect
dopamine: Antagonized vasopressor activity of dopamine
epinephrine, methoxamine, norepinephrine, phenylephrine: Inhibited alpha-adrenergic effects of these drugs
metaraminol: Possibly decreased vasopressor effect of metaraminol

ACTIVITIES

alcohol use: Additive vasodilation, increased risk of hypotension and tachycardia

Adverse Reactions

CNS: Dizziness
CV: Angina; arrhythmias, including tachycardia; hypotension
EENT: Nasal congestion
GI: Diarrhea, nausea, vomiting
GU: Ejaculation disorders, priapism
MS: Muscle weakness
SKIN: Flushing

Nursing Considerations

- Reconstitute each 5-mg vial of phentolamine with 1 ml of sterile water for injection.
- Use reconstituted solution immediately; don't store unused portion.
- Dilute 5 to 10 mg of reconstituted solution in 500 ml of D_5W.
- Inspect drug for particles and discoloration before administering it.
- When using drug to diagnose pheochromocytoma, withhold all nonessential drugs, as ordered, for at least 24 hours (preferably 48 to 72 hours) before test.
- Before giving an I.V. test dose for pheochromocytoma, place patient in supine position and determine baseline blood pressure by taking blood pressure readings every 10 minutes for at least 30 minutes.
- Expect patient with pheochromocytoma to have excessive hypotension after receiving drug.
- Take safety precautions according to facility policy if patient experiences dizziness.
- Store drug at 15° to 30° C (59° to 86° F).

PATIENT TEACHING

- Instruct patient to move slowly after phentolamine administration to minimize dizziness and avoid falls.

phenylephrine hydrochloride

Neo-Synephrine

Class and Category

Chemical: Sympathomimetic amine
Therapeutic: Antiarrhythmic, vasoconstrictor, vasopressor
Pregnancy category: C

Indications and Dosages

▶ *To manage mild to moderate hypotension*

I.V. INJECTION

Adults. *Initial:* 0.1 to 0.5 mg. *Usual:* 0.2 mg, repeated no more often than q 10 to 15 min, as prescribed.

▶ *To treat severe hypotension or shock*

I.V. INFUSION

Adults. *Initial:* 100 to 180 mcg/min (0.1 to 0.18 mg/min) until blood pressure is stable. *Maintenance:* 40 to 60 mcg/min (0.04 to 0.06 mg/min). Infusion concentration and flow rate, adjusted as prescribed, based on patient response.

▶ *To treat hypotension during spinal anesthesia*

I.V. INJECTION

Adults. *Initial:* 0.2 mg, increased by no more than 0.2 mg, as prescribed. *Maximum:* 0.5 mg/dose.

Children. 0.5 to 1 mg for each 11.3 kg (25 lb).

▶ *To treat paroxysmal supraventricular tachycardia*

I.V. INJECTION

Adults. *Initial:* Up to 0.5 mg by rapid injection; later doses increased to 0.1 to 0.2 mg above preceding dose, as prescribed. *Maximum:* 1 mg/dose.

Route	Onset	Peak	Duration
I.V.	Immediately	Unknown	15 to 20 min

Mechanism of Action

Directly stimulates alpha-adrenergic receptors and inhibits activity of the intracellular enzyme adenyl cyclase, which then inhibits production of cAMP. The inhibition of cAMP causes arterial and venous constriction and increases peripheral vascular resistance and systolic blood pressure. With greater-than-therapeutic doses, phenylephrine directly stimulates beta-adrenergic receptors in the myocardium, which increases the activity of adenyl cyclase and produces positive inotropic and chronotropic effects.

Contraindications

Hypersensitivity to bisulfites, phenylephrine, or their components; severe coronary artery disease or hypertension; use within 14 days of MAO inhibitor therapy; ventricular tachycardia

Interactions

DRUGS

alpha blockers, haloperidol, loxapine, phenothiazines, thioxanthenes: Possibly decreased vasoconstrictor effect of phenylephrine
antihypertensives, diuretics: Possibly decreased antihypertensive effects
atropine, methylphenidate: Possibly enhanced vasopressor effect of phenylephrine
beta blockers: Decreased therapeutic effects of both drugs
bretylium: Possibly potentiated vasopressor effect and arrhythmias
doxapram: Increased vasopressor effect of both drugs
ergot alkaloids: Possibly cerebral blood vessel rupture, increased vasopressor effect, peripheral vascular ischemia, and gangrene (with ergotamine)
guanadrel, guanethidine: Increased vasopressor effect of phenylephrine, increased risk of severe hypertension and arrhythmias
hydrocarbon inhalation anesthetics: Increased risk of serious arrhythmias
MAO inhibitors: Increased and prolonged cardiac stimulation, increased vasopressor effect, increased risk of severe cardiovascular and cerebrovascular effects, hyperpyrexia, vomiting
maprotiline, tricyclic antidepressants: Increased risk of severe cardiovascular effects (including arrhythmias, hyperpyrexia, severe hypertension); possibly increased or decreased sensitivity to phenylephrine
mecamylamine, methyldopa: Decreased hypotensive effects of these drugs, increased vasopressor effect of phenylephrine
nitrates: Possibly decreased vasopressor effect of phenylephrine and decreased antianginal effect of nitrates
other sympathomimetics (such as dopamine and isoproterenol): Possibly increased cardiovascular effects or adverse reactions
oxytocin: Possibly severe, persistent hypertension
phenoxybenzamine: Decreased vasoconstrictor effect of phenylephrine, possibly hypotension and tachycardia
thyroid hormones: Increased cardiovascular effects of both drugs

Adverse Reactions

CNS: Dizziness, headache, insomnia, nervousness, paresthesia, restlessness, tremor, weakness

CV: Angina, bradycardia, hypertension, hypotension, palpitations, peripheral vasoconstriction that may lead to necrosis or gangrene, tachycardia, ventricular arrhythmias
GI: Nausea, vomiting
RESP: Dyspnea
SKIN: Extravasation with tissue necrosis and sloughing, pallor
Other: Allergic reaction

Nursing Considerations

- Be aware that phenylephrine may not be prescribed for patients with occlusive vascular disease, such as atherosclerosis, Buerger's disease, diabetic endarteritis, or Raynaud's disease, because of the risk of decreased peripheral circulation.
- For I.V. use, dilute with D_5W or sodium chloride for injection and prepare as prescribed—usually 10 mg/500 ml. Administer infusions using an infusion pump to ensure appropriate administration rate.
- Assess for signs and symptoms of angina, arrhythmias, and hypertension because phenylephrine may increase myocardial oxygen demand and the risk of proarrhythmias and blood pressure changes.
- **WARNING** Monitor patient with thyroid disease for increased sensitivity to catecholamines and, possibly, thyrotoxicity or cardiotoxicity.
- **WARNING** Be aware that extravasation may cause tissue necrosis, gangrene, and other reactions around injection site. If extravasation occurs, expect to use phentolamine to antagonize vasoconstriction and minimize sloughing and tissue necrosis.
- Store drug at 15° to 30° C (59° to 86° F); protect from freezing and light.

PATIENT TEACHING

- Advise patient to avoid potentially hazardous activities until phenylephrine's CNS effects are known.

phenytoin sodium

Dilantin

Class and Category

Chemical: Hydantoin derivative
Therapeutic: Anticonvulsant
Pregnancy category: C

Indications and Dosages

▶ *To treat status epilepticus*

I.V. INJECTION

Adults and adolescents. *Initial:* 15 to 20 mg/kg by slow push in 50 ml of sodium chloride for injection at a rate not to exceed 50 mg/min. *Maintenance:* Beginning within 12 to 24 hr of initial dose, 100 mg q 6 to 8 hr or 5 mg/kg daily P.O. in divided doses b.i.d. to q.i.d.

Children. 15 to 20 mg/kg at no more than 1 mg/kg/min. *Maximum:* 50 mg/min.

DOSAGE ADJUSTMENT For elderly or very ill patients and those with cardiovascular or hepatic disease, dosage reduced to 25 mg/min, as prescribed, or possibly to as low as 5 to 10 mg/min to reduce the risk of adverse reactions.

▶ *To prevent or treat seizures during neurosurgery*

I.V. INJECTION

Adults. 100 to 200 mg q 4 hr at a rate not to exceed 50 mg/min during or immediately after neurosurgery.

Mechanism of Action

Limits the spread of seizure activity and the start of new seizures by regulating voltage-dependent sodium and calcium channels in neurons, inhibiting calcium movement across neuronal membranes, and enhancing sodium–potassium–adenosine triphosphatase activity in neurons and glial cells. These actions all help stabilize the neurons.

Incompatibilities

Don't mix phenytoin in same syringe with any other drugs or with any I.V. solutions other than sodium chloride for injection because a precipitate will form.

Contraindications

Adams-Stokes syndrome, hypersensitivity to phenytoin or its components, SA block, second- or third-degree heart block, sinus bradycardia

Interactions

DRUGS

acetaminophen: Possibly hepatoxicity, decreased acetaminophen effects

activated charcoal, antacids, calcium salts, enteral feedings, sucralfate: Decreased absorption of oral phenytoin
allopurinol, benzodiazepines, chloramphenicol, cimetidine, disulfiram, fluconazole, isoniazid, itraconazole, methylphenidate, metronidazole, miconazole, omeprazole, phenacemide, ranitidine, sulfonamides, trazodone, trimethoprim: Decreased metabolism and increased effects of phenytoin
amiodarone, ticlopidine: Possibly increased blood phenytoin level
antifungals (azole): Increased blood phenytoin level, decreased blood antifungal level
antineoplastics, nitrofurantoin, pyridoxine: Decreased phenytoin effects
barbiturates: Variable effects on blood phenytoin level
bupropion, clozapine, loxapine, MAO inhibitors, maprotiline, molindone, phenothiazines, pimozide, thioxanthenes, tricyclic antidepressants: Decreased seizure threshold, decreased anticonvulsant effect of phenytoin
calcium channel blockers: Increased metabolism and decreased effects of these drugs, possibly increased blood phenytoin level
carbamazepine: Decreased blood level and effects of carbamazepine, possibly phenytoin toxicity
carbonic anhydrase inhibitors: Increased risk of osteopenia from phenytoin
chlordiazepoxide, diazepam: Possibly increased blood phenytoin level, decreased effects of these drugs
clonazepam: Possibly decreased blood level and effects of clonazepam, possibly phenytoin toxicity
corticosteroids, cyclosporine, dicumarol, digoxin, disopyramide, doxycycline, estrogens, furosemide, lamotrigine, levodopa, methadone, metyrapone, mexiletine, oral contraceptives, quinidine, sirolimus, tacrolimus, theophylline: Increased metabolism and decreased effects of these drugs
dopamine: Increased risk of severe hypotension and bradycardia
fluoxetine: Increased blood phenytoin level and risk of phenytoin toxicity
folic acid, leucovorin: Decreased blood phenytoin level, increased risk of seizures
haloperidol: Decreased effects of haloperidol, decreased anticonvulsant effect of phenytoin
halothane anesthetics: Increased risk of hepatotoxicity and phenytoin toxicity
ifosfamide: Decreased phenytoin effects, possibly increased toxicity
influenza virus vaccine: Possibly decreased phenytoin effects

insulin, oral antidiabetic drugs: Possibly hyperglycemia, increased blood phenytoin level (with tolbutamide)
levonorgestrel, mebendazole, streptozocin, sulfonylureas: Decreased effects of these drugs
lidocaine, propranolol (possibly other beta blockers): Increased cardiac depressant effects, possibly decreased blood level and increased adverse effects of phenytoin
lithium: Increased risk of lithium toxicity, increased risk of neurologic symptoms with normal blood lithium level
meperidine: Increased metabolism and decreased effects of meperidine, possibly meperidine toxicity
methadone: Possibly increased metabolism of methadone and withdrawal symptoms
neuromuscular blockers: Shorter duration of action and decreased effects of neuromuscular blockers
oral anticoagulants: Decreased metabolism and increased effects of phenytoin; early increase in anticoagulant effect followed by decrease
paroxetine: Decreased bioavailability of both drugs
phenylbutazone, salicylates: Increased phenytoin effects, possibly phenytoin toxicity
primidone: Increased primidone effects, possibly primidone toxicity
rifampin: Increased hepatic metabolism of phenytoin
valproic acid: Possibly decreased phenytoin metabolism, resulting in increased phenytoin effects; possibly decreased blood valproic acid level
vitamin D: Possibly decreased vitamin D effects, resulting in rickets or osteomalacia (with long-term use of phenytoin)
ACTIVITIES
alcohol use: Additive CNS depression, increased phenytoin clearance

Adverse Reactions

CNS: Ataxia, confusion, depression, dizziness, drowsiness, excitement, fever, headache, involuntary motor activity, lethargy, nervousness, peripheral neuropathy, restlessness, slurred speech, tremor, weakness
CV: Cardiac arrest, hypotension, vasculitis
EENT: Amblyopia, conjunctivitis, diplopia, earache, epistaxis, eye pain, gingival hyperplasia, hearing loss, loss of taste, nystagmus, pharyngitis, photophobia, rhinitis, sinusitis, taste perversion, tinnitus
ENDO: Gynecomastia, hyperglycemia
GI: Abdominal pain, anorexia, constipation, diarrhea, epigastric

pain, hepatic dysfunction, hepatic necrosis, hepatitis, nausea, vomiting
GU: Glycosuria, priapism, renal failure
HEME: Acute intermittent porphyria (exacerbation), agranulocytosis, anemia, eosinophilia, leukopenia, pancytopenia, thrombocytopenia
MS: Arthralgia, arthropathy, bone fractures, muscle twitching, osteomalacia, polymyositis
RESP: Apnea, asthma, bronchitis, cough, dyspnea, hypoxia, increased sputum production, pneumonia, pneumothorax, pulmonary fibrosis
SKIN: Exfoliative dermatitis, jaundice, maculopapular or morbilliform rash, purpuric dermatitis, Stevens-Johnson syndrome, toxic epidermal necrolysis, unusual hair growth, urticaria
Other: Facial feature enlargement, injection site pain, lupuslike symptoms, lymphadenopathy, polyarteritis, weight gain or loss

Nursing Considerations

- Be aware that preferred administration routes for phenytoin are I.V. injection and oral. Phenytoin has a variable absorption rate when administered by I.M. route.
- Inspect I.V. form for particles and discoloration before administering.
- Administer I.V. injection through a large vein, using a large-gauge needle or an I.V. catheter.
- **WARNING** Avoid rapid I.V. injection because it may cause cardiac arrest, CNS depression, or severe hypotension. Administer at a rate not to exceed 50 mg/minute.
- To decrease vein irritation, follow I.V. injection with flush of sodium chloride for injection through same I.V. catheter.
- Continuously monitor ECG tracings and blood pressure when administering I.V. phenytoin.
- Frequently assess I.V. site for signs of extravasation because drug can cause tissue necrosis.
- Administer oral phenytoin at least 2 hours before or after antacids and calcium salts.
- If patient has difficulty swallowing, open prompt (rapid-release) capsules and mix contents with food or fluid.
- Shake oral suspension before measuring dose, and use a calibrated measuring device.
- To minimize GI distress, give phenytoin with or just after meals.
- If patient has an NG tube in place, minimize drug absorption by polyvinyl chloride tubing by diluting suspension threefold with

sodium chloride for injection, D_5W, or sterile water. After administering drug, flush tube with at least 20 ml of diluent.
- Expect continuous enteral feedings to disrupt phenytoin absorption and, possibly, reduce blood phenytoin level. Discontinue tube feedings 1 to 2 hours before and after phenytoin administration, as prescribed. Anticipate increasing phenytoin dosage, as prescribed, to compensate for reduced bioavailability during continuous tube feedings.
- Monitor blood phenytoin level. Therapeutic level ranges from 10 to 20 mg/L.
- **WARNING** Monitor hematologic status during therapy because phenytoin can cause blood dyscrasias. Patients with a history of agranulocytosis, leukopenia, or pancytopenia may have an increased risk of infection because phenytoin can cause myelosuppression.
- Anticipate that drug may worsen intermittent porphyria.
- Frequently monitor blood glucose level of patient with diabetes mellitus because drug can stimulate glucagon and impair insulin secretion, either of which can raise blood glucose level.
- Monitor blood thyroid hormone levels of patients receiving thyroid replacement therapy, as appropriate, because phenytoin may decrease circulating thyroid hormone levels and increase thyroid-stimulating hormone level.
- Be aware that long-term phenytoin therapy may increase patient's requirements for folic acid or vitamin D supplements. However, keep in mind that a diet high in folic acid may decrease seizure control.
- Store drug at 15° to 30° C (59° to 86° F); don't freeze.

PATIENT TEACHING
- Caution patient to avoid potentially hazardous activities until phenytoin's CNS effects are known.
- Explain to patient with diabetes mellitus that she may be at increased risk for hyperglycemia and may need an increased dosage of antidiabetic drug during phenytoin therapy. Inform her that her blood glucose level will be monitored frequently.
- Instruct patient to crush or thoroughly chew phenytoin chewable tablets or to shake oral solution well before swallowing.
- Advise patient to take drug exactly as prescribed and not to change brands or dosage or stop taking drug unless instructed by prescriber.
- Instruct patient to avoid taking antacids or calcium products within 2 hours of oral phenytoin.

- Urge patient to avoid alcohol during phenytoin therapy.
- Stress the importance of good oral hygiene, and encourage patient to inform her dentist that she's taking phenytoin.
- Encourage patient to carry medical identification indicating her diagnosis and drug therapy.

physostigmine salicylate

Antilirium

Class and Category

Chemical: Salicylic acid derivative
Therapeutic: Anticholinergic antidote, cholinesterase inhibitor
Pregnancy category: Not rated

Indications and Dosages

▶ *To counteract toxic anticholinergic effects (anticholinergic syndrome)*

I.V. INJECTION

Adults and adolescents. 0.5 to 2 mg at no more than 1 mg/min; then 1 to 4 mg, repeated q 20 to 30 min as needed and as prescribed.

Children. 0.02 mg/kg at a rate not to exceed 0.5 mg/min, repeated q 5 to 10 min as needed and as prescribed. *Maximum:* 2 mg/dose.

Route	Onset	Peak	Duration
I.V.	3 to 8 min	5 min	30 to 60 min

Mechanism of Action

Inhibits the destruction of acetylcholine by acetylcholinesterase. This action increases the concentration of acetylcholine at cholinergic transmission sites and prolongs and exaggerates the effects of acetylcholine that are blocked by toxic doses of anticholinergics.

Contraindications

Asthma; cardiovascular disease; diabetes mellitus; gangrene; GI or GU obstruction; hypersensitivity to physostigmine, sulfites, or their components

Interactions

DRUGS

choline esters: Enhanced effects of carbachol and bethanechol with

concurrent use of physostigmine, enhanced effects of acetylcholine and methacholine with prior use of physostigmine
succinylcholine: Prolonged neuromuscular paralysis

Adverse Reactions

CNS: CNS stimulation, fatigue, hallucinations, restlessness, seizures (with too-rapid administration), weakness
CV: Bradycardia (with too-rapid administration), irregular heartbeat, palpitations
EENT: Increased salivation, lacrimation, miosis
GI: Abdominal pain, diarrhea, nausea, vomiting
GU: Urinary urgency
MS: Muscle twitching
RESP: Bronchospasm, chest tightness, dyspnea (with too-rapid administration), increased bronchial secretions, wheezing
SKIN: Diaphoresis

Nursing Considerations

- Avoid rapid administration of physostigmine because it may lead to bradycardia, respiratory distress, or seizures.
- Frequently monitor pulse and respiratory rates, blood pressure, and neurologic status during therapy.
- Monitor ECG tracing during drug administration. Patients with a history of bradycardia may be at increased risk for drug-induced bradycardia.
- Closely monitor patients with asthma for an asthma attack; drug may precipitate an attack by causing bronchoconstriction.
- Monitor for drug-induced seizures due to drug's CNS-stimulating effects in patients with a history of seizures.
- Assess patients with Parkinson's disease for increased tremors, akinesia, or rigidity.
- **WARNING** Be alert for signs of a life-threatening cholinergic crisis, which may indicate a physostigmine overdose: confusion, diaphoresis, hypotension, miosis, muscle weakness, nausea, paralysis (including respiratory paralysis), salivation, seizures, sinus bradycardia, and vomiting. If you detect such signs, prepare to give atropine (the antidote) and use resuscitation equipment. Keep in mind that atropine counteracts only muscarinic cholinergic effects; paralytic effects may continue.
- Store drug at 15° to 30° C (59° to 86° F); protect from freezing and light.

PATIENT TEACHING

- Reassure patient that her vital signs will be monitored frequently during physostigmine administration to help prevent or detect adverse reactions.
- Instruct patient to notify prescriber immediately about signs of cholinergic crisis.

piperacillin sodium

Pipracil

Class and Category

Chemical: Piperazine derivative of ampicillin, acylureidopenicillin
Therapeutic: Antibiotic
Pregnancy category: B

Indications and Dosages

▶ *To treat moderate to severe bacterial infections, including bone and joint infections, gynecologic infections, intra-abdominal infections, lower respiratory tract infections, septicemia, and skin and soft-tissue infections, caused by susceptible strains of* Acinetobacter *sp., anaerobic cocci,* Bacteroides *sp.,* Enterobacter *sp.,* Escherichia coli, Haemophilus influenzae, Klebsiella *sp.,* Proteus *sp.,* Pseudomonas aeruginosa, *and* Serratia *sp.*

I.V. INFUSION

Adults and adolescents. 12 to 18 g daily or 200 to 300 mg/kg daily in divided doses q 4 to 6 hr. *Maximum:* 24 g daily.

▶ *To treat bacterial meningitis*

I.V. INFUSION

Adults and adolescents. 4 g q 4 hr or 75 mg/ kg q 6 hr. *Maximum:* 24 g daily.

▶ *To treat uncomplicated UTI and community-acquired pneumonia caused by susceptible organisms, including* E. coli, Klebsiella *sp., and* Serratia *sp.*

I.V. INFUSION

Adults. 6 to 8 g daily or 100 to 125 mg/kg daily in divided doses q 6 to 12 hr.

▶ *To treat complicated UTI caused by susceptible organisms, including* Acinetobacter *sp.,* Klebsiella *sp., and* Serratia *sp.*

I.V. INFUSION

Adults. 8 to 16 g daily or 125 to 200 mg/kg daily in divided doses q 6 to 8 hr.

I.V. INFUSION

Adults. 2 g 20 to 30 min before anesthesia, 2 g during surgery, and 2 g q 6 hr for 24 hr after surgery.

▶ *To provide surgical prophylaxis in abdominal hysterectomy*

I.V. INFUSION

Adults. 2 g 20 to 30 min before anesthesia, 2 g just after surgery, and 2 g 6 hr later.

▶ *To provide surgical prophylaxis in vaginal hysterectomy*

I.V. INFUSION

Adults. 2 g 20 to 30 min before anesthesia, then 2 g 6 and 12 hr after initial dose.

▶ *To provide surgical prophylaxis in cesarean section*

I.V. INFUSION

Adults. 2 g after cord is clamped, then 2 g 4 and 8 hr after initial dose.

Mechanism of Action

Binds to specific penicillin-binding proteins and inhibits the third and final stage of bacterial cell wall synthesis by interfering with an autolysin inhibitor. Uninhibited autolytic enzymes destroy the cell wall and result in cell lysis.

Incompatibilities

Don't mix piperacillin sodium in same container with aminoglycosides because of chemical incompatibility (depending on concentrations, diluents, pH, and temperature). Don't mix with solutions that contain only sodium bicarbonate because of chemical instability.

Contraindications

Hypersensitivity to cephalosporins, penicillins, or their components

Interactions

DRUGS

aminoglycosides: Additive or synergistic effects against some bacteria, possibly mutual inactivation

anti-inflammatory drugs (including aspirin and NSAIDs), heparin, oral anticoagulants, platelet aggregation inhibitors, sulfinpyrazone, thrombolytics: Increased risk of bleeding

hepatotoxic drugs (including labetalol and rifampin): Increased risk of hepatotoxicity

methotrexate: Increased blood methotrexate level and risk of toxicity
probenecid: Increased blood piperacillin level and risk of toxicity
vecuronium: Possibly prolonged perioperative neuromuscular blockade of vecuronium

Adverse Reactions

CNS: CVA, dizziness, fever, hallucinations, headache, lethargy, seizures
CV: Cardiac arrest, hypotension, palpitations, tachycardia, vasodilation, vasovagal reactions
EENT: Oral candidiasis, pharyngitis
GI: Diarrhea, epigastric distress, intestinal necrosis, nausea, pseudomembranous colitis, vomiting
GU: Hematuria, impotence, nephritis, neurogenic bladder, priapism, proteinuria, renal failure, vaginal candidiasis
HEME: Agranulocytosis, eosinophilia, hemolytic anemia, leukopenia, neutropenia, pancytopenia, prolonged bleeding time, thrombocytopenia
MS: Arthralgia
RESP: Dyspnea, pulmonary embolism, pulmonary hypertension
SKIN: Exfoliative dermatitis, mottling, rash, toxic epidermal necrolysis, urticaria
Other: Anaphylaxis; facial edema; hypokalemia; hyponatremia; injection site pain, phlebitis, and skin ulcer; superinfection

Nursing Considerations

- Obtain blood, sputum, or other samples for culture and sensitivity testing, as ordered, before giving piperacillin. Expect to begin piperacillin therapy before results are available.
- Be aware that sunlight may darken powder for dilution but won't alter drug potency.
- For initial dilution for I.V. infusion, reconstitute each gram of drug with at least 5 ml of sterile water for injection, sodium chloride for injection, D_5W, dextrose 5% in normal saline solution, or bacteriostatic water that contains parabens or benzyl alcohol. Shake solution vigorously after adding diluent to help drug dissolve, and inspect for particles and discoloration before giving.
- For further dilution, use sodium chloride for injection, D_5W, dextrose 5% in normal saline solution, lactated Ringer's solution, or dextran 6% in normal saline solution. Solutions diluted with lactated Ringer's solution should be given within 2 hours.
- For intermittent infusion, infuse dose over 20 to 30 minutes.

- Give aminoglycosides 1 hour before or after piperacillin; use a separate site, I.V. bag, and tubing.
- Watch for bleeding or excessive bruising because drug can decrease platelet aggregation. If bleeding occurs, notify prescriber and expect to stop piperacillin.
- Monitor CBC regularly, as ordered, to detect hematologic abnormalities, such as leukopenia and neutropenia.
- Monitor serum potassium level to detect hypokalemia from urinary potassium loss.
- Check for diarrhea (possible pseudomembranous colitis) during and after therapy.
- Watch closely for hypersensitivity reactions, especially if patient has cystic fibrosis. Notify prescriber, and expect to stop drug.

PATIENT TEACHING

- Advise patient to consult prescriber before using OTC drugs during piperacillin therapy because of the risk of interactions.
- Inform patient that increased bruising may occur if she takes anti-inflammatory drugs during piperacillin therapy.
- Advise patient to report signs of superinfection, such as severe diarrhea or white patches on tongue or in mouth.
- Instruct patient to complete full course of therapy, even if symptoms subside.

piperacillin sodium and tazobactam sodium

Tazocin (CAN), Zosyn

Class and Category

Chemical: Piperazine derivative of ampicillin, acylureidopenicillin (piperacillin); penicillinate sulfone (tazobactam)
Therapeutic: Antibiotic
Pregnancy category: B

Indications and Dosages

▶ *To treat moderate to severe gram-negative or anaerobic infections, such as appendicitis, community-acquired pneumonia, diabetic foot ulcers, intra-abdominal infections, pelvic inflammatory disease, peritonitis, postpartum endometritis, and uncomplicated or complicated skin or soft-tissue infections caused by susceptible organisms, such as* Bacteroides *sp. (including many strains of* Bacteroides fragilis*),* Clostridium *sp.,* Enterobacter *sp.,* Enterococcus faecalis, Escherichia coli, Haemophilus influenzae, Klebsiella pneumoniae, Morganella morganii, Neisseria gonorrhoeae, Proteus mirabilis, Proteus vulgaris, Pseudomonas aeruginosa, *and* Serratia *sp.*

I.V. INFUSION

Adults and adolescents. 3.375 g q 6 hr. *Maximum:* 4.5 g q 6 to 8 hr.

▶ *To treat nosocomial pneumonia caused by susceptible organisms*

I.V. INFUSION

Adults and adolescents. 4.5 g q 6 hr in addition to aminoglycoside therapy for 7 to 14 days.

DOSAGE ADJUSTMENT Dosage possibly decreased to 2.25 g q 6 hr for patients with creatinine clearance of 20 to 40 ml/min/1.73 m^2; to 2.25 g q 8 hr for those with creatinine clearance of less than 20 ml/min/1.73 m^2.

Mechanism of Action

Binds to specific penicillin-binding proteins and inhibits the third and final stage of bacterial cell wall synthesis. Piperacillin does this by interfering with an autolysin inhibitor. Uninhibited autolytic enzymes destroy the cell wall and result in cell lysis.

Tazobactam doesn't change piperacillin's action, but it protects piperacillin against Richmond and Sykes types II, III, IV, and V beta-lactamases; staphylococcal beta-lactamases; and extended-spectrum beta-lactamases.

Incompatibilities

Don't mix piperacillin and tazobactam in same container with aminoglycosides because of chemical incompatibility (depending on concentrations, diluents, pH, and temperature), except when using reformulated piperacillin and tazobactam containing EDTA with amikacin and gentamicin.

Contraindications

Hypersensitivity to beta-lactamase inhibitors, cephalosporins, penicillins, piperacillin, tazobactam, or their components

Interactions

DRUGS

aminoglycosides: Additive or synergistic effects against some bacteria, possibly mutual inactivation

anti-inflammatory drugs (including aspirin and NSAIDs), heparin, oral anticoagulants, platelet aggregation inhibitors, sulfinpyrazone, thrombolytics: Increased risk of bleeding

hepatotoxic drugs (including labetalol and rifampin): Increased risk of hepatotoxicity
methotrexate: Increased blood methotrexate level and risk of toxicity
probenecid: Increased blood piperacillin level and risk of toxicity
vecuronium: Possibly prolonged neuromuscular blockade in perioperative period

Adverse Reactions

CNS: Chills, CVA, dizziness, fever, hallucinations, headache, lethargy, seizures
CV: Cardiac arrest, hypotension, palpitations, tachycardia, vasodilation, vasovagal reactions
EENT: Epistaxis, oral candidiasis, pharyngitis
GI: Cholestatic jaundice, diarrhea, elevated liver function test results, epigastric distress, hepatitis, intestinal necrosis, nausea, pseudomembranous colitis, vomiting
GU: Hematuria, impotence, nephritis, neurogenic bladder, priapism, proteinuria, renal failure, vaginal candidiasis
HEME: Agranulocytosis, anemia, eosinophilia, hemolytic anemia, leukopenia, neutropenia, pancytopenia, thrombocytopenia, thrombocytosis
MS: Arthralgia, prolonged muscle relaxation
RESP: Dyspnea, pulmonary embolism, pulmonary hypertension
SKIN: Erythema multiforme, exfoliative dermatitis, mottling, rash, Stevens-Johnson syndrome, toxic epidermal necrolysis
Other: Anaphylaxis, facial edema, hypokalemia, hyponatremia

Nursing Considerations

- Expect to obtain blood, sputum, or other samples for culture and sensitivity testing before giving piperacillin and tazobactam. Therapy may start before tests are complete.
- Be aware that sunlight may darken powder for dilution but won't alter drug potency.
- Reconstitute with sterile water for injection, sodium chloride for injection, D_5W, or bacteriostatic water or normal saline solution that contains parabens or benzyl alcohol.
- For additional dilution (50 to 150 ml except as noted), use appropriate solution, such as sodium chloride for injection, sterile water for injection (no more than 50 ml), D_5W, or dextran 6% in normal saline solution.
- Shake solution vigorously after adding diluent to help drug dissolve, and inspect for particles and discoloration before giving.
- Administer over at least 30 minutes.

- Assess for bleeding or excessive bruising because drug can decrease platelet aggregation, especially in patients with renal failure. If bleeding occurs, notify prescriber and expect to discontinue piperacillin.
- Monitor serum potassium level; hypokalemia may result from urinary potassium loss.
- Monitor patients who need to limit salt intake for fluid retention and unexplained sudden weight gain because piperacillin and tazobactam contains 64 mg of sodium/gram of the drug; at the usual dose, a patient would receive between 768 and 1024 mg of sodium daily. Also monitor elderly patients closely because they may exhibit a blunted natriuresis to excessive salt intake.
- Monitor for diarrhea during or shortly after drug therapy; diarrhea may signal pseudomembranous colitis.
- Give aminoglycosides 1 hour before or after piperacillin and tazobactam; use a separate site, I.V. bag, and tubing.

PATIENT TEACHING

- Instruct patient to take drug for as long as prescribed, even after feeling better.
- Inform diabetic patients who test urine glucose level that drug may alter results of copper reduction tests, such as Clinitest. Advise using a test based on enzymatic glucose oxidase reaction, such as Diastix or TesTape.
- Advise patient to consult prescriber before using OTC drugs during treatment with piperacillin and tazobactam because of the risk of interactions.
- Inform patient that increased bruising may occur if she takes anti-inflammatory drugs, such as aspirin and NSAIDs, during piperacillin and tazobactam therapy.
- Advise patient to notify prescriber about signs of superinfection, such as severe diarrhea or white patches on tongue or in mouth.

polymyxin B sulfate

Aerosporin

Class and Category

Chemical: Bacillus polymyxa derivative
Therapeutic: Antibiotic
Pregnancy category: Not rated

Indications and Dosages

▶ *To treat infections that are resistant to less toxic drugs, such as bacteremia, septicemia, and UTI caused by susceptible organisms, including* Enterobacter aerogenes, Escherichia coli, Haemophilus influenzae, *and* Klebsiella pneumoniae

I.V. INFUSION

Adults and children age 2 and over. 15,000 to 25,000 units/kg daily in divided doses q 12 hr or as a continuous infusion. *Maximum:* 2 million units daily.

Infants and children under age 2. Up to 40,000 units/kg daily in divided doses q 12 hr or as a continuous infusion.

DOSAGE ADJUSTMENT Dosage reduced by 50% for patients with creatinine clearance of 5 to 20 ml/min/1.73 m^2 and by 85% for patients with creatinine clearance of less than 5 ml/min/1.73 m^2.

▶ *To treat meningitis caused by susceptible strains of* Pseudomonas aeruginosa *or* H. influenzae

INTRATHECAL INJECTION

Adults and children age 2 and over. 50,000 units daily for 3 to 4 days; then 50,000 units q other day for at least 2 wk after CSF cultures are negative and glucose content is normal.

Infants and children under age 2. 20,000 units daily for 3 to 4 days, then 25,000 units q other day for at least 2 wk after CSF cultures are negative and glucose content is normal.

Mechanism of Action

Binds to cell membrane phospholipids in gram-negative bacteria, increasing the permeability of the bacterial cell membrane. Polymyxin B also acts as a cationic detergent, altering the osmotic barrier of the cell membrane and causing essential intracellular metabolites to leak out. Both actions lead to cell death.

Incompatibilities

Don't mix polymyxin B sulfate with amphotericin B, calcium salts, chloramphenicol, chlorothiazide, heparin sodium, magnesium salts, nitrofurantoin, penicillins, prednisolone, or tetracyclines because these drugs are incompatible.

Contraindications

Hypersensitivity to polymyxin B or its components

Interactions

DRUGS

general anesthetics, neuromuscular blockers, skeletal muscle relaxants: Increased or prolonged skeletal muscle relaxation, possibly respiratory paralysis

nephrotoxic and neurotoxic drugs (such as aminoglycosides, amphotericin B, colistin, sodium citrate, streptomycin, tobramycin, and vancomycin): Increased risk of nephrotoxicity and neurotoxicity

Adverse Reactions

CNS: Ataxia, confusion, dizziness, drowsiness, fever, giddiness, headache, increased leukocyte and protein levels in CSF, neurotoxicity, paresthesia (circumoral or peripheral), slurred speech
CV: Thrombophlebitis
EENT: Blurred vision, nystagmus
GU: Albuminuria, azotemia, cylindruria, decreased urine output, hematuria, nephrotoxicity
HEME: Eosinophilia
RESP: Respiratory muscle paralysis
SKIN: Rash, urticaria
Other: Anaphylaxis, drug-induced fever, facial flushing, injection site pain, stiff neck (with intrathecal injection), superinfection

Nursing Considerations

- Be aware that patients receiving polymyxin B sulfate are hospitalized to allow appropriate supervision.
- Obtain blood, urine, or other specimens for culture and sensitivity tests, as ordered, before giving drug. Expect to begin polymyxin B therapy before results are known. Keep in mind that baseline renal function tests should have been performed before administration. Check these test results, if available, and notify prescriber of abnormalities.
- For I.V. infusion, dissolve polymyxin B in 300 to 500 ml of D_5W and infuse over 60 to 90 minutes.
- For intrathecal administration, add 10 ml of sodium chloride for injection to vial of polymyxin B.
- Inspect for particles and discoloration before giving drug.
- Monitor renal function, including BUN and serum creatinine levels, during therapy, especially in patients with a history of renal insufficiency.
- **WARNING** Be aware that declining urine output and rising BUN level suggest nephrotoxicity, which also is characterized by albuminuria, azotemia, cylindruria, excessive excretion of

electrolytes, hematuria, leukocyturia, and rising blood drug level. Notify prescriber immediately if you detect any of these signs.

- **WARNING** Notify prescriber immediately if patient experiences blurred vision, circumoral or peripheral paresthesia, confusion, dizziness, drowsiness, facial flushing, giddiness, myasthenia, nystagmus, or slurred speech. These may be signs of neurotoxicity, a serious adverse reaction that may lead to respiratory arrest or paralysis if untreated.
- Assess for signs of superinfection, such as mouth sores, severe diarrhea, and white patches on tongue or in mouth, especially in debilitated or elderly patients.
- Monitor fluid intake and output, and provide adequate fluids to reduce the risk of nephrotoxicity.

PATIENT TEACHING

- Encourage patient to maintain adequate fluid intake during polymyxin B therapy.
- Instruct patient to immediately report diarrhea, mouth sores, or vaginitis, which may be early signs of superinfection.

potassium acetate

(contains 2 or 4 mEq of elemental potassium per 1 ml of injection)

potassium chloride

(contains 0.1, 0.2, 0.3, 0.4, 1.5, 2, 3, or 10 mEq of elemental potassium per 1 ml of injection)

Class and Category

Chemical: Electrolyte cation
Therapeutic: Electrolyte replacement
Pregnancy category: C

Indications and Dosages

▶ *To prevent or treat hypokalemia in patients who can't ingest sufficient dietary potassium or who are losing potassium because of certain conditions (such as hepatic cirrhosis and prolonged vomiting) or drugs (such as potassium-wasting diuretics and certain antibiotics)*

I.V. INFUSION (POTASSIUM ACETATE AND POTASSIUM CHLORIDE)

Adults and adolescents with serum potassium level above 2.5 mEq/L. Up to 10 mEq/hr. *Maximum:* 200 mEq daily.

Adults and adolescents with serum potassium level below 2 mEq/L, ECG changes, or paralysis. Up to 20 mEq/hr. *Maximum:* 400 mEq daily.

Children. 3 mEq/kg daily.

DOSAGE ADJUSTMENT Dosage adjusted as prescribed based on patient's ECG patterns and serum potassium level.

Mechanism of Action

Acts as the major cation in intracellular fluid, activating many enzymatic reactions that are essential for physiologic processes, including nerve impulse transmission and cardiac and skeletal muscle contraction. Potassium also helps maintain electroneutrality in cells by controlling the exchange of intracellular and extracellular ions. It also helps maintain normal renal function and acid-base balance.

Incompatibilities

Don't mix potassium chloride for injection in same syringe with amino acid solutions, lipid solutions, or mannitol because these drugs may precipitate from solution. Administration with blood or blood products can cause lysis of infused RBCs.

Contraindications

Acute dehydration, Addison's disease (untreated), concurrent use of potassium-sparing diuretics, crush syndrome, heat cramps, hyperkalemia, hypersensitivity to potassium salts or their components, renal impairment with azotemia or oliguria, severe hemolytic anemia

Interactions

DRUGS

ACE inhibitors, beta blockers, blood products, cyclosporine, heparin, NSAIDs, potassium-containing drugs, potassium-sparing diuretics: Increased risk of hyperkalemia

amphotericin B, corticosteroids (glucocorticoids or mineralocorticoids), gentamicin, penicillins, polymyxin B: Possibly hypokalemia

anticholinergics, drugs with anticholinergic activity: Increased risk of GI ulceration, stricture, and perforation

calcium salts (parenteral): Possibly arrhythmias

digoxin: Increased risk of digitalis toxicity

insulin, laxatives, sodium bicarbonate: Decreased serum potassium level

sodium polystyrene sulfonate: Possibly decreased serum potassium level and fluid retention

thiazide diuretics: Possibly hyperkalemia when diuretic is discontinued

FOODS

low-salt milk, salt substitutes: Increased risk of hyperkalemia

Adverse Reactions

CNS: Confusion, paralysis, paresthesia, weakness
CV: Arrhythmias, ECG changes
EENT: Throat pain when swallowing
GI: Abdominal pain; bloody stools; diarrhea; flatulence; GI bleeding, perforation, or ulceration; intestinal obstruction; nausea; vomiting
RESP: Dyspnea
SKIN: Rash
Other: Hyperkalemia

Nursing Considerations

- **WARNING** Be aware that direct injection of potassium concentrate may be immediately fatal. Dilute potassium for injection with an adequate volume of solution before I.V. use. Maximum recommended concentration is 40 mEq/L, although concentrations up to 80 mEq/L may be used for severe hypokalemia. Inappropriate solutions or improper technique may cause extravasation, fever, hyperkalemia, hypervolemia, I.V. site infection, phlebitis, venospasm, and venous thrombosis.
- Infuse potassium slowly to avoid phlebitis and decrease the risk of adverse cardiac reactions. Keep in mind that different forms of potassium salts contain different amounts of elemental potassium per gram and that not all forms are dosage equivalent.
- Monitor serum potassium level before and during administration of I.V. potassium.
- **WARNING** Be aware that some forms of potassium contain tartrazine, which may cause an allergic reaction, such as asthma. Some forms may also contain aluminum, which may become toxic in a patient with impaired renal function.
- Regularly assess patient for evidence of hypokalemia (such as arrhythmias, fatigue, and weakness) or hyperkalemia (such as arrhythmias, confusion, dyspnea, and paresthesia).
- Because adequate renal function is needed for potassium supplementation, monitor serum creatinine level and urine output during administration. Notify prescriber about signs of decreased renal function.

PATIENT TEACHING

- Teach patient how to take her radial pulse, and advise her to notify prescriber about significant changes in heart rate or rhythm.

- Advise patient to watch stools for changes in color and consistency and to notify prescriber if they become black or tarry or bright red from blood.
- Tell patient her serum potassium level will be checked regularly.

potassium phosphates
sodium phosphates

Class and Category
Chemical: Anion, soluble salts
Therapeutic: Electrolyte replenisher
Pregnancy category: C

Indications and Dosages
▶ *To prevent or treat hypophosphatemia*
I.V. INFUSION (POTASSIUM PHOSPHATES)
Adults and adolescents. 10 mmol (310 mg) daily.
Children. 1.5 to 2 mmol (46.5 to 62 mg) daily.
I.V. INFUSION (SODIUM PHOSPHATES)
Adults and adolescents. 10 to 15 mmol (310 to 465 mg) daily.
Children. 1.5 to 2 mmol (46.5 to 62 mg) daily.

Mechanism of Action
Reverses symptoms of hypophosphatemia by replenishing the body's supply of phosphate.

Incompatibilities
Don't add potassium or sodium phosphates to calcium- or magnesium-containing solutions because a precipitate may form.

Contraindications
Hyperkalemia (potassium formulations only), hypernatremia (sodium formulations only), hyperphosphatemia, magnesium ammonium phosphate urolithiasis accompanied by infection, severe renal insufficiency, UTIs caused by urea-splitting organisms

Interactions
DRUGS
ACE inhibitors, cyclosporine, heparin (long-term use), NSAIDs, potassium-containing drugs, potassium-sparing diuretics: Increased risk of hyperkalemia (potassium formulations only)

anabolic steroids, androgens, corticosteroids, estrogens: Increased risk of edema (sodium formulations only)
calcium-containing drugs: Increased risk of calcium deposition in soft tissues
phosphate-containing drugs, vitamin D: Increased risk of hyperphosphatemia
salicylates: Increased blood salicylate level
zinc supplements: Reduced zinc absorption
FOODS
low-salt milk, salt substitutes: Increased risk of hyperkalemia

Adverse Reactions

CNS: Anxiety, confusion, dizziness, fatigue, headache, paresthesia, seizures, tremor, weakness
CV: Arrhythmias, edema of legs, tachycardia
GI: Thirst
GU: Decreased urine output
MS: Muscle cramps or weakness
RESP: Dyspnea
Other: Hyperkalemia, hypernatremia, hyperphosphatemia, hypocalcemia, weight gain

Nursing Considerations

- Avoid mixing potassium or sodium phosphates with solutions containing calcium or magnesium to prevent the formation of precipitates. Dilute phosphates, as prescribed, before administration.
- Monitor serum phosphorus level, as appropriate, of patients with a condition that may be associated with an elevated phosphorus level, such as chronic renal disease, hypoparathyroidism, and rhabdomyolysis; phosphates may further increase serum phosphorus level.
- Monitor serum calcium level, as appropriate, of patients with a condition that may be associated with a low calcium level, such as acute pancreatitis, chronic renal disease, hypoparathyroidism, osteomalacia, rhabdomyolysis, and rickets; phosphates may further decrease serum calcium level.
- Monitor serum potassium level, as appropriate, of patients who receive potassium phosphates and have a condition that may be associated with an elevated potassium level, such as acute dehydration, adrenal insufficiency, extensive tissue breakdown (as in severe burns), myotonia congenita, pancreatitis, rhabdomyolysis, and severe renal insufficiency; they may be at increased risk for hyperkalemia.

- Monitor serum sodium level of patients who receive sodium phosphates and have a condition that may be exacerbated by sodium excess, such as heart failure, hypernatremia, hypertension, peripheral or pulmonary edema, preeclampsia, renal impairment, and severe hepatic disease.
- Monitor ECG tracing frequently during I.V. infusion of sodium phosphates to detect arrhythmias.
- Store drug at 15° to 30° C (59° to 86° F); don't freeze.

PATIENT TEACHING

- Urge patient receiving potassium or sodium phosphates to immediately report muscle weakness or cramps, unexplained weight gain, or shortness of breath.
- Encourage increased intake of fluids (8 oz/hour, if not contraindicated) to prevent kidney stones.

pralidoxime chloride
(2-PAM chloride, 2-pyridine aldoxime methochloride)

Protopam Chloride

Class and Category

Chemical: Quaternary ammonium oxime
Therapeutic: Anticholinesterase antidote
Pregnancy category: C

Indications and Dosages

▶ *As adjunct to reverse organophosphate pesticide toxicity*

I.V. INFUSION, I.M. OR S.C. INJECTION

Adults. *Initial:* 1 to 2 g in 100 ml of normal saline solution infused over 15 to 30 min, given with atropine 2 to 6 mg q 5 to 60 min until muscarinic signs and symptoms disappear; may be repeated in 1 hr and then q 3 to 8 hr if muscle weakness persists. If I.V. route isn't feasible, give I.M. or S.C.
Children. *Initial:* 20 mg/kg in 100 ml of normal saline solution infused over 15 to 30 min, given with atropine (dosage individualized); may be repeated in 1 hr and then q 3 to 8 hr if muscle weakness persists. If I.V. route isn't feasible, give I.M. or S.C.

▶ *To treat anticholinesterase overdose secondary to myasthenic drugs (including ambenonium, neostigmine, and pyridostigmine)*

I.V. INJECTION

Adults. *Initial:* 1 to 2 g, followed by 250 mg q 5 min.

▶ *To treat exposure to nerve agents*

I.V. INJECTION

Adults. *Initial:* 1 atropine-containing autoinjector followed by 1 pralidoxime-containing autoinjector as soon as atropine's effects are evident; both injections repeated q 15 min for 2 additional doses if nerve agent symptoms persist.

DOSAGE ADJUSTMENT Dosage reduced for patients with renal insufficiency.

Mechanism of Action

Reverses muscle paralysis by removing the phosphoryl group from inhibited cholinesterase molecules at the neuromuscular junction of skeletal and respiratory muscles. Reactivation of cholinesterase restores the body's ability to metabolize acetylcholine, which is inhibited by the effects of organophosphate pesticides, anticholinesterase overdose, or nerve agent poisoning.

Contraindications

Hypersensitivity to pralidoxime chloride or its components

Interactions

DRUGS

aminophylline, morphine, phenothiazines, reserpine, succinylcholine, theophylline: Increased symptoms of organophosphate poisoning

barbiturates: Potentiated barbiturate effects

Adverse Reactions

CNS: Dizziness, drowsiness, headache
CV: Increased systolic and diastolic blood pressure, tachycardia
EENT: Accommodation disturbances, blurred vision, diplopia
GI: Nausea, vomiting
MS: Muscle weakness
RESP: Hyperventilation
Other: Injection site pain

Nursing Considerations

- Be aware that pralidoxime must be administered within 36 hours of toxicity to be effective.
- Use drug with extreme caution in patients with myasthenia gravis who are being treated for organophosphate poisoning because pralidoxime may precipitate myasthenic crisis.
- Reconstitute drug according to manufacturer's guidelines and administration route.

- For intermittent infusion, further dilute with normal saline solution to a volume of 100 ml and infuse over 15 to 30 minutes.
- Avoid too-rapid administration, which may cause hypertension, laryngospasm, muscle spasms, neuromuscular blockade, and tachycardia. Also be sure to avoid intradermal injection.
- Closely monitor neuromuscular status during therapy.
- Monitor BUN and serum creatinine levels, as appropriate, in patients with renal insufficiency because pralidoxime is excreted in urine.
- When pralidoxime is administered with atropine, expect signs of atropinization, such as dry mouth and nose, flushing, mydriasis, and tachycardia, to occur earlier than when atropine is given alone.
- Store drug at room temperature.

PATIENT TEACHING

- Inform patient receiving I.M. pralidoxime that she'll experience pain at the injection site for 40 to 60 minutes afterward.
- Reassure patient that she'll be closely monitored throughout therapy.

procainamide hydrochloride

Pronestyl

Class and Category

Chemical: Ethyl benzamide monohydrochloride
Therapeutic: Antiarrhythmic
Pregnancy category: C

Indications and Dosages

▶ *To treat life-threatening ventricular arrhythmias, to treat ventricular extrasystoles and arrhythmias associated with anesthesia and surgery*

I.V. INFUSION OR INJECTION

Adults. *Initial:* 100 mg diluted in D_5W and administered at no more than 50 mg/min. Dosage repeated q 5 min until arrhythmia is controlled or maximum total dose of 1 g is reached. Alternatively, 10 to 15 mg/kg I.V. bolus administered at 25 to 50 mg/min. *Maintenance:* 1 to 4 mg/min by continuous infusion.

DOSAGE ADJUSTMENT For elderly patients or patients with cardiac or hepatic insufficiency, dosage possibly reduced or dosing intervals increased. For patients with creatinine clearance less than 50 ml/min/1.73 m^2, initial dosage reduced to 1 to 2 mg/min.

Route	Onset	Peak	Duration
I.V.	Unknown	Immediate	Unknown

Mechanism of Action

Prolongs the recovery period after myocardial repolarization by inhibiting sodium influx through myocardial cell membranes. This action prolongs the refractory period, causing myocardial automaticity, excitability, and conduction velocity to decline.

Contraindications

Complete heart block, hypersensitivity to procainamide or its components, systemic lupus erythematosus, torsades de pointes

Interactions

DRUGS

antiarrhythmics: Additive cardiac effects
anticholinergics, antidyskinetics, antihistamines: Possibly intensified atropine-like adverse effects, increased risk of ileus
antihypertensives: Additive hypotensive effects
antimyasthenics: Possibly antagonized effect of antimyasthenic on skeletal muscle
bethanechol: Possibly antagonized cholinergic effect of bethanechol
bone marrow depressants: Possibly increased leukopenic or thrombocytopenic effects
bretylium: Possibly decreased inotropic effect of bretylium and enhanced hypotension
neuromuscular blockers: Possibly increased or prolonged neuromuscular blockade
pimozide: Possibly prolonged QT interval, leading to life-threatening arrhythmias

Adverse Reactions

CNS: Chills, disorientation, dizziness, light-headedness
CV: Heart block (second-degree), hypotension, pericarditis, prolonged QT interval, tachycardia
EENT: Bitter taste
GI: Abdominal distress, anorexia, diarrhea, nausea, vomiting
HEME: Agranulocytosis, neutropenia, thrombocytopenia
MS: Arthralgia, myalgia
RESP: Pleural effusion
SKIN: Pruritus, rash
Other: Drug-induced fever, lupuslike symptoms

Nursing Considerations

- Place patient in a supine position before administering procainamide to minimize hypotensive effects. Monitor blood pressure frequently and ECG tracings continuously during administration and for 30 minutes afterward.
- Inspect parenteral solution for particles and discoloration before administering; discard if particles are present or solution is darker than light amber.
- Dilute procainamide with D_5W according to manufacturer's instructions.
- For I.V. infusion, dilute 200 to 1,000 mg of procainamide with 50 to 500 ml of D_5W, respectively, to yield a concentration of 2 or 4 mg/ml.
- Administer I.V. infusion with an infusion pump or other controlled-delivery device.
- Don't administer more than 500 mg in 30 minutes by I.V. infusion or 50 mg/minute by I.V. injection because heart block or cardiac arrest may occur.
- Anticipate that patient has reached maximum clinical response when ventricular tachycardia resolves, hypotension develops, or QRS complex is 50% wider than it was originally.
- If patient is switching to oral form, expect to administer first oral dose 3 or 4 hours after last I.V. dose.
- Before diluting procainamide, store it at 15° to 30° C (59° to 86° F).

PATIENT TEACHING

- Advise patient receiving procainamide to immediately report bruising, chills, diarrhea, fever, or rash.
- Urge patient to obtain needed dental work before therapy starts or after blood count returns to normal, if possible, because drug can cause myelosuppression and increase the risk of bleeding and infection. Stress the need for good oral hygiene during therapy, and urge patient to consult prescriber before scheduling dental procedures.

prochlorperazine edisylate

Compazine

Class and Category

Chemical: Phenothiazine, piperazine
Therapeutic: Antianxiety agent, antiemetic
Pregnancy category: Not rated

Indications and Dosages

▶ *To control nausea and vomiting related to surgery*

I.V. INFUSION OR INJECTION

Adults and adolescents. 5 to 10 mg at no more than 5 mg/ml 15 to 30 min before anesthesia or during or after surgery, as needed. Dosage repeated once, if necessary. *Maximum:* 10 mg/ dose, 40 mg daily.

▶ *To control severe nausea and vomiting*

I.V. INFUSION OR INJECTION

Adults and adolescents. 2.5 to 10 mg at no more than 5 mg/ min. *Maximum:* 40 mg daily.

▶ *To provide short-term treatment of anxiety*

I.V. INFUSION OR INJECTION

Adults and adolescents. 2.5 to 10 mg at no more than 5 mg/ min. *Maximum:* 40 mg daily.

DOSAGE ADJUSTMENT Initial dose usually reduced and subsequent dosage increased more gradually for elderly, emaciated, and debilitated patients.

Route	Onset	Peak	Duration
I.V.	Unknown	Up to 6 mo	Unknown

Mechanism of Action

Alleviates nausea and vomiting by centrally blocking dopamine receptors in the medullary chemoreceptor trigger zone and by peripherally blocking the vagus nerve in the GI tract. In addition, prochlorperazine's anticholinergic effects and alpha-adrenergic blockade reduce anxiety by decreasing arousal and filtering internal stimuli to the reticular activating system.

Incompatibilities

Don't mix prochlorperazine in same syringe with other drugs. A precipitate may form when prochlorperazine edisylate is mixed in same syringe with morphine sulfate.

Contraindications

Age younger than 2 years, blood dyscrasias, bone marrow depression, cerebral arteriosclerosis, coma, coronary artery disease, hepatic dysfunction, hypersensitivity to phenothiazines, myeloproliferative disorders, pediatric surgery, severe CNS depression, severe hypertension or hypotension, subcortical brain damage, use of large quantities of CNS depressants, weight less than 9 kg (20 lb)

Interactions

DRUGS

amantadine, anticholinergics, antidyskinetics, antihistamines: Possibly intensified anticholinergic adverse effects, increased risk of prochlorperazine-induced hyperpyretic effect
amphetamines: Decreased stimulant effect of amphetamines, decreased antipsychotic effect of prochlorperazine
anticonvulsants: Lowered seizure threshold
antithyroid drugs: Increased risk of agranulocytosis
apomorphine: Possibly decreased emetic response to apomorphine, additive CNS depression
appetite suppressants: Possibly antagonized anorectic effect of appetite suppressants (except for phenmetrazine)
astemizole, cisapride, disopyramide, erythromycin, pimozide, probucol, procainamide: Additive QT interval prolongation, increased risk of ventricular tachycardia
beta blockers: Increased risk of additive hypotensive effects, irreversible retinopathy, arrhythmias, and tardive dyskinesia
bromocriptine: Decreased effectiveness of bromocriptine
CNS depressants: Additive CNS depression
dopamine: Possibly antagonized peripheral vasoconstriction (with high doses of dopamine)
ephedrine, epinephrine: Decreased vasopressor effects of these drugs
hepatotoxic drugs: Increased incidence of hepatotoxicity
hypotension-producing drugs: Possibly severe hypotension with syncope
levodopa: Inhibited antidyskinetic effect of levodopa
lithium: Reduced absorption of oral prochlorperazine, increased excretion of lithium, increased extrapyramidal effects, possibly masking of early symptoms of lithium toxicity
MAO inhibitors, maprotiline, tricyclic antidepressants: Possibly prolonged and intensified anticholinergic and sedative effects, increased blood antidepressant levels, inhibited prochlorperazine metabolism, and increased risk of neuroleptic malignant syndrome
mephentermine: Possibly antagonized antipsychotic effect of prochlorperazine and vasopressor effect of mephentermine
metrizamide: Increased risk of seizures
opioid analgesics: Increased risk of CNS and respiratory depression, orthostatic hypotension, severe constipation, and urine retention
ototoxic drugs: Possibly masking of some symptoms of ototoxicity, such as dizziness, tinnitus, and vertigo

phenytoin: Possibly inhibited phenytoin metabolism and increased risk of phenytoin toxicity
thiazide diuretics: Possibly potentiated hyponatremia and water intoxication
ACTIVITIES
alcohol use: Additive CNS depression

Adverse Reactions

CNS: Akathisia, altered temperature regulation, dizziness, drowsiness, extrapyramidal reactions (such as dystonia, pseudoparkinsonism, tardive dyskinesia)
CV: Hypotension, orthostatic hypotension, tachycardia
EENT: Blurred vision, dry mouth, nasal congestion, ocular changes, pigmentary retinopathy
ENDO: Galactorrhea, gynecomastia
GI: Constipation, epigastric pain, nausea, vomiting
GU: Dysuria, ejaculation disorders, menstrual irregularities, urine retention
SKIN: Decreased sweating, photosensitivity, pruritus, rash
Other: Weight gain

Nursing Considerations

- Wear gloves when working with prochlorperazine because the parenteral solution may cause contact dermatitis.
- Be aware that I.V. form may be administered undiluted as an injection or diluted in isotonic solution as an infusion. Don't administer more than 10 mg as a single dose or exceed a rate of 5 mg/minute.
- Be aware that parenteral solution may develop a slight yellowing that won't affect potency. Don't use if discoloration is pronounced or precipitate is present.
- **WARNING** Monitor closely for numerous adverse reactions that may be serious.
- **WARNING** Monitor patients with chronic respiratory disorders (such as severe asthma or emphysema) or acute respiratory tract infections for exacerbations of these conditions caused by prochlorperazine's CNS depressant effects. Be alert for possible suppressed cough reflex, which increases patient's risk of aspirating vomitus.
- Be aware that patients with cardiovascular or renal disease are at increased risk for developing hypotension, heart failure, and arrhythmias.
- **WARNING** If patient develops neuroleptic malignant syndrome (hyperpyrexia, muscle rigidity, altered mental status,

autonomic instability), notify prescriber immediately and expect to discontinue drug and begin intensive medical treatment.

- Be aware that patients with impaired hepatic function are at risk for decreased prochlorperazine metabolism or further hepatic dysfunction. Monitor patients with a history of hepatic encephalopathy from cirrhosis for increased sensitivity to drug's CNS effects.
- Because prochlorperazine may have anticholinergic effects, monitor patients with a history of, or predisposition to, glaucoma for signs and symptoms of this disorder, such as eye pain, vision changes, or nausea and vomiting from increased intraocular pressure.
- Be aware that drug should be used cautiously in those who are exposed to organophosphorus insecticides.
- Monitor patients who have been exposed to extreme heat for heatstroke due to drug-induced suppression of temperature regulation. Symptoms include tachycardia, fever, and confusion.
- Be aware that pediatric and elderly patients are at increased risk for developing hypotension and extrapyramidal reactions, especially if they're acutely ill or debilitated.
- Store drug at less than 30° C (86° F); protect from freezing and light.

PATIENT TEACHING

- Advise patient to rise slowly from a lying or sitting position during prochlorperazine therapy to minimize effects of orthostatic hypotension.
- Instruct patient to avoid potentially hazardous activities because of the risk of drowsiness and impaired judgment and coordination.
- Urge patient to report involuntary movements and restlessness.
- Advise patient to report sudden sore throat or other signs of infection.
- Inform patient that drug may reduce body's response to heat and cold; advise her to avoid temperature extremes, such as very cold or hot showers.
- Suggest sugarless chewing gum, hard candy, and fluids to relieve dry mouth.
- Urge patient to avoid alcohol and OTC drugs that may contain CNS depressants.
- Instruct patient to avoid excessive sun exposure and to wear sunscreen when outdoors.

promethazine hydrochloride

Anergan 25, Anergan 50, Antinaus 50, Histantil (CAN), Pentazine, Phenazine 25, Phenazine 50, Phencen-50, Phenergan, Phenerzine, Phenoject-50, Pro-50, Promacot, Pro-Med 50, Promet, Prorex-25, Prorex-50, Prothazine, Shogan, V-Gan-25, V-Gan-50

Class and Category

Chemical: Phenothiazine derivative
Therapeutic: Antiemetic, antihistamine, antivertigo, sedative-hypnotic
Pregnancy category: C

Indications and Dosages

▶ *To prevent or treat nausea and vomiting in certain types of anesthesia and surgery*

I.V. INJECTION

Adults and adolescents. 12.5 to 25 mg q 4 hr, p.r.n. *Maximum:* 150 mg daily.

▶ *To treat signs and symptoms of allergic response*

I.V. INJECTION

Adults and adolescents. 25 mg, repeated within 2 hr, if needed.

▶ *To provide nighttime, preoperative, or postoperative sedation*

I.V. INJECTION

Adults and adolescents. 25 to 50 mg as a single dose. Alternatively, for preoperative and postoperative sedation, 25 to 50 mg combined with appropriately reduced dosages of analgesics and anticholinergics.

DOSAGE ADJUSTMENT Dosage usually decreased for elderly patients.

▶ *To provide obstetric sedation*

I.V. INJECTION

Adults and adolescents. 50 mg for early stages of labor, followed by 1 or 2 doses of 25 to 75 mg after labor is definitely established, repeated q 4 hr during normal labor.

Route	Onset	Peak	Duration
I.V.	3 to 5 min	Unknown	4 to 6 hr

Contraindications

Age younger than 2; angle-closure glaucoma; benign prostatic hyperplasia; bladder neck obstruction; bone marrow depression;

breast-feeding; coma; hypersensitivity or history of idiosyncratic reaction to promethazine, other phenothiazines, or their components; hypertensive crisis; lower respiratory tract disorders (including asthma) when used as an antihistamine; pyloroduodenal obstruction; stenosing peptic ulcer; use of large quantities of CNS depressants

Mechanism of Action

Competes with histamine for H_1-receptor sites, thereby antagonizing many histamine effects and reducing allergy signs and symptoms. Promethazine also prevents motion sickness, nausea, and vertigo by acting centrally on the medullary chemoreceptive trigger zone and by decreasing vestibular stimulation and labyrinthine function in the inner ear. In addition, it promotes sedation and relieves anxiety by blocking receptor sites within the CNS, directly reducing stimuli to the brain.

Interactions

DRUGS

amphetamines: Decreased stimulant effect of amphetamines
anticholinergics: Possibly intensified anticholinergic adverse effects
anticonvulsants: Lowered seizure threshold
appetite suppressants: Possibly antagonized anorectic effect of appetite suppressants
beta blockers: Increased risk of additive hypotensive effects, irreversible retinopathy, arrhythmias, and tardive dyskinesia
bromocriptine: Decreased effectiveness of bromocriptine
CNS depressants: Additive CNS depression
dopamine: Possibly antagonized peripheral vasoconstriction (with high doses of dopamine)
ephedrine, metaraminol, methoxamine: Decreased vasopressor response to these drugs
epinephrine: Blocked alpha-adrenergic effects of epinephrine, increased risk of hypotension
guanadrel, guanethidine: Decreased antihypertensive effects of these drugs
hepatotoxic drugs: Increased risk of hepatotoxicity
hypotension-producing drugs: Possibly severe hypotension with syncope
levodopa: Inhibited antidyskinetic effects of levodopa

MAO inhibitors: Possibly prolonged and intensified anticholinergic and CNS depressant effects of promethazine
metrizamide: Increased risk of seizures
ototoxic drugs: Possibly masking of some symptoms of ototoxicity, such as dizziness, tinnitus, and vertigo
quinidine: Additive cardiac effects
riboflavin: Increased riboflavin requirements
ACTIVITIES
alcohol use: Additive CNS depression

Adverse Reactions

CNS: Akathisia, CNS stimulation, confusion, dizziness, drowsiness, dystonia, euphoria, excitation, fatigue, hallucinations, hysteria, incoordination, insomnia, irritability, nervousness, neuroleptic malignant syndrome, paradoxical stimulation, pseudoparkinsonism, restlessness, sedation, seizures, syncope, tardive dyskinesia, tremor
CV: Bradycardia, hypertension, hypotension, tachycardia
EENT: Blurred vision; diplopia; dry mouth, nose, and throat; nasal congestion; tinnitus; vision changes
ENDO: Hyperglycemia
GI: Anorexia, cholestatic jaundice, ileus, nausea, vomiting
GU: Dysuria
HEME: Agranulocytosis, leukopenia, thrombocytopenia, thrombocytopenic purpura
RESP: Apnea, respiratory depression, tenacious bronchial secretions
SKIN: Dermatitis, diaphoresis, jaundice, photosensitivity, rash, urticaria
Other: Angioedema, paradoxical reactions

Nursing Considerations

- Use promethazine cautiously in children because they may be more sensitive to drug effects, especially respiratory effects, which may include life-threatening respiratory depression and apnea despite weight-calculated dosage. Also use cautiously in elderly patients and patients with cardiovascular disease or hepatic dysfunction.
- Use drug cautiously in patients with asthma because of its anticholinergic effects and in patients with seizure disorders or those who use medication that may affect seizure threshold because drug may lower patient's seizure threshold.
- **WARNING** Avoid inadvertent intra-arterial injection of promethazine because it can cause arteriospasm; gangrene

may develop from impaired circulation.
- Give I.V. injection at a rate not to exceed 25 mg/min; rapid I.V. administration may produce a transient fall in blood pressure.
- **WARNING** Monitor respiratory function because drug may suppress cough reflex and cause thickening of bronchial secretions, aggravating such conditions as asthma and COPD, and, in rare cases, may depress respirations and induce apnea.
- Monitor patient's hematologic status as ordered because promethazine may cause bone marrow depression, especially when used with other marrow-toxic agents. Assess patient for evidence of infection or bleeding.
- **WARNING** Monitor patient for evidence of neuroleptic malignant syndrome, such as fever, hypertension or hypotension, involuntary motor activity, mental changes, muscle rigidity, tachycardia, and tachypnea. Be prepared to provide supportive treatment and additional drug therapy, as prescribed.
- Be aware that patient shouldn't have intradermal allergen tests within 72 hours of receiving promethazine because drug may significantly alter flare response.

PATIENT TEACHING
- Advise patient to avoid OTC drugs unless approved by prescriber.
- Instruct patient to notify prescriber immediately if she experiences involuntary movements and restlessness.
- Urge patient to avoid alcohol and other CNS depressants while taking promethazine.
- Instruct patient to avoid hazardous activities until drug's CNS effects are known.
- Suggest frequent rinsing and use of sugarless gum or hard candy to relieve dry mouth.
- Advise patient to avoid excessive sun exposure and to use sunscreen when outdoors.

propofol
(disoprofol)
Diprivan

Class and Category
Chemical: 2,6-Diisopropylphenol derivative
Therapeutic: Sedative-hypnotic
Pregnancy category: B

Indications and Dosages

▶ *To provide sedation for critically ill patients in intensive care*

I.V. INFUSION

Adults. 2.8 to 130 mcg/kg/min. *Usual:* 27 mcg/kg/min.

Route	Onset	Peak	Duration
I.V.	Within 40 sec	Unknown	3 to 5 min

Mechanism of Action

Decreases cerebral blood flow, cerebral metabolic oxygen consumption, and ICP and increases cerebrovascular resistance, which may play a role in propofol's hypnotic effects.

Incompatibilities

Don't mix propofol with other drugs before administration. Don't administer propofol through same I.V. line as blood or plasma products because globular component of emulsion will aggregate.

Contraindications

Hypersensitivity to propofol or its components

Interactions

DRUGS

CNS depressants: Additive CNS depressant, respiratory depressant, and hypotensive effects; possibly decreased emetic effects of opioids
droperidol: Possibly decreased control of nausea and vomiting

ACTIVITIES

alcohol use: Additive CNS depressant, respiratory depressant, and hypotensive effects

Adverse Reactions

CV: Bradycardia, hypotension
GI: Nausea, vomiting
MS: Involuntary muscle movements (transient)
RESP: Apnea
Other: Injection site burning, pain, or stinging

Nursing Considerations

- If ordered to dilute propofol before administration, use only D_5W to yield a final concentration of 2 mg/ml or more.
- Consult prescriber about pretreating injection site with 1 ml of 1% lidocaine to minimize pain, burning, or stinging that may occur with propofol administration. Administering drug through

a larger vein in the forearm or antecubital fossa may also minimize injection site discomfort.
- Shake container well before using, and administer drug promptly after opening.
- Use a drop counter, syringe pump, or volumetric pump to safely control infusion rate. Don't infuse drug through filter with a pore size of less than 5 microns because doing so could cause emulsion to break down.
- Discard all unused portions of propofol solution as well as reservoirs, I.V. tubing, and solutions immediately after or within 12 hours of administration (6 hours if propofol was transferred from original container) to prevent bacterial growth in stagnant solution. Also, protect solution from light.
- Be aware that dosage may be reduced for debilitated or hypovolemic patients and in those older than age 55. Propofol is not approved to treat sedation in children.
- Expect patient to recover from sedation within 8 minutes.
- Monitor patients with cardiac disease, peripheral vascular disease, impaired cerebral circulation, or increased ICP for signs of exacerbation because drug may aggravate these disorders.
- Store drug at 4° to 22° C (40° to 72° F); don't refrigerate. Protect from light.

PATIENT TEACHING
- Encourage patient and family to voice concerns and ask questions before propofol administration.
- Reassure patient that she'll be closely monitored throughout drug administration and that her vital functions, including breathing, will be supported as needed.

propranolol hydrochloride

Inderal

Class and Category

Chemical: Beta-adrenergic blocker
Therapeutic: Antiarrhythmic,
Pregnancy category: C

Indications and Dosages

▶ *To treat supraventricular arrhythmias and ventricular tachycardia*

I.V. INJECTION

Adults. 1 to 3 mg at a rate not to exceed 1 mg/min; repeated after 2 min and again after 4 hr, if needed.

Children. 0.01 to 0.1 mg/kg at no more than 1 mg/min; repeated q 6 to 8 hr, as needed. *Maximum:* 1 mg/dose.
DOSAGE ADJUSTMENT Dosage decreased for patients with hepatic insufficiency

Mechanism of Action

Exerts the following effects through its beta-blocking actions:

- prevents arterial dilation and inhibits renin secretion, resulting in decreased blood pressure (in hypertension and pheochromocytoma) and relief of migraine headaches
- decreases the heart rate, which helps resolve tachyarrhythmias
- improves myocardial contractility, which helps ease the symptoms of hypertrophic cardiomyopathy
- decreases myocardial oxygen demand, which helps prevent angina pain and death of myocardial tissue.

In addition, peripheral beta-adrenergic blockade may play a role in propranolol's ability to alleviate tremor.

Contraindications

Asthma, cardiogenic shock, greater than first-degree AV block, heart failure (unless secondary to tachyarrhythmia that's responsive to propranolol), hypersensitivity to propranolol or its components, sinus bradycardia

Interactions

DRUGS

allergen immunotherapy, allergenic extracts for skin testing: Increased risk of serious systemic adverse reactions or anaphylaxis
amiodarone: Additive depressant effects on conduction, negative inotropic effects
anesthetics (hydrocarbon inhalation): Increased risk of myocardial depression and hypotension
antidepressants such as tricyclic agents: Increased risk of hypotension
beta blockers: Additive beta blockade effects
calcium channel blockers, clonidine, diazoxide, guanabenz, resperpine, other hypotension-producing drugs: Additive hypotensive effect and, possibly, other beta blockade effects
cimetidine: Possibly interference with propranolol clearance
estrogens: Decreased antihypertensive effect of propranolol
fentanyl, fentanyl derivatives: Possibly increased risk of initial brady-

cardia after induction doses of fentanyl or a derivative (with long-term propranolol use)
glucagon: Possibly blunted hyperglycemic response
haloperidol: Possibly increased risk of hypotension and cardiac arrest
indomethacin: Possibly reduced effect of propranolol to reduce blood pressure and heart rate
insulin, oral antidiabetic drugs: Possibly impaired glucose control, masking of tachycardia in response to hypoglycemia
lidocaine: Decreased lidocaine clearance, increased risk of lidocaine toxicity
MAO inhibitors: Increased risk of significant hypertension
neuromuscular blockers: Possibly potentiated and prolonged action of these drugs
NSAIDs: Possibly decreased hypotensive effects
phenothiazines: Increased blood levels of both drugs
phenytoin: Additive cardiac depressant effects (with parenteral phenytoin)
propafenone: Increased blood level and half-life of propranolol
sympathomimetics, xanthines: Possibly mutual inhibition of therapeutic effects
thyroxine: Decreased T_3 concentration
warfarin: Increased concentration of warfarin increasing risk of bleeding
ACTIVITIES
nicotine chewing gum, smoking cessation, smoking deterrents: Increased therapeutic effects of propranolol

Adverse Reactions

CNS: Anxiety, depression, disorientation, dizziness, drowsiness, emotional lability, fatigue, fever, hallucinations, insomnia, lethargy, light headedness, nervousness, paresthesia of hands, short term memory loss, weakness
CV: Arterial insufficiency, AV conduction disorders, bradycardia, cardiac arrest, cold extremities, heart failure, hypotension, sinus bradycardia
EENT: Laryngospasm, nasal congestion, pharyngitis, sore throat, visual disturbances
GI: Abdominal pain, constipation, diarrhea, epigastric distress, ischemic colitis, mesenteric arterial thrombosis, nausea, vomiting
GU: Sexual dysfunction
HEME: Agranulocytosis, thrommbocytopenia
MS: Muscle weakness

RESP: Bronchospasm, dyspnea, respiratory distress, wheezing
SKIN: Cutaneous ulcers, erythema multiforme, erythematous rash, exfoliative dermatitis, Stevens-Johnson syndrome, toxic epidermal necrolysis, urticaria
Other: Anaphylaxis, flulike symptoms, systemic lupus erythematosus

Nursing Considerations

- Monitor blood pressure, apical and radial pulses, fluid intake and output, daily weight, respiration, and circulation in extremities before and during propranolol therapy.
- Give I.V. injection at no more than 1 mg/ minute.
- **WARNING Monitor ECG continuously, as ordered, when giving I.V. injection. Have emergency drugs and equipment available in case of hypotension or cardiac arrest.**
- Protect injection solution from light.
- Because drug's negative inotropic effect can depress cardiac output, monitor cardiac output in patients with heart failure, particularly those with severely compromised left ventricular dysfunction.
- Be aware that propranolol can mask tachycardia in hyperthyroidism and that abrupt withdrawal of drug in patients with hyperthyroidism or thyrotoxicosis can precipitate thyroid storm.
- Monitor diabetic patient who is receiving antidiabetic drugs because propranolol can prolong hypoglycemia or promote hyperglycemia. Propranolol also can mask signs of hypoglycemia, especially tachycardia, palpitations, and tremor, but it doesn't suppress diaphoresis or hypertensive response to hypoglycemia.
- **WARNING Be aware that abruptly stopping drug may cause myocardial ischemia, MI, ventricular arrhythmias, or severe hypertension, especially in patients with cardiac disease.**

PATIENT TEACHING

- Advise patient to notify prescriber immediately if she experiences shortness of breath.
- Instruct diabetic patient to regularly monitor blood glucose level and urine for ketones.
- Advise patient to consult prescriber before taking OTC drugs, especially cold remedies.
- Urge patient to avoid potentially hazardous activities until drug's CNS effects are known.
- Advise smoker to notify prescriber immediately if she stops smoking because smoking cessation may decrease drug metabolism, calling for dosage adjustments.

protamine sulfate

Class and Category

Chemical: Simple low-molecular-weight protein
Therapeutic: Heparin antagonist
Pregnancy category: C

Indications and Dosages

▶ *To treat heparin toxicity or hemorrhage associated with heparin therapy*

I.V. INJECTION

Adults and children. 1 mg for each 100 units of heparin to be neutralized, or as indicated by coagulation test results. *Maximum:* 100 mg (within 2-hr period).

Route	Onset	Peak	Duration
I.V.	5 min	Unknown	2 hr

Mechanism of Action

Combines with strongly acidic heparin complex to form an inactive stable salt, thereby neutralizing the anticoagulant activity of both drugs.

Incompatibilities

Don't mix protamine sulfate in same syringe with other drugs unless they're known to be compatible. Several cephalosporins, penicillins, and other antibiotics are incompatible with protamine.

Contraindications

Allergy to fish, hypersensitivity to protamine or its components

Interactions

DRUGS

heparin: Neutralized anticoagulant effect of both drugs

Adverse Reactions

CNS: Weakness
CV: Bradycardia, hypertension, hypotension, shock
GI: Nausea, vomiting
HEME: Unusual bleeding or bruising
RESP: Dyspnea, pulmonary edema (noncardiogenic), pulmonary hypertension
SKIN: Flushing, sensation of warmth
Other: Anaphylaxis

Nursing Considerations

- Expect to administer protamine undiluted. However, dilute drug if needed (for patients other than neonates) with 5 ml of bacteriostatic water for injection containing 0.9% benzyl alcohol.
- **WARNING** When administering drug to neonates or premature infants, reconstitute with preservative-free sterile water for injection. Avoid using solutions that contain benzyl alcohol because they can cause a fatal toxic syndrome in infants, characterized by CNS, respiratory, circulatory, and renal impairment and metabolic acidosis.
- Inject drug slowly at a rate of 5 mg/minute; administer no more than 50 mg in 10 minutes or 100 mg in 2 hours.
- Discard any unused portion because protamine contains no preservatives.
- **WARNING** Be aware that rapid administration may cause severe hypotension and anaphylaxis.
- Be prepared to obtain coagulation studies (APTT, activated clotting time) 5 to 15 minutes after administering drug and to repeat studies in 2 to 8 hours to assess for heparin-rebound hypotension, shock, and bleeding.
- Monitor vital signs, hemodynamic parameters, and fluid intake and output, and assess for flushing sensation.
- Have fluids—epinephrine 1:1,000, dobutamine, or dopamine—available for allergic or hypotensive reactions.
- Be aware that vasectomized males have an increased risk of hypersensitivity reaction because of possible accumulation of antiprotamine antibodies.
- Store drug at 2° to 8° C (36° to 46° F); don't freeze.

PATIENT TEACHING

- Instruct patient receiving protamine to report adverse reactions immediately.

pyridostigmine bromide

Mestinon, Mestinon-SR (CAN), Mestinon Timespans, Regonol (CAN)

Class and Category

Chemical: Bromide dimethylcarbamate
Therapeutic: Antimyasthenic
Pregnancy category: Not rated

Indications and Dosages

▶ *To treat symptoms of myasthenia gravis*

I.V. INJECTION

Adults and adolescents. 2 mg q 2 to 3 hr.

▶ *To reverse the effects of neuromuscular blockers*

I.V. INJECTION

Adults and adolescents. 10 to 20 mg after 0.6 to 1.2 mg of I.V. atropine has been given.

DOSAGE ADJUSTMENT Dosage possibly reduced for patients with renal impairment.

Route	Onset	Peak	Duration
I.V.	2 to 5 min	Unknown	2 to 4 hr

Mechanism of Action

Improves muscle strength compromised by myasthenia gravis or neuromuscular blockade by competing with acetylcholine for its binding site on acetylcholinesterase. This action potentiates the effects of acetylcholine on skeletal muscle and the GI tract. Inhibited destruction of acetylcholine allows freer transmission of nerve impulses across the neuromuscular junction.

Contraindications

Hypersensitivity to pyridostigmine or its components, mechanical obstruction of GI or urinary tract

Interactions

DRUGS

aminoglycosides (systemic), capreomycin, hydrocarbon inhalation anesthetics, lidocaine (I.V.), lincomycins, polymyxins, quinine: Possibly antagonized effect of pyridostigmine on skeletal muscle; possibly decreased neuromuscular blocking activity of these drugs (with large doses of pyridostigmine)

anticholinergics: Possibly masking of signs of pyridostigmine overdose and reduced intestinal motility

cholinesterase inhibitors: Increased risk of additive toxicity

edrophonium: Possibly worsening of patient's condition

guanadrel, guanethidine, mecamylamine, neuromuscular blockers, procainamide: Possibly prolonged phase I blocking effect or reversal of nondepolarization blockade

local anesthetics: Inhibited neuronal transmission, increased anesthesia effects

quinidine, trimethaphan: Possibly antagonized effects of pyridostigmine

Adverse Reactions

CV: Thrombophlebitis
EENT: Increased salivation, lacrimation, miosis
GI: Abdominal cramps, diarrhea, increased peristalsis, nausea, vomiting
GU: Urinary frequency, incontinence, or urgency
MS: Fasciculations, muscle spasms or weakness
RESP: Increased tracheobronchial secretions
SKIN: Diaphoresis, rash

Nursing Considerations

- **WARNING** Maintain a rigid dosing schedule because a missed or late dose of pyridostigmine can precipitate myasthenic crisis.
- Observe for cholinergic reactions, such as muscle weakness, during drug administration.
- Monitor BUN and serum creatinine levels, as ordered, in patients with renal disease because pyridostigmine is mainly excreted unchanged by the kidneys.
- **WARNING** Be aware that pyridostigmine overdose may obscure the diagnosis of myasthenic crisis because the primary symptom in both is muscle weakness. Respiratory muscle involvement can lead to death. Be prepared to treat cholinergic crisis by immediately stopping pyridostigmine therapy, administering atropine as prescribed, and assisting with endotracheal intubation and mechanical ventilation, if needed.
- Be aware that reversal of neuromuscular blockade usually occurs in 15 to 30 minutes. Be prepared to maintain patent airway and ventilation until normal voluntary respiration returns completely. Assess respiratory measurements and muscle tone with peripheral nerve stimulator device, as indicated.
- Store drug at 15° to 30° C (59° to 86° F); protect from freezing and light.

PATIENT TEACHING

- Instruct patient receiving pyridostigmine to report muscle weakness, difficulty breathing, diarrhea, nausea, or vomiting.
- Ask patient to record pyridostigmine dosage, times taken, and effects to help determine optimal dosage and schedule for her needs.
- Urge patient to carry medical identification describing her condition and drug regimen.

pyridoxine hydrochloride (vitamin B_6)

Beesix, Doxine, Nestrex, Pyri, Rodex, Vitabee 6

Class and Category

Chemical: Water-soluble B complex vitamin
Therapeutic: Nutritional supplement
Pregnancy category: A

Indications and Dosages

▶ *To prevent vitamin B_6 deficiency based on U.S. and Canadian recommended daily allowances (RDAs)*

I.V. INFUSION

Adults and children. Dosage individualized as part of total parenteral nutrition.

▶ *To treat pyridoxine dependency syndrome*

I.V. INJECTION

Adults and children age 11 and over. 30 to 600 mg daily.
Infants with seizures. *Initial:* 10 to 100 mg; then individualized based on severity of deficiency, as prescribed.

▶ *To treat drug-induced pyridoxine deficiency*

I.V. INJECTION

Adults and children age 11 and over. 50 to 200 mg daily for 3 wk; then 25 to 100 mg daily as needed.

Mechanism of Action

Replaces vitamin in pyridoxine deficiency. In erythrocytes, pyridoxine breaks down to pyridoxal and pyridoxamine, which act as coenzymes in fat, protein, and carbohydrate metabolism. Pyridoxine is used to help convert tryptophan to niacin or serotonin, to break down glycogen to glucose-1-phosphate, and to convert oxalate to glycine. It's also essential in the synthesis of both gamma-aminobutyric acid (within the CNS) and heme.

Contraindications

Hypersensitivity to pyridoxine or its components

Interactions

DRUGS

azathioprine, chlorambucil, corticosteroids, cyclophosphamide, cycloserine, cyclosporine, ethionamide, hydralazine, isoniazid, mercaptopurine, penicillamine: Possibly anemia or peripheral neuritis
estrogens, oral contraceptives: Possibly increased RDA of pyridoxine

levodopa: Reversal of levodopa's antiparkinsonian effects

Adverse Reactions

CNS: Sensory neuropathy

Nursing Considerations

- Assess patient's daily intake of pyridoxine, including any OTC sources. If patient has been ingesting high doses (2 to 6 g daily) for several months, assess for sensory neuropathy, characterized by unstable gait and numbness in feet and hands. If symptoms occur, notify prescriber and expect to discontinue drug.
- Evaluate drug's effectiveness in reversing deficiency by assessing for resolution of signs and symptoms, including xanthurenic aciduria, sideroblastic anemia, neurologic problems, seborrheic dermatitis, and cheilosis.
- Store drug at 15° to 30° C (59° to 86° F); protect from freezing and light.

PATIENT TEACHING

- Instruct patient to report unsteadiness while walking or numbness of hands or feet during pyridoxine therapy.
- Inform patient that vitamin is not a substitute for proper diet. Inform her that best sources of dietary pyridoxine include bananas, egg yolks, lima beans, meat, peanuts, and whole grain cereals.

Q·R·S

quinidine gluconate

Class and Category

Chemical: Dextrorotatory isomer of quinine
Therapeutic: Class IA antiarrhythmic
Pregnancy category: C

Indications and Dosages

▶ *To prevent or treat cardiac arrhythmias, including established atrial fibrillation, atrial flutter, paroxysmal atrial fibrillation, paroxysmal atrial tachycardia, paroxysmal AV junctional rhythm, paroxysmal ventricular tachycardia not associated with complete heart block, and premature atrial and ventricular contractions*

I.V. INFUSION

Adults. 800 mg in 40 ml of D_5W at up to 0.25 mg/kg/min.

Mechanism of Action

Depresses excitability, conduction velocity, and contractility of the myocardium and increases the effective refractory period to suppress arrhythmic activity in the atria, ventricles, and His-Purkinje system.

Contraindications

Digitalis toxicity; history of quinidine-induced thrombocytopenic purpura or torsades de pointes; hypersensitivity to quinidine, other cinchona derivatives, or their components; long QT syndrome; myasthenia gravis; pacemaker-dependent conduction disturbances

Interactions

DRUGS

antiarrhythmics, phenothiazines, rauwolfia alkaloids, and other drugs that prolong QT interval: Additive cardiac effects
anticholinergics: Possibly intensified atropine-like adverse effects
antimyasthenics: Antagonized antimyasthenic effects on skeletal muscle

barbiturates, rifampin: Possibly accelerated elimination and decreased effectiveness of quinidine
cimetidine: Increased elimination half-life, possibly leading to quinidine toxicity
digoxin: Possibly digitalis toxicity
hepatic enzyme inducers: Possibly decreased blood quinidine level
hepatic enzyme inhibitors: Possibly increased blood quinidine level
neuromuscular blockers: Possibly potentiated neuromuscular blockade
oral anticoagulants: Additive hypoprothrombinemia, increased risk of bleeding
pimozide: Risk of arrhythmias
quinine: Increased risk of quinidine toxicity
urinary alkalizers (such as antacids, carbonic anhydrase inhibitors, citrates, sodium bicarbonate, and thiazide diuretics): Increased renal tubular reabsorption of quinidine, possibly leading to quinidine toxicity
verapamil: Possibly AV block, bradycardia, pulmonary edema, significant hypotension, and ventricular tachycardia

Adverse Reactions

CNS: Anxiety, asthenia, ataxia, confusion, delirium, difficulty speaking, dizziness, drowsiness, extrapyramidal reactions, fever, headache, hypertonia, syncope, vertigo
CV: Complete heart block, orthostatic hypotension, palpitations, peripheral edema, prolonged QT interval, torsades de pointes, vasculitis, ventricular arrhythmias, widening QRS complex
EENT: Blurred vision, change in color perception, diplopia, dry mouth, hearing loss (high-frequency), pharyngitis, photophobia, rhinitis, tinnitus
GI: Abdominal pain, anorexia, constipation, diarrhea, indigestion, nausea, vomiting
HEME: Agranulocytosis, hemolytic anemia, leukopenia, neutropenia, thrombocytopenia, thrombocytopenic purpura
MS: Arthralgia, myalgia
RESP: Dyspnea
SKIN: Diaphoresis, eczema, exfoliative dermatitis, flushing, hyperpigmentation, photosensitivity, pruritus, psoriasis, purpura, rash, urticaria
Other: Angioedema, flulike symptoms, weight gain

Nursing Considerations

- For intermittent I.V. infusion, dilute quinidine in 40 ml of D_5W and administer using an infusion pump at a rate of 0.25 mg/kg/

minute or less. Rapid administration may cause hypotension. Use diluted solutions within 24 hours if stored at room temperature or within 48 hours if refrigerated. Monitor ECG tracings and blood pressure throughout administration.
- Monitor therapeutic blood level of quinidine, as ordered, in all patients receiving drug.
- Monitor heart rate and rhythm closely because quinidine may cause serious adverse reactions and can be cardiotoxic, especially at dosages exceeding 2.4 g daily. Implement continuous cardiac monitoring, as ordered.
- Monitor serum electrolyte levels, especially potassium, as prescribed to identify electrolyte imbalances, which increase patient's risk of developing adverse cardiac reactions such as torsades de pointes.
- Assess for early signs and symptoms of cinchonism, including blurred vision, change in color perception, confusion, diplopia, headache, and tinnitus, which may indicate quinidine toxicity.
- Before diluting quinidine, store it at 15° to 30° C (59° to 86° F).

PATIENT TEACHING
- Urge patient receiving quinidine to immediately report blurred or double vision, change in color perception, confusion, diarrhea, fever, headache, loss of hearing, or tinnitus.

quinupristin and dalfopristin

Synercid

Class and Category

Chemical: Pristinamycin I and IIa derivative, streptogramin
Therapeutic: Antibiotic
Pregnancy category: B

Indications and Dosages

▶ *To treat serious or life-threatening infections, such as bacteremia, caused by vancomycin-resistant* Enterococcus faecium

I.V. INFUSION

Adults and adolescents age 16 and over. 7.5 mg/kg q 8 hr.

▶ *To treat complicated skin and soft-tissue infections caused by methicillin-susceptible strains of* Staphylococcus aureus *or* Streptococcus pyogenes

I.V. INFUSION

Adults and adolescents age 16 and over. 7.5 mg/kg q 12 hr for at least 7 days.

Mechanism of Action

Inhibits bacterial protein synthesis by irreversibly blocking ribosome functioning. Quinupristin inhibits the late phase of protein synthesis by binding to the 50S ribosomal subunit. Dalfopristin inhibits the early phase of protein synthesis by binding to the 70S or 50S ribosomal subunit. This combined activity also inhibits transfer RNA (tRNA) synthetase activity, which decreases the amount of free tRNA within the cell. Without tRNA, the bacterial cell cannot incorporate amino acids into peptide chains and eventually dies.

Incompatibilities

Don't mix quinupristin and dalfopristin in saline solutions, including normal saline solution, 0.45 normal saline solution, 3% sodium chloride, and 5% sodium chloride, because drug is physically incompatible with these solutions.

Contraindications

Hypersensitivity to quinupristin or dalfopristin, other streptogramin antibiotics, or their components

Interactions

DRUGS

alfentanil, alprazolam, carbamazepine, delavirdine, diazepam, diltiazem, disopyramide, dofetilide, donepezil, erythromycin, ethinyl estradiol, felodipine, fexofenadine, indinavir, lidocaine, lovastatin, methylprednisolone, nevirapine, norethindrone, quinidine, ritonavir, saquinavir, simvastatin, tacrolimus, triazolam, trimetrexate, verapamil, vinblastine: Decreased elimination of these drugs, possibly resulting in toxicity

astemizole, cisapride: Decreased elimination of these drugs, possibly prolonged QT interval

cyclosporine, midazolam, nifedipine: Possibly increased blood levels of these drugs

terfenadine: Decreased elimination and increased blood level of terfenadine, possibly prolonged QT interval

Adverse Reactions

CNS: Anxiety, confusion, dizziness, fever, headache, hypertonia, insomnia, paresthesia

CV: Chest pain, palpitations, peripheral edema, thrombophlebitis, vasodilation

EENT: Oral candidiasis, stomatitis

GI: Abdominal pain, constipation, diarrhea, elevated liver func-

tion test results, indigestion, nausea, pancreatitis, pseudomembranous colitis, vomiting
GU: Hematuria, vaginitis
MS: Arthralgia, gout, muscle spasms, myalgia, myasthenia
RESP: Dyspnea, pleural effusion
SKIN: Diaphoresis, pruritus, rash, urticaria
Other: Injection site edema, inflammation, pain, or thrombophlebitis

Nursing Considerations

- **WARNING** Reconstitute and further dilute quinupristin and dalfopristin only with dextrose in water or sterile water for injection. Don't use saline solutions because drug is physically incompatible with them.
- Reconstitute 500-mg vial (150 mg quinupristin and 350 mg dalfopristin) only with 5 ml of 5% dextrose for injection or sterile water for injection to yield a concentration of 100 mg/ml.
- Swirl gently to mix; don't shake. Let foam dissipate until solution is clear.
- Further dilute reconstituted solution within 30 minutes. Vials are for single use only. Discard any unused portion.
- Dilute prescribed dose in 250 ml of D_5W. Use diluted solution as soon as possible to avoid possible microbial contamination—within 5 hours if stored at room temperature or within 54 hours if refrigerated; don't freeze. Infuse drug over 1 hour through a peripheral I.V. line. If administered by central venous catheter, dilute prescribed dose in 100 ml of D_5W. Central venous administration may decrease incidence of infusion site reaction. Use an infusion pump or device to control rate of infusion.
- Don't flush I.V. catheter with saline or heparin flush solution because of possible incompatibility. Flush I.V. catheter only with D_5W before and after drug administration.
- Monitor patient for diarrhea, a possible indication of overgrowth of normal intestinal flora, such as *Clostridium difficile*. Be aware that pseudomembranous colitis may result from a toxin produced by *C. difficile*.
- If you suspect that patient has pseudomembranous colitis, notify prescriber and expect to stop drug immediately.
- If patient develops pseudomembranous colitis, be aware that drugs that inhibit peristalsis are contraindicated because of the risk of toxic megacolon.
- Assess infusion area for redness or swelling, and ask patient if he feels discomfort. If irritation occurs, expect to change infusion

site, increase amount of diluent to 500 or 750 ml, or administer drug by peripherally inserted central catheter, if ordered.
- Store unopened vials of quinupristin and dalfopristin in refrigerator.

PATIENT TEACHING
- Advise patient receiving quinupristin and dalfopristin to immediately report diarrhea or abdominal pains.
- Emphasize the importance of completing the full course of quinupristin and dalfopristin therapy, as prescribed.
- Inform patient that if he requires long-term therapy, drug will be administered either in the hospital or clinic or by a home health care nurse.

ranitidine hydrochloride

Zantac

Class and Category

Chemical: Aminoalkyl-substituted puran derivative
Therapeutic: Antiulcer agent, gastric acid secretion inhibitor
Pregnancy category: B

Indications and Dosages

▶ *To provide short-term treatment of active duodenal and benign gastric ulcers*

CONTINUOUS I.V. INFUSION

Adults and adolescents. 6.25 mg/hr. *Maximum:* 400 mg daily.

INTERMITTENT I.V. INFUSION

Adults and adolescents. 50 mg diluted to total volume of 100 ml and infused over 15 to 20 min q 6 to 8 hr. *Maximum:* 400 mg daily.

Children. 2 to 4 mg/kg daily diluted to a suitable volume and infused over 15 to 20 min.

I.V. INJECTION

Adults and adolescents. 50 mg diluted to total volume of 20 ml and injected slowly, over no less than 5 min, q 6 to 8 hr. *Maximum:* 400 mg daily.

▶ *To treat acute gastroesophageal reflux disease*

INTERMITTENT I.V. INFUSION

Children. 2 to 8 mg/kg diluted to suitable volume and infused over 15 to 20 min t.i.d.

▶ *To treat hypersecretory GI conditions, such as Zollinger-Ellison syndrome, systemic mastocytosis, and multiple endocrine adenoma syndrome*

CONTINUOUS I.V. INFUSION

Adults and adolescents. *Initial:* 1 mg/kg/hr, increased by 0.5 mg/kg/hr up to 2.5 mg/kg/hr. *Maximum:* 400 mg daily.

INTERMITTENT I.V. INFUSION

Adults. 50 mg diluted to total volume of 100 ml and infused over 15 to 20 min q 6 to 8 hr. *Maximum:* 400 mg daily.

I.V. INJECTION

Adults and adolescents. 50 mg diluted to total volume of 20 ml and injected slowly, over no less than 5 min, q 6 to 8 hr. *Maximum:* 400 mg daily.

DOSAGE ADJUSTMENT For adult patients with creatinine clearance of less than 50 ml/min/1.73 m^2, 50 mg q 18 to 24 hr; dosage interval increased to q 12 hr as needed. Dosage reduction may also be necessary for patients with hepatic dysfunction.

Route	Onset	Peak	Duration
I.V.	Unknown	1 to 3 hr	13 hr

Mechanism of Action

Inhibits basal and nocturnal secretion of gastric acid and pepsin by competitively inhibiting the action of histamine at H_2 receptors on gastric parietal cells. This action reduces total volume of gastric juices and, thus, irritation of GI mucosa.

Contraindications

Acute porphyria, hypersensitivity to ranitidine or its components

Interactions

DRUGS

bone marrow depressants: Increased risk of neutropenia or other blood dyscrasias

diazepam, itraconazole, ketoconazole, sucralfate: Decreased absorption of these drugs

glipizide, glyburide, metoprolol, midazolam, nifedipine, phenytoin, theophylline, warfarin: Increased effects of these drugs, possibly leading to toxic reactions

Adverse Reactions

CNS: Dizziness, drowsiness, headache, insomnia

GI: Abdominal distress, constipation, diarrhea, nausea, vomiting

GU: Impotence

MS: Arthralgia, myalgia

Nursing Considerations

- Be aware that ranitidine must be diluted for I.V. administration if premixed solution is not being used. For I.V. injection, dilute to total volume of 20 ml with normal saline solution, D_5W, $D_{10}W$, lactated Ringer's solution, or 5% sodium bicarbonate. For I.V. infusion, dilute to total volume of 100 ml with any of the above solutions. Use diluted solution within 48 hours if stored at room temperature.
- Administer I.V. injection at no more than 4 ml/minute, intermittent I.V. infusion at 5 to 7 ml/minute, and continuous I.V. infusion at 6.25 mg/hour (except in patients with hypersecretory conditions, for whom initial infusion rate is 1 mg/kg/hour and then gradually increased after 4 hours, as needed, in increments of 0.5 mg/kg/hour).
- Don't introduce additives into premixed solution.
- Stop primary I.V. solution infusion during piggyback administration.
- Store undiluted ranitidine below 30° C (86° F); store premixed form at 2° to 25° C (36° to 77° F). Protect drug from freezing and light.

PATIENT TEACHING

- Instruct patient to report discomfort at ranitidine infusion site.
- Inform patient about potential adverse reactions, such as dizziness, headache, and myalgia, and advise her to report them.
- Inform patient that healing of an ulcer may require 4 to 8 weeks of therapy.

remifentanil hydrochloride

Ultiva

Class, Category, and Schedule

Chemical: Fentanyl analogue
Therapeutic: Anesthesia adjunct
Pregnancy category: C
Controlled substance: Schedule II

Indications and Dosages

▶ *As adjunct to induce general anesthesia*

INTERMITTENT I.V. INFUSION

Adults and children age 2 and over. 0.5 to 1 mcg/kg in addition to inhalation or I.V. anesthetic.

▶ *To maintain general anesthesia*

INTERMITTENT I.V. INFUSION

Adults and children age 2 and over. 0.05 to 0.2 mcg/kg, followed by 0.5 to 1 mcg/kg q 2 to 5 min, as needed.

▶ *To continue analgesic effect in immediate postoperative period*

CONTINUOUS I.V. INFUSION

Adults and children age 2 and over. *Initial:* 0.1 mcg/kg/min, adjusted by 0.025 mcg/kg/min q 5 min, as prescribed, to balance the level of analgesia and the respiratory rate. *Maximum:* 0.2 mcg/kg/min.

▶ *To supplement local or regional anesthesia in a monitored anesthetic setting*

I.V. INFUSION

Adults and children age 2 and over. With a benzodiazepine: 0.05 mcg/kg/min, beginning 5 min before placement of local or regional block; after placement of block, decreased to 0.025 mcg/kg/min and then further adjusted q 5 min in increments of 0.025 mcg/kg/min, as needed. Without a benzodiazepine: 0.1 mcg/kg/min, beginning 5 min before placement of local or regional block; after placement of block, decreased to 0.05 mcg/kg/min and then further adjusted q 5 min in increments of 0.025 mcg/kg/min, as needed.

I.V. INJECTION

Adults and children age 2 and over. With a benzodiazepine: 0.5 mcg/kg administered over 30 to 60 sec as a single dose 60 to 90 sec before local anesthetic is administered. Without a benzodiazepine: 1 mcg/kg administered over 30 to 60 sec as a single dose 60 to 90 sec before local anesthetic is administered.

DOSAGE ADJUSTMENT For elderly patients, starting dose possibly reduced by half. If patient is more than 30% over ideal body weight, starting dose should be based on ideal body weight.

Route	Onset	Peak	Duration
I.V.	1 min	1 to 2 min	5 to 10 min

Incompatibilities

Don't administer remifentanil through same I.V. line as blood because nonspecific esterases in blood products may inactivate drug.

Contraindications

Epidural or intrathecal administration, hypersensitivity to fentanyl analogues

Mechanism of Action

Remifentanil decreases the transmission and perception of pain by stimulating mu-opioid receptors in neurons. This action decreases the activity of adenyl cyclase in neurons, which in turn decreases cAMP production. With less cAMP available, potassium (K^+) is forced out of neurons, and calcium (Ca^{++}) is prevented from entering neurons. As a result, neuron excitability declines, and fewer neurotransmitters (such as substance P) leave the neurons, thereby decreasing pain transmission.

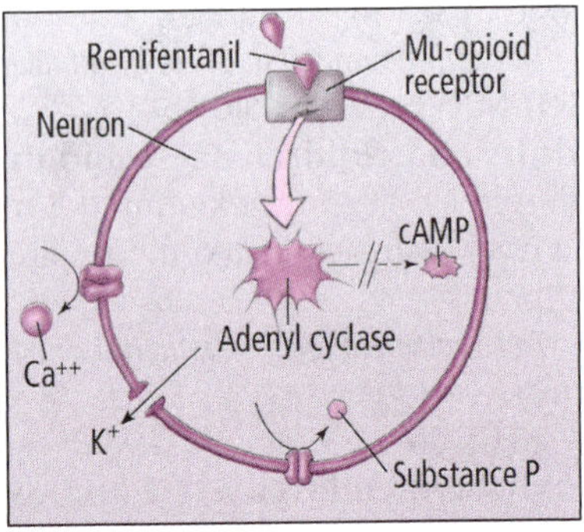

Interactions

DRUGS

anesthetics (barbiturate, inhalation), benzodiazepines, propofol: Possibly synergistic effects, increasing risk of hypotension and respiratory depression
atropine, glycopyrrolate: Possibly reversal of remifentanil-induced bradycardia
ephedrine, epinephrine, norepinephrine: Possibly reversal of remifentanil-induced hypotension
neuromuscular blockers: Prolonged remifentanil-induced skeletal muscle rigidity
opioid antagonists: Possibly reversal of remifentanil's effects

Adverse Reactions

CNS: Headache, shivering
CV: Asystole, bradycardia, hypotension
GI: Nausea, vomiting
MS: Skeletal muscle rigidity
RESP: Apnea, cough, dyspnea, respiratory depression, stridor, wheezing
Other: Anaphylaxis

Nursing Considerations

- Inject remifentanil into I.V. tubing at or as close as possible to venous cannula.
- Use infusion device for continuous infusion.

- Monitor vital signs and oxygenation continuously during administration.
- Expect analgesic effects to dissipate rapidly when drug is discontinued. Expect to start adequate postoperative analgesia, as prescribed, before stopping drug.
- **WARNING** After stopping drug, clear I.V. tubing to prevent inadvertent later administration.
- Monitor respiratory status continuously because of risk of respiratory depression from residual effects of other anesthetics for up to 30 minutes after infusion stops.

PATIENT TEACHING

- Explain expected drug effects to patient, and reassure her that she'll be monitored continuously during drug administration.

reteplase

Retavase

Class and Category

Chemical: Recombinant plasminogen activator (r-PA)
Therapeutic: Thrombolytic
Pregnancy category: C

Indications and Dosages

▶ *To improve ventricular function, prevent heart failure, and reduce mortality after acute MI*

I.V. INJECTION

Adults. 10 units over 2 min; repeated after 30 min.

Mechanism of Action

Converts plasminogen to plasmin, which works to break up fibrin clots that have formed in the coronary arteries. Elimination of the clots improves cardiac blood and oxygen flow to the area, thus improving ventricular function.

Incompatibilities

Don't add other drugs to, or administer them through same I.V. line as, reteplase injection solution.

Contraindications

Active internal bleeding, aneurysm, arteriovenous malformation, bleeding diathesis, brain tumor, history of CVA or other cerebrovascular disease, hypersensitivity to reteplase or its components, intracranial or intraspinal surgery or trauma during previous 2 months, severe uncontrolled hypertension (systolic blood pressure of 200 mm Hg or higher, diastolic blood pressure of 110 mm Hg or higher)

Interactions

DRUGS

antifibrinolytics (including aminocaproic acid, aprotinin, and tranexamic acid): Decreased effectiveness of reteplase

antineoplastics, antithymocyte globulin, certain cephalosporins (such as cefamandole, cefoperazone, and cefotetan), heparin, oral anticoagulants, platelet aggregation inhibitors (such as abciximab, aspirin, and dipyridamole), strontium-89 chloride, sulfinpyrazone, valproic acid: Increased risk of bleeding

Adverse Reactions

CNS: Intracranial hemorrhage
GI: GI bleeding, nausea, vomiting
HEME: Thrombocytopenia
RESP: Hemoptysis
SKIN: Bleeding from wounds, ecchymosis, hematoma, purpura
Other: Anaphylaxis, injection site bleeding

Nursing Considerations

- Expect to begin reteplase therapy, as prescribed, as soon as possible after MI symptoms begin.
- Closely monitor patient with atrial fibrillation, severe hypertension, or other cardiac disease for signs and symptoms of cerebral embolism.
- Reconstitute drug using diluent, syringe, needle, and dispensing pin provided. Withdraw 10 ml of preservative-free sterile water for injection. Remove and discard needle from syringe, and connect dispensing pin to syringe. Remove protective cap from spike end of dispensing pin, and insert spike into reteplase vial. Inject 10 ml of sterile water into the vial. With the spike still in the vial, swirl gently—don't shake—to dissolve the powder. Expect to see slight foaming. Let vial stand for several minutes. When bubbles dissipate, withdraw 10 ml of reconstituted solution into syringe (about 0.7 ml may remain in vial). Now detach syringe from dispensing pin and attach 20G needle.
- Use solution within 4 hours. Discard if it appears discolored or contains particles.
- Don't administer heparin and reteplase in same solution. Instead, flush heparin line with normal saline solutin or D_5W before and after reteplase injection.

- Because fibrin is lysed during therapy, closely monitor all possible bleeding sites (catheter insertions, arterial and venous punctures, cutdowns, and needle punctures).
- Avoid I.M. injections, venipunctures, and nonessential handling of patient during therapy.
- If arterial puncture is necessary, use an arm vessel that can be compressed, if possible. After sample is obtained, apply pressure for at least 30 minutes, and then apply a pressure dressing. Check site frequently for bleeding.
- If bleeding occurs and can't be controlled by local pressure, notify prescriber immediately. Be prepared to stop concurrent anticoagulant therapy immediately and to discontinue second reteplase bolus, as prescribed.
- Anticipate that reperfusion arrhythmias—premature ventricular contractions, ventricular tachycardia—may follow coronary thrombolysis.
- Store drug at 2° to 25° C (36° to 77° F), and protect from light.

PATIENT TEACHING

- Advise patient to immediately report adverse reactions to reteplase, including bleeding or bruising, headache, rash, or difficulty breathing.
- Instruct patient to maintain strict bed rest while receiving reteplase to prevent or minimize bleeding.

rifampin
(rifampicin)

Rifadin, Rifadin IV, Rimactane, Rofact (CAN)

Class and Category

Chemical: Semisynthetic antibiotic derivative of rifamycin
Therapeutic: Antimycobacterial antitubercular
Pregnancy category: C

Indications and Dosages

▶ *As adjunct to treat tuberculosis caused by all strains of* Mycobacterium tuberculosis

I.V. INFUSION

Adults. 10 mg/kg daily in combination with other antitubercular drugs for 2 mo. *Maximum:* 600 mg daily.
Infants and children. 10 to 20 mg/kg daily in combination with other antitubercular drugs for 2 mo. *Maximum:* 600 mg daily.

▶ *To eliminate meningococci from nasopharynx of asymptomatic carriers*

of Neisseria meningitidis
I.V. INFUSION
Adults. 600 mg q 12 hr for 2 days (total of 4 doses).
Infants age 1 month and over and children. 10 mg/kg q 12 hr for 2 days (total of 4 doses). *Maximum:* 600 mg daily.
Infants under age 1 month. 5 mg/kg q 12 hr for 2 days (total of 4 doses). *Maximum:* 600 mg daily.
DOSAGE ADJUSTMENT For patients with hepatic impairment, maximum dosage of 8 mg/kg daily. For patients with creatinine clearance of 10 ml/min/1.73 m^2 or less, recommended dosage usually decreased by 50%.

Mechanism of Action

Inhibits bacterial and mycobacterial RNA synthesis by binding to DNA-dependent RNA polymerase, thereby blocking RNA transcription. Exhibits dose-dependent bactericidal or bacteriostatic action. Rifampin is highly effective against rapidly dividing bacilli in extracellular cavitary lesions, such as those found in the nasopharynx.

Incompatibilities

Don't administer rifampin in the same I.V. line as diltiazem.

Contraindications

Concurrent use of nonnucleoside reverse transcriptase inhibitors or protease inhibitors by patients with HIV, hypersensitivity to rifamycins

Interactions

DRUGS
aminophylline, oxtriphylline, theophylline: Increased metabolism and clearance of these theophylline preparations
anesthetics (hydrocarbon inhalation, except isoflurane), hepatotoxic drugs, isoniazid: Increased risk of hepatotoxicity
beta blockers, chloramphenicol, clofibrate, corticosteroids, cyclosporine, dapsone, digitalis glycosides, disopyramide, hexobarbital, itraconazole, ketoconazole, mexiletine, oral anticoagulants, oral antidiabetic drugs, phenytoin, propafenone, quinidine, tocainide, verapamil (oral): Increased metabolism, resulting in lower blood levels of these drugs
bone marrow depressants: Increased leukopenic or thrombocytopenic effects

clofazimine: Reduced absorption of rifampin, delaying its peak concentration and increasing its half-life
diazepam: Enhanced elimination of diazepam, resulting in decreased drug effectiveness
estramustine, estrogens, oral contraceptives: Decreased estrogenic effects
methadone: Possibly impaired absorption of methadone, leading to withdrawal symptoms
probenecid: Increased blood level or prolonged duration of rifampin, increasing risk of toxicity
nonnucleoside reverse transcriptase inhibitors, protease inhibitors (indinavir, nelfinavir, ritonavir, saquinavir): Accelerated metabolism of these drugs (by patients with HIV), resulting in subtherapeutic levels; delayed metabolism of rifampin, increasing risk of toxicity
trimethoprim: Increased elimination and shortened elimination half-life of trimethoprim
vitamin D: Increased metabolism and decreased efficacy of vitamin D, leading to decreased serum calcium and phosphate levels and increased parathyroid hormone levels
ACTIVITIES
alcohol use: Increased risk of hepatotoxicity

Adverse Reactions

CNS: Chills, dizziness, drowsiness, fatigue, headache, paresthesia
EENT: Discolored saliva, tears, and sputum; mouth or tongue soreness; periorbital edema
GI: Abdominal cramps, anorexia, diarrhea, discolored feces, elevated liver function test results, epigastric discomfort, flatulence, heartburn, hepatitis, nausea, pseudomembranous colitis, vomiting
GU: Discolored urine
MS: Arthralgia, myalgia
SKIN: Discolored skin and sweat
Other: Facial edema, flulike symptoms

Nursing Considerations

- Obtain blood samples or other specimens for culture and sensitivity testing, as ordered, before giving rifampin and throughout therapy to monitor response to drug.
- Expect to monitor liver function test results before and every 2 to 4 weeks during therapy. Immediately report abnormalities.
- For I.V. infusion, reconstitute by adding 10 ml of sterile water for injection to 600-mg vial of rifampin. Swirl gently to dissolve. Withdraw appropriate dose and add to 500 ml of D_5W

(preferred solution) or normal saline solution and infuse over 3 hours. Alternatively, withdraw appropriate dose and add to 100 ml of D_5W (preferred solution) or normal saline solution and infuse over 30 minutes. Use reconstituted drug promptly because rifampin may precipitate out of D_5W solution after 4 hours. Normal saline solution solution is stable for up to 24 hours at room temperature.

- Be aware that patient receiving intermittent therapy (once or twice weekly) is at increased risk for adverse reactions.
- Expect drug to discolor skin and body fluids reddish orange to reddish brown.
- Be aware that rifampin can cause myelosuppression and increase risk of infection. Notify prescriber immediately if signs of infection, such as fever, develop.

PATIENT TEACHING

- Explain that drug may turn urine, feces, saliva, sputum, sweat, tears, and skin reddish orange to reddish brown.
- Caution patient against wearing soft contact lenses during therapy because drug may permanently stain them.
- Advise patient who takes an oral contraceptive to use an additional form of birth control during rifampin therapy.
- Urge patient to notify prescriber about flulike symptoms, anorexia, darkened urine, fever, joint pain or swelling, malaise, nausea, vomiting, and yellowish skin or eyes, which may indicate hepatitis.
- Advise patient to avoid alcohol during rifampin therapy.
- Instruct patient to notify prescriber if no improvement occurs within 2 to 3 weeks.

rituximab

Rituxan

Class and Category

Chemical: Chimeric murine-human monoclonal antibody
Therapeutic: Antirheumatic
Pregnancy category: C

Indications and Dosages

▶ *To reduce signs and symptoms in patients with moderate to severe active rheumatoid arthritis who take methotrexate and had an inadequate response to one or more tumor necrosis factor antagonists*

I.V. INFUSION

Adults. 1,000 mg at an initial rate of 50 mg/hr and then increased if no hypersensitivity or infusion reaction occurs in increments of 50 mg/hr q 30 minutes to a maximum of 400 mg/hr. Dosage repeated in 2 wk at an initial rate of 100 mg/hr and then increased in increments of 100 mg/hr q 30 minutes to a maximum of 400 mg/hr if no reaction occurrs with first infusion given 2 wks prior.

DOSAGE ADJUSTMENT For patients experiencing a hypersensitivity or infusion reaction with first dose, infusion temporarily slowed or stopped until symptoms are alleviated and then infusion restarted at one-half the previous rate. For patients who had experienced a hypersensitivity or infusion reaction with first dose, second dose given in the same manner as first dose.

Mechanism of Action

Binds to the CD20 antigen on pre-B and mature B lymphocytes. B lymphocytes may play a role in autoimmune and inflammatory processes, including the pathogenesis of rheumatoid arthritis. Processes may include production of rheumatoid factor and other autoantibodies, antigen presentation, T-cell activation, and production of pro-inflammatory cytokines. Interference with these activities hinders the autoimmune and inflammatory processes, reducing signs and symptoms of rheumatoid arthritis.

Contraindications

Hepatitis, history of anaphylaxis or IgE-mediated hypersensitivity to murine proteins, hypersensitivity to rituximab or its components, renal impairment

Interactions

DRUGS

anticoagulants: Additive risk of bleeding in thrombocytopenic patients

antihypertensives: Inreased risk of hypotension

cisplatin: Possibly increased risk of renal toxicity

fludarabine: Additive cytotoxic effects

vaccines: Suboptimal antibody response, particularly to live virus vaccines

Adverse Reactions

CNS: Anxiety, asthenia, chills, fever, insomnia, migraine headaches, paresthesia, rigors, vertigo
CV: Angina, cardiogenic shock, hypercholesterolemia, hypertension, hypotension, MI, supraventricular tachycardia, ventricular tachycardia or fibrillation
EENT: Nasopharyngitis, rhinitis, sneezing, sinusitis, throat irritation
GI: Anorexia, dyspepsia, nauseaupper abdominal pain
GU: UTI
MS: Arthralgia
RESP: Acute respiratory distress syndrome, bronchitis, bronchospasm, cough, hypoxia, pulmonary infiltrates, upper respiratory tract infection
SKIN: Flushing, paraneoplastic pemphigus, Stevens-Johnson syndrome, lichenoid or vesiculobullous dermatitis, toxic epidermal necrolysis, pruritus, urticaria
Other: Anaphylaxis, angioedema, injection site reaction, weight loss

Nursing Considerations

- Expect to administer methylprednisolone 100 mg IV or its equilvalent 30 minutes prior to each rituximab dose to reduce the risk and severity of infusion reactions.
- Expect to administer methotrexate concomitantly with rituximab therapy.
- Dilute drug before giving it by withdrawing prescribed amount of rituximab from the vial to an infusion bag containing either normal saline solution or D_5W to make a final concentration of 1 to 4 mg/ml. Gently invert the bag to mix the contents. If solution will not be administered immediately, refrigerate and use within 48 hours.
- Administer drug only as an I.V. infusion and not as an I.V. push or bolus.
- **WARNING** Monitor patient closely for a potentially life-threatening infusion reaction manifested by fever, chills, rigors, pruritus, urticaria, rash, angioedema, sneezing, throat irritation, cough and or bronchospasm with possibly hypertension or hypotension. If present, notify prescriber and expect to slow or stop infusion and provide supportive care.
- Monitor patient's blood pressure and cardiac function throughout rituximab therapy and afterwards to detect abnormalities because drug-induced infusion reaction may also cause adverse

cardiac effects. Discontinue infusion if a serious event such as a life-threatening arrhythmia or angina occurs, notify prescriber, and provide supportive care.
- Inspect patient's skin regularly for abnormalities because rituximab therapy may cause serious to life-threatening adverse dermatological effects.

PATIENT TEACHING
- Inform patient that infusion reactions may occur with rituximab therapy. Review what signs and symptoms to report immediately if experienced. Reassure patient know that he will receive a steroid preparation 30 minutes prior to the infusion to reduce the risk and severity of infusion reactions.
- Tell patient that drug will be administered twice two weeks apart.
- Alert patient that adverse effects may appear after infusion is completed and after patient is at home. Emphasize need to report any unusual or serious adverse effects immediately to prescriber.

scopolamine hydrobromide

Class and Category

Chemical: Belladonna alkaloid, tertiary amine
Therapeutic: Anesthesia adjunct, anticholinergic, antiemetic, antispasmodic, antivertigo agent
Pregnancy category: C

Indications and Dosages

▶ *To treat biliary tract disorders, enuresis, nausea and vomiting, and nocturia*

I.V. INJECTION

Adults and adolescents. 300 to 600 mcg (0.3 to 0.6 mg) as a single dose.

Children. 6 mcg (0.006 mg)/kg as a single dose.

▶ *As adjunct to anesthesia to induce sleep and calmness*

I.V. INJECTION

Adults and adolescents. 0.6 mg t.i.d. or q.i.d.

▶ *As adjunct to anesthesia to induce amnesia*

I.V. INJECTION

Adults and adolescents. 0.32 to 0.65 mg.

DOSAGE ADJUSTMENT Dosage reduction possible for elderly patients because of their increased sensitivity to scopolamine.

Route	Onset	Peak	Duration
I.V.*	10 min	50 to 80 min	2 hr

Mechanism of Action

Competitively inhibits acetylcholine at autonomic postganglionic cholinergic receptors. Because the most sensitive receptors are in the salivary, bronchial, and sweat glands, this action reduces secretions from these glands. Scopolamine also decreases nasal and oropharyngeal secretions, GI smooth-muscle tone and bladder detrusor muscle tone, and gastric secretions and GI motility. It also relaxes smooth muscles in the bronchi and bronchioles, resulting in decreased airway resistance.

In addition, scopolamine blocks neural pathways in the inner ear. This action relieves motion sickness and depresses the cerebral cortex to produce sedation and hypnotic effects.

Contraindications

Angle-closure glaucoma; hemorrhage with hemodynamic instability; hepatic dysfunction; hypersensitivity to barbiturates, scopolamine, other belladonna alkaloids, or their components; ileus; intestinal atony; myasthenia gravis; myocardial ischemia; obstructive GI disease, such as pyloric stenosis; obstructive uropathy, as in prostatic hyperplasia; renal impairment; tachycardia; toxic megacolon; ulcerative colitis

Interactions

DRUGS

antimyasthenics: Possibly reduced intestinal motility
CNS depressants: Possibly potentiated effects of either drug, resulting in additive sedation
cyclopropane: Increased risk of ventricular arrhythmias
haloperidol: Decreased antipsychotic effect of haloperidol
ketoconazole: Decreased absorption of ketoconazole
lorazepam (parenteral): Possibly hallucinations, irrational behavior, and sedation
metoclopramide: Possibly antagonized effect of metoclopramide on GI motility
opioid analgesics: Increased risk of severe constipation and ileus
other anticholinergics: Possibly intensified anticholinergic effects

* For amnesia.

potassium chloride: Possibly increased severity of potassium chloride–induced GI lesions
urinary alkalizers (antacids, carbonic anhydrase inhibitors, citrates, sodium bicarbonate): Delayed excretion of scopolamine, possibly leading to increased therapeutic and adverse effects
ACTIVITIES
alcohol use: Additive CNS effects

Adverse Reactions
CNS: Dizziness, drowsiness, euphoria, insomnia, memory loss, paradoxical stimulation
CV: Palpitations, tachycardia
EENT: Blurred vision; dry eyes, mouth, nose, and throat; mydriasis
GI: Constipation, dysphagia
GU: Urinary hesitancy, urine retention
SKIN: Decreased sweating, dry skin, flushing
Other: Injection site irritation or redness

Nursing Considerations
- Dilute scopolamine with sterile water for injection.
- Assess for bladder distention and monitor urine output because drug's antimuscarinic effects on ureters and bladder can cause urine retention.
- Monitor for pain. In presence of pain, drug may act as a stimulant and produce delirium if used without morphine or meperidine.
- Monitor heart rate for transient tachycardia, which may occur with high doses of scopolamine. Expect normal rate to return within 30 minutes.
- Store scopolamine at 15° to 30° C (59° to 86° F) in a light-resistant container; don't freeze.

PATIENT TEACHING
- Advise patient to avoid potentially hazardous activities until scopolamine's CNS effects are known.
- Instruct patient to avoid alcohol while receiving scopolamine.
- Suggest lubricating drops to relieve dry eyes.

sodium bicarbonate

Class and Category
Chemical: Electrolyte
Therapeutic: Electrolyte replenisher, systemic and urinary alkalizer
Pregnancy category: C

Indications and Dosages

▶ *To provide urinary alkalization*

I.V. INFUSION

Adults and children. 2 to 5 mEq/kg over 4 to 8 hr.

▶ *To treat metabolic acidosis during cardiac arrest*

I.V. INJECTION

Adults and children. *Initial:* 1 mEq/kg, followed by 0.5 mEq/kg q 10 min while arrest continues.

▶ *To treat less urgent forms of metabolic acidosis*

I.V. INFUSION

Adults and children. 2 to 5 mEq/kg over 4 to 8 hr.

DOSAGE ADJUSTMENT Dosage reduction possible for elderly patients because of age-related renal impairment.

Mechanism of Action

Increases plasma bicarbonate level, buffers excess hydrogen ions, and raises blood pH, thereby reversing metabolic acidosis. Sodium bicarbonate also increases the excretion of free bicarbonate ions in urine, raising urine pH; increased alkalinity of urine may help to dissolve uric acid calculi.

Incompatibilities

Don't mix sodium bicarbonate in same solution or give through same I.V. line as other drugs because a precipitate may form.

Contraindications

Hypocalcemia in which alkalosis may lead to tetany; hypochloremic alkalosis secondary to vomiting, diuretics, or nasogastric suction; preexisting metabolic or respiratory alkalosis

Interactions

DRUGS

amphetamines, quinidine: Decreased urinary excretion of these drugs, possibly resulting in toxicity

anticholinergics: Decreased anticholinergic absorption and effectiveness

chlorpropamide, lithium, salicylates, tetracyclines: Increased renal excretion of these drugs

ciprofloxacin, norfloxacin, ofloxacin: Decreased solubility of these drugs, leading to crystalluria and nephrotoxicity

citrates: Increased risk of systemic alkalosis; increased risk of calcium calculus formation and hypernatremia in patients with history of uric acid calculi

digoxin: Possibly elevated blood digoxin level
ephedrine: Increased ephedrine half-life and duration of action
mecamylamine: Decreased excretion and prolonged effect of mecamylamine
methenamine: Decreased methenamine effectiveness
mexiletine: Possibly mexiletine toxicity
potassium supplements: Decreased serum potassium level
urinary acidifiers (ammonium chloride, ascorbic acid, potassium and sodium phosphates): Counteracted effects of urinary acidifiers

Adverse Reactions

CNS: Mental or mood changes
CV: Irregular heartbeat, peripheral edema (with large doses), weak pulse
EENT: Dry mouth
GI: Abdominal cramps, thirst
MS: Muscle spasms, myalgia
SKIN: Extravasation with necrosis, tissue sloughing, or ulceration

Nursing Considerations

- Dilute sodium bicarbonate with normal saline solution, D_5W, or other standard electrolyte solution before administration.
- **WARNING** Avoid rapid I.V. infusion, which can cause severe alkalosis. However, be aware that during cardiac arrest, the risk of death from acidosis may outweigh the risks associated with rapid infusion. In addition, rapid administration in children under age 2 poses a risk of hypernatremia with decreased CSF pressure and, possibly, intracranial hemorrhage.
- Monitor urine pH, as ordered, to determine drug's effectiveness as urinary alkalizer.
- Be aware that parenteral formulations are hypertonic and that increased sodium intake can produce edema and weight gain. Patients with impaired renal function, heart failure, or other conditions that predispose them to sodium retention or edema are at increased risk.
- Assess I.V. site often for evidence of extravasation. If it occurs, notify prescriber immediately and remove I.V. catheter. Elevate the extremity, apply warm compresses, and expect prescriber to administer a local injection of hyaluronidase or lidocaine.
- When calculating sodium intake for patients on a sodium-restricted diet, keep in mind that sodium bicarbonate contains varying amounts of sodium, depending on concentration of solution used; check label to calculate amount of sodium that patient is receiving.

• Store drug at 15° to 30° C (59° to 86° F); don't freeze.

PATIENT TEACHING

• Advise patient receiving sodium bicarbonate to report pain, swelling, or redness at I.V. insertion site.
• Instruct patient to avoid taking OTC drugs without prescriber's approval because many drugs interact with sodium bicarbonate.

sodium ferric gluconate

(contains 62.5 mg of elemental iron per 5 ml)
Ferrlecit

Class and Category

Chemical: Iron salt, mineral
Therapeutic: Antianemic
Pregnancy category: B

Indications and Dosages

▶ *To treat iron deficiency anemia in patients receiving long-term hemodialysis and erythropoietin*

I.V. INFUSION OR INJECTION

Adults. 125 mg of elemental iron. *Usual:* Minimum cumulative dose of 1 g of elemental iron given over eight sequential dialysis treatment. Dosage repeated at lowest dosage necessary to maintain target levels of hemoglobin and hematocrit and acceptable limits of blood iron levels.

Mechanism of Action

Acts to replenish iron stores lost during hemodialysis because of increased blood loss or increased iron utilization from epoetin therapy. Iron is an essential component of hemoglobin, myoglobin, and several enzymes, including cytochromes, catalase, and peroxidase, and is needed for catecholamine metabolism and normal neutrophil function. Sodium ferric gluconate also normalizes RBC production by binding with hemoglobin or being stored as ferritin in the reticuloendothelial cells of the liver, spleen, and bone marrow.

Incompatibilities

Don't mix sodium ferric gluconate with other drugs or parenteral nutrition solutions for I.V. infusion.

Contraindications

Anemia other than iron deficiency, hypersensitivity to iron salts or their components, iron overload

Interactions

DRUGS

oral iron preparations: Possibly reduced absorption of oral iron

Adverse Reactions

CNS: Asthenia, dizziness, fatigue, fever, headache, hypertonia, hypoesthesia, loss of consciousness, nervousness, paresthesia, seizures, syncope
CV: Chest pain, generalized edema, hypertension, hypotension, phlebitis, shock, tachycardia
EENT: Dry mouth
GI: Abdominal pain, diarrhea, nausea, vomiting
HEME: Hemorrhage
MS: Back pain, leg cramps
RESP: Cough, dyspnea, upper respiratory tract infection, wheezing
SKIN: Discoloration, diaphoresis, pallor, pruritus
Other: Generalized pain, hyperkalemia, hypersensitivity, infusion or injection site reaction

Nursing Considerations

- To reconstitute sodium ferric gluconate for I.V. infusion, dilute prescribed dose in 100 ml of normal saline solution immediately before infusion. Infuse over 1 hour. Discard any unused diluted solution.
- Inspect drug for particles and discoloration before administration and discard if present.
- Administer undiluted drug by slow I.V. injection at a rate up to 12.5 mg/min, not to exceed 125 mg per injection.
- Be aware that most patients need a minimum cumulative dose of 1 gram of elemental iron administered over eight sequential dialysis treatments.
- **WARNING** Assess patient for signs and symptoms of an allergic reaction, including chills, facial flushing, pruritus, and rash, and of a hypersensitivity reaction, including diaphoresis, dyspnea, nausea, severe lower back pain, vomiting, and wheezing. Discontinue drug and notify prescriber immediately if patient develops an allergic or hypersensitivity reaction, and be prepared to provide emergency interventions.
- **WARNING** Assess blood pressure often after drug administration because hypotension may occur and may be related to infusion rate or total cumulative dose. Avoid rapid infusion and be prepared to provide I.V. fluids for volume expansion.
- Expect to monitor blood hemoglobin level, hematocrit, serum ferritin level, and transferrin saturation, as ordered, before, dur-

ing, and after sodium ferric gluconate therapy. Make sure that serum iron level is tested 48 hours after last dose. To prevent iron toxicity, notify prescriber and expect to discontinue therapy if blood iron level is normal or elevated.
- Assess patient for possible iron overload (bleeding in GI tract and lungs, decreased activity, pale conjunctivae, and sedation).

PATIENT TEACHING
- Warn patient not to take oral iron preparations during sodium ferric gluconate therapy without first consulting prescriber.
- Inform patient that iron deficiency may cause decreased stamina, learning problems, shortness of breath, and fatigue.

sodium thiosalicylate

Rexolate, Tusal

Class and Category

Chemical: Salicylic acid derivative
Therapeutic: Analgesic, anti-inflammatory
Pregnancy category: Not rated

Indications and Dosages

▶ *To relieve symptoms of acute gout*

I.V. INJECTION

Adults. *Initial:* 100 mg q 3 to 4 hr for 2 days, followed by 100 mg daily.

▶ *To relieve pain from musculoskeletal conditions*

I.V. INJECTION

Adults. 50 to 100 mg daily or q other day.

▶ *To relieve symptoms of osteoarthritis*

I.V. INJECTION

Adults. 100 mg 3 times/wk for several wk, followed by 100 mg once/wk, usually up to a total dose of 2.5 g. After 1 to 2 wk, another course of treatment may be given.

▶ *To treat rheumatic fever*

I.V. INJECTION

Adults. *Initial:* 100 to 150 mg q 4 to 8 hr for 3 days, followed by 100 mg b.i.d.

Mechanism of Action

Exerts peripherally induced analgesic and anti-inflammatory effects by blocking pain impulses and inhibiting prostaglandin synthesis.

Contraindications

GI bleeding; hemophilia; hemorrhage; hypersensitivity to sodium thiosalicylate, NSAIDs, or their components; Reye's syndrome

Interactions

DRUGS

ACE inhibitors, beta blockers: Decreased antihypertensive effect
activated charcoal: Decreased sodium thiosalicylate absorption
antacids, urinary alkalizers: Increased sodium thiosalicylate excretion, leading to reduced effectiveness and shortened half-life
carbonic anhydrase inhibitors (such as acetazolamide): Increased risk of salicylate toxicity; possibly displacement of acetazolamide from protein-binding sites, resulting in toxicity
corticosteroids: Possibly increased sodium thiosalicylate excretion
insulin, oral antidiabetic drugs: Altered glucose control (with large doses of sodium thiosalicylate)
loop diuretics: Possibly decreased effectiveness of loop diuretics in patients with renal or hepatic impairment
methotrexate: Increased risk of methotrexate toxicity
nizatidine: Increased blood sodium thiosalicylate level
probenecid, sulfinpyrazone: Decreased uricosuric effects
spironolactone: Possibly inhibited diuretic effect of spironolactone
urinary acidifiers (including ammonium chloride, ascorbic acid, and methionine): Decreased sodium thiosalicylate excretion, possibly leading to salicylate toxicity

ACTIVITIES

alcohol use: Increased risk of GI ulceration

Adverse Reactions

GI: Anorexia, diarrhea, GI bleeding, heartburn, hepatotoxicity, indigestion, nausea, thirst, vomiting
HEME: Leukopenia, platelet dysfunction, prolonged bleeding time, thrombocytopenia
RESP: Bronchospasm
SKIN: Rash, urticaria
Other: Angioedema

Nursing Considerations

- Inspect vial before administration. If drug contains slight precipitate from oxidation, shake well. Discard if precipitate persists.
- Administer sodium thiosalicylate by slow injection.
- Watch for evidence of a hypersensitivity reaction, such as angioedema, bronchospasm, and rash. Patients with asthma, chronic urticaria, or nasal polyps are more prone to drug hypersensitivity.

- Expect to monitor hepatic and renal function during long-term drug therapy.
- After repeated administration or large doses, assess for signs of salicylate toxicity: CNS depression, confusion, diaphoresis, diarrhea, difficulty hearing, dizziness, headache, hyperventilation, lassitude, tinnitus, and vomiting.
- Be aware that tinnitus usually means blood sodium thiosalicylate has reached or exceeded upper limit of therapeutic effects.
- Store drug at 15° to 30° C (59° to 86° F).

PATIENT TEACHING

- Instruct patient to report bleeding or symptoms of salicylate toxicity immediately.

streptokinase

Kabikinase, Streptase

Class and Category

Chemical: Purified beta-hemolytic *Streptococcus* filtrate
Therapeutic: Thrombolytic
Pregnancy category: C

Indications and Dosages

▶ *To lyse coronary artery thrombi*

I.V. INFUSION

Adults. 1,500,000 international units within 60 min of event.

INTRACORONARY INFUSION

Adults. 20,000–international unit bolus, followed by 2,000 international units/min for 60 min for total dose of 140,000 international units.

▶ *To lyse acute arterial thromboembolism or thrombosis, acute pulmonary embolism, or deep vein thrombosis*

I.V. INFUSION

Adults. 250,000–international unit bolus over 30 min, followed by 100,000 international units/hr for 24 to 72 hr.

▶ *To clear occluded arteriovenous cannula*

I.V. INJECTION

Adults. 100,000 to 250,000 international units instilled slowly into each occluded lumen.

Route	Onset	Peak	Duration
I.V.	Immediate	20 to 120 min	4 hr

Mechanism of Action
Binds to fibrin in a thrombus and converts trapped plasminogen to plasmin. Plasmin breaks down fibrin, fibrinogen, and other clotting factors, thereby dissolving the thrombus.

Incompatibilities
Don't mix streptokinase in same syringe or administer through same I.V. line as other drugs.

Contraindications
Active internal bleeding, arteriovenous malformation or aneurysm, bleeding diathesis, CVA or intracranial or intraspinal surgery within the past 2 months, hypersensitivity to streptokinase or its components, intracranial cancer, severe uncontrolled hypertension

Interactions
DRUGS
anticoagulants, enoxaparin, heparin, NSAIDs, platelet aggregation inhibitors: Increased risk of bleeding
antifibrinolytics: Antagonized effects of both drugs
antihypertensives: Increased risk of severe hypotension, especially when streptokinase is give rapidly for coronary artery occlusion
cefamandole, cefoperazone, cefotetan, plicamycin, valproic acid: Possibly hypoprothrombinemia and increased risk of severe hemorrhage
corticosteroids, ethacrynic acid, salicylates: Possibly GI ulceration or bleeding

Adverse Reactions
CNS: Chills, fever
CV: Arrhythmias, hypotension
HEME: Unusual bleeding or bruising
Other: Allergic reaction

Nursing Considerations
- Obtain hematocrit, platelet count, APTT, PT, and INR, as ordered, before, during, and after streptokinase therapy.
- Consult manufacturer's instructions for reconstituting and diluting drug for I.V. and intracoronary infusions. If drug will be used to clear occluded arteriovenous cannula, slowly reconstitute 250,000-international unit vial with 2 ml of sodium chloride injection or 5% dextrose injection.
- To prevent foaming, don't shake drug during reconstitution.

- Watch for bleeding at I.V. site and for blood in urine and stools. Perform neurologic assessment to detect intracranial bleeding.
- Monitor the following patients for signs and symptoms of bleeding or hemorrhage because they're at increased risk during streptokinase therapy: pregnant women and patients with acute pericarditis (risk of hemopericardium, possibly leading to cardiac tamponade); cerebrovascular disease; hemorrhagic ophthalmic conditions; history of major surgery, GI or GU bleeding, or trauma within past 10 days; hypertension; mitral stenosis with atrial fibrillation (risk of embolism); septic thrombophlebitis; severe hepatic or renal disease; or subacute bacterial endocarditis.
- Closely monitor all puncture sites, such as catheter insertion and needle puncture sites, for bleeding.
- If serious spontaneous bleeding occurs and can't be controlled by local pressure, stop streptokinase infusion immediately and notify prescriber.
- Monitor for signs of a hypersensitivity reaction, such as nausea, pruritus, rash, or wheezing. Keep equipment and drugs used to treat anaphylaxis, such as epinephrine, glucocorticoids, and antihistamines, nearby.
- Monitor heart rate and rhythm by continuous ECG, as ordered.
- Avoid giving I.M. injections and handling patient unnecessarily during streptokinase therapy. Perform venipuncture only when necessary, using a 23G or smaller needle.
- If an arterial puncture is needed after streptokinase administration, use an arm vessel that allows easy manual compression. Apply manual pressure for 30 minutes. Then apply a pressure dressing and check puncture site frequently for bleeding.
- Treat fever with acetaminophen, as prescribed, rather than aspirin to reduce the risk of bleeding.
- Store drug at 15° to 30° C (59° to 86° F).

PATIENT TEACHING

- Explain to patient that he'll be on bed rest during therapy.
- Inform patient that minor bleeding may occur at arterial puncture or surgical sites. Reassure him that appropriate care measures will be taken if bleeding occurs.
- Advise patient to obtain medical alert identification stating that he's receiving streptokinase.
- If patient experiences chest pain within 12 months of receiving streptokinase, instruct him to inform health care providers about his streptokinase therapy because repeated administration within 12 months may be ineffective.

T·U·V

tenecteplase

TNKase

Class and Category

Chemical: Purified glycoprotein
Therapeutic: Thrombolytic
Pregnancy category: C

Indications and Dosages

▶ *To reduce mortality in acute MI*

I.V. INJECTION

Adults. Single bolus given over 5 sec in individualized dosage based on patient's weight, as follows: 30 mg (6 ml) for patients weighing less than 60 kg; 35 mg (7 ml) for patients weighing 60 to 69 kg; 40 mg (8 ml) for patients weighing 70 to 79 kg; 45 mg (9 ml) for patients weighing 80 to 89 kg; 50 mg (10 ml) for patients weighing 90 kg or more. *Maximum:* 50 mg total dose.

Mechanism of Action

Activates plasminogen, a naturally occurring substance secreted by endothelial cells in response to arterial wall injury that contributes to clot formation. Plasminogen is converted into plasmin, which breaks down the fibrin mesh that binds the clot together, resulting in dissolution of the clot.

Incompatibilities

Don't administer tenecteplase through an I.V. line containing dextrose because precipitation may occur.

Contraindications

Active internal bleeding, aneurysm, arteriovenous malformation, bleeding diathesis, brain tumor, history of CVA, hypersensitivity to tenecteplase or its components, intracranial or intraspinal surgery or trauma within past 2 months, severe uncontrolled hypertension

Interactions

DRUGS

abciximab, aspirin, clopidogrel, dipyridamole, heparin, oral anticoagulants, ticlopidine: Possibly increased risk of bleeding

Adverse Reactions

CNS: Intracranial hemorrhage
EENT: Epistaxis, gingival bleeding, pharyngeal bleeding
GI: GI and retroperitoneal bleeding
GU: Genitourinary bleeding, prolonged or heavy menstrual bleeding
HEME: Hematoma
RESP: Hemoptysis
SKIN: Bleeding at puncture sites, surgical incision sites, or venous cutdown sites

Nursing Considerations

- **WARNING** Reconstitute tenecteplase for injection immediately before use because drug contains no antibacterial preservatives. If reconstituted drug isn't used immediately, refrigerate vial at 2° to 8° C (36° to 46° F). Discard solution if not used within 8 hours.
- To reconstitute and administer drug, use supplied 10-ml syringe with dual cannula device. Withdraw 10 ml of supplied (preservative-free) sterile water for injection into syringe, and inject entire contents into vial containing tenecteplase dry powder, directing stream of diluent into powder. Gently swirl—don't shake—vial until contents are completely dissolved. If slight foaming occurs during reconstitution, allow drug to stand undisturbed for a few minutes to allow large bubbles to dissipate. Then, using supplied syringe, withdraw prescribed dose of tenecteplase from reconstituted drug in vial. Make sure that reconstituted preparation is a colorless to pale yellow transparent solution. Discard any unused portion.
- Administer drug as a single I.V. bolus over 5 seconds. Although supplied syringe is intended for use with needleless I.V. systems, be aware that it is also compatible with a conventional needle. Follow manufacturer's directions for use with each system. Flush any dextrose-containing I.V. lines with saline solution before and after administering tenecteplase.
- **WARNING** Monitor patient for signs and symptoms of GI bleeding, including bloody or black, tarry stools; bloody or coffee-ground vomitus; and severe stomach pain. Notify pre-

scriber at once if patient develops any of these signs or symptoms.

- Assess tenecteplase injection site for signs and symptoms of hematoma, including deep, dark purple bruises under skin and itching, pain, redness, or swelling. Also monitor for superficial bleeding, delayed bleeding at puncture sites, and bleeding from surgical incisions.
- Assess for signs and symptoms of intracranial bleeding (such as decreased LOC), retroperitoneal bleeding (such as abdominal pain or swelling and back pain), genitourinary bleeding (such as hematuria), or respiratory tract bleeding (such as hemoptysis). Notify prescriber immediately if patient develops any of these signs or symptoms.
- If serious bleeding (not controllable by local pressure) occurs, expect to discontinue concomitant heparin or oral antiplatelet therapy immediately.
- If possible, avoid I.M. injections and nonessential handling of patient for first few hours after drug administration.
- If arterial puncture becomes necessary during first few hours after tenecteplase administration, expect to use an upper extremity that is accessible to manual compression. Apply pressure for at least 30 minutes after procedure, use a pressure dressing, and frequently monitor puncture site for signs of bleeding.
- Before reconstituting tenecteplase, store it at controlled room temperature or refrigerate it.

PATIENT TEACHING

- Instruct patient to limit physical activity during tenecteplase administration to reduce the risk of injury or bleeding.
- Advise patient to immediately report any bleeding, including from nose or gums.

theophylline in dextrose injection

Class and Category

Chemical: Xanthine derivative
Therapeutic: Bronchodilator
Pregnancy category: C

Indications and Dosages

▶ *As loading dose to treat reversible airway obstruction in patients not currently receiving theophylline*

I.V. INFUSION

Adults and children. 5 mg/kg infused over 20 to 30 min.

▶ *As partial loading dose to treat reversible airway obstruction in patients currently receiving theophylline*
I.V. INFUSION
Adults and children. Dosage individualized based on blood theophylline level, as prescribed. Loading dose based on principle that 0.5 mg/kg of theophylline will produce a 1-mcg/ml increase in blood theophylline level.
▶ *To provide maintenance treatment of reversible airway obstruction associated with asthma or COPD*
I.V. INFUSION
Adults and adolescents age 16 and over. 0.4 mg/kg/hr for nonsmokers, 0.7 mg/kg/hr for smokers.
Children ages 9 to 16. 0.7 mg/kg/hr.
Children ages 1 to 9. 0.8 mg/kg/hr.
Full-term infants up to age 1. Dosage highly individualized, as prescribed.
DOSAGE ADJUSTMENT For elderly patients and adults with cardiac decompensation, cor pulmonale, or hepatic impairment, dosage reduced to 0.2 mg/kg/hr.

Mechanism of Action

Inhibits phosphodiesterase enzymes, causing bronchodilation. Normally, these enzymes inactivate cAMP and cGMP, which are responsible for bronchial smooth-muscle relaxation. Theophylline also may cause calcium translocation, antagonize prostaglandins and adenosine receptors, stimulate catecholamines, and inhibit cGMP metabolism.

Incompatibilities

Don't mix parenteral theophylline solution with any additives. Don't infuse theophylline through same I.V. line as Hetastarch (Hespan), a colloidal plasma volume expander, which is incompatible with theophylline.

Contraindications

Hypersensitivity to theophylline or its components, peptic ulcer disease, uncontrolled seizure disorder

Interactions

DRUGS
adenosine: Decreased adenosine effectiveness
allopurinol, cimetidine, ciprofloxacin, clarithromycin, disulfiram, enoxacin, erythromycin, fluvoxamine, interferon alfa (human recombi-

nant), methotrexate, mexiletine, pentoxifylline, propafenone, propranolol, tacrine, thiabendazole, ticlopidine, troleandomycin, verapamil: Increased blood theophylline level and risk of toxicity
aminoglutethimide, carbamazepine, isoproterenol (I.V.), moricizine, oral contraceptives (containing estrogen), phenobarbital, phenytoin, rifampin: Decreased blood level and possibly effectiveness of theophylline
benzodiazepines: Possibly reversal of benzodiazepine sedation
beta blockers: Possibly decreased bronchodilator effect of theophylline
ephedrine: Increased adverse effects, including insomnia, nausea, and nervousness
halothane anesthetics: Increased risk of ventricular arrhythmias
ketamine: Lowered seizure threshold
lithium: Decreased lithium effectiveness
neuromuscular blockers: Possibly antagonized neuromuscular blockade
FOODS
caffeine: Possibly increased risk of adverse CNS effects
high-carbohydrate, low-protein diet: Possibly decreased theophylline elimination
low-carbohydrate, high-protein diet; daily intake of charbroiled beef: Possibly increased theophylline elimination
ACTIVITIES
alcohol use: Increased blood theophylline level and risk of toxicity
smoking: Increased drug clearance, decreased drug effectiveness
smoking cessation: Possibly decreased drug clearance

Adverse Reactions

CNS: Agitation, anxiety, behavioral changes, confusion, disorientation, headache, insomnia, nervousness, seizures, tremor
CV: Hypotension, tachycardia, ventricular arrhythmias
ENDO: Hyperglycemia
GI: Abdominal pain, diarrhea, heartburn, nausea, vomiting
GU: Increased urine output

Nursing Considerations

- Be aware that ideal body weight is used to calculate theophylline dosages because drug doesn't bind well in body fat.
- Discard unused portions of theophylline and dextrose solutions because they contain no preservatives.
- Infuse theophylline loading dose, bolus, or intermittent infusion at a rate not exceeding 25 mg/minute.
- Administer continuous theophylline infusion with a rate-controlled infusion device.
- Frequently assess heart rate and rhythm because theophylline can exacerbate existing arrhythmias.

- Monitor blood theophylline level, as ordered, to gauge therapeutic level and detect toxicity.
- Be especially alert for signs of toxicity in patients with acute pulmonary edema, hypothyroidism, prolonged fever, sepsis with multiple organ failure, shock, or viral pulmonary infection and those who have recently received an influenza vaccine because drug clearance is decreased in these patients. Patients with uncorrected acidemia also have an increased risk of toxicity.
- Suspect toxicity if patient experiences vomiting; be prepared to obtain blood theophylline level.
- Expect patients with cystic fibrosis or hyperthyroidism to experience increased theophylline clearance and decreased drug effectiveness. Monitor blood theophylline level, as ordered.
- Store drug at 15° to 30° C (59° to 86° F); don't freeze.

PATIENT TEACHING

- Advise patient to report if she develops a fever, makes a significant dietary change, or starts or stops smoking or taking other drugs because these factors may alter blood theophylline level.
- Urge patient to avoid excessive intake of caffeine (found in coffee, tea, cola, and chocolate), which can increase her risk of developing adverse CNS reactions, such as agitation and nervousness.

thiamine hydrochloride
(vitamin B_1)

Betaxin (CAN), Biamine

Class and Category

Chemical: Water-soluble B-complex vitamin
Therapeutic: Nutritional supplement
Pregnancy category: A (parenteral)

Indications and Dosages

▶ *To provide nutritional supplementation based on U.S. and Canadian recommended daily allowances (RDAs), to prevent thiamine deficiency*

I.V. INFUSION

Adults and children. Dosage individualized and added to total parenteral nutrition solution.

▶ *To treat beriberi*

I.V. INJECTION

Adults. *Initial:* 5 to 100 mg q 8 hr, then switched to P.O. therapy as soon as possible and continued for 1 mo.

Children and infants. 10 to 25 mg daily.

▶ *To treat Wernicke's encephalopathy*

I.V. INJECTION

Adults. *Initial:* 100 mg. *Maintenance:* 50 to 100 mg daily until normal RDA is achieved.

Mechanism of Action

Replaces vitamin in thiamine deficiency, which can lead to beriberi or Wernicke's encephalopathy. Thiamine combines with ATP to produce thiamine pyrophosphate, a coenzyme needed for carbohydrate metabolism. Thiamine is necessary for the conversion of pyruvic acid to acetyl-CoA so that it can enter the Krebs cycle; in patients without adequate thiamine, pyruvic acid accumulates in the blood, where it's converted to lactic acid.

Incompatibilities

Don't add thiamine to alkaline or neutral solutions or mix it with oxidizing and reducing agents, including barbiturates, carbonates, citrates, and copper ions.

Contraindications

Hypersensitivity to thiamine preparations or their components

Interactions

None known.

Adverse Reactions

CNS: Restlessness, weakness
EENT: Sneezing, throat tightness
GI: Nausea, vomiting
SKIN: Diaphoresis, pruritus, sensation of warmth, urticaria

Nursing Considerations

- Be aware that symptoms of thiamine deficiency may appear as a syndrome of nonspecific symptoms that include headache, malaise, myalgia, and nausea.
- **WARNING** Severe thiamine deficiency causes beriberi, which can affect the CNS and cardiovascular system. Monitor patient for neurologic effects, such as ataxia, confabulation, impaired ability to learn, neuropathy, and retrograde amnesia, as well as cardiovascular effects, such as biventricular failure, edema, and peripheral vasodilation.
- Expect an intradermal test dose to be prescribed before I.V. administration of thiamine.

- Use thiamine immediately if mixed in solutions containing sodium bisulfite as an antioxidant or preservative because drug stability is poor in such solutions.
- Be aware that a high-carbohydrate diet and dextrose-containing I.V. solutions may increase thiamine requirements and worsen symptoms of thiamine deficiency.
- Be aware that thiamine absorption is decreased in patients with alcoholism, cirrhosis, or GI disease.
- Assess patient and laboratory test results for signs of lactic acidosis. In patients with a thiamine deficiency, pyruvic acid accumulates in the blood and is converted to lactic acid.
- Keep in mind that thiamine is a water-soluble vitamin that won't accumulate in the body.
- Store drug at 15° to 30° C (59° to 86° F); protect from freezing and light.

PATIENT TEACHING

- Inform breast-feeding patient that she and her infant must be treated with thiamine if infant has beriberi.
- Encourage patient to improve diet to prevent disease recurrence.

ticarcillin disodium

Ticar

Class and Category

Chemical: Penicillin
Therapeutic: Antibiotic
Pregnancy category: B

Indications and Dosages

▶ *To treat moderate to severe infections, such as bacteremia, diabetic foot ulcers, empyema, intra-abdominal infections, lower respiratory tract infections (including pneumonia), lung abscess, peritonitis, pulmonary infections due to complications of cystic fibrosis (including bronchiectasis and pneumonia), septicemia, and skin and soft-tissue infections (including cellulitis) caused by susceptible organisms*

I.V. INFUSION

Adults and children. 200 to 300 mg/kg daily in divided doses q 4 to 6 hr. *Usual:* 3 g q 4 hr or 4 g q 6 hr.

▶ *To treat severe infections (including sepsis) caused by susceptible strains of* Pseudomonas *sp.,* Proteus *sp., and* Escherichia coli

Neonates during first week of life weighing less than 2 g. 75 mg/kg q 12 hr.

Neonates during first week of life weighing more than 2 g. 75 mg/kg q 8 hr.
Neonates after first week of life weighing less than 2 g. 75 mg/kg q 8 hr.
Neonates after first week of life weighing more than 2 g. 100 mg/kg q 8 hr or 75 mg/kg q 6 hr.

▶ *To treat uncomplicated UTI*

I.V. INFUSION

Adults and children weighing 40 kg (88 lb) or more. 1 g q 6 hr.
Children over age 1 month weighing less than 40 kg. 50 to 100 mg/kg daily in divided doses q 6 to 8 hr.

▶ *To treat complicated UTI*

I.V. INFUSION

Adults and children. 150 to 200 mg/kg in equally divided doses q 4 to 6 hr. *Usual:* 3 g q 6 hr.

DOSAGE ADJUSTMENT Adult patients with renal impairment given a loading dose of 3 g, then dosage adjusted as follows: for creatinine clearance of 30 to 60 ml/min/1.73 m^2, 2 g q 4 hr; for creatinine clearance of 10 to 30 ml/min/1.73 m^2, 2 g q 8 hr; for creatinine clearance of less than 10 ml/min/1.73 m^2, 2 g q 12 hr; for creatinine clearance of less than 10 ml/min/1.73 m^2 *and* impaired hepatic function, 2 g q 24 hr; for patients who undergo hemodialysis, 2 g q 12 hr and 3 g after each dialysis session; for patients who undergo peritoneal dialysis, 3 g q 12 hr.

Mechanism of Action

Inhibits bacterial cell wall synthesis by binding to specific penicillin-binding proteins located inside the bacterial cell wall. Ultimately, this leads to cell wall lysis and death.

Incompatibilities

Don't administer ticarcillin through same I.V. line as amikacin, gentamicin, or tobramycin or within 1 hour of aminoglycosides.

Contraindications

Hypersensitivity to ticarcillin, other penicillins, or their components

Interactions

DRUGS

aminoglycosides: Additive or synergistic activity against some bacteria, possibly mutual inactivation

anticoagulants: Possibly interference with platelet aggregation, prolonged PT
methotrexate: Prolonged blood methotrexate level, increased risk of methotrexate toxicity
probenecid: Prolonged blood ticarcillin level

Adverse Reactions

CV: Thrombophlebitis, vasculitis
GI: Elevated liver function test results, nausea, pseudomembranous colitis, vomiting
GU: Proteinuria
HEME: Anemia, eosinophilia, hemorrhage, leukopenia, neutropenia, prolonged bleeding time, thrombocytopenia
SKIN: Erythema nodosum, exfoliative dermatitis, pruritus, rash, toxic epidermal necrolysis, urticaria
Other: Anaphylaxis, hypernatremia, hypokalemia, superinfection

Nursing Considerations

- Obtain body fluid or tissue specimens for culture and sensitivity testing, as ordered. Review test results, if possible, before giving first dose of ticarcillin.
- Before starting ticarcillin therapy, make sure patient has had no previous hypersensitivity reactions to ticarcillin or other penicillins.
- Reconstitute each gram of ticarcillin with 4 ml of a compatible diluent, such as 5% dextrose injection or 0.9% sodium chloride injection. Further dilute reconstituted I.V. solution to 10 to 100 mg/ml with a compatible I.V. solution. To minimize vein irritation, don't exceed concentration of 100 mg/ml (concentrations of 50 mg/ml or greater are preferred). Infuse appropriate adult or children's dose over 30 to 120 minutes; infuse neonatal dose over 10 to 20 minutes.
- Assess for local injection site reaction, including thrombophlebitis, during therapy.
- **WARNING** Monitor patient's platelet count, PT, and APTT because ticarcillin may increase bleeding time and, in rare cases, may induce thrombocytopenia.
- Be aware that ticarcillin may exacerbate symptoms in patients with a history of GI disease or colitis.
- Implement seizure precautions according to facility policy for patients with renal impairment because they're at increased risk for seizures.
- Assess patient for signs of pseudomembranous colitis, such as abdominal cramps and severe watery diarrhea. Also assess for

other signs of superinfection, such as oral candidiasis and rash in breast-feeding infant.
- Monitor serum electrolyte levels for hypernatremia due to drug's high sodium content and for hypokalemia due to increased urinary potassium loss.
- When calculating sodium intake for patients on a sodium-restricted diet, keep in mind that each gram of ticarcillin contains approximately 5.2 to 6.5 mEq of sodium.
- Before reconstituting drug, store it at 15° to 30° C (59° to 86° F).

PATIENT TEACHING
- Instruct patient receiving ticarcillin to immediately report adverse reactions, including rash, difficulty breathing, or fever.
- Advise patient to decrease sodium intake to reduce the risk of electrolyte imbalance.
- Advise patient to report diarrhea and to check with prescriber before taking an antidiarrheal because it may mask symptoms of pseudomembranous colitis.

ticarcillin disodium and clavulanate potassium

Timentin

Class and Category

Chemical: Penicillin
Therapeutic: Antibiotic combination
Pregnancy category: B

Indications and Dosages

▶ *To treat moderate to severe infections, such as appendicitis, bacteremia, bone and joint infections (including osteomyelitis), diabetic foot ulcers, diverticulitis, gynecologic infections (including endometritis), infectious arthritis, intra-abdominal infections, lower respiratory tract infections (including pneumonia), peritonitis, septicemia, skin and soft-tissue infections (including cellulitis), and UTI caused by susceptible organisms; to manage febrile neutropenia*

I.V. INFUSION

Adults and children age 12 and older weighing 60 kg (132 lb) or more. 3.1 g (3 g of ticarcillin and 100 mg of clavulanic acid) infused over 30 min q 4 to 6 hr.

Adults and children age 12 and older weighing less than 60 kg. 200 to 300 mg/kg daily (based on ticarcillin content) in divided doses q 4 to 6 hr.

Children and infants over age 3 months. For mild to moderate infections, 200 mg/kg daily (based on ticarcillin content) in divided doses q 6 hr; for severe infections, 300 mg/kg daily (based on ticarcillin content) in divided doses q 4 to 6 hr.
DOSAGE ADJUSTMENT Adult patients with renal impairment given loading dose of 3.1 g (3 g of ticarcillin and 100 mg of clavulanic acid), then dosage adjusted as follows: for creatinine clearance of 30 to 60 ml/min/1.73 m^2, 2 g q 4 hr; for creatinine clearance of 10 to 30 ml/min/1.73 m^2, 2 g q 8 hr; for creatinine clearance of less than 10 ml/min/1.73 m^2, 2 g q 12 hr; for creatinine clearance of less than 10 ml/min/1.73 m^2 *and* impaired hepatic function, 2 g q 24 hr; for patients who undergo hemodialysis, 2 g q 12 hr and 3.1 g after each dialysis; for patients who undergo peritoneal dialysis, 3.1 g q 12 hr.

▶ *To treat pulmonary infections caused by complications of cystic fibrosis, such as bronchiectasis or pneumonia*

I.V. INFUSION

Children. 350 to 450 mg/kg daily (based on ticarcillin content) in divided doses.

Mechanism of Action

Inhibits bacterial cell wall synthesis by binding to specific penicillin-binding proteins located inside bacterial cell walls. In this way, ticarcillin ultimately leads to cell wall lysis and death. Clavulanic acid, which doesn't alter the action of ticarcillin, binds with bound and extracellular beta-lactamase, preventing beta-lactamase from inactivating ticarcillin.

Incompatibilities

Don't administer ticarcillin and clavulanate through same I.V. line as amikacin, gentamicin, or tobramycin. Don't combine with sodium bicarbonate or administer within 1 hour of aminoglycosides.

Contraindications

Hypersensitivity to ticarcillin or other penicillins, clavulanic acid, or their components

Interactions

DRUGS

aminoglycosides: Additive or synergistic activity against some bacteria, possibly mutual inactivation
anticoagulants: Possibly interference with platelet aggregation

methotrexate: Prolonged blood methotrexate level, increased risk of methotrexate toxicity
probenecid: Prolonged blood ticarcillin level

Adverse Reactions

CV: Thrombophlebitis, vasculitis
GI: Elevated liver function test results, nausea, pseudomembranous colitis, vomiting
GU: Proteinuria
HEME: Anemia, eosinophilia, hemorrhage, leukopenia, neutropenia, prolonged bleeding time, thrombocytopenia
SKIN: Erythema nodosum, exfoliative dermatitis, pruritus, rash, toxic epidermal necrolysis, urticaria
Other: Anaphylaxis, hypernatremia, hypokalemia, infusion site pain

Nursing Considerations

- Obtain body fluid or tissue specimens for culture and sensitivity testing, as ordered. Review test results, if possible, before giving first dose of ticarcillin and clavulanate.
- Before starting drug, make sure patient has had no previous hypersensitivity reactions to ticarcillin, other penicillins, or clavulanic acid.
- Keep in mind that 3.1 g of combination drug ticarcillin and clavulanate corresponds to 3 g of ticarcillin and 100 mg of clavulanic acid.
- Dilute reconstituted I.V. solution to concentration of 10 to 100 mg/ml with compatible I.V. solution. To minimize vein irritation, don't exceed concentration of 100 mg/ml. Concentrations of 50 mg/ml or greater are preferred. Infuse appropriate I.V. dose over 30 to 120 min.
- Be aware that premixed minibags are available for use in concentration of 3.1 g (3 g of ticarcillin and 100 mg of clavulanic acid) in 100 ml. Before using minibags, store them below −10° C (14° F). Allow them to thaw at room temperature. Examine contents closely before administration to make sure that ice crystals have melted. When administering minibags, don't use I.V. lines with series connections because they may cause air embolism.
- Know that ticarcillin and clavulanate may exacerbate symptoms in patients with a history of GI disease, especially colitis.
- Assess patient for signs of pseudomembranous colitis, such as abdominal cramps and severe watery diarrhea. Also assess for

other signs of superinfection, such as oral candidiasis and rash in breast-feeding infant.
- Implement seizure precautions, according to facility policy, for patients with renal impairment because they're at increased risk for seizures.
- Monitor serum electrolyte levels for hypernatremia due to drug's high sodium content and for hypokalemia due to increased urinary potassium loss.
- **WARNING Monitor patient's platelet count, PT, and APTT because drug may increase bleeding time and, in rare cases, may induce thrombocytopenia.**
- Be aware that patient receiving high doses of ticarcillin may develop pseudoproteinuria.
- When calculating sodium intake for patients on a sodium-restricted diet, keep in mind that each gram of ticarcillin contains approximately 4.75 mEq of sodium.
- Before reconstituting drug, store it at 15° to 30° C (59° to 86° F). Store premixed minibags below −10° C (14° F) before thawing.

PATIENT TEACHING
- Instruct patient receiving ticarcillin and clavulanate to immediately report adverse reactions, including fever, rash, and difficulty breathing.
- Advise patient to decrease sodium intake to reduce the risk of electrolyte imbalance.
- Advise patient to report diarrhea and to check with prescriber before taking an antidiarrheal because it may mask symptoms of pseudomembranous colitis.

tigecycline

Tygacil

Class and Category

Chemical: Glycylcycline
Therapeutic: Antibiotic
Pregnancy category: D

Indications and Dosages

▶ *To treat complicated skin and skin structure infections caused by* Escherichia coli, Enterococcus faecalis *(vancomycin-susceptible isolates only),* Staphylococcus aureus *(methicillin-susceptible and -resistant isolates),* Streptococcus agalactiae, Streptococcus anginosus *group (includes* S. anginosus, S. intermedius, *and* S. constellatus*),* Streptococcus pyogenes, *and* Bacteroides fragilis; *to treat complicated intra-abdominal infections caused by* Citrobacter freundii, Enterobacter cloacae, Escherichia coli, Klebsiella oxytoca, Klebsiella pneumoniae, Enterococcus faecalis *(vancomycin-suseptible isolates only),* Staphylococcus aureus *(methicillin-susceptible isolates only),* Streptococcus anginosus *group,* Bacteroides fragilis, Bacteroides thetaiotaomicron, Bacteroides uniformis, Bacteroides vulgatus, Clostridium perfringens, *and* Peptostreptococcus micros

I.V. INFUSION

Adults. *Initial:* 100 mg infused over 30 to 60 min followed by 50 mg infused over 30 to 60 min q 12 hr for 5 to 14 days.

DOSAGE ADJUSTMENT For patients with severe hepatic impairment, initial dosage of 100 mg should be followed by a reduced maintenance dosage of 25 mg q 12 hr.

Mechanism of Action

Inhibits protein translation in bacteria by binding to the 30S ribosomal subunit, which prevents binding of amino-acyl tRNA molecules to the ribosome complex, thus interfering with protein synthesis. Through this bacteriostatic action, bacteria are weakened.

Incompatibilities

Don't give amphotericin B, chlorpromazine, methylprednisolone, or voriconazole simultaneously through the same Y-site.

Contraindications

Hypersensitivity to tigecycline or its components

Interactions

None known

Adverse Reactions

CNS: Asthenia, chills, dizziness, fever, headache, insomnia, somnolence

CV: Bradycardia, hypertension, hypotension, peripheral edema, phlebitis, septic shock, tachycardia, thrombophlebitis, vasodilation

EENT: Dry mouth, taste perversion

ENDO: Hyperglycemia, hypoglycemia

GI: Abdominal pain, acute pancreatitis, anorexia, constipation, diarrhea, dyspepsia, elevated liver enzyme levels, jaundice, nausea, vomiting

GU: Acute pancreatitis, elevated BUN and creatinine levels, vaginal candidiasis
HEME: Anemia, leukocytosis, thrombocythemia
MS: Back pain
RESP: Increased cough, dyspnea
SKIN: Diaphoresis, photosensitivity, pruritus, rash
Other: Hypersensitivity reaction, hypocalcemia; hypokalemia; hyponatremia; hypoproteinemia; injection site reaction, such as edema, phlebitis, inflammation, and pain

Nursing Considerations

- Obtain body tissue and fluid samples for culture and sensitivity tests as ordered before giving first dose. Expect to begin drug therapy before test results are known.
- Avoid giving tigecycline to children younger than age 8 because drug may cause permanent brown or yellow tooth discoloration and enamel hypoplasia.
- Use tigecycline cautiously in patients hypersensitive to tetracycline class antibiotics because glycylcycline class antibiotics are structurally similar to tetracycline class antibiotics.
- Also use cautiously in patients with complicated intra-abdominal infections secondary to intestinal perforation because of the risk of septic shock.
- Determine whether female patients could be pregnant before starting tigecycline therapy because the drug may cause harm to fetus.
- Reconstitute each vial of tigecycline with 5.3 ml of normal saline injection or 5% dextrose injection to achieve a concentration of 10 mg/ml. Note that the color will be yellow to orange. If not, the solution should be discarded. Immediately withdraw reconstituted solution from the vial and add to a 100-ml I.V. bag for infusion. Drug may be stored in the I.V. bag at room temperature for up to 6 hours or refrigerated up to 24 hours before use.
- If I.V. line is used to infuse other drugs, flush the line with either normal saline injection or 5% dextrose injection before and after tigecycline infusion.
- Infuse tigecycline over 30 to 60 minutes.
- Monitor patient closely for diarrhea, which may indicate pseudomembranous colitis, which is known to occur with many antibiotics. If diarrhea occurs during therapy, notify prescriber and expect to withhold drug. Expect to treat psuedomembra-

nous colitis, if confirmed, with fluids, electrolytes, protein, and an antibiotic effective against *Clostridium difficile*.

- Monitor patient for adverse reactions, keeping in mind the similarity between tigecycline and tetracycline.
- Assess patient for superinfection, such as vaginal candiasis, that may result from overgrowth of nonsusceptible organisms, including fungi. If signs of infection are present, notify prescriber and provide supportive care, as prescribed.

PATIENT TEACHING

- Instruct patient to report adverse reactions to prescriber, especially hypersensitivity reactions, such as a rash or itching, as well as diarrhea.
- Tell patient to report discomfort at infusion site because site may need to be changed.

tirofiban hydrochloride

Aggrastat

Class and Category

Chemical: Tyrosine derivative
Therapeutic: Platelet aggregation inhibitor
Pregnancy category: B

Indications and Dosages

▶ *To treat acute coronary syndrome*

I.V. INFUSION

Adults. 0.4 mcg/kg/min for 30 min, followed by 0.1 mcg/kg/min. **DOSAGE ADJUSTMENT** For patients with creatinine clearance of less than 30 ml/min/1.73 m^2, infusion rate reduced by one-half.

Route	Onset	Peak	Duration
I.V.	Immediate	30 min	4 to 8 hr

Mechanism of Action

Binds to glycoprotein IIb/IIIa receptor sites on the surface of activated platelets. Circulating fibrinogen can bind to these receptor sites and link platelets together, forming a clot that eventually blocks a coronary artery. By binding to receptor sites, tirofiban prevents the normal binding of fibrinogen and other factors and inhibits platelet aggregation.

Incompatibilities

Don't infuse tirofiban in same I.V. line with any drug other than atropine sulfate, dobutamine, dopamine, epinephrine hydrochloride, furosemide, heparin, lidocaine, midazolam hydrochloride, morphine sulfate, nitroglycerin, potassium chloride, propranolol hydrochloride, or famotidine (Pepcid injection).

Contraindications

Acute pericarditis; arteriovenous malformation; coagulopathy; CVA that occurred within previous 30 days or a history of hemorrhagic CVA; GI or GU bleeding; hemophilia; history of thrombocytopenia after tirofiban use; hypersensitivity to tirofiban or its components; intracranial aneurysm or mass, intracranial bleeding, retinal bleeding, aortic dissection, or any evidence of active abnormal bleeding within previous 30 days; major surgery or trauma within previous 6 weeks; severe uncontrolled hypertension (systolic blood pressure above 180 mm Hg, diastolic blood pressure above 110 mm Hg)

Interactions

DRUGS

antineoplastics, antithymocyte globulin, NSAIDs, oral anticoagulants, platelet aggregation inhibitors, strontium-89 chloride, thrombolytics: Increased risk of bleeding

levothyroxine, omeprazole: Increased rate of tirofiban clearance

porfimer: Decreased effectiveness of porfimer photodynamic therapy

salicylates: Increased risk of bleeding, possibly hypoprothrombinemia

Adverse Reactions

CNS: Chills, dizziness, fever, headache, intracranial hemorrhage

CV: Edema, hemopericardium, peripheral edema, sinus bradycardia

GI: Hematemesis, nausea, retroperitoneal bleeding, vomiting

GU: Hematuria, pelvic pain

HEME: Severe thrombocytopenia with chills, fever, and possibly fatal bleeding complications

RESP: Pulmonary hemorrhage

SKIN: Diaphoresis, rash, urticaria

Other: Allergic reaction, anaphylaxis, infusion site bleeding

Nursing Considerations

- **WARNING** Dilute 50-ml vial of tirofiban before use; don't dilute 500-ml container because it holds premixed solution ready for I.V. infusion. Don't use solution unless it's clear and the seal is intact.

- If prescribed, administer tirofiban with heparin for 48 to 108 hours. Expect to continue infusion throughout angiography and for 12 to 24 hours after angioplasty or ather-ectomy.
- **WARNING** If patient is also receiving a heparin infusion, expect to monitor APTT before treatment, 6 hours after heparin infusion starts, and regularly thereafter. Expect to adjust heparin dosage to maintain APTT at about two times the control. Notify prescriber immediately if patient develops an abnormally high APTT. Also, assess patient for signs and symptoms of abnormal bleeding and report them to prescriber immediately because potentially life-threatening bleeding may occur.
- After cardiac catheterization or percutaneous transluminal coronary angioplasty, maintain patient on bed rest and keep head of bed elevated. Ensure percutaneous site hemostasis at least 4 hours before discharge. Minimize invasive procedures, including epidural procedures, to reduce the risk of bleeding.
- Monitor patient's platelet count, hemoglobin level, and hematocrit, as ordered. Expect to discontinue tirofiban if patient's platelet count is less than 90,000/mm^3. Expect to administer a platelet transfusion, as prescribed, if patient's platelet count falls below 50,000/mm^3.

PATIENT TEACHING

- Advise patient to immediately report any bleeding, bruising, headache, pain, or swelling during I.V. infusion of tirofiban.

tobramycin sulfate

Tobi

Class and Category

Chemical: Aminoglycoside
Therapeutic: Antibiotic
Pregnancy category: D

Indications and Dosages

▶ *To treat bacteremia; bone and joint, gynecologic, intra-abdominal, lower respiratory tract, skin and soft-tissue, and urinary tract infections; endocarditis; meningitis; neonatal sepsis; pyelonephritis; and septicemia caused by susceptible strains of* Acinetobacter *sp.,* Aeromonas *sp.,* Citrobacter *sp.,* Enterobacter *sp.,* Escherichia coli, Haemophilus influenzae *(beta-lactamase–negative and –positive),* Klebsiella *sp.,* Morganella morganii, Proteus mirabilis, Proteus vulgaris, Providencia rettgeri, Pseudomonas aeruginosa, Salmonella *sp.,* Serratia *sp.,* Shigella *sp.,* Staphylococcus aureus, *and* Staphylococcus epidermidis; *to treat febrile neutropenia*

I.V. INFUSION

Adults. 3 to 6 mg/kg daily in divided doses q 8 to 12 hr.

Children over age 5. 2 to 2.5 mg/kg q 8 hr.

Children under age 5. 2.5 mg/kg q 8 to 16 hr.

Neonates over age 7 days weighing more than 2 kg (4.4 lb). 2.5 mg/kg q 8 hr.

Neonates over age 7 days weighing 1.2 to 2 kg (2.6 to 4.4 lb). 2.5 mg/kg q 8 to 12 hr.

Neonates age 7 days and under weighing 2 kg or more. 2.5 mg/kg q 12 hr.

Neonates age 7 days and under weighing 1.2 to 2 kg. 2.5 mg/kg q 12 to 18 hr.

Preterm neonates weighing 1 to 1.2 kg (2.2 to 2.6 lb). 2.5 mg/kg q 18 to 24 hr.

Preterm neonates weighing less than 1 kg. 3.5 mg/kg q 24 hr.

▶ *To treat pulmonary infection caused by* P. aeruginosa *in patients with cystic fibrosis*

I.V. INFUSION

Adults and children. 2.5 to 3.3 mg/kg q 8 hr; dosage adjusted to achieve peak blood drug level of 8 to 12 mcg/ml and trough blood drug level below 2 mcg/ml.

DOSAGE ADJUSTMENT For patients with renal impairment, dosage possibly reduced.

Mechanism of Action

Inhibits bacterial protein synthesis by binding irreversibly to one of two aminoglycoside-binding sites on the 30S ribosomal subunit, resulting in bacteriostatic effects. Bactericidal effects may stem from tobramycin's ability to accumulate within cells so that the intracellular drug level exceeds the extracellular level.

Incompatibilities

Don't mix tobramycin in same solution with parenteral aminoglycosides or beta-lactam antibiotics because mutual inactivation may result. Don't dilute or mix inhalation solution in nebulizer with dornase alfa.

Contraindications

Concurrent cidofovir therapy; hypersensitivity to tobramycin, aminoglycosides, sodium bisulfite, or their components

Interactions

DRUGS

acyclovir, aminoglycosides, amphotericin B, carboplatin, cisplatin, NSAIDs, vancomycin: Additive nephrotoxicity
carbenicillin, ticarcillin: Possibly inactivation of tobramycin
dimenhydrinate: Possibly masking of symptoms of ototoxicity
ethacrynic acid, furosemide: Additive ototoxicity
general anesthetics, neuromuscular blockers: Possibly exaggerated neuromuscular blockade

Adverse Reactions

CNS: Confusion, dizziness, headache, lethargy, neurotoxicity, vertigo
EENT: Hearing loss, tinnitus
GI: Diarrhea, elevated liver function test results, nausea, vomiting
GU: Elevated BUN and serum creatinine levels, nephrotoxicity, oliguria, proteinuria, renal failure
HEME: Anemia, leukocytosis, leukopenia, neutropenia, thrombocytopenia
SKIN: Exfoliative dermatitis, pruritus, rash, urticaria
Other: Hypocalcemia, hypokalemia, hypomagnesemia, hyponatremia, injection site pain

Nursing Considerations

- Obtain body fluid and tissue samples for culture and sensitivity testing before and during tobramycin treatment, as ordered. Review test results, if available, before therapy begins.
- After reconstituting drug with 30 ml of sterile or bacteriostatic water for injection, dilute further with normal saline solution or D_5W.
- Give each I.V. dose over 20 to 60 minutes.
- **WARNING** Don't infuse tobramycin over less than 20 minutes because doing so may result in neuromuscular blockade and excessive peak blood drug level.
- Because drug can cause bilateral and irreversible hearing loss, assess for early signs of cochlear and vestibular ototoxicity, including high-frequency hearing loss and vertigo.

- Monitor serum calcium, magnesium, potassium, and sodium levels to detect electrolyte imbalances.
- **WARNING** Be alert for allergic reactions, including anaphylaxis, because some forms of drug contain sodium bisulfite.
- Discontinue tobramycin therapy 7 days before starting cidofovir therapy, as prescribed.
- Assess for signs of nephrotoxicity, such as elevated BUN and serum creatinine levels.
- Expect dehydration to increase the risk of nephrotoxicity.
- **WARNING** Monitor patient with myasthenia gravis or parkinsonism for increased muscle weakness because of tobramycin's potential curare-like effect.

PATIENT TEACHING

- Urge patient to immediately report high-frequency hearing loss and vertigo.
- Instruct female patient to notify prescriber immediately about known or suspected pregnancy because drug poses danger to fetus.

torsemide

Demadex

Class and Category

Chemical: Anilinopyridine sulfonylurea derivative
Therapeutic: Antihypertensive, diuretic
Pregnancy category: B

Indications and Dosages

▶ *To treat edema in heart failure*

I.V. INJECTION

Adults. *Initial:* 10 to 20 mg daily, adjusted by doubling, as prescribed, to achieve desired effect. *Maximum:* 200 mg daily.

▶ *To treat edema in chronic renal failure*

I.V. INJECTION

Adults. *Initial:* 20 mg daily, adjusted by doubling, as prescribed, to achieve desired effect. *Maximum:* 200 mg daily.

▶ *To treat ascites, alone or with amiloride or spironolactone*

I.V. INJECTION

Adults. *Initial:* 5 to 10 mg daily. *Maximum:* 40 mg daily.

Route	Onset	Peak	Duration
I.V.	10 min	1 hr	6 to 8 hr

Mechanism of Action

Blocks active sodium and chloride reabsorption in the ascending loop of Henle by promoting rapid excretion of water, sodium, and chloride. Torsemide also increases the production of renal prostaglandins, increasing the plasma renin level and renal vasodilation. As a result, systolic and diastolic blood pressures fall, reducing preload and afterload.

Contraindications

Hypersensitivity to torsemide, sulfonamides, or their components

Interactions

DRUGS

ACE inhibitors, other antihypertensives: Additive hypotension
amiloride, spironolactone, triamterene: Possibly counteraction of torsemide-induced hypokalemia
amphotericin B: Increased risk of nephrotoxicity and severe, prolonged hypokalemia or hypomagnesemia
cisplatin: Increased risk of significant hypokalemia or hypomagnesemia, possibly permanent ototoxicity
cortisone, hydrocortisone: Increased risk of sodium retention and hypokalemia
digoxin: Increased risk of arrhythmias and digitalis toxicity due to hypokalemia or hypomagnesemia
indomethacin: Possibly decreased diuretic and antihypertensive effects of torsemide and increased risk of renal failure
lithium: Possibly lithium toxicity
metolazone, thiazide diuretics: Increased risk of severe fluid and electrolyte loss
neuromuscular blockers: Possibly increased neuromuscular blockade due to hypokalemia
probenecid: Possibly decreased diuretic effect of torsemide
quinidine and other ototoxic drugs: Increased risk of ototoxicity
salicylates: Increased risk of salicylate toxicity

ACTIVITIES

alcohol use: Additive diuresis and, possibly, dehydration

Adverse Reactions

CNS: Dizziness, drowsiness, fatigue, headache, insomnia, lethargy, nervousness, restlessness, weakness
CV: Chest pain, ECG abnormalities, edema, hypotension, tachycardia

EENT: Dry mouth, hearing loss, ototoxicity, pharyngitis, rhinitis, tinnitus
GI: Constipation, diarrhea, indigestion, nausea, thirst, vomiting
GU: Azotemia (prerenal), oliguria, urinary frequency
MS: Muscle spasms, myalgia
RESP: Cough
Other: Hypochloremia, hypokalemia, hypomagnesemia, hyponatremia, hypovolemia

Nursing Considerations

- Examine torsemide before administering it; discard if it contains particles or is discolored.
- Inject drug slowly over 2 minutes. Flush I.V. line with normal saline solution before and after administration.
- Don't exceed 200 mg in a single dose.
- Monitor serum electrolyte levels, as ordered, and fluid intake and output to detect hypovolemia.
- **WARNING** Expect drug-induced electrolyte imbalances, such as hypokalemia and hypomagnesemia, to increase the risk of toxicity and fatal arrhythmias in a patient who takes a digitalis glycoside. Hypokalemia also potentiates neuromuscular blockade effects of nondepolarizing neuromuscular blockers.
- Store drug at 15° to 30° C (59° to 86° F); don't freeze.

PATIENT TEACHING

- Advise patient to change position slowly during torsemide therapy to minimize effects of orthostatic hypotension.
- Instruct patient to immediately report drowsiness, dry mouth, hearing changes, lethargy, muscle cramps or pain, nausea, restlessness, thirst, vomiting, and weakness.
- Inform diabetic patient that her blood glucose level will be monitored frequently because torsemide may increase it.

trastuzumab

Herceptin

Class and Category

Chemical: Recombinant DNA-derived humanized monoclonal antibody
Therapeutic: Antineoplastic
Pregnancy category: B

Indications and Dosages

▶ *To treat metastatic breast cancer in patients whose tumors overexpress the protein human epidermal growth factor receptor 2 (HER2), either as a single agent (for those who have previously received at least one chemotherapy regimen for metastatic disease) or in combination with paclitaxel (for those who have not previously received chemotherapy for metastatic disease)*

I.V. INFUSION

Adults. *Initial:* 4 mg/kg infused over 90 min. *Maintenance:* 2 mg/kg infused over 30 min if initial dose was well tolerated.

Route	Onset	Peak	Duration
I.V.	Unknown	16 to 32 wk	Unknown

Mechanism of Action

Preferentially binds to the HER2 protein, which is associated with more aggressive forms of breast cancer. In this way, trastuzumab inhibits the proliferation of tumor cells and mediates antibody-dependent cellular toxicity in cancer cells that overexpress HER2.

Incompatibilities

Don't mix trastuzumab with dextrose solutions or any other drug.

Contraindications

None known.

Interactions

DRUGS

cyclophosphamide, doxorubicin, epirubicin: Increased risk of cardiac dysfunction

paclitaxel: Possibly increased blood level and effects of trastuzumab

Adverse Reactions

CNS: Asthenia, headache, insomnia, paresthesia

CV: Cardiomyopathy, cardiotoxicity (including heart failure), hypotension, ventricular dysfunction

EENT: Rhinitis

GI: Anorexia, diarrhea, nausea, vomiting

HEME: Anemia, leukopenia

RESP: Adult respiratory distress syndrome, bronchospasm, cough, dyspnea, hypoxia, pleural effusion, pulmonary edema (noncardiogenic), pulmonary infiltrates, pulmonary insufficiency, sinusitis, wheezing

SKIN: Rash, urticaria

Other: Allergic reaction, anaphylaxis, angioedema, infection, infusion reaction

Nursing Considerations

- Perform baseline cardiac assessment before beginning trastuzumab therapy. Expect patient to receive an echocardiogram, an ECG, or a multigated acquisition (MUGA) scan before initiation of therapy. Be aware that patients with a history of cardiac disease, including preexisting cardiac dysfunction, are at increased risk for developing cardiomyopathy. In addition, patients who have previously received a cardiotoxic drug or radiation therapy to the chest wall are at increased risk for cardiotoxicity.
- Be aware that adverse reactions can vary when trastuzumab is administered in combination therapy. Review information for all drugs administered as part of a specific regimen, including drug interactions and adverse effects.
- **WARNING** Reconstitute trastuzumab with 20 ml of the 30 ml of bacteriostatic water for injection (containing benzyl alcohol) provided by manufacturer to produce a multidose vial of 21 mg/ml. Discard the remaining 10 ml of diluent; using all of it would result in a lower-than-intended dose. Label vial with "DO NOT USE AFTER" and insert date that is 28 days after date of reconstitution. Use contents within 28 days if stored at 2° to 8° C (36° to 46° F).
- If patient is hypersensitive to benzyl alcohol, prepare initial dilution using 20 ml of sterile water for injection *without* preservative. Use immediately.
- When reconstituting drug, slowly inject the stream of diluent directly into lyophilized cake of trastuzumab. Swirl gently; don't shake. Let vial stand for about 5 minutes to allow slight foaming that may have formed to dissipate. Expect solution to be clear to slightly opalescent and colorless to pale yellow. Discard if solution contains particles.
- Dilute reconstituted trastuzumab with a 250-ml infusion bag of normal saline solution; use within 24 hours if stored at 2° to 8° C.
- Administer trastuzumab by I.V. infusion, *not* by I.V. push or bolus.
- **WARNING** Monitor patient for possibly life-threatening infusion reaction, pulmonary complications, or allergic reaction. Assess for such signs as dizziness, fever or chills, headache, nausea, rash, shortness of breath, vomiting, or weakness, particularly during administration and for at least 24 hours afterward. Be aware that infusion reaction typically occurs with

the first dose but may occur with subsequent doses. Patients with preexisting pulmonary compromise from lung disease or pulmonary malignancy are at increased risk for pulmonary complications.

- Continue to assess cardiac function, including left ventricular function, in all patients during trastuzumab treatment. Prescriber may discontinue drug if patient develops a clinically significant decrease in left ventricular function. Patients who receive trastuzumab in combination with anthracyclines and cyclophosphamide are at increased risk.
- Expect to discontinue infusion if patient experiences dyspnea or clinically significant hypotension. Assess patient until signs and symptoms completely resolve. Prescriber may discontinue drug if patient develops anaphylaxis, angioedema, or acute respiratory distress syndrome.
- Before reconstituting trastuzumab, store it at 2° to 8° C.

PATIENT TEACHING

- Advise patient to immediately report signs of an infusion or allergic reaction or pulmonary complications, including difficulty breathing, rash, and facial swelling. Inform her that such reactions may occur 24 hours or longer after infusion.
- Instruct female patients not to breast-feed during trastuzumab therapy and for 6 months afterward.
- Stress the importance of complying with the dosage regimen and of keeping follow-up medical appointments and appointments for laboratory tests.

treprostinil sodium

Remodulin

Class and Category

Chemical: Prostaglandin, tricyclic benzidene analogue
Therapeutic: Vasodilator
Pregnancy category: B

Indications and Dosages

▶ *To treat pulmonary artery hypertension in patients who have New York Heart Association Class II to IV symptoms in order to diminish exercise-induced symptoms*

I.V. INFUSION

Adults. *Initial:* 1.25 nanograms/kg/min. *Maintenance:* Infusion rate increased in increments of no more than 1.25 nanograms/kg/min each wk for first 4 wk, and in increments of no more

than 2.5 nanograms/kg/min each wk thereafter, as needed. *Maximum:* 40 nanograms/kg/min.
DOSAGE ADJUSTMENT If initial dosage isn't tolerated or if patient has mild to moderate hepatic insufficiency, decrease initial dose to 0.625 nanogram/kg/min (using ideal body weight).

Mechanism of Action

Acts directly on pulmonary and systemic arterial vascular beds to produce vasodilation. The vasodilatory effects reduce right and left ventricular afterload and increase cardiac output and stroke volume. These effects improve symptoms of pulmonary hypertension, such as dyspnea, and enable patients with pulmonary hypertension to walk greater distances with less discomfort.

Contraindications

Hypersensitivity to treprostinil, its components, or structurally related compounds

Interactions

DRUGS

anticoagulants: Increased risk of bleeding
antihypertensives, diuretics, other vasodilators: Increased risk of hypotension

Adverse Reactions

CNS: Anxiety, dizziness, headache, restlessness
CV: Edema, hypotension, vasodilatation
EENT: Jaw pain
GI: Diarrhea, nausea, vomiting
SKIN: Cellulitis, pruritus, rash
Other: Infusion site pain or reaction (erythema, induration, rash)

Nursing Considerations

- Use treprostinil cautiously in patients with hepatic or renal impairment.
- Assess patient's ability to care for an I.V. catheter and to use an infusion pump. Discuss findings with prescriber before starting treprostinil therapy.
- For I.V. use, dilute with sterile water for injection or normal saline solution according to manufacturer's instructions.
- Calculate infusion rate using the formula provided in the package insert, or refer to charts in package insert to find infusion delivery rate for prescribed dosage and administration route.

- **WARNING** Don't abruptly stop treprostinil infusion or make sudden large reductions in dose because symptoms of pulmonary hypertension may worsen.
- Assess patient frequently for drug effectiveness and for adverse reactions. Know that the goal of chronic dosage adjustments is to find a dose that will improve symptoms of pulmonary hypertension, such as dyspnea and fatigue, while minimizing the drug's adverse effects, such as headache, nausea, vomiting, restlessness, anxiety, and infusion site pain or reaction.
- Monitor patients with mild to moderate hepatic insufficiency closely for adverse reactions, especially after dosage increases, because treprostinil is metabolized primarily by the liver.
- Be aware that patient must be discharged with a backup infusion pump. It should be one that's adjustable to about 0.002 ml/hr and has alarms that indicate occlusion/no delivery, low battery, programming error, and motor malfunction. Also, the pump should have a delivery accuracy of 66% or better, be positive-pressure driven, and have a reservoir made of polyvinyl chloride, polypropylene, or glass. Make sure patient has additional I.V. or S.C. infusion sets to prevent potential interruptions in drug delivery.

PATIENT TEACHING

- Explain to patient that treprostinil is infused continuously through an I.V. catheter via an infusion pump.
- Teach patient to operate and maintain the I.V. infusion pump and to recognize the drug's adverse effects.
- To reduce the risk of infection, caution patient to always use aseptic technique when preparing and giving drug.
- Tell patient that a single vial of the drug shouldn't be used beyond 14 days after opening and that once the drug is placed in the pump's reservoir, it shouldn't be used after 72 hours.
- Instruct patient to store treprostinil vials at room temperature (about 25° C [77° F]).
- Inform patient that drug will be needed for prolonged periods, possibly years. Stress the importance of not stopping drug abruptly or making sudden large reductions in dosage without consulting prescriber because symptoms could worsen.
- Make sure patient understands that treprostinil use doesn't preclude the subsequent use of an alternative I.V. prostacyclin therapy such as epoprostenol.
- Make sure patient has emergency contact information for problems or questions about giving treprostinil at home.

triflupromazine hydrochloride

Vesprin

Class and Category

Chemical: Phenothiazine
Therapeutic: Antiemetic, antipsychotic
Pregnancy category: Not rated

Indications and Dosages

▶ *To treat nausea and vomiting*

I.V. INJECTION

Adults. 1 mg p.r.n. *Maximum:* 3 mg daily.

Mechanism of Action

Prevents nausea and vomiting by inhibiting or blocking dopamine receptors in the medullary chemoreceptor trigger zone and, peripherally, by blocking the vagus nerve in the GI tract. Triflupromazine also blocks postsynaptic dopamine receptors, increasing dopamine turnover and decreasing dopamine neurotransmission. This action may depress the areas of the brain that control activity and aggression, including the cerebral cortex, hypothalamus, and limbic system.

Contraindications

Blood dyscrasias, bone marrow depression, cerebral arteriosclerosis, coma or severe CNS depression, concurrent use of large quantity of CNS depressants, coronary artery disease, hepatic dysfunction, hypersensitivity to phenothiazines, severe hypertension or hypotension, subcortical brain damage

Interactions

DRUGS

amantadine, anticholinergics, antidyskinetics, antihistamines: Possibly intensified adverse anticholinergic effects, increased risk of triflupromazine-induced hyperpyrexia
amphetamines: Decreased stimulant effect of amphetamines, decreased antipsychotic effect of triflupromazine
anticonvulsants: Lowered seizure threshold
antithyroid drugs: Increased risk of agranulocytosis
apomorphine: Possibly decreased emetic response to apomorphine, additive CNS depression
appetite suppressants: Decreased anorectic effect of appetite suppressants

astemizole, cisapride, disopyramide, erythromycin, pimozide, probucol, procainamide, quinidine: Prolonged QT interval, increased risk of ventricular tachycardia
beta blockers: Increased blood levels of both drugs, possibly leading to additive hypotensive effect, arrhythmias, irreversible retinopathy, and tardive dyskinesia
bromocriptine: Impaired therapeutic effects of bromocriptine
CNS depressants: Additive CNS depression
ephedrine: Decreased vasopressor response to ephedrine
epinephrine: Blocked alpha-adrenergic effects of epinephrine
extrapyramidal reaction–causing drugs (droperidol, haloperidol, metoclopramide, metyrosine, risperidone): Increased severity and frequency of extrapyramidal reactions
hepatotoxic drugs: Increased risk of hepatotoxicity
hypotension-producing drugs: Possibly severe hypotension with syncope
levodopa: Decreased antidyskinetic effect of levodopa
lithium: Possibly encephalopathy and additive extrapyramidal effects
MAO inhibitors, maprotiline, tricyclic antidepressants: Increased CNS depression, impaired triflupromazine metabolism, increased risk of neuroleptic malignant syndrome
mephentermine: Possibly antagonized antipsychotic effect of triflupromazine and vasopressor effect of mephentermine
metaraminol: Decreased vasopressor effect of metaraminol
methoxamine, phenylephrine: Decreased vasopressor effect and shortened duration of action of these drugs
metrizamide: Increased risk of seizures
opioid analgesics: Increased risk of CNS and respiratory depression, orthostatic hypotension, severe constipation, and urine retention
ototoxic drugs: Possibly masking of symptoms of ototoxicity, such as dizziness, tinnitus, and vertigo
phenytoin: Lowered seizure threshold; inhibited phenytoin metabolism, possibly leading to phenytoin toxicity
photosensitizing drugs: Possibly additive photosensitivity and intraocular photochemical damage to choroid, lens, or retina
thiazide diuretics: Possibly hyponatremia and water intoxication

ACTIVITIES

alcohol use: Increased CNS and respiratory depression, increased hypotensive effect

Adverse Reactions

CNS: Akathisia, altered temperature regulation, dizziness, drowsi-

ness, extrapyramidal reactions (dystonia, pseudoparkinsonism, tardive dyskinesia), neuroleptic malignant syndrome
CV: Hypotension, orthostatic hypotension, tachycardia
EENT: Blurred vision, dry mouth, nasal congestion, ocular changes (deposits of fine particles in cornea and lens), pigmentary retinopathy
ENDO: Galactorrhea, gynecomastia
GI: Constipation, epigastric pain, nausea, vomiting
GU: Ejaculation disorders, menstrual irregularities, urine retention
SKIN: Decreased sweating, photosensitivity, pruritus, rash
Other: Injection site irritation and sterile abscess, weight gain

Nursing Considerations

- Be aware that I.V. triflupromazine is not recommended for use in children because of its hypotensive and severe, rapid-onset extrapyramidal effects.
- Before administering triflupromazine, observe parenteral solution, which may turn slightly yellow without altering potency. Don't use solution if discoloration is pronounced or precipitate is present.
- Don't let solution come in contact with your skin because contact dermatitis may result.
- **WARNING Monitor patient closely for tardive dyskinesia, which may continue after treatment stops. Notify prescriber if patient exhibits such signs as uncontrolled movements of arms, body, cheeks, jaw, legs, mouth, or tongue.**
- Closely monitor elderly patients and severely ill or dehydrated children because they're at increased risk for certain adverse CNS reactions. Elderly patients are also at increased risk for developing hypotension amd extrapyramidal reactions, especially if they're acutely ill or debilitated.
- Monitor patients with glaucoma for signs and symptoms of this disorder, such as eye pain, vision changes, and nausea or vomiting from increased intraocular pressure, because of drug's anticholinergic effects.
- Monitor patients with chronic respiratory disorders (such as asthma and emphysema) or acute respiratory tract infections for exacerbations due to drug's CNS depressant effects.
- Monitor patients with cardiovascular, hepatic, or renal disease because they're at increased risk for developing hypotension, heart failure, and arrhythmias.
- Be aware that triflupromazine should be used cautiously in patients who will be exposed to organophosphate insecticides.

- **WARNING** If patient develops neuroleptic malignant syndrome (hyperpyrexia, muscle rigidity, altered mental status, autonomic instability), notify prescriber immediately and expect to discontinue drug and begin intensive medical treatment.
- **WARNING** Be alert for suppressed cough reflex, which increases patient's risk of aspirating vomitus.
- Monitor patients with a history of hepatic encephalopathy due to cirrhosis for increased sensitivity to drug's CNS effects.
- Monitor patients who have been exposed to extreme heat for heatstroke due to drug-induced suppression of temperature regulation. Symptoms include tachycardia, fever, and confusion.
- Before using triflupromazine, store it at 15° to 30° C (59° to 86° F); protect from freezing and light.

PATIENT TEACHING

- Instruct patient to change position slowly during triflupromazine therapy to minimize effects of orthostatic hypotension.
- Urge patient to avoid potentially hazardous activities until drug's CNS effects are known.
- Instruct patient to immediately report difficulty swallowing or speaking and tongue protrusion.
- Caution patient to avoid alcohol during therapy.
- Urge patient to avoid exposure to the sun and extreme heat because drug may cause photosensitivity and interfere with thermoregulation. Encourage her to wear sunscreen when outdoors.

tromethamine

Tham

Class and Category

Chemical: Organic amine
Therapeutic: Alkalinizer
Pregnancy category: C

Indications and Dosages

▶ *To treat metabolic acidosis associated with cardiac arrest*

I.V. INFUSION

Adults and children. 3.6 to 10.8 g (111 to 333 ml) of 0.3 M solution.

▶ *To treat metabolic acidosis during cardiac bypass surgery*

I.V. INFUSION

Adults and children. 9 ml (2.7 mEq or 0.32 g) of 0.3 M solution/

kg as a single dose. *Usual:* 500 ml (150 mEq or 18 g) infused over 1 hr. *Maximum:* 500 mg/kg over 1 hr.

Mechanism of Action

Combines with hydrogen ions and their associated acid anions, including lactic, pyruvic, and carbonic acid, to form salts that are excreted in urine. Tromethamine exerts additional alkalinizing effects by acting as an osmotic diuretic, promoting the excretion of alkaline urine that contains increased amounts of carbon dioxide and electrolytes.

Contraindications

Anuria, chronic respiratory acidosis, hypersensitivity to tromethamine or its components, uremia

Interactions

DRUGS

amphetamines, quinidine, other pH-dependent drugs: Altered excretion of these drugs

Adverse Reactions

CNS: Fever
CV: Vasospasm
ENDO: Hypoglycemia
GI: Hepatic necrosis (hemorrhagic)
RESP: Respiratory depression
Other: Hypervolemia; infusion site infection, phlebitis, or venous thrombosis; metabolic alkalosis

Nursing Considerations

- Evaluate blood pH, blood glucose, and serum bicarbonate and electrolyte levels, and partial pressure of arterial carbon dioxide before, during, and after tromethamine therapy, as ordered.
- Administer infusion by an indwelling catheter inserted into a large vein, such as one in the antecubital area.
- **WARNING** Be aware that exceeding the recommended dosage can cause alkalosis, respiratory depression, and reduced carbon dioxide level. Because of the risk of alkalosis, tromethamine therapy is limited to 1 day, except in life-threatening situations.
- Be aware that I.V. administration of tromethamine increases the risk of hypervolemia and subsequent pulmonary edema.

- Assess infusion site frequently for signs of infiltration, which may cause inflammation, necrosis, thrombosis, tissue sloughing, and vasospasm.
- Be aware that patients with renal failure have an increased risk of hyperkalemia. For such patients, be prepared to monitor ECG continuously and assess serum potassium level often.
- Monitor blood glucose level often during and after therapy because rapid administration can cause hypoglycemia for several hours.
- Protect drug from freezing and extreme heat.

PATIENT TEACHING

- Inform family members that patient's vital signs and laboratory test results will be evaluated frequently to monitor her progress.

urea
(carbamide)

Ureaphil

Class and Category

Chemical: Carbonic acid diamide salt
Therapeutic: Antiglaucoma agent, diuretic
Pregnancy category: C

Indications and Dosages

▶ *To reduce cerebral edema and intracranial pressure (ICP)*

I.V. INFUSION

Adults and children age 2 and over. 500 mg to 1.5 g/kg as 30% solution in D_5W, $D_{10}W$, or 10% invert sugar solution infused over 30 min to 2 hr at 4 ml/min or as ordered, according to manufacturer's instructions. *Maximum:* 2 g/kg daily.

Children under age 2. 100 mg to 1.5 g/kg as 30% solution in D_5W, $D_{10}W$, or 10% invert sugar solution infused over 30 min to 2 hr at 4 ml/min or as ordered, according to manufacturer's instructions.

▶ *To treat malignant or secondary glaucoma*

I.V. INFUSION

Adults. 500 mg to 1.5 g/kg as 30% solution in D_5W, $D_{10}W$, or 10% invert sugar solution infused over 30 min to 2 hr at 4 ml/min or as ordered, according to manufacturer's instructions. *Maximum:* 2 g/kg daily.

DOSAGE ADJUSTMENT Dosage reduced or drug withheld for patients with renal impairment if BUN level rises to 75 mg/

dl or more or if diuresis fails to occur within 2 hr after administration.

Route	Onset	Peak	Duration
I.V.	10 min	1 to 2 hr	3 to 10 hr*

Mechanism of Action

Elevates blood plasma osmolality, creating an osmotic effect that increases the movement of water from the brain, CSF, and anterior portion of the eyes into interstitial fluid and plasma. This action reduces cerebral edema, ICP, CSF volume, and intraocular pressure. Large doses of urea inhibit the reabsorption of water and solutes in the renal tubules and induce diuresis by affecting the osmotic pressure gradient of the glomerular filtrate.

Incompatibilities

If patient is receiving blood simultaneously, don't administer urea through same administration set.

Contraindications

Active intracranial bleeding, hepatic failure, hypersensitivity to urea or its components, renal impairment, severe dehydration

Interactions

DRUGS

carbonic anhydrase inhibitors, other diuretics: Additive diuretic and intraocular pressure–reducing effects

lithium: Increased renal excretion of lithium

Adverse Reactions

CNS: Agitation, confusion, fever, headache, hyperthermia, nervousness, subarachnoid hemorrhage, subdural hematoma, syncope

CV: Tachycardia

EENT: Dry mouth, intraocular hemorrhage

GI: Nausea, thirst, vomiting

GU: Elevated BUN level

HEME: Hemolysis

SKIN: Blemishes, extravasation with tissue necrosis and sloughing

* For diuresis; 5 to 6 hr for reduction of intraocular pressure in malignant or secondary glaucoma.

Other: Dehydration, hypokalemia, hyponatremia, infusion site phlebitis or thrombosis

Nursing Considerations

- Expect to administer urea 60 minutes before intracranial or ocular surgery to obtain maximum reduction of ICP or intraocular pressure.
- Don't mix urea with invert sugar solution if patient has fructose intolerance from aldolase deficiency.
- Avoid infusing drug into leg veins to reduce the risk of phlebitis and thrombosis.
- Discard unused portion of drug after 24 hours.
- Be aware that rapid administration may cause hemolysis, increased capillary bleeding, and, in patients with glaucoma, intraocular hemorrhage.
- Maintain adequate hydration to minimize adverse reactions. Assess for signs of dehydration, including dry mucous membranes or tenting.
- Monitor BUN and serum electrolyte levels as well as fluid intake and output during urea therapy because prolonged use can cause diuresis.
- Store drug at 15° to 30° C (59° to 86° F); don't freeze.

PATIENT TEACHING

- Instruct patient to immediately report difficulty breathing or shortness of breath because urea can cause transient increases in circulatory volume, leading to circulatory overload, exacerbations of heart failure, or pulmonary edema.
- Advise patient to expect increased urine output.
- Encourage patient to remain on bed rest during urea therapy.

urokinase

Abbokinase, Abbokinase Open-Cath

Class and Category

Chemical: Renal enzymatic protein
Therapeutic: Thrombolytic
Pregnancy category: B

Indications and Dosages

▶ *To treat acute coronary artery thrombosis*

INTRACORONARY INFUSION

Adults. 6,000 international units/min until artery is maximally opened (up to 2 hr may be required). *Usual:* 500,000 international units.

▶ *To treat acute pulmonary thromboembolism including massive events*

I.V. INFUSION

Adults. *Initial:* 4,400 international units/kg over 10 min, followed by 4,400 international units/kg/hr for 12 hr.

▶ *To clear I.V. catheter occlusion*

INSTILLATION

Adults and children. 5,000 international units/ml instilled into occluded line.

Route	Onset	Peak	Duration
I.V.	Unknown	20 min to 2 hr	4 hr
Intracoronary	Unknown	Unknown	4 hr

Mechanism of Action

Indirectly promotes conversion of plasminogen to plasmin, an enzyme that breaks down fibrin clots, fibrinogen, and other plasma proteins, including procoagulant factors V and VIII.

Incompatibilities

Don't administer I.V. urokinase through the same I.V. line as other drugs or add other drugs to urokinase solution.

Contraindications

Arteriovenous malformation, bleeding disorder, CVA during previous 2 months, hypersensitivity to urokinase or its components, internal bleeding, intracranial aneurysm, intracranial or intraspinal surgery during previous 2 months, intracranial tumor, recent cardiopulmonary resuscitation, recent trauma, severe uncontrolled hypertension (systolic blood pressure of 200 mm Hg or higher, or diastolic blood pressure of 110 mm Hg or higher)

Interactions

DRUGS

antifibrinolytics (aminocaproic acid, aprotinin): Mutual antagonism

antihypertensives: Increased risk of severe hypotension

cefamandole, cefoperazone, cefotetan, plicamycin, valproic acid: Increased risk of hypoprothrombinemia and severe hemorrhage

corticosteroids, ethacrynic acid, salicylates (nonacetylated): Increased risk of GI ulceration and bleeding

enoxaparin, heparin, NSAIDs, oral anticoagulants, platelet-aggregation inhibitors: Increased risk of hemorrhage
thiotepa: Increased therapeutic effects of thiotepa

Adverse Reactions

CNS: Chills, CVA, fever, headache
CV: Arrhythmias, including tachycardia; chest pain; cholesterol embolization, hypertension; hypotension
EENT: Orolingual edema
GI: Nausea, vomiting
HEME: Unusual bleeding
MS: Back pain, myalgia
RESP: Bronchospasm, dyspnea, hypoxemia, wheezing
SKIN: Cyanosis, ecchymosis, flushing, pruritus, rash, urticaria
Other: Anaphylaxis, infusion site reactions, metabolic acidosis

Nursing Considerations

- To prevent foaming, don't shake urokinase when reconstituting. Consult with pharmacist about giving drug through 0.45-micron or smaller cellulose membrane filter.
- Assess baseline hematocrit, platelet count, thrombin time, APTT, PT, and INR as ordered.
- Monitor heart rate and rhythm by continuous ECG during therapy, especially during rapid lysis of coronary thrombi, because arrhythmias can occur with reperfusion.
- Monitor blood pressure for hypotension. If hypotension occurs, notify prescriber and expect to reduce infusion rate.
- Check for bleeding at puncture sites and in urine and stool. Check for intracranial bleeding by performing frequent neurologic assessments.
- After arterial puncture is performed, apply pressure for at least 30 minutes and then apply pressure dressing. Check often for bleeding during therapy.
- To prevent bleeding and associated complications, avoid venipunctures; use an external blood pressure cuff to measure blood pressure; give acetaminophen (not aspirin), as prescribed, for fever; and handle patient as little as possible.
- **WARNING** If serious bleeding begins and can't be controlled with local pressure, stop infusion immediately and notify prescriber.

PATIENT TEACHING

- Instruct patient to remain on bed rest during urokinase therapy.
- Inform patient that minor bleeding may occur at wounds or puncture sites.

valproic acid

Alti-Valproic (CAN), Depakene, Deproic (CAN), Dom-Proic (CAN), Med-Valproic (CAN), Novo-Valproic (CAN), Nu-Valproic (CAN), PMS-Valproic Acid (CAN)

valproate sodium

Depacon

divalproex sodium

Depakote, Epival (CAN)

Class and Category

Chemical: Carboxylic acid derivative
Therapeutic: Anticonvulsant
Pregnancy category: D

Indications and Dosages

▶ *To treat simple or complex absence seizures, complex partial seizures, myoclonic seizures, and generalized tonic-clonic seizures as monotherapy*

I.V. INFUSION

Adults and adolescents. *Initial:* 10 to 15 mg/kg daily in divided doses b.i.d. or t.i.d., increased by 5 to 10 mg/kg daily q wk, as needed and as prescribed. *Maximum:* 60 mg/kg daily.

Children. *Initial:* 15 to 45 mg/kg daily in divided doses b.i.d. or t.i.d., increased by 5 to 10 mg/kg daily q wk, as needed and as prescribed.

▶ *As adjunct to treat simple or complex absence seizures, complex partial seizures, myoclonic seizures, and generalized tonic-clonic seizures*

I.V. INFUSION

Adults and adolescents. 10 to 30 mg/kg daily in divided doses, increased by 5 to 10 mg/kg daily q wk, as needed and as prescribed.

Children. 30 to 100 mg/kg daily in divided doses, as prescribed.

DOSAGE ADJUSTMENT For adults being converted from immediate-release divalproex tablets to delayed-release tablets, dosage increased to 8% to 20% more than total daily dose of immediate-release tablets and given once daily.

Mechanism of Action

May decrease seizure activity by blocking the reuptake of gamma-aminobutyric acid (GABA), the most common inhibitory neurotransmitter in the brain. GABA is known to suppress the rapid firing of neurons by inhibiting voltage-sensitive sodium channels.

Contraindications

Hepatic dysfunction; hypersensitivity to valproic acid, valproate sodium, divalproex sodium, or their components; urea cycle disorders

Interactions

DRUGS

aspirin, heparin, NSAIDs, oral anticoagulants, thrombolytics: Increased inhibition of platelet aggregation and risk of bleeding
barbiturates, primidone: Increased blood levels of both drugs, additive CNS effects
carbamazepine: Possibly decreased valproic acid effectiveness
cholestyramine: Decreased bioavailability of valproic acid
clonazepam: Increased risk of absence seizures
CNS depressants: Increased CNS depression
diazepam: Inhibited diazepam metabolism
ethosuximide: Unpredictable blood ethosuximide level
felbamate: Impaired valproic acid metabolism and increased blood drug level
haloperidol, loxapine, MAO inhibitors, maprotiline, phenothiazines, thioxanthenes, tricyclic antidepressants: Increased CNS depression, lowered seizure threshold
lamotrigine: Decreased lamotrigine clearance
mefloquine: Decreased blood levels of valproic acid, divalproex, and valproate sodium; increased risk of seizures
phenytoin: Increased risk of phenytoin toxicity, loss of seizure control
topiramate: Increased risk of hyperammonemia and encephalopathy

ACTIVITIES

alcohol use: Additive CNS depression

Adverse Reactions

CNS: Agitation, ataxia, confusion, depression, dizziness, drowsiness, euphoria, hallucinations, headache, hyperesthesia, lack of coordination, lethargy, loss of seizure control, paresthesia, psychosis, sedation, tremor, vertigo, weakness
EENT: Diplopia, nystagmus, pharyngitis, spots before eyes
ENDO: Galactorrhea, hyperglycemia
GI: Abdominal pain, anorexia, constipation, diarrhea, elevated liver function test results, hepato-renal syndrome, hepatotoxicity, increased appetite, indigestion, nausea, pancreatitis, vomiting
GU: Menstrual irregularities, nephritis, oliguria

HEME: Eosinophilia, hematoma, leukopenia, neutropenia, prolonged bleeding time, thrombocytopenia
MS: Arthralgia, dysarthria
SKIN: Alopecia, diaphoresis, erythema multiforme, jaundice, petechiae, photosensitivity, pruritus, rash, Stevens-Johnson syndrome
Other: Facial edema, hyperammonemia, injection site pain, lympadenopathy, multi-organ hypersensitivity reaction, weight gain or loss

Nursing Considerations

- For I.V. administration, dilute prescribed dose with at least 50 ml of compatible diluent and infuse over 60 minutes.
- Be aware that patient should be switched from I.V. to P.O. form of valproic acid as soon as possible.
- **WARNING** Although rare, life-threatening multi-organ hypersensitivity reaction have occurred, during initiation of valproic acid therapy. Monitor patient closely for fever and rash accompanied by organ involvement such as lymphadenopathy, hepatitis, liver function test abnormalities, eosinophilia, thrombocytopenia, neutropenia, nephritis, pruritis, oliguria, hepato-renal syndrome, arthralgia, and asthenia. Notify prescriber immediately if present, discontinue drug, as ordered, and be prepared to provide supportive care.
- Be aware that patient with hypoalbuminemia or another protein-binding deficiency is at increased risk for valproic acid toxicity.
- Assess for signs and symptoms of decreased hepatic function, including anorexia, facial edema, jaundice, lethargy, loss of seizure control, malaise, vomiting, and weakness.
- Monitor liver function test results, as or dered. Assess for signs and symptoms of hepatotoxicity during first 6 months of treatment, especially in children under age 2. Notify prescriber immediately if you suspect hepatotoxicity.
- Monitor platelet count, as ordered, for signs of thrombocytopenia, and notify prescriber if they appear.
- **WARNING** Be aware that hyperammonemia may occur even if patient's liver function test results are normal. Monitor ammonia levels, as ordered. If patient develops unexplained lethargy, vomiting, or changes in mental status with an increase in ammonia level or if asymptomatic ammonia elevations are detected and persist, expect valproic acid to be discontinued.

PATIENT TEACHING

- Instruct patient to report any unusual, persistent or severe signs and symptoms to prescriber, especially unexplained fever and rash accompanied by other complaints.
- Advise patient to avoid potentially hazardous activities during therapy because drug may affect mental and motor performance.
- Urge patient to avoid alcohol during therapy.
- Urge female patient to notify prescriber immediately about suspected or known pregnancy.
- Advise patient to notify prescriber if tremor develops during therapy; occurrence of tremor may be dose-related.

vancomycin hydrochloride

Vancocin

Class and Category

Chemical: Tricyclic glycopeptide derivative
Therapeutic: Antibiotic
Pregnancy category: C (parenteral)

Indications and Dosages

▶ *To treat bacterial endocarditis caused by methicillin-resistant* Staphylococcus aureus

I.V. INFUSION

Adults. 30 mg/kg daily in equally divided doses b.i.d. for 4 to 6 wk. *Maximum:* 2 g daily.

▶ *As adjunct to treat bacterial endocarditis caused by methicillin-resistant* S. aureus *in patients with prosthetic heart valve*

I.V. INFUSION

Adults. 30 mg/kg daily in equally divided doses b.i.d. to q.i.d. for 6 wk or longer in conjunction with rifampin and gentamicin. *Maximum:* 2 g daily.

▶ *To treat bacterial endocarditis caused by* Streptococcus bovis *or* Streptococcus viridans

I.V. INFUSION

Adults. 30 mg/kg daily in equally divided doses b.i.d. for 4 wk. *Maximum:* 2 g daily.

▶ *As adjunct to treat bacterial endocarditis caused by enterococci*

I.V. INFUSION

Adults. 30 mg/kg daily in equally divided doses b.i.d. for 4 to 6 wk in conjunction with gentamicin. *Maximum:* 2 g daily.

▶ *To treat bacterial septicemia, bone and joint infections, pneumonia, and skin and soft-tissue infections caused by* Staphylococcus, *including methicillin-resistant strains, and life-threatening infections*

I.V. INFUSION

Adults and children age 12 and over. 500 mg q 6 hr or 1 g q 12 hr infused over at least 60 min. *Maximum:* 4 g daily.

Children ages 1 month to 12 years. 10 mg/kg q 6 hr or 20 mg/kg q 12 hr infused over at least 60 min.

Neonates ages 1 week to 1 month. *Initial:* 15 mg/kg followed by 10 mg/kg q 8 hr infused over at least 60 min.

Neonates under age 1 week. *Initial:* 15 mg/kg followed by 10 mg/kg q 12 hr infused over at least 60 min.

Mechanism of Action

Inhibits bacterial RNA and cell wall synthesis; alters permeability of bacterial membranes, causing cell wall lysis and cell death.

Incompatibilities

Don't give I.V. vancomycin through the same I.V. line as other drugs. Don't add vancomycin to albumin-containing solutions, alkaline solutions, aminophylline, amobarbital sodium, aztreonam, cefepime, ceftazidime, chloramphenicol sodium succinate, chlorothiazide sodium, dexamethasone sodium phosphate, foscarnet sodium, heparin sodium, methicillin sodium, penicillin G, pentobarbital sodium, phenobarbital sodium, piperacillin sodium and tazobactam sodium, secobarbital sodium, and sodium bicarbonate. Drug may precipitate with heavy metals.

Contraindications

Hypersensitivity to vancomycin or its components, hypersensitivity to corn or corn products when vancomycin is given with dextrose solutions

Interactions

DRUGS

aminoglycosides (amikacin, gentamicin, tobramycin), amphotericin B, bacitracin (parenteral), bumetanide, capreomycin, carmustine, cidofovir, cisplatin, cyclosporine, ethacrynic acid, furosemide, paromomycin, pentamidine (parenteral), polymyxins, salicylates (parenteral), streptozocin: Additive nephrotoxicity or ototoxicity

antihistamines, buclizine, cyclizine, meclizine, phenothiazines, thioxanthenes, trimethobenzamide: Masked symptoms of ototoxicity

cholestyramine, colestipol: Decreased antibacterial activity of oral vancomycin
dexamethasone: Decreased penetration of vancomycin into CSF
nephrotoxic drugs: Increased risk of nephrotoxicity

Adverse Reactions

CNS: Chills, dizziness, vertigo
CV: Hypotension
EENT: Ototoxicity
GI: Nausea
GU: Nephrotoxicity
HEME: Eosinophilia, neutropenia
RESP: Dyspnea, wheezing
SKIN: Exfoliative dermatitis; extravasation with pain, tenderness, thrombophlebitis, and tissue necrosis; pruritus; rash; toxic epidermal necrolysis; urticaria
Other: Anaphylaxis, drug-induced fever, injection site inflammation, superinfection

Nursing Considerations

- To reconstitute 500-mg vial of vancomycin for I.V. use, add 10 ml of sterile water for injection; further dilute with at least 100 ml of compatible I.V. solution. For 1-g vial of dry, sterile powder, add 20 ml of sterile water for injection; further dilute with at least 200 ml of compatible I.V. solution.
- **WARNING Infuse over at least 1 hour. Rapid administration may cause hypotension or transient "red man syndrome," characterized by chills; fainting; fever; flushing of face, neck, upper arms, and torso; hypotension; nausea; tachycardia; and vomiting.**
- Monitor blood vancomycin levels, as ordered; be aware that therapeutic levels are 10 to 15 mcg/ml trough and 30 to 40 mcg/ml peak.
- If patient has an inflammatory intestinal disorder, assess him often for adverse reactions because vancomycin absorption may be increased in these conditions.
- Monitor CBC results and serum creatinine and BUN levels during therapy, especially if patient has renal impairment or takes an aminoglycoside.
- Monitor I.V. infusion site for signs and symptoms of extravasation, including necrosis, pain, tenderness, and thrombophlebitis. If extravasation occurs, discontinue infusion immediately and notify prescriber.

- Monitor hearing during therapy. Transient or permanent ototoxicity may occur if patient receives an excessive amount of drug, has an underlying hearing loss, or receives concurrent aminoglycosides.
- Monitor patient receiving prolonged therapy for signs and symptoms of superinfection, such as severe diarrhea and white patches on tongue.

PATIENT TEACHING
- Advise patient to notify prescriber if no improvement occurs after a few days.
- Caution patient that she should consult prescriber before taking any drug to control diarrhea because that condition may signal superinfection.
- Instruct patient to keep follow-up appointments during and after treatment.

verapamil hydrochloride

Isoptin

Class and Category

Chemical: Phenylalkylamine derivative
Therapeutic: Antianginal, antiarrhythmic, antihypertensive
Pregnancy category: C

Indications and Dosages

▶ *To prevent or treat supraventricular tachycardia*

I.V. INJECTION

Adults and adolescents age 15 and over. *Initial:* 5 to 10 mg slowly over 2 min; then 10 mg, as prescribed, if response isn't adequate after 30 min.

Children ages 1 to 15. *Initial:* 100 to 300 mcg/kg slowly over 2 min, up to maximum of 5 mg; then 10 mg, as prescribed, if response isn't adequate after 30 min.

Infants up to age 1. *Initial:* 100 to 200 mcg/kg slowly over 2 min.

DOSAGE ADJUSTMENT I.V. drug administered over 3 minutes in elderly patients.

Route	Onset	Peak	Duration
I.V.	1 to 5 min	3 to 5 min	10 min to 6 hr

Mechanism of Action

Inhibits calcium movement into coronary and vascular smooth-muscle cells by blocking slow calcium channels in cell membranes. The resulting decrease in the intracellular calcium level has the following effects:

- inhibits smooth-muscle cell contractions
- decreases myocardial oxygen demand by relaxing coronary and vascular smooth muscle, reducing peripheral vascular resistance, and decreasing systolic and diastolic pressures
- slows AV conduction time and prolongs AV nodal refractoriness
- interrupts reentry circuit in AV nodal reentrant tachycardias.

Incompatibilities

Don't mix I.V. verapamil with albumin, amphotericin B injection, hydralazine hydrochloride injection, nafcillin, or sulfamethoxazole and trimethoprim injection. Solutions with pH above 6.0 cause precipitation.

Contraindications

Cardiogenic shock, concomitant use of beta blockers (with I.V. verapamil), hypersensitivity to verapamil or its components, hypotension, severe heart failure unless secondary to supraventricular tachycardia that responds to verapamil, severe left ventricular dysfunction, sick sinus syndrome or second- or third-degree heart block unless artificial pacemaker is in place, ventricular tachycardia (with I.V. verapamil)

Interactions

DRUGS

alpha blockers, antihypertensives, general anesthetics (hydrocarbon), prazosin: Hypotensive effects

aspirin: Increased bleeding time

beta blockers: Increased risk of heart failure, hypotension, and severe bradycardia

calcium supplements: Decreased response to verapamil

carbamazepine, cyclosporine, theophylline, valproate: Increased risk of toxicity from these drugs

cimetidine: Decreased metabolism and increased blood level of verapamil

dantrolene: Increased risk of hyperkalemia and myocardial depression

digoxin: Increased blood digoxin level and risk of digitalis toxicity
disopyramide, flecainide: Additive negative inotropic effects
erythromycin, ritonavir: Increased blood verapamil level
lithium: Increased risk of neurotoxicity
neuromuscular blockers: Prolonged recovery from neuromuscular blockade
NSAIDs, sympathomimetics: Decreased antihypertensive effect of verapamil
phenobarbital: Increased verapamil clearance
procainamide: Increased Q-T interval, additive negative inotropic effects
protein-bound drugs (hydantoins, salicylates, sulfonamides, sulfonylureas, and warfarin and other oral anticoagulants): Altered blood levels of these drugs
quinidine: Increased risk of quinidine toxicity, increased Q-T interval, additive negative inotropic effects
rifampin: Decreased bioavailability of oral verapamil
FOODS
grapefruit juice: Increased concentrations of verapamil
ACTIVITIES
alcohol use: Increased blood alcohol level and prolonged CNS effects

Adverse Reactions

CNS: Confusion, CVA, disequilibrium, dizziness, extrapyramidal reactions, fatigue, headache, insomnia, paresthesia, psychosis, shakiness, somnolence
CV: Angina, AV conduction disorders, bradycardia, claudication, heart failure, hypotension, peripheral edema, tachycardia
GI: Constipation, elevated liver function test results, nausea
GU: Galactorrhea, menstrual irregularities
MS: Muscle spasms
RESP: Dyspnea, pulmonary edema, wheezing
SKIN: Flushing, rash

Nursing Considerations

- Administer I.V. verapamil with compatible solutions, including Ringer's injection, D_5W, or normal saline solution.
- Maintain continuous ECG monitoring and keep emergency resuscitative equipment and drugs readily available during I.V. therapy.

- Assess patient with hypertrophic cardiomyopathy for early development of hypotension and pulmonary edema because second-degree AV block and sinus arrest can result.
- Assess for bradycardia and hypotension, and notify prescriber if heart rate or blood pressure declines significantly.
- Be aware that disopyramide or flecainide shouldn't be given within 48 hours before or 24 hours after verapamil because additive negative inotropic effects can result.
- Institute measures to prevent constipation, including a high-fiber diet and a stool softener, as prescribed.

PATIENT TEACHING

- Direct patient to check her pulse rate before taking verapamil and to notify prescriber if it's below 50 beats/minute or as instructed by prescriber.
- Caution patient about possible dizziness and the need to avoid potentially hazardous activities until drug's CNS effects are known.
- Inform patient that adverse skin reactions may subside with continued use. Advise her to notify prescriber about persistent rash.
- Encourage patient to increase dietary fiber intake to help prevent constipation. Advise her to notify prescriber if problem becomes persistent or severe.

vinblastine sulfate

Velban, Velbe (CAN)

Class and Category

Chemical: Vinca alkaloid
Therapeutic: Antimicrotubule antineoplastic
Pregnancy category: D

Indications and Dosages

▶ *To treat breast or testicular cancer, gestational trophoblastic tumors, histiocytosis X, Hodgkin's disease or non-Hodgkin's lymphoma, Kaposi's sarcoma, or mycosis fungoides*

I.V. INJECTION

Adults. *Initial:* 100 mcg (0.1mg)/kg or 3.7 mg/m^2 over 1 min q 7 days, increased in weekly increments of 50 mcg (0.05 mg)/kg or 1.8 to 1.9 mg/m^2 until leukocyte count falls to 3,000/mm^3. *Maintenance:* 50 mcg (0.05 mg/kg) or 1.8 to 1.9 mg/m^2 less than final initial dose. *Maximum:* 500 mcg (0.5 mg)/kg or 18.5 mg/m^2.

Adolescents and children. *Initial:* 2.5 mg/m^2 over 1 min q 7 days, increased in weekly increments of 1.25 mg/m^2 until leukocyte count falls to 3,000/mm^3. *Maintenance:* 1.25 mg/m^2 less than final initial dose. *Maximum:* 7.5 mg/m^2.

DOSAGE ADJUSTMENT Dosage decreased by 50% for patients who have a direct serum bilirubin concentration above 3 mg/dl.

Mechanism of Action

Binds to tubulin, a protein component of microtubules, which normally contribute to cell structure and movement, thereby inhibiting microtubule assembly and arresting cells in metaphase. Vinblastine may also interfere with amino acid metabolism. This drug is cell-cycle–phase specific for the M phase of cell division.

Incompatibilities

Prepare vinblastine solution using normal saline solution. Don't mix solution with any other drug.

Contraindications

Bacterial infection; granulocytopenia resulting from condition other than disease being treated

Interactions

DRUGS

blood-dyscrasia–causing drugs (such as cephalosporins and sulfasalazine): Increased risk of leukopenia and thrombocytopenia

bone marrow depressants (such as carboplatin and lomustine): Possibly additive bone marrow depression

hepatic enzyme inhibitors (such as allopurinol and cimetidine): Possibly earlier onset or increased severity of vinblastine adverse effects

itraconazole: Possibly earlier onset or increased severity of neuromuscular adverse effects

phenytoin: Possibly decreased blood phenytoin level and increased risk of seizures

vaccines, killed virus: Possibly decreased antibody response to vaccine

vaccines, live virus: Possibly decreased antibody response to vaccine, increased adverse effects of vaccine, and severe infection

Adverse Reactions

CNS: Malaise, neurotoxicity, weakness

CV: Hypertension
EENT: Jaw pain, stomatitis
GI: Anorexia, constipation, nausea, vomiting
GU: Uric acid nephropathy
HEME: Anemia, leukopenia, thrombocytopenia (transient)
MS: Bone pain, tissue pain at tumor site
SKIN: Alopecia
Other: Hyperuricemia, injection site pain or redness

Nursing Considerations

- Follow facility protocols for preparation and handling of antineoplastic drugs and for appropriate disposal of used equipment.
- Be aware that vinblastine dosage may vary, depending on dosage schedule and regimen being used.
- Be aware that adverse reactions can vary when vinblastine is administered in combination therapy. Review information for all drugs administered as part of a specific regimen, including drug interactions and adverse effects.
- Monitor liver function test results; hematocrit, hemoglobin, and platelet count; and leukocyte count (total and differential) before and periodically during treatment, as ordered.
- Monitor blood uric acid level of patients with a history of gout or renal calculi before and periodically during vinblastine therapy to detect hyperuricemia. Expect to give allopurinol, as ordered, to patients with elevated blood uric acid levels to prevent uric acid nephropathy. Be aware that patients already receiving antigout drugs, such as allopurinol, colchicine, probenecid, or sufinpyrazone, may require an adjustment in antigout drug dosage.
- Be aware that vinblastine is available in a 1-mg/ml preparation or as a powder for reconstitution. To reconstitute vinblastine, add 10 ml of 0.9% sodium chloride injection to a vial containing 10 mg/ml to yield a final concentration of 1 mg/ml. If the diluent contains a preservative, such as benzyl alcohol, use diluted solution within 28 days if stored at 2° to 8° C (36° to 46° F). If the diluent doesn't contain a preservative, use solution immediately and discard unused portion.
- **WARNING** When preparing vinblastine for neonates or premature infants, don't use a diluent that contains benzyl alcohol because this preservative has been linked to a fatal toxic syndrome characterized by CNS, respiratory, circulatory, and renal impairment and metabolic acidosis.

- If vinblastine solution comes in contact with your skin or mucosa, wash if off thoroughly with warm water. If drug comes in contact with your eye, irrigate eye thoroughly with water to prevent irritation or corneal ulceration.
- **WARNING** Clearly label syringe containing prepared dose "FATAL IF GIVEN INTRATHECALLY. FOR I.V. USE ONLY" and place in overwrap. Label overwrap with the same warning and the additional statement "DO NOT REMOVE COVERING UNTIL THE MOMENT OF INJECTION." Don't administer drug intrathecally because potentially fatal paralysis may occur.
- Inspect I.V. site for signs of infiltration and leakage into surrounding tissues. If extravasation occurs, stop injection immediately and notify prescriber. Then resume injection in another vein. Apply warm heat to affected area, and expect to administer a local injection of hyaluronidase, if ordered, to help decrease discomfort and reduce the risk of cellulitis.
- Be aware that subsequent doses of vinblastine shouldn't be administered until leukocyte count after previous dose has returned to at least 4,000/mm^3, even if 7 days has passed.
- Monitor patients who have, or have recently been exposed to, chicken pox or who have herpes zoster for signs and symptoms of severe generalized disease.
- Be aware that patients who have previously received cytotoxic therapy and those who are receiving concurrent or consecutive radiation therapy are at risk for additive bone marrow depression.
- If patient develops thrombocytopenia, implement protective precautions according to facility policy.
- Assess for signs of infection, such as fever, if patient develops leukopenia. Expect to obtain appropriate specimens for culture and sensitivity testing and implement protective precautions according to facility policy.
- Before reconstituting powder form or using diluted form, store vinblastine at 2° to 8° C (36° to 46° F).

PATIENT TEACHING

- Advise patient to have any needed dental work completed before beginning vinblastine treatment, if possible, or to defer such work until blood counts return to normal because vinblastine can delay healing and cause gingival bleeding. Teach patient proper oral hygiene, and advise her to use a soft-bristled toothbrush.

- Advise patient to immediately report burning at injection site or other signs of extravasation.
- Instruct patient who develops bone marrow depression to avoid people with infections. Advise her to report fever, chills, cough, hoarseness, lower back or side pain, or painful or difficult urination because these signs and symptoms may indicate an infection.
- Instruct patient to avoid touching her eyes or inside of her nose unless she washes her hands immediately beforehand.
- Caution patient to avoid receiving immunizations unless approved by prescriber. Instruct her to avoid people who have recently received vaccines or to wear a protective mask over her nose and mouth if she must be around them.
- Instruct patient to immediately report unusual bleeding or bruising, black or tarry stools, blood in urine or stools, or red pinpoint spots on skin.
- Stress the importance of avoiding accidental cuts from sharp objects, such as razor blades or fingernail clippers, because excessive bleeding or infection may occur.
- Encourage patient to drink plenty of fluids to increase urine output and help excrete uric acid.
- Suggest that patient with stomatitis eat bland, soft foods served cold or at room temperature to decrease irritation.
- Caution patient to avoid contact sports or other situations that put her at risk for bruising or injury.
- Stress the importance of complying with the dosage regimen and of keeping follow-up medical appointments and appointments for laboratory tests.
- Reassure patient that her hair should grow back after vinblastine therapy has been completed.
- Urge patient to use contraception because of the risk of fetal harm from vinblastine therapy. Instruct her to notify prescriber immediately if she becomes pregnant.

vincristine sulfate

Oncovin, Vincasar PFS

Class and Category

Chemical: Vinca alkaloid
Therapeutic: Antineoplastic
Pregnancy category: D

Indications and Dosages

▶ *To treat acute lymphocytic leukemia, Hodgkin's disease or non-Hodgkin's lymphoma, neuroblastoma, or Wilms' tumor*

I.V. INJECTION

Adults. 10 to 30 mcg (0.01 to 0.03 mg)/kg or 400 mcg (0.4 mg) to 1.4 mg/m^2 over 1 min q wk. Dosage adjusted based on patient's clinical response and presence or severity of toxicity.

Children weighing more than 10 kg. 1.5 to 2 mg/m^2 over 1 min q wk.

Children weighing 10 kg and less. 50 mcg (0.05 mg)/kg over 1 min q wk.

DOSAGE ADJUSTMENT Dosage decreased by 50% for patients with direct serum bilirubin concentration above 3 mg/dl.

Mechanism of Action

Inhibits the formation of microtubules, which normally contribute to cell structure and movement, thus arresting cells in metaphase. Vincristine is cell-cycle–phase specific for the M phase of cell division.

Incompatibilities

Don't administer vincristine with solutions that lower or raise pH outside the range of 3.5 to 5.5. Administer only with normal saline solution or D_5W.

Contraindications

Demyelinating form of Charcot-Marie-Tooth syndrome

Interactions

DRUGS

asparaginase, itraconazole, neurotoxic drugs: Possibly additive neurotoxic effects

bleomycin: Increased susceptibility of cancer cells to bleomycin

blood-dyscrasia–causing drugs (such as cephalosporins and sulfasalazine): Increased risk of leukopenia and thrombocytopenia

bone marrow depressants (such as carboplatin and lomustine): Possibly additive bone marrow depression

doxorubicin: Increased risk of myelosuppression when used in combination with vincristine and prednisone

phenytoin: Possibly decreased blood phenytoin level and increased risk of seizures

vaccines, killed virus: Possibly decreased antibody response to vaccine

vaccines, live virus: Possibly decreased antibody response to vaccine, increased adverse effects of vaccine, and severe infection

Adverse Reactions

CNS: Fever, headache, progressive neurotoxicity (including blurred or double vision, decreased reflexes, difficulty walking, neuritic pain, and paresthesia)
CV: Hypertension, hypotension
EENT: Stomatitis
ENDO: Syndrome of inappropriate ADH secretion (SIADH)
GI: Bloating, constipation (severe), diarrhea, nausea, vomiting
GU: Dysuria, polyuria, uric acid nephropathy, urine retention
HEME: Anemia, leukopenia, thrombocytopenia
RESP: Bronchospasm, dyspnea
SKIN: Alopecia, rash
Other: Allergic reaction, hyperuricemia, injection site pain or redness, weight loss

Nursing Considerations

- Follow facility protocols for preparation and handling of antineoplastic drugs and for appropriate disposal of used equipment.
- Be aware that vincristine dosage may vary, depending on dosage schedule and regimen being used.
- Be aware that adverse reactions can vary when vincristine is given in combination therapy. Review information for all drugs administered as part of a specific regimen, including drug interactions and adverse effects.
- Monitor liver function test results; hematocrit, hemoglobin, and platelet count; and leukocyte count (total and differential) before and periodically during treatment, as ordered.
- Monitor the blood uric acid level of patients with a history of gout or renal calculi before and periodically during therapy to detect hyperuricemia. Expect to administer allopurinol, as ordered, to patients with elevated blood uric acid levels to prevent uric acid nephropathy. Be aware that patients already receiving antigout drugs, such as allopurinol, colchicine, probenecid, or sufinpyrazone, may require an adjustment in antigout drug dosage.
- If vincristine solution comes in contact with your skin or mucosa, wash it off thoroughly with warm water. If drug comes in contact with your eye, irrigated the eye thoroughly with water to prevent irritation or corneal ulceration.

- **WARNING** After withdrawing appropriate amount of drug from vial, as ordered, clearly label syringe "FATAL IF GIVEN INTRATHECALLY. FOR I.V. USE ONLY" and place in overwrap. Label overwrap with the same warning and the additional statement "DO NOT REMOVE COVERING UNTIL THE MOMENT OF INJECTION." Don't administer drug intrathecally because potentially fatal paralysis may occur.
- Administer vincristine over a 1-minute period by I.V. bolus, or inject it into a free-flowing I.V. infusion of normal saline solution or D_5W.
- Inspect I.V. site for signs of infiltration and leakage into surrounding tissues. If extravasation occurs, stop the vincristine injection immediately and notify prescriber. Then resume the injection in another vein. Apply warm heat to affected area, and expect to administer a local injection of hyaluronidase, if ordered, to help decrease discomfort and reduce the risk of cellulitis.
- Administer a prophylactic enema or laxative, if ordered, to prevent ileus.
- Monitor patient for hypotension and signs of neurotoxicity, such as paresthesia, decreased reflexes, and weakness. If such signs occur, notify prescriber and expect to decrease dosage or discontinue therapy, as ordered.
- Monitor patients who have, or have recently been exposed to, chicken pox or who have herpes zoster for signs and symptoms of severe generalized disease.
- Be aware that patients who have previously received cytotoxic therapy and those who are receiving concurrent or consecutive radiation therapy are at risk for additive bone marrow depression.
- If patient develops thrombocytopenia, implement protective precautions according to facility policy.
- Assess for signs of infection, such as fever, if patient develops leukopenia. Expect to obtain appropriate specimens for culture and sensitivity testing.
- Store vincristine at 2° to 8° C (36° to 46° F) in a light-resistant container.

PATIENT TEACHING

- Advise patient to immediately report burning at the injection site or other signs or symptoms of extravasation during vincristine therapy.

- Instruct patient who develops bone marrow depression to avoid people with infections. Advise her to report fever, chills, cough, hoarseness, lower back or side pain, or painful or difficult urination because these signs and symptoms may indicate an infection.
- Instruct patient to avoid touching her eyes or the inside of her nose unless she has washed her hands immediately before doing so.
- Caution patient to avoid receiving immunizations unless approved by prescriber. Urge her to avoid people who have recently received vaccines or to wear a protective mask over her nose and mouth if she must be around them.
- Instruct patient to immediately report unusual bleeding or bruising, black or tarry stools, blood in urine or stool, or red pinpoint spots on skin during vincristine therapy.
- Stress the importance of avoiding accidental cuts from sharp objects, such as razor blades or fingernail clippers, because excessive bleeding or infection may occur.
- Caution patient to avoid contact sports or other situations that put her at risk for bruising or injury.
- Encourage patient to drink fluids to increase urine output and help excrete uric acid; however, caution her not to drink excessive amounts because of the risk of SIADH.
- Suggest that patient with stomatitis eat bland, soft foods served cold or at room temperature to decrease irritation.
- Advise patient to consult prescriber about using a laxative if she develops constipation.
- Reassure patient that her hair should grow back after vincristine therapy has been completed.
- Urge patient to use contraception because of the risk of fetal harm from vincristine therapy. Instruct her to notify prescriber immediately if she becomes pregnant.
- Stress the importance of complying with the dosage regimen and of keeping follow-up medical appointments and appointments for laboratory tests.

voriconazole

Vfend

Class and Category

Chemical: Triazole
Therapeutic: Antifungal

Pregnancy category: D

Indications and Dosages

▶ *To treat invasive aspergillosis; to treat serious fungal infections caused by* Scedosporium apiospermum *and* Fusarium *sp., including* Fusarium solani, *in patients intolerant of or refractory to other therapy*

I.V. INFUSION

Adults and children age 12 and over. *Initial:* 6 mg/kg over 1 to 2 hr at a rate not to exceed 3 mg/kg/hr q 12 hr for 2 doses. *Maintenance:* 4 mg/kg over 1 to 2 hr at a rate not to exceed 3 mg/kg/hr q 12 hr.

▶ *To treat candidemia in nonneutropenic patients and other deep-tissue disseminatinated* Candida *infections involving the abdomen, kidney, bladder wall, skin, or a wound*

I.V. INFUSION

Adults. *Initial:* 6 mg/kg over 1 to 2 hr at no more than 3 mg/kg/hr q 12 hr for two doses. *Maintenance:* 3 to 4 mg/kg over 1 to 2 hr at no more than 3 mg/kg/hr q 12 hr for at least 14 days after symptoms resolve or last positive culture, whichever takes longer.

DOSAGE ADJUSTMENT If patient can't tolerate drug, I.V. maintenance dose may be reduced to 3 mg/kg q 12 hr. For use with phenytoin, maintenance dose may be increased to 5 mg/kg I.V. q 12 hr. For patients with mild to moderate hepatic cirrhosis, standard loading dose should be used but maintenance dose halved for I.V. use.

Incompatibilities

Don't infuse into the same line or cannula with other drugs, including parenteral nutrition, to prevent an increase in subvisible particulate matter. Avoid infusion with blood products and any electrolyte supplements. Don't dilute with 4.2% sodium bicarbonate infusion because the mildly alkaline nature of the diluent causes slight degradation of voriconazole after 24 hours of storage at room temperature.

Mechanism of Action

Prevents fungal ergosterol biosynthesis by inhibiting fungal cytochrome P450–mediated 14 alpha-lanosterol demethylation. The loss of ergosterol in the fungal cell wall renders the fungal cell inactive.

Contraindications

Coadministration with long-acting barbiturates, carbamazepine, CYP3A4 substrates (astemizole, cisapride, pimozide, quinidine, or terfenadine), efavirenz, ergot alkaloids, rifabutin, rifampin, ritonavir, or sirolimus; hypersensitivity to voriconazole or its components; galactose intolerance, glucose-galactose malabsorption, or Lapp lactase deficiency (oral form only contains lactose)

Interactions

DRUGS

benzodiazepines: Possibly prolonged sedative effect of benzodiazepines

calcium channel blockers; HMG-CoA reductase inhibitors, such as lovastatin; omeprazole; sirolimus: Possibly increased plasma concentrations of these drugs, leading to increased risk of adverse reactions and toxicity

carbamazepine, long-acting barbiturates, phenytoin, rifampin: Decreased plasma voriconazole concentration

coumarin, warfarin: Possibly increased PTT

cyclosporine, sirolimus, tacrolimus: Increased serum concentrations of these drugs and increased risk of toxicity, especially nephrotoxicity

CYP3A4 substrates (astemizole, cisapride, pimozide, quinidine, terfenadine): Increased plasma concentrations of CYP3A4 substrates, which may lead to prolonged QT interval and, rarely, torsades de pointes

ergot alkaloids (ergotamine, dihydroergotamine): May increase plasma concentration of ergot alkaloids leading to ergotism

HIV protease inhibitors (amprenavir, nelfinavir, ritonavir, saquinavir), non-nucleoside reverse transcriptase inhibitors (delavirdine, efavirenz): Possibly inhibited metabolism of these drugs and voriconazole

methadone: Increased plasma concentration of methadone, possibly leading to toxicity, including QT-interval prolongation

oral contraceptives: Increased plasma concentration of voriconazole

rifabutin: Increased rifabutin plasma concentration; decreased voriconazole plasma concentrations

sulfonylureas: Possibly increased plasma concentrations of sulfonylureas and increased risk of hypoglycemia

vinca alkaloids: Possibly increased risk of neurotoxicity

Adverse Reactions

CNS: Chills, dizziness, fever, hallucinations, headache
CV: Chest pain, hypertension, hypotension, peripheral edema, tachycardia, vasodilation
EENT: Abnormal or blurred vision, altered or enhanced visual perception, change in color perception, chromatopsia, dry mouth, eye hemorrhage, photophobia, visual disturbances
GI: Abdominal pain, diarrhea, elevated liver function test results, nausea, vomiting
GU: Abnormal kidney function, acute renal failure, elevated serum creatinine level
HEME: Anemia, leukopenia, pancytopenia, thrombocytopenia
RESP: Respiratory disorders
SKIN: Cholestatic jaundice, erythema multiforme, jaundice, maculopapular rash, photosensitivity, pruritus, rash, Stevens-Johnson syndrome, toxic epidermal necrolysis
Other: Anaphylaxis (I.V. form), elevated alkaline phosphatase, hypokalemia, hypomagnesemia, sepsis

Nursing Considerations

- Use voriconazole cautiously in patients with known hypersensitivity to other azoles and in patients at risk for proarrhythmic events (such as those receiving cardiotoxic chemotherapy or those who have cardiomyopathy or hypokalemia) because some azoles may cause prolong QT interval.
- Obtain specimens for fungal culture and other relevant laboratory studies (including histopathology), as ordered, before giving first dose. Expect to begin drug before test results are known.
- Assess patient's liver function, including bilirubin, as ordered, at the start of voriconazole therapy and periodically thereafter. Be aware that drug may be discontinued if liver abnormalities occur.
- Check patient's electrolyte levels before start of therapy, as ordered, and correct any imbalances, as prescribed, before administering voriconazole because electrolyte imbalances increase the risk of adverse reactions.
- For I.V. infusion, reconstitute powder with 19 ml of water for injection to obtain 20 ml of concentrate that contains 10 mg/ml of voriconazole. Use a standard 10-ml nonautomated syringe to ensure that exact amount of water is injected into vial.
- Shake the vial until all powder is dissolved.

- Further dilute so that final concentration is not less than 0.5 mg/ml nor more than 5 mg/ml. This requires withdrawing and discarding at least an equal volume of diluent from the infusion bag or bottle before instillation of concentrate.
- Discard partially used vials after mixing. If infusion isn't administered immediately, store at 2° to 8° C (37° to 46° F) for no longer than 24 hours.
- Administer I.V. infusion over 1 to 2 hours at a rate that doesn't exceed 3 mg/kg/hr.
- Monitor renal function, especially serum creatinine level, when administering I.V. form of voriconazole because drug may accumulate in body when creatinine clearance is less than 50 ml/min, increasing the risk of adverse reactions.
- **WARNING Observe patient receiving I.V. voriconazole closely for anaphylactoid-type reactions—such as flushing, fever, sweating, tachycardia, chest tightness, dyspnea, faintness, nausea, pruritus and rash—which may occur immediately after starting the infusion. Stop the infusion if these reactions occur, and notify prescriber immediately.**
- Monitor patient closely throughout therapy for skin rash, which may indicate a serious cutaneous reaction, such as Stevens-Johnson syndrome. If a rash occurs, notify prescriber, and expect that drug may be discontinued.
- Monitor patient closely for elevated levels of cyclosporine, tacrolimus, and warfarin when voriconazole is given with any of these drugs.
- Watch closely for hypoglycemia in diabetic patients who also take sulfonylureas, and check their blood glucose levels regularly.
- Be aware that voriconazole dosage will need to be adjusted when given with phenytoin. Expect to monitor plasma phenytoin levels and observe patient closely for phenytoin-related adverse reactions.
- Assess patient's visual function, including visual acuity, visual field, and color perception, if voriconazole therapy continues longer than 28 days.

PATIENT TEACHING

- Inform female patient of possible risk to fetus, and stress the importance of avoiding pregnancy. Tell her to use an effective form of contraception throughout voriconazole therapy and to notify the prescriber immediately if she is or could be pregnant or of she plans to become pregnant.

- Caution patient not to drive at night and to avoid potentially hazardous activities because drug may cause visual disturbances, including blurring or photophobia.
- Advise patient to avoid exposure to direct sunlight or UV light and to wear sunscreen when outdoors.

W·X·Y·Z

warfarin sodium

Coumadin

Class and Category

Chemical: Coumarin derivative
Therapeutic: Anticoagulant
Pregnancy category: X

Indications and Dosages

▶ *To prevent or treat pulmonary embolism; recurrent MI; thromboembolic complications from atrial fibrillation, heart valve replacement, or MI; and venous thrombosis (and its extension)*

I.V. INJECTION

Adults. *Initial:* 2 to 5 mg daily infused over 1 to 2 min. *Usual:* 2 to 10 mg daily infused over 1 to 2 min. *Maximum:* Determined by target PT and INR results, as prescribed.

DOSAGE ADJUSTMENT For patients with hepatic dysfunction, dosage reduced to 0.1 mg/kg, as prescribed. For elderly patients, dosage possibly reduced based on PT and INR results.

Route	Onset	Peak	Duration
I.V.	Unknown	3 to 4 days	2 to 5 days

Mechanism of Action

Interferes with the liver's ability to synthesize vitamin K-dependent clotting factors, depleting clotting factors II (prothrombin), VII, IX, and X. This action, in turn, interferes with the clotting cascade. By depleting vitamin K-dependent clotting factors and interfering with the clotting cascade, warfarin prevents coagulation.

Incompatibilities

Don't mix warfarin in solution with amikacin sulfate, epinephrine hydrochloride, metaraminol tartrate, oxytocin, promazine hydrochloride, tetracycline hydrochloride, or vancomycin hydrochloride.

Contraindications

Bleeding or bleeding tendencies; blood dyscrasias; cerebral or dissecting aneurysm; cerebrovascular hemorrhage; diverticulitis; eclampsia or preeclampsia; history of warfarin-induced necrosis; hypersensitivity to warfarin or its components; malignant or severe uncontrolled hypertension; malnutrition and emaciation; mental state or condition that leads to lack of patient cooperation; pericardial effusion; pericarditis; polyarthritis; pregnancy; prostatectomy; recent or planned neurosurgery, ophthalmic surgery, or spinal puncture; severe hepatic or renal disease

Interactions

DRUGS

acetaminophen, aminoglycosides, amiodarone, androgens, argatroban, beta blockers, bivalirudin, capecitabine, cephalosporins, chloral hydrate, chloramphenicol, chlorpropamide, cimetidine, clofibrate, corticosteroids, cyclophosphamide, dextrothyroxine, diflunisal, disulfiram, erythromycin, ezetimibe, fluconazole, gemfibrozil, glucagon, hydantoins, ifosfamide, influenza virus vaccine, isoniazid, ketoconazole, lepirudin, loop diuretics, lovastatin, metronidazole, miconazole, mineral oil, moricizine, nalidixic acid, NSAIDs, omeprazole, penicillins, phenylbutazones, propafenone, propoxyphene, proton pump inhibitors, quinidine, quinine, quinolones, salicylates, streptokinase, sulfamethoxazole-trimethoprim, sulfinpyrazone, sulfonamides, tamoxifen, tetracyclines, thyroid hormones, urokinase, valdecoxib, vitamin E: Increased anticoagulant effect of warfarin, increased risk of bleeding

aminoglutethimide, barbiturates, carbamazepine, cholestyramine, dicloxacillin, estrogens, ethchlorvynol, etretinate, glutethimide, griseofulvin, nafcillin, oral contraceptives, rifampin, spironolactone, sucralfate, thiazide diuretics, trazodone, vitamin C, vitamin K: Decreased anticoagulant effect of warfarin

atorvastatin, pravastatin: Increased or decreased anticoagulant effect of warfarin

herbal remedies (including bromelains, danshen, dong quai, garlic, ginkgo biloba, and ginseng): Increased anticoagulant effect of warfarin, increased risk of bleeding

I.V. lipid emulsion, other medical products that contain soybean oil: Possibly decreased vitamin K absorption and increased anticoagulant effect of warfarin

nicotine patch: Altered response to warfarin

FOODS

certain multivitamins, enteral feedings, vitamin-K–rich foods: Decreased effects of warfarin

ACTIVITIES

alcohol use: Increased risk of hypoprothrombinemia

smoking, smoking cessation: Altered response to warfarin

Adverse Reactions

CNS: Coma, intracranial hemorrhage, loss of consciousness, syncope, weakness

CV: Angina, hypotension

EENT: Epistaxis, intraocular hemorrhage

GI: Abdominal cramps and pain, diarrhea, hepatitis, nausea, vomiting

GU: Hematuria, vaginal bleeding (abnormal)

HEME: Anemia, potentially fatal hemorrhage (from any tissue or organ)

SKIN: Alopecia, ecchymosis, jaundice, pallor, petechiae, pruritus, purple-toe syndrome, tissue necrosis

NURSING CONSIDERATIONS

- Reconstitute parenteral warfarin just before administration with 2.7 ml of sterile water for injection to yield 2 mg/ml. Then administer slowly over 1 to 2 minutes through peripheral I.V.
- Avoid I.M. injections during warfarin therapy, if possible, because they can result in bleeding, bruising, and hematoma.
- Monitor international normalized ratio (INR) (daily in acute care setting) and assess for therapeutic effects, as prescribed. Therapeutic INR levels are 2.0 to 3.0 for bioprosthetic heart valve, nonvalvular atrial fibrillation, and venous thromboembolism, and 2.5 to 3.5 after MI and for mechanical heart valve.
- Expect treatment to last up to 12 weeks for bioprosthetic heart valve, 1 to 3 months for nonvalvular atrial fibrillation or venous thromboembolism, and for rest of life after MI and for mechanical heart valve replacement.
- **WARNING** Be aware of the increased risk for intracranial hemorrhage if patient has cerebral ischemia (such as recent transient ischemic attack or minor ischemic CVA) and INR of 3 to 4.5. As prescribed, withhold next warfarin dose and give vitamin K if INR exceeds 4 because of the risk of bleeding.
- Assess for occult bleeding if patient receives I.V. lipid emulsion or other medical product that contains soybean oil. Such products can decrease vitamin K absorption and increase warfarin's anticoagulant effect.

PATIENT TEACHING

- Explain that warfarin therapy aims to prevent thrombosis by decreasing clotting ability while avoiding the risk of spontaneous bleeding.
- Urge patient to keep weekly follow-up appointments for blood tests after discharge until PT and INR levels are stabilized.
- Advise patient to avoid alcohol during warfarin therapy.
- Urge patient to take precautions against bleeding, such as using an electric shaver and a soft-bristled toothbrush. Advise him to continue these precautions for 2 to 5 days after therapy stops, as directed, because anticoagulant effect may persist during this time.
- Caution patient to avoid activities that could cause traumatic injury and bleeding.
- Advise patient to eat consistent amounts of vitamin K–rich foods, such as dark green, leafy vegetables.
- Urge patient to notify prescriber immediately about unusual bleeding and any unexplained symptoms, such as abnormal vaginal bleeding; dizziness; easy bruising; gum bleeding; headache; nosebleeds; prolonged bleeding from cuts; red, black, or tarry stool; red or dark brown urine; swelling; and weakness.
- Advise patient to consult prescriber before taking other drugs—including OTC drugs and herbal remedies—during therapy.
- Instruct female patient of childbearing age to stop taking warfarin and notify prescriber immediately about known or suspected pregnancy.
- Explain that drug may cause reversible purple-toe syndrome and that this syndrome isn't harmful.
- Urge patient to carry medical identification that reveals he's taking warfarin therapy.

zidovudine

Retrovir

Class and Category

Chemical: Synthetic pyrimidine nucleoside analogue
Therapeutic: Antiviral
Pregnancy category: C

Indications and Dosages

▶ *To treat HIV infection*

I.V. INFUSION

Adults and children over age 12 (United States). 1 mg/kg

infused over 1 hr five or six times a day. *Maximum pediatric dose:* 160 mg.
Adults and children over age 12 (Canada). 1 to 2 mg/kg infused over 1 hr q 4 hr. *Maximum pediatric dose:* 160 mg.
DOSAGE ADJUSTMENT Adult dosage reduced to 1 mg/kg q 6 to 8 hr for patients with end-stage renal disease.

▶ *To prevent maternal-fetal HIV transmission*

I.V. INFUSION

Mother. 2 mg/kg infused over 1 hr at the start of labor and delivery, followed by 1 mg/kg/hr by continuous infusion until umbilical cord is clamped.
Neonate. 1.5 mg/kg infused over 30 min q 6 hr.

Mechanism of Action

Ultimately converted by thymidine kinase and other cellular enzymes to zidovudine triphosphate. Zidovudine triphosphate is incorporated into growing chains of viral DNA polymerase, an enzyme used in the viral DNA replication process, thus inhibiting DNA viral replication of HIV.

Incompatibilities

Don't mix zidovudine with biological or colloidal solutions, such as blood products or protein-containing solutions.

Contraindications

Hypersensitivity to zidovudine or its components

Interactions

DRUGS

atovaquone: Possibly decreased zidovudine clearance and increased blood zidovudine level
blood-dyscrasia–causing drugs (such as cephalosporins and sulfasalazine), bone marrow depressants (such as carboplatin and lomustine): Increased risk of additive myelosuppressive effects
clarithromycin: Decreased blood zidovudine level and time to peak zidovudine concentration
cytotoxic drugs, ganciclovir, interferon alfa: Increased risk of hematologic toxicities
hepatic glucuronidation–metabolized drugs (such as acetaminophen, aspirin, benzodiazepines, cimetidine, indomethacin, morphine, and sulfonamides): Possibly decreased clearance and toxicity of both drugs
interferons, ribavirin: Increased risk of hepatic decompensation, neutropenia, and anemia

methadone, rifampin: Possibly altered blood zidovudine level
phenytoin: Possibly decreased blood phenytoin level and decreased zidovudine clearance
probenecid: Possibly increased blood ziduvodine level and flulike symptoms
ribovirin, stavudine: Possibly antagonized antiviral effect

Adverse Reactions

CNS: Chills, fever, headache, insomnia, tiredness, weakness
EENT: Pharyngitis
GI: Nausea
HEME: Anemia, bone marrow depression, granulocytopenia, leukopenia, neutropenia, platelet count changes
MS: Myalgia
SKIN: Altered skin pigmentation, hyperpigmentation (bluish-brown bands) of nails, pallor
Other: Immune reconstitution syndrome

Nursing Considerations

- Be aware that I.V. infusion of zidovudine is ordered only until oral drug can be administered.
- Dilute ziduvodine with D_5W to a maximum concentration of 4 mg/ml. Use within 8 hours if stored at room temperature or within 24 hours if stored at 2° to 8° C (36° to 46° F) to decrease the risk of microbial contamination. Discard solution if you observe particles or discoloration before administration.
- Administer zidovudine by I.V. infusion at a constant rate over 1 hour; don't administer drug by rapid infusion or by I.M. injection.
- Monitor CBC periodically during zidovudine therapy. Be aware that anemia most commonly occurs after 4 to 6 weeks of therapy and that patient may require dosage adjustment, discontinuation of drug, blood transfusions, or epoetin treatment if hemoglobin level is less than 7.5 g/dl or if granulocyte count is less than $750/mm^3$.
- Assess patient for dyspnea, tachypnea, or decreased blood bicarbonate level; if she exhibits such findings, expect zidovudine to be discontinued until a diagnosis of lactic acidosis can be ruled out.
- Monitor patient for immune reconstitution syndrome, which may occur during combination antiretroviral therapy that includes zidovudine. During the initial phase of treatment, the syndrome is exhibited by patients developing an inflammatory response to certain infections such as *Mycobactgerium avium* in-

fection, cytomegalovirus, *Pneumocystits jirovecii* (formerly *carinii*) pneumonia or tuberculosis that may require additional therapy.
- Before diluting drug, store it at 15° to 25° C (59° to 77° F) and protect from light.

PATIENT TEACHING
- Advise mothers being treated for HIV infection not to breast-feed infant to prevent transmission of virus.
- Instruct patient to use a condom to decrease the risk of transmitting HIV. Also, urge patient not to share needles with anyone.
- Teach patient proper oral hygiene, and advise her to use a soft-bristled toothbrush to decrease the risk of infection or delayed healing.
- Inform patient who is also receiving cidofovir that zidovudine dosage may need to be adjusted or therapy temporarily discontinued on the day of cidofovir therapy.
- Explain to patient that zidovudine is not a cure for HIV infection. Stress the importance of complying with dosage regimen and of keeping follow-up medical appointments and appointments for laboratory tests.

zinc chloride

(contains 1 mg of elemental zinc per ml for I.V. infusion)

zinc sulfate

1 or 5 mg of elemental zinc per ml for I.V. infusion)
Zinca-Pak

Class and Category

Chemical: Trace element, mineral
Therapeutic: Copper absorption inhibitor, nutritional supplement
Pregnancy category: C

Indications and Dosages

▶ *To prevent zinc deficiency based on U.S. and Canadian recommended daily allowances (RDAs)*

I.V. INFUSION

Adults and children. 2.5 to 4 mg daily added to total parenteral nutrition (TPN) solution. *Maximum:* 12 mg daily.
Children from birth to age 5. 100 mcg/kg daily added to TPN solution.
Premature infants weighing up to 3 kg. 300 mcg/kg daily added to TPN solution.

▶ *To treat zinc deficiency*

I.V. INFUSION

Adults and adolescents. 2.5 to 4 mg daily added to TPN solution. *Maximum:* 12 mg daily.

Children from birth to age 5. 100 mcg/kg daily added to TPN solution.

Premature infants weighing up to 3 kg. 300 mcg/kg daily added to TPN solution.

Mechanism of Action

Needed for proper functioning of more than 200 metalloenzymes (those containing tightly bound zinc atoms as an integral part of their structure), including carbonic anhydrase, carboxypeptidase A, alcohol dehydrogenase, alkaline phosphatase, and RNA polymerase. Zinc also helps maintain nucleic acid, protein, and cell membrane structure and is essential for certain physiologic functions, including cell growth and division, sexual maturation and reproduction, dark adaptation and night vision, wound healing, host immunity, and taste acuity. This mineral also provides cellular antioxidant protection by scavenging free radicals.

In addition, zinc acetate interferes with intestinal absorption of copper and produces a protein that binds with copper, preventing its transfer to the blood. Bound copper is then excreted in stools, thus decreasing copper toxicity in Wilson's disease.

Contraindications

Hypersensitivity to zinc or its components

Interactions

DRUGS

copper supplements: Impaired copper absorption (with large doses of zinc)

oral iron supplements, oral phosphate salts, penicillamine, phosphorus-containing drugs: Decreased zinc absorption

quinolones, tetracyclines: Decreased absorption and possibly decreased effectiveness of these antibiotics

thiazide diuretics: Increased urinary excretion of zinc

zinc-containing preparations: Increased blood zinc level

FOODS

fiber- or phylate-containing foods (such as bran, whole-grain breads, cereal), phosphorus-containing foods (including milk, poultry): Decreased zinc absorption

Adverse Reactions

None with usual dosages

Nursing Considerations

- **WARNING** Don't administer I.V. zinc preparations that contain benzyl alcohol to neonates or premature infants because this preservative may cause a fatal toxic syndrome characterized by metabolic acidosis and CNS, respiratory, circulatory, and renal function impairment.
- Monitor patient receiving long-term zinc therapy for sideroblastic anemia, which may result from zinc-induced copper deficiency and is characterized by anemia, leukopenia, neutropenia, granulocytopenia, and bone marrow problems. Be aware that these effects are reversible after zinc is discontinued.
- Monitor patient with preexisting copper deficiency for exacerbation of this condition; zinc can decrease serum copper level.
- Assess patient for evidence of zinc deficiency, such as growth retardation, hypogonadism, delayed sexual maturation, alopecia, impaired wound healing, skin lesions, immune deficiencies, behavioral disturbances, night blindness, and taste impairment.
- Monitor blood alkaline phosphatase level monthly, as ordered; it may increase.
- Be aware that zinc chloride contains aluminum, which may accumulate to the point of toxicity if the patient's kidney function is impaired. Assess kidney function regularly.

PATIENT TEACHING

- Inform patient that I.V. therapy is only necessary until she is able to take zinc orally.

zoledronic acid

Zometa

Class and Category

Chemical: Bisphosphonate
Therapeutic: Antihypercalcemic, bone resorption inhibitor
Pregnancy category: D

Indications and Dosages

▶ *To treat hypercalcemia caused by cancer*

I.V. INFUSION

Adults. 4 mg infused over at least 15 min. After 7 days, retreatment with 4 mg if serum calcium level doesn't remain at or return to normal. *Maximum:* 4 mg/dose.

▶ *As adjunct treatment for patients with multiple myeloma or bony metastasis who are receiving standard antineoplastic therapy and have a creatinine clearance above 60 ml/min/1.73 m^2*

I.V. INFUSION

Adults. 4 mg infused over at least 15 min q 3 to 4 wk.
DOSAGE ADJUSTMENT If creatinine clearance is 50 to 60 ml/min/1.73 m^2, dosage decreased to 3.5 mg; if it's 40 to 49 ml/min/1.73 m^2, dosage decreased to 3.3 mg; and if it's 30 to 39 ml/min/1.73 m^2, dosage decreased to 3 mg.

Mechanism of Action

Inhibits resorption of mineralized bone and cartilage by osteoclasts and induces osteoclast breakdown. In cancer-related hypercalcemia, hyperactive osteoclasts cause bone resorption and release of calcium into the blood, which causes polyuria, GI disruption, progressive dehydration, and decreasing GFR. This, in turn, increases renal calcium resorption and worsens hypercalcemia. Zoledronic acid interrupts this process.

Incompatibilities

Don't mix zoledronic acid with calcium-containing I.V. solutions, such as LR.

Contraindications

Hypersensitivity to zoledronic acid, other bisphosphonates, or their components

Interactions

DRUGS

aminoglycosides: Possibly additive serum calcium–lowering effect
loop diuretics, such as furosemide: Possibly increased risk of hypocalcemia

Adverse Reactions

CNS: Chills, fever, hyperesthesia, tremor
CV: Bradycardia, hypertension, hypotension
EENT: Blurred vision, conjunctivitis, dry mouth, episcleritis, taste disturbance, uveitis
GI: Nausea, vomiting
GU: Elevated serum creatinine level, hematuria, proteinuria, renal insufficiency or failure
MS: Arthralgia, myalgia; severe bone, joint, and muscle pain
SKIN: Diaphoresis, flushing

Other: Angioedema, hyperkalemia, hypernatremia, hypocalcemia, hypomagnesemia, hypophosphatemia, infusion site redness and swelling, weight gain

Nursing Considerations

- Be aware that zoledronic acid isn't indicated for hypercalcemia from hyperparathyroidism or other nontumor conditions.
- Make sure patient has had a dental checkup before zoledronic acid starts, especially if patient has cancer; is receiving chemotherapy, head or neck radiation, or a corticosteroid; or has poor oral hygiene because the risk of osteonecrosis is increased in these patients, and invasive dental procedures during zoledronic acid therapy may worsen osteonecrosis.
- Expect to aggressively hydrate hypercalcemic patient with I.V. normal saline solution before and throughout zoledronic acid therapy, as prescribed, to achieve and maintain a urine output of about 2 L daily.
- **WARNING** During hydration, monitor fluid intake and output often and assess patient, especially one with heart failure, for evidence of life-threatening overhydration.
- Reconstitute zoledronic acid by adding 5 ml of sterile water for injection to drug vial to yield a solution that contains 4 mg of zoledronic acid. Make sure drug is completely dissolved before withdrawing prescribed dose. Further dilute in 100 ml of normal saline solution or 5% dextrose injection, and infuse over no less than 15 minutes.
- Before giving drug, inspect the reconstituted and diluted solution and discard if particles or discoloration are present.
- Refrigerate reconstituted drug at 2° to 8° C (36° to 46° F) and discard it after 24 hours.
- Give drug as a single I.V. solution in a separate I.V. line.
- **WARNING** Be aware that a single dose of zoledronic acid shouldn't exceed 4 mg and shouldn't be infused over less than 15 minutes because this may lead to significant renal function deterioration, which may progress to renal failure.
- **WARNING** Assess patient's renal function, as ordered, before and during zoledronic acid therapy to detect deterioration. For patient with a normal serum creatinine level who develops an increase of 0.5 mg/dl within 2 weeks of receiving drug, expect to withhold next dose until serum creatinine level is within 10% of patient's baseline value. For patient with an abnormal serum creatinine level who develops an increase of 1 mg/dl within 2 weeks of receiving drug, expect to withhold

next dose until serum creatinine level is within 10% of baseline value.

- Monitor patient's serum calcium, magnesium, and phosphate levels, as ordered, throughout therapy. If hypocalcemia, hypomagnesemia, or hypophosphatemia occurs, expect to give short-term supplemental therapy, as ordered.
- Assess aspirin-sensitive asthma patients for worsening of respiratory symptoms during zoledronic acid therapy because other bisphosphonates have caused bronchoconstriction in these patients.
- Store drug at 25° C (77° F).

PATIENT TEACHING

- Teach patient the importance of consuming a nutritious diet, including adequate amounts of calcium and vitamin D.
- Advise patient to alert prescriber about muscle or bone pain.
- Instruct patient on proper oral hygiene and on need to notify prescriber before undergoing invasive dental procedures.

EQUIANALGESIC DOSES FOR OPIOID AGONISTS

An equianalgesic dose of a synthetic opioid agonist is the dose that produces the same level of analgesia as 10 mg of I.M. or S.C. morphine, the principal opioid obtained from opium poppies. If your patient is switched from one opioid to another, expect to use the equianalgesic dose to decrease the risk of adverse reactions while increasing the likelihood of adequate pain relief. The chart below compares equianalgesic doses (oral and parenteral) for adults and children who weigh 50 kg (110 lb) or more.

Opioid agonist	Oral dose	Parenteral dose
codeine	200 mg (not recommended dose)	120 to 130 mg
hydrocodone	30 mg	Not applicable
hydromorphone	7.5 mg	1.5 mg
levorphanol	4 mg	2 mg
meperidine	300 mg	75 to 100 mg
morphine (around-the-clock dosing)	30 mg	10 mg
morphine (single or intermittent dosing)	60 mg	10 mg
oxycodone	30 mg	Not applicable

CALCULATING THE STRENGTH OF A SOLUTION

Most solutions come prepared in the required strength by the pharmacy or medical supply source. But sometimes only the concentrated form is available, and you'll need to dilute the solution or solid to administer the prescribed strength.

When a solid form of a drug is used to prepare a solution, the drug must be completely dissolved. Solid drug forms, such as tablets, crystals, and powders, are considered 100% strength. (An exception to this is boric acid, which is only 5% at full strength.) The final diluted solution is stated in terms of liquid measurement. To prepare a solution, you'll need to add the prescribed solid or liquid form of the drug (the solute) to the prescribed amount of diluent (the solvent). Two of the most common diluents used in the clinical setting are normal saline solution and sterile water.

You can use either of two formulas to calculate the strength of a solution, as shown in the examples below.

Method 1: Calculating percentage and volume

Use the following formula:

$$\frac{\text{Weaker solution}}{\text{Stronger solution}} = \frac{\text{Solute}}{\text{Solvent}}$$

Example: You need to dilute a stock solution of 100% strength to a 5% solution. How much solute will you need to add to obtain 500 ml of the 5% solution?

Calculate as follows:

$$\frac{5\ (\%)\ (\text{Weaker solution})}{100\ (\%)\ (\text{Stronger solution})} = \frac{X\ (\text{g})\ (\text{Solute})}{500\ \text{ml}\ (\text{Solvent})}$$

$$100\,X = (500)(5) \text{ or } 2{,}500$$

$$X = 25\ \text{g}$$

Answer: You'll need to add 25 g of solute to each 500 ml of solvent to prepare a 5% solution.

(continued)

CALCULATING THE STRENGTH OF A SOLUTION *(continued)*

Method 2: Calculating percentage and volume

Use the following formula:

$$\frac{\text{(Desired strength)}}{\text{(Available strength)}} \times \begin{matrix}\text{Total amount}\\ \text{of desired}\\ \text{solution}\end{matrix} = X \begin{matrix}\text{(Amount of undiluted}\\ \text{drug needed to}\\ \text{make solution)}\end{matrix}$$

Example: You need to make 100 ml of a 20% solution, using an 80% solution. How much of the 80% solution must you add to the sterile water to yield a final volume of 100 ml of a 20% solution?

Calculate as follows:

$$\frac{\text{20 (\%) (Desired strength)}}{\text{80 (\%) (Available strength)}} \times \text{100 ml} \begin{matrix}\text{(Total amount of}\\ \text{desired solution)}\end{matrix} = X$$

$$\frac{0.20}{0.80} = 0.25$$

$$0.25 \times 100\ \text{(ml)} = X$$

$$X = 25\ \text{ml of 80\% solution}$$

Answer: You'll need to add 25 ml of the 80% solution to the water to yield a final volume of 100 ml of a 20% solution.

CALCULATING PARENTERAL DRUG DOSAGES

You may need to calculate drug dosages when you're asked to administer a drug that is available in one measure, but prescribed in another. To make such calculations, you can use any of the three common methods of ratio and proportion shown in the examples below.

Example: You need to administer a prescribed dose of 1 mg morphine sulfate from a unit-dose cartridge that contains 4 mg per 2 ml. How many milliliters will you need to give to equal the prescribed dose of 1 mg?

Method 1: Using labeled amount of drug

In this method, the proportions between the drug label and the prescribed dose are used to determine ratio and proportion. The drug label, which states the amount of drug in one unit of measure (in this case, 4 mg in 2 ml), is the first ratio and is expressed as follows:

milligrams : milliliter = milligrams : milliliter
4 mg (amount of drug) : 2 ml (unit of measure)

The prescribed dose—in this case, 1 mg—is the second ratio; it must be expressed in the same order and units of measure as the first, as follows:

$$4 \text{ mg} : 2 \text{ ml} = 1 \text{ mg} : X \text{ ml}$$

Calculate as follows:

$$4X = 2$$

$$X = \frac{2}{4}$$

$$X = 0.5 \text{ ml}$$

Answer: You'll need to give 0.5 ml of morphine sulfate to equal the prescribed dose of 1 mg.

CALCULATING PARENTERAL DRUG DOSAGES *(continued)*

Method 2: Using an established formula

Use this formula:

$$\frac{\text{Prescribed dose}}{\text{Dose available}} \times \text{Quantity (unit of measure)} = \text{X (unknown quantity to be given)}$$

Calculate as follows:

$$\frac{1\text{ mg}}{4\text{ mg}} \times 2\text{ ml} = \text{X (number of ml)}$$

$$\frac{4}{2} = 0.5$$

Answer: You'll need to give 0.5 ml of morphine sulfate to equal the prescribed dose of 1 mg.

Method 3: Calculating according to proportion size

To determine the correct amount of morphine sulfate to give using this method, use the following formula:

smaller : greater = smaller : greater
milligrams : milligrams = milliliters : milliliters

Critical thinking leads us to believe that 1 mg is less than 4 mg and that you'll need less than 2 ml to give 1 mg of the drug; therefore, 1 mg goes into the smaller part of the first ratio, and X goes into the smaller part of the second ratio. Set up the proportion as follows:

$$1\text{ mg} : 4\text{ mg} = \text{X (ml)} : 2\text{ ml}$$

$$4X = 2$$

$$X = \frac{2}{4}$$

$$X = 0.5$$

Answer: You'll need to give 0.5 ml of morphine sulfate to equal the prescribed dose of 1 mg.

CALCULATING I.V. FLOW RATES

When an I.V. solution is delivered by gravity, you must calculate the number of drops needed per minute for proper infusion. To calculate I.V. flow rates, you need to know three things:

- the drip factor—or the number of drops contained in 1 ml for the type of I.V. set you'll be using—which is provided on the individual package label
- the amount and type of fluid that you'll infuse, as prescribed on the physician's order sheet
- the infusion duration time in minutes.

Once you've gathered this information, you can calculate the I.V. flow rate using the following equation:

$$\frac{\text{Total number of ml}}{\text{Total number of min}} \times \text{drip factor (gtt/ml)} = \text{flow rate (gtt/min)}$$

Example 1: If the physician prescribes 1,000 ml of D_5W to infuse over 10 hours, and the drip rate for your administration set is 15 drops (gtt)/ml, calculate as follows:

$$\frac{1{,}000 \text{ ml}}{10 \text{ hr} \times 60 \text{ min}} \times 15 \text{ gtt/ml} = \text{X gtt/min}$$

$$\frac{1{,}000 \text{ ml}}{600 \text{ min}} \times 15 \text{ gtt/ml} = \text{X gtt/min}$$

$$1.67 \text{ ml/min} \times 15 \text{ gtt/ml} = \text{X gtt/min}$$

$$25.05 \text{ gtt/min} = \text{X}$$

Answer: To infuse, round off 25.05 to 25 gtt/min or according to your institution's policy.

CALCULATING I.V. FLOW RATES *(continued)*

Example 2: If the physician prescribes 500 ml of 0.45NS to infuse over 2 hours, and the drip rate for your administration set is 10 gtt/ml, calculate as follows:

$$\frac{500 \text{ ml}}{2 \text{ hr} \times 60 \text{ min}} \times 10 \text{ gtt/ml} = \text{X gtt/min}$$

$$\frac{500 \text{ ml}}{120 \text{ min}} \times 10 \text{ gtt/ml} = \text{X gtt/min}$$

$$4.17 \text{ ml/min} \times 10 \text{ gtt/ml} = \text{X gtt/min}$$

$$41.7 \text{ gtt/min} = \text{X}$$

Answer: To infuse, round off 41.7 to 42 gtt/min or according to your institution's policy.

Note: When a controlled infusion device is being used for I.V. administration, the electronic flow-regulator will either count drops using an electronic eye or use a controlled pumping action to deliver the fluid in milliliters. Your final calculation will be based on the unit of measure used by the device: drops per minute, or milliliters per hour.

I.V. ANTINEOPLASTIC DRUGS

Antineoplastic drugs have become the standard of treatment for most types of cancer today. Most of these drugs work by inhibiting cell proliferation, thereby leading to cell death. They're most effective at killing cells that are actively dividing. Cell-specific antineoplastics exert their actions during one or more phases of the cell cycle. S-phase antineoplastics interfere with DNA synthesis; M-phase drugs interfere with the formation of microtubules and disrupt mitosis. Most antineoplastics impair DNA in one of the following four ways:

- preventing separation of DNA strands
- inhibiting DNA repair
- mimicking DNA bases
- disrupting the triplicate codons or producing oxygen free radicals that damage the DNA.

Antineoplastic drugs are cytotoxic, which means that they affect both neoplastic cells and normal cells. As a result, they may cause serious and sometimes life-threatening adverse reactions. Antineoplastics are most harmful to normal cells that exhibit rapid activity and growth, such as bone marrow tissue, the epithelium of the GI mucosa, and hair follicles. When they suppress bone marrow activity, the patient may develop leukopenia, thrombocytopenia, or anemia. When the drugs affect the GI mucosa, the patient may experience nausea, vomiting, anorexia, bowel dysfunction, and mucosal ulcerations. When they affect the hair follicles, the result is hair loss (alopecia), one of the most common adverse reactions; although not life-threatening, hair loss can be emotionally traumatic for patients, especially women.

Drug Classification

Antineoplastics are classified according to their mechanism of action.

Alkylating drugs, the first drugs developed to fight cancer, are most effective against slow-growing tumors. These agents can damage tissue at the injection site and produce systemic toxicity. They can damage cells during all stages of growth, causing mitotic arrest. Because their actions are not limited to neoplastic cells, they also cause myelosuppression, a predictable adverse reaction. They can also result in secondary tumor development, even years after the initial therapy.

I.V. ANTINEOPLASTIC DRUGS *(continued)*

Antibiotic antineoplastics originated from a genus of fungus-like bacteria called *Streptomyces*. Their classification is based on their origin, not on mechanism of action, toxicity, pharmacokinetics, or varying clinical indications. Many of these drugs bind to specific bases and block DNA synthesis, thus interfering with cell replication.

Antimetabolites are cell-cycle-phase–specific drugs that act by preventing synthesis of nucleotides or inhibiting enzymes by mimicking nucleotides. These drugs tend to be more effective when used in combination.

Antimitotic antineoplastics disrupt the formation of microtubule structures within the cell during mitosis. This breakdown of microtubule production stops the formation of the mitotic spindle, inhibiting cellular reproduction.

Biological response modifiers alter tumor-host metabolic and immunologic relationships.

Antineoplastic enzymes interfere with the breakdown of extracellular asparagine, an endogenous enzyme that leukemic cells depend on for their survival. The rapid depletion of asparagine eventually kills leukemic cells by fragmenting them into membrane-bound particles that are eliminated by phagocytosis.

Hormonal antineoplastics act as agonists to inhibit tumor cell growth or as antagonists to compete with endogenous growth-promoting hormones. Steroid hormones form specific receptor complexes that bind to certain nuclear proteins necessary for DNA transcription.

Miscellaneous antineoplastics act in a variety of ways, such as by destroying microtubules that are essential for tumor cell structure before mitosis and by inhibiting topoisomerase, the enzyme that affects the degree of supercoiling in DNA by cutting one or both strands. This inhibition causes DNA strands to break and synthesizes toxic compounds that inhibit DNA strand repair.

You'll find complete entries for some of the most common I.V. antineoplastics in this book. The following chart lists the generic and common trade names of additional I.V. antineoplastics, which are grouped according to mechanism of action. It also includes FDA-approved indications and the usual adult I.V. dosage for each drug.

(continued)

I.V. ANTINEOPLASTIC DRUGS *(continued)*

Generic and Trade Names	Indications	Usual Adult Dosages
Alkylating drugs		
busulfan Busulfex, Myleran	To prepare for hematopoietic progenitor cell transplantation for chronic myelogenous leukemia	0.8 mg/kg I.V. over 2 hr q 6 hr for 4 days for a total of 16 doses as an adjunct with cyclophosphamide
carmustine (BCNU) BiCNU, Gliadel Wafer	To treat primary brain tumors, Hodgkin's disease, non-Hodgkin's lymphoma, and multiple myeloma	150 to 200 mg/m^2 by slow I.V. infusion as a single dose q 6 to 8 wk; or 75 to 100 mg/m^2 by slow I.V. infusion q.d. for 2 days q 6 wk
ifosfamide IFEX	To treat germ cell testicular tumors	1.2 g/m^2 daily by I.V. infusion for 5 days q 3 wk
melphalan (L-phenylalanine mustard) **melphalan hydrochloride** Alkeran	To treat multiple myeloma	16 mg/m^2 I.V. over 15 min q 2 wk for 4 doses; then at 4 wk
mechlorethamine hydrochloride (nitrogen mustard) Mustargen	To treat Hodgkin's disease, non-Hodgkin's lymphoma, and mycosis fungoides	0.4 mg/kg I.V. as a single dose or in divided doses over 2 to 4 days
streptozocin Zanosar	To treat islet cell or pancreatic carcinoma	500 mg/m^2 I.V. for 5 days q 6 wk, or 1,000 mg/m^2 I.V. q wk for 2 wk
thiotepa (TESPA, triethylenethiophosphoramide, TSPA) Thioplex	To treat breast cancer, epithelial ovarian cancer, and Hodgkin's disease	0.3 to 0.4 mg/kg I.V. q 1 to 4 wk, or 0.2 mg/kg for 4 to 5 days q 2 to 3 wk

I.V. ANTINEOPLASTIC DRUGS *(continued)*

Generic and Trade Names	Indications	Usual Adult Dosages
Antibiotic antineoplastics		
bleomycin sulfate Blenoxane	To treat non-Hodgkin's lymphoma, squamous cell carcinoma, and testicular cancer	0.25 to 0.5 unit/kg or 10 to 20 units/m^2 1 or 2 times/wk I.V., or 0.25 unit/kg or 15 units/m^2 daily by I.V. infusion over 24 hr
	To treat Hodgkin's disease	0.25 to 0.5 unit/kg I.V. or 10 to 20 units/m^2 1 or 2 times/wk
dactinomycin (actinomycin-D) Cosmegen	To treat Ewing's sarcoma, gestational trophoblastic or Wilms' tumor, rhabdomyosarcoma, sarcoma botryoides, and testicular cancer or tumors	15 to 500 mcg/kg daily I.V. for 5 days; may repeat after 3 wk
daunorubicin hydrochloride Cerubidine	To treat acute lymphocytic leukemia	45 mg/m^2 I.V. daily for first 3 days of a 32-day course with vincristine, prednisone, and asparaginase
	To treat acute nonlymphocytic leukemia	45 mg/m^2 I.V. q.d. for first 3 days of first course of combination therapy with cytarabine and first 2 days of second course of combination therapy with cytarabine
daunorubicin, liposomal DaunoXome	To treat AIDS-related Kaposi's sarcoma	40 mg/m^2 I.V. over 60 min q 2 wk

(continued)

I.V. ANTINEOPLASTIC DRUGS *(continued)*

Generic and Trade Names	Indications	Usual Adult Dosages
Antibiotic antineoplastics *(continued)*		
epirubicin hydrochloride Ellence	To treat breast cancer	100 to 120 mg/m^2 by I.V. infusion over 3 to 5 min by a free-flowing I.V. solution as a single dose on day 1 or in divided doses on days 1 and 8; repeated q 3 to 4 wk for 6 cycles in combination with other chemotherapeutic drugs
idarubicin hydrochloride Idamycin	To treat acute nonlymphocytic leukemia	12 mg/m^2/day I.V. over 10 to 15 min for 3 days in combination with cytarabine
mitomycin (mitomycin-C) Mutamycin	To treat gastric or pancreatic cancer	20 mg/m^2 I.V. as a single dose q 6 to 8 wk
pentostatin (2′-deoxycoformycin) Nipent	To treat hairy cell leukemia	4 mg/m^2 by rapid I.V. injection or diluted for infusion over 20 to 30 min as a single dose q other wk
plicamycin (mithramycin) Mithracin	To treat testicular cancer	0.025 to 0.03 mg/kg I.V. q.d. over 4 to 6 hr for 8 to 10 days
	To treat hypercalcemia and hypercalciuria	0.015 to 0.025 mg/kg I.V. q.d. over 4 to 6 hr for 3 to 4 days; may repeat dose q wk as needed
Antimetabolites		
cladribine (2-CdA, 2-chlorodeoxyadenosine) Leustatin	To treat hairy cell leukemia	0.1 mg/kg/day by continuous I.V. infusion for 7 days

I.V. ANTINEOPLASTIC DRUGS *(continued)*

Generic and Trade Names	Indications	Usual Adult Dosages
Antimetabolites *(continued)*		
cytarabine (ARA-C, cytosine arabinoside) Cytosar, Cytosar-U	To treat acute nonlymphocytic leukemia	Initially, 100 mg/m^2/day by continuous I.V. infusion for 7 days, alone or in combination with other drugs; or 100 mg/m^2 I.V. q 12 hr on days 1 to 7, then consult manufacturer's literature for specific dosage; or high-dose therapy of 2 to 3 g/m^2 I.V over 1 to 3 hr for 2 to 6 days, then consult manufacturer's literature for specific dosage.
	To prevent or treat acute lymphocytic leukemia and chronic myelocytic leukemia	Consult manufacturer's literature for specific dosage.
fludarabine phosphate Fludara	To treat chronic lymphocytic leukemia	25 mg/m^2 I.V. infused over 30 min for 5 days; cycle repeated q 28 days
Antimitotic antineoplastics		
docetaxel Taxotere	To treat breast cancer	60 to 100 mg/m^2 by I.V. infusion over 1 hr q 3 wk
	To treat non–small-cell lung carcinoma	75 mg/m^2 by I.V. infusion over 1 hr q 3 wk
vinorelbine tartrate Navelbine	To treat non–small-cell lung carcinoma	30 mg/m^2 I.V. over 6 to 10 min q wk; or, 25 mg/m^2 I.V. over 6 to 10 min q wk when combined with cisplatin 100 mg/m^2 q 4 wk

(continued)

I.V. ANTINEOPLASTIC DRUGS *(continued)*

Generic and Trade Names	Indications	Usual Adult Dosages
Antineoplastic enzymes		
asparaginase Colaspase, Elspar, Kidrolase (CAN)	To treat acute lymphocytic leukemia	200 international units/kg I.V. daily for 28 days
pegaspargase (PEG-L-asparaginase) Oncaspar	To treat acute lymphoblastic leukemia in adults up to age 21	2,500 international units/m^2 I.V. q 14 days
Biological response modifiers		
aldesleukin (IL-2, interleukin-2) Proleukin	To treat renal cancer and metastatic melanoma	600,000 international units/kg by I.V. infusion over 15 min q 8 hr for 14 doses, followed by 9 days of no drug; then course of 14 doses repeated for total of 28 doses
alemtuzumab Campath	To treat B-cell chronic lymphocytic leukemia	Initially, 3 mg I.V. over 2 hr daily; then 10 mg I.V. over 2 hr daily. For maintenance, 30 mg I.V. over 2 hr three times/wk q other day for up to 12 wk.
denileukin diftitox Ontak	To treat cutaneous or T-cell lymphomas, including mycosis fungoides	9 or 18 mcg/kg/day by I.V. infusion over at least 15 min for 5 days; repeated q 21 days
Miscellaneous antineoplastics		
arsenic trioxide Trisenox	To treat acute promyelocytic leukemia	Induction: 0.15 mg/kg I.V. daily until bone marrow remission. Maximum, 60 doses. Consolidation: Starting 3 to 6 wk after induction is complete, 0.15 mg/kg I.V. daily for 25 doses over up to 5 wk

I.V. ANTINEOPLASTIC DRUGS *(continued)*

Generic and Trade Names	Indications	Usual Adult Dosages
Miscellaneous antineoplastics *(continued)*		
dacarbazine DTIC (CAN), DTIC-Dome	To treat Hodgkin's disease	150 mg/m² I.V. daily for 5 days with other drugs, possibly repeated q 28 days; or 375 mg/m² q 15 days with other drugs
	To treat malignant melanoma	2 to 4.5 mg/kg I.V. daily for 10 days and q 28 days thereafter; or, 250 mg/m² I.V. daily for 5 days and q 21 days thereafter
gemcitabine hydrochloride Gemzar	To treat non–small-cell lung carcinoma	1,000 mg/m² by I.V. infusion over 30 min daily on days 1, 8, and 15 q 28 days with cisplatin 100 mg/m² on day 28; or 1,250 mg/m² I.V. q.d. on days 1 and 8 q 21 days with cisplatin 100 mg/m² I.V. on day 21
	To treat pancreatic cancer	1,000 mg/m² by I.V. infusion over 30 min q wk for 7 wk, followed by 1 wk of no drug; then q wk for 3 wk, followed by 1 wk of no drug; then 4-wk cycle repeated
gemtuzumab ozogamicin Mylotarg	To treat first relapse in patients with CD33-positive acute myeloid leukemia who are age 60 or over and who are not candidates for cytotoxic therapy	9 mg/m² by I.V. infusion over 2 hr; repeated in 24 days

(continued)

I.V. ANTINEOPLASTIC DRUGS *(continued)*

Generic and Trade Names	Indications	Usual Adult Dosages
Miscellaneous antineoplastics *(continued)*		
mitoxantrone hydrochloride Novantrone	To treat hormone-refractory prostate cancer	12 to 14 mg/m^2 I.V. q 21 days
	To treat acute nonlymphocytic leukemia	12 mg/m^2 by I.V. infusion through free-flowing norml saline solution or D_5W over 3 min daily on days 1 and 3 in with cytarabine 100 mg/m^2 daily by continuous I.V. infusion on days 1 to 7; if response is inadequate, second course of same dosage may be given
porfimer sodium Photofrin	To treat esophageal cancer and non–small-cell lung carcinoma	2 mg/kg I.V. over 3 to 5 min, followed by laser light illumination and debridement of tumor; course may be repeated q 30 days three times

ANTINEOPLASTIC DRUGS *(continued)*

Generic and Trade Names	Indications	Usual Adult Dosages
Miscellaneous antineoplastics *(continued)*		
topotecan hydrochloride Hycamtin	To treat ovarian cancer and small-cell lung carcinoma	1.5 mg/m^2 I.V. over 30 min q.d. for 5 days; repeated q 21 days
trastuzumab Herceptin	To treat breast cancer	4 mg/kg I.V. over 90 min, followed by 2 mg/kg I.V. over 30 min q 7 days
velcade Bortezomib	To treat multiple myeloma	1.3 mg/m^2 by I.V. bolus on days 1, 4, 8, and 11 for 2 wk, followed by rest on days 12 through 21. Then repeat 3-wk cycle

BODY MASS INDEX CALCULATION

Body mass index (BMI) is a formula used to determine obesity; it's calculated by dividing a person's weight in kilograms by his height in meters squared (kg/m^2). A BMI of 25 or higher increases your patient's risk of developing hypertension, cardiovascular disease, type 2 diabetes mellitus, and stroke. It also increases the risk that he won't respond effectively to the usual drug dosages. If your patient has an abnormal BMI, be prepared to make dosage adjustments that are individualized based on body weight, as prescribed.

WEIGHT (POUNDS)

HEIGHT (INCHES)																		
58	91	96	100	105	110	115	119	124	129	134	138	143	148	153	158	162	167	172
59	94	99	104	109	114	119	124	128	133	138	143	148	153	158	163	168	173	178
60	97	102	107	112	118	123	128	133	138	143	148	153	158	163	168	174	179	184
61	100	106	111	116	122	127	132	137	143	148	153	158	164	169	174	180	185	190
62	104	109	115	120	126	131	136	142	147	153	158	164	169	175	180	186	191	196
63	107	113	118	124	130	135	141	146	152	158	163	169	175	180	186	191	197	203
64	110	116	122	128	134	140	145	151	157	163	169	174	180	186	192	197	204	209
65	114	120	126	132	138	144	150	156	162	168	174	180	186	192	198	204	210	216
66	118	124	130	136	142	148	155	161	167	173	179	186	192	198	204	210	216	223
67	121	127	134	140	146	153	159	166	172	178	185	191	198	204	211	217	223	230
68	125	131	138	144	151	158	164	171	177	184	190	197	203	210	216	223	230	236
69	128	135	142	149	155	162	169	176	182	189	196	203	209	216	223	230	236	243
70	132	139	146	153	160	167	174	181	188	195	202	209	216	222	229	236	243	250
71	136	143	150	157	165	172	179	186	193	200	208	215	222	229	236	243	250	257
72	140	147	154	162	169	177	184	191	199	206	213	221	228	235	242	250	258	265
73	144	151	159	166	174	182	189	197	204	212	219	227	235	242	250	257	265	272
74	148	155	163	171	179	186	194	202	210	218	225	233	241	249	256	264	272	280
75	152	160	168	176	184	192	200	208	216	224	232	240	248	256	264	272	279	287
76	156	164	172	180	189	197	205	213	221	230	238	246	254	263	271	279	287	295
BODY MASS INDEX	**19**	**20**	**21**	**22**	**23**	**24**	**25**	**26**	**27**	**28**	**29**	**30**	**31**	**32**	**33**	**34**	**35**	**36**

The table below will help you find your patient's BMI easily. It converts pounds to kilograms and inches to meters, and then it shows the BMI. To use it, simply find the patient's height on either side of the table; then move across the row to the weight that most closely matches your patient's. At the bottom of the column containing the weight, you'll find the BMI for that patient. For example, the BMI for a patient who is 70″ tall and weighs 208 lb is 30.

WEIGHT (POUNDS)

																		HEIGHT (INCHES)
177	181	186	191	196	201	205	210	215	220	224	229	234	239	244	248	253	258	**58**
183	188	193	198	203	208	212	217	222	227	232	237	242	247	252	257	262	267	**59**
189	194	199	204	209	215	220	225	230	235	240	245	250	255	261	266	271	276	**60**
195	201	206	211	217	222	227	232	238	243	248	254	259	264	269	275	280	285	**61**
202	207	213	218	224	229	235	240	246	251	256	262	267	273	278	284	289	295	**62**
208	214	220	225	231	237	242	248	254	259	265	270	278	282	287	293	299	304	**63**
215	221	227	232	238	244	250	256	262	267	273	279	285	291	296	302	308	314	**64**
222	228	234	240	246	252	258	264	270	276	282	288	294	300	306	312	318	324	**65**
229	235	241	247	253	260	266	272	278	284	291	297	303	309	315	322	328	334	**66**
236	242	249	255	261	268	274	280	287	293	299	306	312	319	325	331	338	344	**67**
243	249	256	262	269	276	282	289	295	302	308	315	322	328	335	341	348	354	**68**
250	257	263	270	277	284	291	297	304	311	318	324	331	338	345	351	358	365	**69**
257	264	271	278	285	292	299	306	313	320	327	334	341	348	355	362	369	376	**70**
265	272	279	286	293	301	308	315	322	329	338	343	351	358	365	372	379	386	**71**
272	279	287	294	302	309	316	324	331	338	346	353	361	368	375	383	390	397	**72**
280	288	295	302	310	318	325	333	340	348	355	363	371	378	386	393	401	408	**73**
287	295	303	311	319	326	334	342	350	358	365	373	381	389	396	404	412	420	**74**
295	303	311	319	327	335	343	351	359	367	375	383	391	399	407	415	423	431	**75**
304	312	320	328	336	344	353	361	369	377	385	394	402	410	418	426	435	443	**76**
37	**38**	**39**	**40**	**41**	**42**	**43**	**44**	**45**	**46**	**47**	**48**	**49**	**50**	**51**	**52**	**53**	**54**	

BODY MASS INDEX

ABBREVIATIONS

The following abbreviations, which are common to nursing practice, are used throughout the book.

ABG	arterial blood gas
a.c.	before meals
ACE	angiotensin-converting enzyme
ADH	antidiuretic hormone
AIDS	acquired immunodeficiency syndrome
ALT	alanine aminotransferase
ANA	antinuclear antibodies
APTT	activated partial thromboplastin time
AST	aspartate aminotransferase
ATP	adenosine triphosphate
AV	atrioventricular
b.i.d.	twice a day
BUN	blood urea nitrogen
°C	degrees Celsius
cAMP	cyclic adenosine monophosphate
(CAN)	Canadian drug trade name
cap	capsule
CBC	complete blood count
cGMP	cyclic guanosine monophosphate
CK	creatine kinase
Cl	chloride
cm	centimeter
CMV	cytomegalovirus
CNS	central nervous system
COPD	chronic obstructive pulmonary disease
C.R.	controlled-release
CSF	cerebrospinal fluid
CV	cardiovascular
CVA	cerebrovascular accident
D_5W	dextrose 5% in water
$D_{10}W$	dextrose 10% in water
$D_{50}W$	dextrose 50% in water
dl	deciliter
DNA	deoxyribonucleic acid
DS	double-strength
EC	enteric-coated
ECG	electrocardiogram
EEG	electroencephalogram
EENT	eyes, ears, nose, and throat
ENDO	endocrine

ABBREVIATIONS *(continued)*

E.R.	extended-release
°F	degrees Fahrenheit
FDA	Food and Drug Administration
g	gram
GFR	glomerular filtration rate
GI	gastrointestinal
GU	genitourinary
H_1	$histamine_1$
H_2	$histamine_2$
HDL	high-density lipoprotein
HEME	hematologic
HIV	human immunodeficiency virus
HPV	human papilloma virus
hr	hour
h.s.	at bedtime
HSV	herpes simplex virus
HZV	herpes zoster virus
ICP	intracranial pressure
I.D.	intradermal
IgA	immunoglobulin A
IgE	immunoglobulin E
I.M.	intramuscular
INR	international normalized ratio
I.V.	intravenous
IVPB	intravenous piggyback
kg	kilogram
KIU	kallikrein inactivator unit
L	liter
LA	long-acting
LD	lactate dehydrogenase
LDL	low-density lipoprotein
LOC	level of consciousness
LR	lactated Ringer's solution
M	molar
m^2	square meter
MAO	monoamine oxidase
mcg	microgram
mEq	milliequivalent
mg	milligram
MI	myocardial infarction
min	minute
ml	milliliter
mm	millimeter

(continued)

ABBREVIATIONS *(continued)*

mm^3	cubic millimeter
mmol	millimole
mo	month
MS	musculoskeletal
Na	sodium
NaCl	sodium chloride
NG	nasogastric
NPH	human isophane insulin
NPO	nothing by mouth
NSAID	nonsteroidal anti-inflammatory drug
OTC	over the counter
p.c.	after meals
PCA	patient-controlled analgesia
P.O.	by mouth
P.R.	by rectum
p.r.n.	as needed
PSVT	paroxysmal supraventricular tachycardia
PT	prothrombin time
PTCA	percutaneous transluminal coronary angioplasty
PVC	premature ventricular contraction
q	every
q.i.d.	four times a day
RBC	red blood cell
REM	rapid eye movement
RESP	respiratory
RNA	ribonucleic acid
RSV	respiratory syncytial virus
SA	sinoatrial
S.C.	subcutaneous
sec	second
S.L.	sublingual
S.R.	sustained-release
stat	immediately
supp	suppository
tab	tablet
T_3	triiodothyronine
T_4	thyroxine
t.i.d.	three times a day
USP	United States Pharmacopeia
UTI	urinary tract infection
VLDL	very low-density lipoprotein
WBC	white blood cell
wk	week

INDEX

- **Generic and alternate names:** lowercase initial letter
- **Trade names:** uppercase initial letter
- **Illustrations:** *i* after page number
- **Tables:** *t* after page number

A

B

C

D

E

I

J

K

L

M

Q

R

S

COMPATIBLE DRUGS IN A SYRINGE

The chart below lets you know at a glance whether particular drugs are compatible for at least 15 minutes when mixed together in a syringe for immediate administration. However, keep in mind that drugs listed as compatible when mixed in a syringe may not be compatible when prepared for other routes of administration. Drug combinations

	atropine	chlorpromazine	dexamethasone	diazepam	diphenhydramine	droperidol	furosemide	glycopyrrolate	haloperidol	heparin	hydromorphone
atropine		C	n/a	n/a	C	C	n/a	C	I	n/a	C
chlorpromazine	C		n/a	n/a	C	C	n/a	C	n/a	I	C
dexamethasone	n/a	n/a		n/a	I	n/a	n/a	n/a	n/a	n/a	C
diazepam	n/a	n/a	n/a		n/a	n/a	n/a	I	n/a	I	n/a
diphenhydramine	C	C	I	n/a		C	n/a	C	I	n/a	C
droperidol	C	C	n/a	n/a	C		I	C	n/a	I	n/a
furosemide	n/a	n/a	n/a	n/a	n/a	I		n/a	n/a	C	n/a
glycopyrrolate	C	C	I	C	C	C	n/a		C	n/a	C
haloperidol	n/a	n/a	n/a	n/a	C	n/a	n/a	n/a		I	C
heparin	C	I	n/a	I	n/a	I	C	n/a	I		n/a
hydromorphone	C	C	n/a	n/a	C	n/a	n/a	C	C	n/a	
hydroxyzine	C	C	n/a	n/a	C	C	n/a	C	I	n/a	C
ketorolac	n/a	n/a	n/a	I	n/a	n/a	n/a	n/a	I	n/a	I
lidocaine	n/a	n/a	n/a	n/a	n/a	n/a	n/a	C	n/a	C	n/a
lorazepam	n/a	n/a	n/a	n/a	n/a	n/a	n/a	n/a	n/a	n/a	C
meperidine	C	C	n/a	C	C	C	n/a	C	n/a	I	n/a
metoclopramide	C	C	n/a	n/a	C	C	I	n/a	n/a	C	C
midazolam	C	C	n/a	n/a	C	n/a	n/a	C	C	n/a	C
morphine	C	C	n/a	n/a	C	C	n/a	C	I	C*	n/a
pentobarbital	C	I	n/a	n/a	I	I	n/a	I	n/a	n/a	C
prochlorperazine	C	n/a	n/a	n/a	C	C	n/a	C	n/a	n/a	I
ranitidine	C	I	C	n/a	C	n/a	n/a	C	n/a	n/a	C
scopolamine	C	C	n/a	n/a	C	C	n/a	C	n/a	n/a	C

* Compatible only with morphine doses of 1 mg, 2 mg, and 5 mg.

prepared for immediate administration usually require a more concentrated solution than those prepared for infusion.

(**Key:** C = Compatible; I = Incompatible; n/a = Compatibility information not available; no recommendations can be given.)

hydroxyzine	ketorolac	lidocaine	lorazepam	meperidine	metoclopramide	midazolam	morphine	pentobarbital	prochlorperazine	ranitidine	scopolamine
C	n/a	n/a	n/a	C	C	C	C	C	C	C	C
C	n/a	n/a	n/a	C	C	C	I	I	C	C	C
n/a	n/a	n/a	n/a	n/a	C	n/a	n/a	n/a	n/a	C	n/a
n/a	I	n/a	n/a	n/a	n/a	n/a	n/a	n/a	n/a	I	n/a
C	n/a	n/a	n/a	C	C	C	C	I	C	C	C
C	n/a	n/a	n/a	C	C	C	C	I	C	n/a	C
n/a	n/a	n/a	n/a	n/a	I	n/a	n/a	n/a	n/a	n	n/a
C	n/a	C	n/a	C	n/a	C	C	I	C	C	C
I	I	n/a	n/a	n/a	n/a	n/a	I	n/a	n/a	n/a	n/a
n/a	n/a	C	n/a	I	C	n/a	C	n/a	n/a	n	n/a
C	I	n/a	C	n/a	n/a	C	n/a	C	I	C	C
	I	C	n/a	C	C	C	C	I	C	C	C
I		n/a	n/a	n/a	n/a	n/a	n/a	n/a	I	n/a	n/a
C	n/a		n/a	n/a	C	n/a	n/a	n/a	n/a	n/a	n/a
n/a	n/a	n/a		n/a	n/a	n/a	n/a	n/a	n/a	I	n/a
C	n/a	n/a	n/a		C	C	I	I	C	C	C
n/a	n/a	C	n/a	C		C	C	n/a	C	C	C
C	n/a	n/a	n/a	C	C		C	I	I	I	C
C	n/a	n/a	n/a	n/a	C	C		I	C	C	C
I	n/a	n/a	n/a	I	I	I	I		I	I	C
C	I	n/a	n/a	C	C	I	C	I		C	C
I	n/a	n/a	I	C	C	I	C	I	C		C
C	n/a	n/a	n/a	C	C	C	C	C	C	C	